Developmental Disabilities in Infancy and Childhood
Second Edition

Volume II:
The Spectrum of Developmental Disabilities

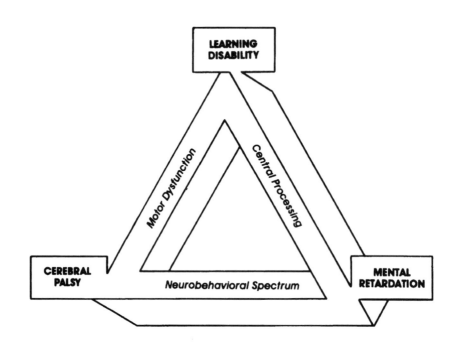

Developmental Disabilities in Infancy and Childhood
Second Edition

Volume II:
The Spectrum of Developmental Disabilities

edited by

Arnold J. Capute, M.D., M.P.H.

and

Pasquale J. Accardo, M.D.

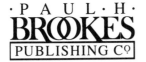

Baltimore • London • Toronto • Sydney

Paul H. Brookes Publishing Co.
Post Office Box 10624
Baltimore, Maryland 21285-0624

Typeset by Brushwood Graphics, Inc., Baltimore, Maryland.
Manufactured in the United States of America by
The Maple Press Co., York, Pennsylvania.

Developmental Disabilities in Infancy and Childhood is a two-volume set:
  Volume I: *Neurodevelopmental Diagnosis and Treatment*
  Volume II: *The Spectrum of Developmental Disabilities*

Library of Congress Cataloging-in-Publication Data

Developmental disabilities in infancy and childhood / edited by Arnold J. Capute and
    Pasquale J. Accardo. — 2nd ed.
        p.   cm.
    Includes bibliographical references and index.
    Contents: v. 1.   Neurodevelopmental diagnosis and treatment — v. 2.   The
spectrum of developmental disabilities.
    ISBN 1-55766-178-2 (v. 1). — ISBN 1-55766-194-4 (v. 2)
    1. Developmental disabilities.   I.   Capute, Arnold J., 1923–
II. Accardo, Pasquale J.
    [DNLM: 1. Child Development Disorders.   WS 350.6 D48884 1995]
    RJ135.D476   1996
    618.92′85889—dc20
    DNLM/DLC
    for Library of Congress   94-34249
                                                                                                         CIP

British Library Cataloguing-in-Publication data are available from the British Library.

Contents
Volume II

Contents

Volume I

Contributors
Volume II

Pasquale J. Accardo, M.D.
Professor of Pediatrics
St. Louis University
School of Medicine
The Knights of Columbus Developmental Center
Cardinal Glennon Children's Hospital
1465 South Grand Boulevard
St. Louis, Missouri 63104

Andrew Robert Adesman, M.D.
Chief, Division of Developmental and Behavioral
  Pediatrics
Associate Professor of Pediatrics
Albert Einstein College of Medicine
Schneider Children's Hospital
Long Island Jewish Medical Center
269-01 76th Avenue
New Hyde Park, NY 11040

Claudine Amiel-Tison, M.D.
Associate Professor of Pediatrics
Port-Royal-Baudelocque
123, Boulevard de Port-Royal
75674 Paris Cedex 14
FRANCE

Marilee C. Allen, M.D.
Associate Professor of Pediatrics
The Johns Hopkins University
School of Medicine
600 North Wolfe Street, CMSC-210
Baltimore, MD 21205

Peter A. Blasco, M.D.
Associate Professor of Pediatrics
Center for Children with Chronic Illness and
  Disability
University of Minnesota
420 Delaware Street, Southeast
Minneapolis, MN 55455

Thomas A. Blondis, M.D.
Assistant Professor of Pediatrics
The University of Chicago School of Medicine
Wyler Children's Hospital
5841 South Maryland Avenue
Mail Code 1051
Chicago, IL 60637-1470

George T. Capone, M.D.
Assistant Professor of Pediatrics
The Johns Hopkins University
School of Medicine
Kennedy Krieger Institute
Department of Pediatrics
707 North Broadway
Baltimore, MD 21205

Arnold J. Capute, M.D., M.P.H.
Professor of Pediatrics
The Johns Hopkins University
School of Medicine
Kennedy Krieger Institute
707 North Broadway
Baltimore, MD 21205

Peter J. Chauvel, M.B., M.P.H.
Director, Department of Developmental Pediatrics
  and Rehabilitation
Princess Margaret Hospital for Children
Box D 184, GPO
Perth, Western Australia 6001
AUSTRALIA

Thomas O. Crawford, M.D.
Assistant Professor of Neurology
The Johns Hopkins Medical Institutions
600 North Wolfe Street, Harvey 811
Baltimore, MD 21287

Larry W. Desch, M.D.
Associate Professor of Pediatrics
University of Wisconsin Medical School
Waisman Center
150 Highland Avenue
Madison, WI 53705-2280

Jon Matthew Farber, M.D.
Alexandria-Lake Ridge Pediatric Centers
4660 Kenmore Avenue, Suite 500
Alexandria, VA 22304

John Freeman, M.D.
Professor of Neurology and Pediatrics
The Johns Hopkins Medical Institutions
Pediatric Epilepsy Center
Meyer 20147
600 North Wolfe Street
Baltimore, MD 21205

Karen Hofman, M.D.
Assistant Professor of Pediatrics and Medicine
The Center for Medical Genetics
The Johns Hopkins Hospital
John Hopkins University
School of Medicine
600 North Wolfe Street
Baltimore, MD 21205

Vanja A. Holm, M.D.
Associate Professor of Pediatrics
University of Washington
School of Medicine
CDMRC WJ 10, Room CD 459
Seattle, WA 98195

Alexander H. Hoon, Jr., M.D., M.P.H.
Assistant Professor of Pediatrics
The Johns Hopkins University
School of Medicine
Department of Developmental Pediatrics
707 North Broadway
Baltimore, MD 21205

Susan L. Hyman, M.D.
Clinical Assistant Professor of Pediatrics
University of Rochester
601 Elmwood Avenue
Box 671
Rochester, NY 14642

Walter E. Kaufmann, M.D.
Assistant Professor of Pathology, Neurology,
    and Pediatrics
The Johns Hopkins University
School of Medicine
Hunterian Building
Room 905
725 North Wolfe Street
Baltimore, MD 21205

Stephen L. Kinsman, M.D.
Assistant Professor of Neurology
Kennedy Krieger Institute
707 North Broadway
Baltimore, MD 21205

Mary Leppert, M.D.
Assistant Professor of Pediatrics
The Johns Hopkins University
School of Medicine
707 North Broadway
Baltimore, MD 21205

Susan E. Levy, M.D.
Assistant Professor of Pediatrics
University of Pennsylvania
Children's Seashore House and Children's Hospital
    of Philadelphia
3405 Civic Center Blvd.
Philadelphia, PA 19104

Ronald L. Lindsay, M.D.
Assistant Professor of Pediatrics
Saint Louis University Health Sciences Center
Knights of Columbus Developmental Center
Cardinal Glennon Children's Hospital
1465 South Grand Boulevard
St. Louis, MO 63104

Thomas M. Lock, M.D.
Clinical Assistant Professor
State University of New York at Buffalo
Robert Warner Rehabilitation Center
Children's Hospital at Buffalo
State University of New York at Buffalo
936 Delaware Avenue
Buffalo, NY 14209-1887

Catherine Lord, Ph.D.
Professor of Psychiatry
Department of Psychiatry
Billings Hospital, AMB S350
950 East 59th Street
Mail Code 3077
Chicago, IL 60637-1470

Beverly A. Myers, M.D.
Clinical Assistant Professor of Psychiatry
    and Pediatrics
Child Development Center
Rhode Island Hospital
593 Eddy Street
Providence, RI 02903

Hugo W. Moser, M.D.
University Professor of Neurology and Pediatrics
The Johns Hopkins University
School of Medicine
Director, Center for Research on Mental Retardation
    and Related Aspects of Human Development
Kennedy Krieger Institute
707 North Broadway
Baltimore, MD 21205

Sakkubai Naidu, M.D.
Associate Professor of Neurology
Department of Neurology and Pediatrics
The Johns Hopkins University
School of Medicine
Director, Neurogenetics Unit
Kennedy Krieger Institute
707 North Broadway
Baltimore, MD 21205

Karin B. Nelson, M.D.
National Institute of Neurological Disorders &
    Stroke
Neuroepidemiology Branch
7550 Wisconsin, Room 714
Bethesda, MD 20892

Rita Panoscha, M.D.
Assistant Professor of Pediatrics
The Johns Hopkins University
School of Medicine
Kennedy Krieger Institute
707 North Broadway
Baltimore, MD 21205

Barbara R. Pober, M.D.
Assistant Professor in Genetics and Pediatrics
Yale University School of Medicine
Post Office Box 208005
New Haven, CT 06520-8005

Brian T. Rogers, M.D.
Clinical Associate Professor of Pediatrics
State University of New York at Buffalo
Robert Warner Rehabilitation Center
Children's Hospital of Buffalo
936 Delaware Avenue
Buffalo, NY 14209

Paul T. Rogers, M.D.
Director, Health Services Letchworth DDSO
Letchworth Village DDSO
Post Office Box 470
Thiels, NY 10984-0470

Nancy J. Roizen, M.D.
Chief, Section Developmental and Behavioral
    Pediatrics
University of Chicago
Pritzker School of Medicine
Chicago, IL 60637-5416

Bruce K. Shapiro, M.D.
Associate Professor of Pediatrics
The Johns Hopkins University School of Medicine
Director of Learning Center
Kennedy Krieger Institute
707 North Broadway
Baltimore, MD 21205

Harvey S. Singer, M.D.
Professor of Neurology and Pediatrics
The Johns Hopkins Hospital
Department of Neurology, Harvey 811
600 North Wolfe Street
Baltimore, MD 21287-8811

Eileen P.G. Vining, M.D.
Associate Professor of Neurology and Pediatrics
The Johns Hopkins Medical Institutions
Pediatric Epilepsy Center
Meyer 20147
600 North Wolfe Street
Baltimore, MD 21287-8811

Foreword

A few years ago this volume could not have been written because the technology did not exist to examine the disturbances in higher cortical function that are addressed here.

Pathophysiology has replaced, to a significant degree, preoccupation with anatomical pathology. An accurate description of functional limitations in cerebral palsy and mental retardation is far more important for therapeutic and educational purposes than precise localization of the neurological injury, which is still necessary for future research. The identification of social barriers to full assimilation into society is also of great significance in view of the recent enactment of the Americans with Disabilities Act (ADA) of 1990 (PL 101-336).

Advances in both chromosomal and DNA genetic analysis also have created a whole new climate regarding etiology of mental retardation and, to a lesser degree, cerebral palsy. The concepts of Mendelian inheritance have been augmented by the discoveries of nontraditional inheritance, such as "triplet repeat" amplification in fragile X syndrome. More than 1,000 causes of mental retardation have been described, and in many the specific gene defect and chromosomal localization have been identified. A wide gap still exists, however, between identifying the defective gene and understanding the mechanisms leading to cognitive disability. Such an understanding will not come easily because cognition is an enormously complex process that is still only imperfectly described by psychological testing. With successful gene therapy for most genetic disorders involving the brain still many years from being realized, intense concentration on the mechanisms of cognition seems warranted. Comparative psychobiology, which examines the relative cognitive processes of species, would seem to be a rich area for research, but the field is almost totally neglected. Certainly, animal behavior has been given considerable study in relation to human behavior, but dissection of the elements of higher cortical function in animals, relative to anatomy, physiology, pharmacology, and biochemistry, is poorly supported. This volume puts appropriate emphasis on higher cortical function. It is hoped that it will stimulate clinical and basic scientists to explore further the fundamental mechanisms of what is called intelligent behavior.

Until biological intervention is possible, the only therapeutic tools for cognitive disabilities lie in the field of childhood education and early intervention. Science has moved from the earlier, rather simplistic belief that generic "stimulation" can accelerate mental development, but there is evidence that specific environmental factors can influence language development. With language as an important element of higher cortical function, efforts to encourage communication by a variety of methods seem reasonable.

As more and more etiologies of mental retardation are identified, education research must be linked more closely to biological research. Differences in learning styles, memory, and problem analysis as well as many other factors require the development of more specific educational approaches to optimize cognition. The individualization of educational approaches to specific functional limitations, as well as to specific abilities, seems to be the next step in the amelioration of cognitive disabilities, while biological research pursues its more distant objectives.

Robert E. Cooke, M.D.
Professor Emeritus of Pediatrics
State University of New York at Buffalo

Preface

Child neurology traditionally has concentrated its efforts on the mechanisms of nervous system impairment, with major focus being placed on localization of dysfunction, the management of rare neurometabolic disorders, and the care of a wide variety of acute neurologic conditions. After a long period of neglect, more chronic neurologic disorders have become the subject of increasing clinical service demands and research attention because societal mandates have required that children with developmental disabilities be removed from institutional settings (i.e., the principle of deinstitutionalization) and instead receive appropriate support services in the community (i.e., the principle of normalization).

As part of this major social revolution, university affiliated programs were established and, along with other postdoctoral fellowship programs, began to produce pediatric subspecialists to meet the specialized medical needs of children with developmental disabilities. Developmental pediatricians were trained in the early diagnosis and assessment, treatment, and management of chronic central nervous system impairments.

Although this new field of developmental pediatrics addresses the total chronic encephalopathic spectrum and shares many areas of interest with neurology and psychiatry, the particular disorders that are of special interest to developmental pediatricians include cerebral palsy; multiple disabilities; impairments of vision and hearing; disorders of higher cortical function, such as mental retardation; learning disabilities; and neurobehavioral syndromes, such as attention deficit disorders. As pediatricians, developmentalists recognize the need for a lifelong, comprehensive, family-centered treatment approach that coordinates an interdisciplinary team composed of primary care medical professionals, medical subspecialists, paramedical professionals, and community-based social agencies to improve function and assist in the care of these children. U.S. society, as well as individual families, has the right to pediatricians with this expertise.

In this second edition of *Developmental Disabilities in Infancy and Childhood*, the contribution of the neurosciences has been highlighted to reflect the significant advances being made in the "decade of the brain." Boundaries that demarcated clinical disciplines previously are becoming more blurred as research in developmental disabilities becomes more interdisciplinary. Neurology is expanding its clinical knowledge base by interfacing with psychiatry, neurosurgery, and physical medicine to form a neuroscience consortium in an increasingly interdisciplinary approach. This neuroscience program has evolved to such an extent that developmental pediatrics and child neurology should join together to improve the care of children with developmental disorders and to cooperate in fostering basic research into such disorders.

Practice also has seen an increasing overlap between developmental pediatrics and child neurology. Developmental pediatricians are exhibiting greater interest in the neuropathologic foundation of functional central nervous system impairments to such an extent that they may be more appropriately identified as neurodevelopmental pediatricians. Much of this overlap is the result of the broad availability of newer techniques for defining mechanisms of central nervous system dysfunction. Child neurologists also have responded to the changing service needs of U.S. society, and, although they may lack formal training in developmental disabilities, they have attempted to incorporate the care of children with disabilities into their practices. Such interfacing and overlapping should be encouraged because shared perspectives will result in higher standards of care and serve to facilitate research endeavors.

Children with chronic neurologic disorders will continue to be served by many different medical professionals, each of whom provides a necessary component of the overall management.

Attempts to carve out clinical turf boundaries and claim exclusivity will prove futile. Children with chronic neurologic disorders and their families deserve formally trained professionals to coordinate their care and deal with their multiple problems, especially because their conditions are lifelong. Given that a decrease in the number of subspecialists in the United States has been declared a national priority, academicians need to focus on training primary health care providers to better assume the care of children with developmental disabilities. In the future, it will most likely be the pediatric generalist or family physician who will be responsible for much of the care delivered to children with disabilities. It is imperative that appropriate resident teaching experiences and consultation services be made available to these physicians.

Failure to interface with one another will diminish the involved specialties. The total spectrum of acute and chronic neurologic disorders is much too broad for a single subspecialty to meet commitments to quality research, teaching, and service. Developmental pediatrics cannot improve the care provided to children with developmental disabilities without better understanding the mechanisms of these disorders. This is the time for an academic "wedding" of developmental pediatrics and child neurology in order to address the total spectrum in an interdisciplinary manner conducive to fostering the needed clinical and basic research. The recent approval by the American Board of Pediatrics of a new subcertificate in neurodevelopmental disabilities and that board's recommendation to negotiate a conjoint arrangement with the American Board of Psychiatry and Neurology to develop combined training programs with child neurology leading to a triple certificate both suggest that this process has finally matured. It is hoped that the third edition of this textbook will address an audience that will include newly evolved developmental neuropediatricians.

Acknowledgments

The production of a second edition twice the size of the first edition has involved much more than twice the time and effort of that earlier work. It could not have been accomplished without the ongoing encouragement and untiring assistance of the staff of Paul H. Brookes Publishing Co. We would especially like to take this opportunity to thank Paul H. Brookes, Melissa A. Behm, Theresa Donnelly, Lyn Tisdale, Kim Collignon, Lynn Weber, Heather Shrestha, Kathy Boyd, and the many others who have worked so hard to see this project through to completion.

Com'anima gentil che non fa scusa,
ma fa sua voglia della voglia altrui,
tosto che'elle'e per segno fuor dischiusa
—Dante

For

Louise, Charles, Arnold, Jr., Allan, and Claiborne

and

Patricia, Jennifer, Matthew, and Claire

Developmental Disabilities in Infancy and Childhood
Second Edition

Volume II:
The Spectrum of Developmental Disabilities

Chapter 1

A Medical History of Developmental Disabilities

Pasquale J. Accardo, M.D.

You may alter the place to which you are going; but you cannot alter the place from which you have come.

G.K. Chesterton

The medical history of developmental disabilities comprises chapters from many other histories: the history of medicine (Accardo, 1992; Gordon, 1959; McGrew, 1985; Mettler, 1947), the history of pediatrics (Garrison, 1923; Ruhrah, 1925, 1932; Still, 1931), and the history of other subspecialties (LeVay, 1990; Weir, 1990), especially psychiatry (Alexander & Selesnick, 1968), neurology (Barbeau, 1981; Clarke & O'Malley, 1968; Denny-Brown, 1980; McHenry, 1969; Neuburger, 1897/1981), and anthropometrics (Boyd, 1980; Tanner, 1981). Many of the earliest contributions to the study of disability on the part of education, psychology, and social work came from physician pioneers.

In their extensive arguments over the nature of humankind, ancient and medieval philosophers debated over the significance of the presence or absence of language to the definition of a human being. Under the general term *infans* ("unable to speak"), Roman law had lumped together persons who were deaf, mute, or insane, those with mental retardation, and minors, because speech was a prerequisite for citizenship. Although many branches of medieval scholastic philosophy acquiesced in this equation, William, Abbot of St. Thierry (d. 1148), influenced by the obvious example of the mandatory silence of his Cistercian order, argued that human beings were unique with regard to both the power of speech and the use of their hands (Gilson, 1955). Because the soul could communicate and express itself through either spoken language or gestures, speech was not essential to humans (Critchley, 1939; O'Neill, 1980; Weiskrantz, 1988).

There was little in the ancient textbooks of medicine relating to disabilities because physicians were encouraged to avoid untreatable or incurable cases, so that chronic diseases typically were given short shrift (Jones, 1923; Spencer, 1938). In the Middle Ages, the charitable impulses of Christianity, Judaism, and Islam led medical philosophers to give somewhat more consideration to these chronic disorders. However, it was more as a philosopher than as a medical scientist, for example, that Avicenna (980–1037) discriminated disorders of locomotion as due to errors in configuration, development, or displacement (Gruner, 1930/1984).

Confusion in the area of diagnosis also was reflected in the primary method of treatment—religion. A number of saints have assumed the role of intercessor for persons with developmental disabilities. St. Dymphna of Gheel became the patroness of persons with mental disorders (including both mental retardation and severe emotional disorders) through such a confusion. Her execution at the hands of an incestuous father—an incomprehensible mixture of moral insanity and madness—contributed to her association with mental disorders. Over the centuries, her cult in Gheel, Belgium, facilitated the evolution of a community-wide, family-oriented, home-based treatment approach for persons with all types of mental disorders—an intervention style that was to anticipate many of the principles of normalization (Wolfensberger, 1972) by six centuries.

The much-neglected patron saint of Valencia, Our Lady of the Unprotected, inspired the

founding in 1413 of the Confraternity of the In-
nocents by Blessed Juan Gilaberto Jofre (Allardyce, 1912). A case also has been made for
Saint Nicholas, the original Santa Claus, as the
patron of children with disabilities, but this appears to reflect a simple generic extension of his
association with children. Systems of religious
belief and a structure of mythology would remain significant components of the way human
beings view developmental disabilities.

Although ancient and medieval medicine
rarely attempted to distinguish between mental
retardation and other forms of mental illness,
ancient and medieval law evolved careful
distinctions between "natural fools" (persons
suffering from permanent idiocy) and "lunatics"
(persons suffering from possibly transient psychiatric disorders). The emphasis of the law was
on the property rights of the person with a disability rather than on the person him- or herself.
Some of the phrasing from jurist Sir Anthony
Fitz-Herbert's 1534 declaration would reappear
in an early formulation by Arnold Gesell almost
four centuries later:

> And he who shall be said to be a sot [i.e., simple-
> ton] and idiot from his birth, is such a person who
> cannot account or number twenty pence, nor can
> tell who was his father or mother, nor how old he
> is, etc., so as it may appear that he hath no under-
> standing of reason what shall be for his profit nor
> what for his loss. But if he hath such understand-
> ing, that he know and understand his letters, and
> do read by teaching or information of another
> man, then it seemeth he is not a sot nor a natural
> idiot. (Doll, 1972, pp. 49–50)

This enumeration of skills not only suggests
something like an early IQ test but also is notable for its emphasis on social and adaptive behaviors. This legal distinction was clear to
philosophers such as John Locke (1632–1704):

> Herein seems to lie the difference between idiots
> and madmen, that madmen put wrong ideas to-
> gether, and so make wrong propositions, but argue
> and reason right from them, but idiots make very
> few or no propositions, and reason scarce at all.
> (1690/1959, Vol. I, p. 210)

The careful clinical description of nine degrees
of cognitive limitation and the relevance of each
of these functional levels to criminal and civil
court decisions found in the physician Isaac

Ray's 1838 (1987) jurisprudence textbook
would not be equaled in the psychological literature for almost another century.

Major advances in the understanding of developmental disorders, especially in the cognitive and motor deficit areas, took place during
the 19th century. Limited but dramatic treatment successes antedated similar advances in
diagnosis. A triphasic movement from apathy
and ignorance through optimism and enthusiasm to pessimism and neglect reflected the impact of the birth and evolution of psychiatry,
neurology, orthopedics, and, in the next century,
genetics. The easy successes and dramatic cures
that resulted largely from misdiagnoses gave
rise to unrealistic dreams that were soon
shattered.

THE 19TH CENTURY

Cerebral Palsy

Prior to the 19th century, physical deformities
were generally lumped together under the single
rubric of "cripple" regardless of whether the
disorder was congenital or acquired, central or
peripheral, or nervous or musculoskeletal in etiology. The absence of any effective intervention
or treatment contributed to this lack of diagnostic discrimination. Because bone setting was not
a recognized part of medicine, orthopedics
started out as a science of positioning and posture (Andry, 1743/1980). In the preanesthesia,
preantisepsis, preantibiotic era, there was little
encouragement to devise novel orthopedic
therapies.

William John Little (1810–1894) is credited
with the first accurate description of cerebral
palsy. In fact, he had first devised a successful
treatment for a major component of both clubfoot and spastic cerebral palsy (adductor tenotomy for talipes equinovarus) before the varying success of the surgical procedure forced
more accurate differential diagnosis—to better
discriminate which patients would benefit from
the procedure—and allowed the evolution of
a clearer understanding of the underlying
brain dysfunction (Accardo, 1980, 1981, 1989;
Schleichkorn, 1987). The smallness of the inci-
sion required for tenotomy and the quickness of

the procedure kept the infection and complication rates relatively low (Little, 1853/1993).

Little's pioneering description of cerebral palsy was of a condition that was more than just a mere motor disorder; it was rather a complex multisystem disorder with motor, cognitive, sensory, and behavioral symptomatology. Indeed, it included the entire continuum of developmental disability. After decades of performing tenotomies, Little ventured to suggest an unexpected etiology for many of his cases of infantile spasmoparalysis: He postulated neonatal asphyxia as a major cause of brain damage that would later present as cerebral palsy (Little, 1861–1862). This hypothesis was revolutionary in that, up to this point in time, the standard textbooks in midwifery and obstetrics held the opinion that there were only two possible outcomes to *asphyxia neonatorum*, either death or complete recovery (Cameron, 1958). Little's "third outcome"—the perception that a cause of brain damage might not have any obvious impact until up to a year or two of age—was the kind of "action at a distance" for which the medical world was not prepared. Yet this was exactly the course of most cases of cerebral palsy, with a latent and even hypotonic period being in evidence during the first 9–18 months of life prior to the development of the classic clinical presentation of spasticity. The etiologic association between later cerebral palsy and perinatal events still remains unclear today (Brown, 1976). Spastic diplegia became known as "Little's disease," even though his original paper includes descriptive case histories of most of the other subtypes of cerebral palsy.

Perceptions implicit in Little's work were to be made explicit later in the writings of the neurologist Sir William Gowers (1845–1915), who espoused "Little's etiology," a causative association between asphyxia neonatorum (and prematurity) with later cerebral palsy (Critchley, 1949; Gowers, 1893/1970). Sir William Osler (1849–1919) also made significant contributions to the clinical description of the various subtypes of cerebral palsy, especially the hemiplegic group. His monograph on the series of patients he had studied at the Elwyn Institute in Pennsylvania (Osler, 1889) gave the disorder the name by which it remains known today.

The Viennese neurologist Sigmund Freud (1856–1939) studied under Jean-Martin Charcot (1825–1893) (Owen, 1971) and devised a classification scheme for the subtypes of cerebral palsy that would provide the basis for all modern nosology. He continued to develop the clinical intuitions that had only been adumbrated by Little. The most striking of these observations was the recognition that three major recognized neurologic impairments of childhood—cerebral palsy, mental retardation, and epilepsy—were closely related and could not be understood independently. Thus, mental retardation could be viewed as cerebral palsy with minimal to no motor component. Epilepsy without seizures could also present as mental retardation. Brain damage, or static encephalopathy, was clearly being interpreted as both a spectrum and a continuum by these pioneers in the developmental disorders of childhood (Accardo, 1982; Freud, 1897/1968). The extremely negative impact of Freud's work in cerebral palsy was the discovery of a relatively complete absence of any correlation between the clinical classification or subtyping of the movement disorder pattern on the one hand and the identifiable neuropathology at autopsy on the other hand. This contributed to a half-century of medical neglect for what was perceived as a wastebasket category of neuromotor conditions that refused to fit into the accepted schema of neuropathologic localization.

It is important to note the peculiar order in which events transpired. An internist devised the first major orthopedic procedure for the correction of a deformity of the human frame in childhood almost a century before differential diagnosis allowed a subtle enough distinction of etiologic classification to apply operative interventions appropriately among this population. Treatment preceded and precipitated accurate diagnosis. This is the reverse of the more typical situation in the evolution of medicine, wherein diagnosis usually precipitates the search for and antedates the discovery of a cure.

Mental Retardation

The pioneering French psychiatrists Philippe Pinel (1745–1826) and Jean Etienne Dominique Esquirol (1772–1840) revolutionized the treatment of persons then labeled as "insane." They considered it imperative to distinguish permanent cognitive deficits (idiocy, imbecility, and feeblemindedness) from possibly ephemeral (and potentially more curable) psychiatric diagnoses, such as insanity, mania, dementia, and melancholy. Pinel (1806/1983) relied on head size and cranial shape (as these differed from the classic norm represented by the Apollo Belvedere) to differentiate these two large groups, and Esquirol (1845/1987, p. 470) stressed the functional use of language to discriminate five levels of mental retardation:

> In the first degree of imbecility, speech is free and easy. In the second, it is less easy, and the vocabulary is more circumscribed. In the first degree of idiocy, properly so called, the idiot uses merely words and short phrases. Idiots of the second degree, articulate only monosyllables, or certain cries. Finally, in the third degree of idiocy, there is neither speech or phrases; words nor monosyllables.

Early in the century, the physician Jean Marc Gaspard Itard (1774–1838), aided with a grant from the French government, undertook the treatment of Victor, the Wild Boy of Aveyron. Itard's "physiologic method" provided his student with a graded series of stimulus discrimination training exercises. The program was derived from the erratic educational speculations of *Emile* (Payne, 1892) by Jean Jacques Rousseau (1712–1778) and the sensationalist philosophy of Etienne Bonnot de Condillac (1715–1780), but had a more solid grounding in Itard's clinical experience with the methods of educating children with deafness and the system of sign language devised by Jacob Rodrigue Pereire (1715–1780). Itard's attempts at educating this feral child created one of the great myths on which 20th century behaviorist psychology is based (Itard, 1801/1806/1962; Lane, 1977). If, on the one hand, Itard's accomplishment was that he succeeded in training a child purportedly raised by wolves to behave in a more socially acceptable manner, his achievement was trivial. On the other hand, if he had been training a youth with brain damage and mental retardation who had been the victim of extreme neglect for a decade, then even his limited success represented a major milestone in the history of special education. Because Itard leaned toward the former interpretation of dismal failure, he devoted the remainder of his career to the founding of otolaryngology as a medical specialty. The whole issue of definite but often limited gains through different interventions has remained a permanent challenge in the field of mental retardation. The myth of feral children has remained as persistently imagined proof for the otherwise unverified assumptions of behaviorist psychology (Malson, 1972).

The physician Edouard Onesmus Seguin (1812–1880) helped formalize Itard's educational techniques (Seguin, 1866/1971). A student of Itard, he nevertheless believed that his mentor's system was too heavily based on sensory input. After immigrating to the United States, Seguin further refined these intervention programs and became one of the founders of the institutional movement, along with such other physician pioneers in the field of mental retardation as Samuel Gridley Howe (1801–1896). Although he described his system as moral training, it retained very close links with the sensory training that formed the basis of Itard's approach (Kraft, 1961). Seguin stressed physical culture and devised a variety of formboards to educate the discriminatory faculties (Talbot, 1964). A number of these educational devices later would find their way into the earliest IQ tests. Of interest with regard to the origin of a popular alternative educational methodology, Maria Montessori (1870–1952) adapted the techniques of Itard and Seguin for use with socioculturally deprived slum children and devised a developmental stimulation curriculum for all children (Montessori, 1972).

This physician-led educational movement evolved before the development of any accurate differential diagnostic capability beyond the psychiatrist's (or other professional's) vague clinical impression as to whether a given patient's slowness might be treatable. As with cerebral palsy, powerful intervention techniques were unleashed in the absence of any very clear diagnostic tools. The next important stage would require a significant improvement in the precision of identifying specific etiologies and subgroups among the broad heterogeneous classification of mental retardation.

William Witherspoon Ireland (1832–1909) wrote the first medical textbook on mental retardation. His 1877 classification of etiologies for "idiocy" was the first attempt at a medical nosology (Table 1). In this classification, genetous referred not to genetics, which did not exist as a discipline at this time (the papers of the Austrian monk Gregor Mendel [1822–1884] still remained undiscovered), but to what would today be called idiopathic; it was Ireland's largest single subgroup and remains so today. Microcephaly was equated with an adult head circumference of less than 17 inches. Both the eclampsic and epileptic subgroups exhibited seizures, but the former subgroup was characterized by convulsions that seemed to disappear with age (as in infantile spasms or hypsarhythmia), whereas the latter experienced seizures throughout the life span. The paralytic group exemplified the strong association between mental retardation and cerebral palsy. Cretinism probably included a mixture of cases of congenital hypothyroidism and patients with Down syndrome. Traumatic idiocy was a sequela to severe head injury, and inflammatory idiocy was postmeningitic or postencephalitic. Idiocy by deprivation referred not to sociocultural retardation but rather to the loss or severe impairment of two or more senses. Under this rubric, persons such as Helen Keller and Laura Dewey Bridgman were presented to the public as typical of the power of the new educational technology to cure mental retardation whenever the appropriate key was found to unlock the mind within. In fact, such cases actually reflected the impact of education on pseudoretardation. The treatment was correct; the diagnosis was erroneous. Ireland's classification would be subsumed into the first major textbook of pediatrics (Holt, 1897/1980).

Much of the material in Ireland's textbook was derived from the pioneering observations of John Langdon Haydon Langdon-Down (1828–1896) in the diagnosis of mental deficiency. In an attempt to produce an ethnic classification of idiots, Down provided the first reasonably accurate depiction of the genetic trisomy that for many years bore his name. Although his delineation of this syndrome as "Mongolian" and the description of patients as "mongoloid" produced much confusion, it was neither unscientific nor derogatory in its time, and was, in fact, but a partial expression of Down's insistence on the breaking up of mental defect into subtypes based in large part on physical dysmorphology. He considered minor malformations to be clear evidence for a prenatal rather than an obstetric etiology of developmental problems, and he was among the first to recognize the importance of correlating brain pathology with behavioral phenotype. He claimed that "the basis of all treatment should be *medical*. Medical, I mean, in an enlarged sense" (Down, 1887/1990, p. 80).

Most surveys of the history of mental retardation (Kanner, 1964; Rosen, Clark, & Kivitz, 1976; Scheerenberger, 1983, 1987) record the decline of enthusiasm for treatment being curative, the genetics scare, and the misguided eugenics and sterilization movements that ended the 19th and opened the 20th centuries. In the early part of the present century, the training schools found themselves left with an increasing hard core residuum of students who could not be trained successfully to enter the community; these institutions transitioned gradually into permanent residential facilities for custodial care. Their initial optimism gradually clouded over into a pseudoscientific pessimism, and they became "institutions" in the modern pejorative sense—warehouses for social outcasts.

Much of this "loss of nerve"—this breaking of faith with the pseudoreligious idealism and worship of progress and of the perfectibility of humans characteristic of the 19th century—is attributed erroneously to the misguided mania

Table 1. Ireland's classification of idiocy

Genetous
Microcephalic
Eclampsic
Epileptic
Hydrocephalic
Paralytic
Cretinism
Traumatic
Inflammatory
Idiocy by deprivation

Adapted from Ireland (1877).

for the abuse and misuse of psychometric tests (a phenomenon highly indigenous to North America) (Chase, 1980) and the related evolution and dominance of a pessimistic medical model of organic deficit. The contribution of the false enthusiasm, if not fraud, generated by such professionals as the revivalist fund-raiser Johann Jacob Guggenbuhl (1816–1863) with his fresh air treatment for cretinism, and numerous other deceptive claims, often is excused politely as well intentioned.

THE 20TH CENTURY

Cerebral Palsy

Progress in cerebral palsy during the first half of the 20th century was excruciatingly slow. Research on the reflex patterns underlying the tone abnormality and movement disorder for each subtype of cerebral palsy was just beginning (Peiper, 1963; Rademaker, 1931/1980). Unproven therapies multiplied with little criticism from the medical and scientific establishments. The first organizational meeting of the American Academy for Cerebral Palsy (AACP; now the American Academy for Cerebral Palsy and Developmental Medicine, AACPDM) was held on November 5, 1947. The founding members included Earl Carlson (1897–1974), Bronson Crothers (1884–1959), George Deaver (1890–1973), Temple Fay (1895–1963), Meyer Perlstein (1902–1969), and Winthrop Phelps (1894–1971); Arnold Gesell was elected to membership at the first meeting. In 1959, Bronson Crothers and Richmond Paine published the first landmark textbook on cerebral palsy. The trend in the first half of the century was toward a more restrictive but more effective use of orthopedic surgery through a tailoring of the surgical procedure to the individual pattern of motor disorder. Such a linking of surgical intervention with the most careful differential diagnosis of the motor disability represents a perfect culmination to the goals originally set by Little.

A pediatrician, Arnold Gesell (1888–1961), was the first professional to document systematically the development of infants and young children; most previous attempts at measuring intelligence or development had ignored the youngest children. His meticulous observations have served as the basis for all succeeding infant tests and remain a useful reservoir of clinical information for the practicing pediatrician (Gesell & Amatruda, 1947). His success in this area stems in part from the fact that many of his test items were derived from parental descriptions of the things in which their children were most interested. Gesell clearly recognized the complexities of development and that it could never be reduced to a single developmental quotient. He saw the developmentalist as the medical professional who would be competent to assess the various areas of development and utilize this information to achieve a comprehensive diagnostic formulation with regard to the child's developmental status. The importance of the developmental pediatrician, the new subspecialist envisioned by Gesell, was slow in finding acceptance. The major obstacle to the training of such personnel was solved in the late 1960s by the establishment of University Affiliated Facilities (UAFs; now University Affiliated Programs, UAPs), with their triple goal of training, service, and research in the area of developmental disabilities. Despite the renewed emphasis on research, successful evaluation of the efficacy of many modes of therapeutic intervention in developmental disabilities remains in the future.

Mental Retardation

The record of the early training schools was impressive with regard to the large numbers of persons with mental retardation that they were able to reintegrate into the community at large. However, the psychologist Alfred Binet (1857–1911) and the physician Theophile Simon (1873–1961) were not to produce the first standardized intelligence test until 1905, and it is both conceivable and probable that many of those persons previously diagnosed as having mental retardation in reality had learning disabilities and language disorders (Binet & Simon, 1916/1973; Peterson, 1926/1969; Wolf, 1973). It is an irony that the modern descendents of this first objective instrument to measure cognitive ability are under attack for the identical reason that first led to its development: distrust of observer bias in identifying cases of mental retardation. Despite its later abuse, the Binet-Simon scale represented a significant step forward, a liberation from otherwise arbitrary and subjective classification.

Ancient and medieval encyclopedists included human monstrosities in their bestiaries, and philosophers pondered on the meaning of such abnormalities for a definition of the human (Warkany, 1971). In his book *Traite des Monstres*, the great surgeon Ambrose Paré (1573/1982) typically described deformities that he had observed personally and also repeated fantastic descriptions of legendary creatures. Until an approach to syndrome identification based on scientific principles could be established, many human deformities would remain medical curiosities (Gould & Pyle, 1896/1956). However, even while the specific nature of the medical disorder remained unclear, by the late 19th century society was able to exhibit empathy toward the plight of individuals such as Joseph Merrick (1862–1890), the so-called elephant man (Howell & Ford, 1980; Treves, 1923/1993). Slowly but surely the scientific foundation for the pseudoscience of physiognomy by Johann Caspar Lavater (1741–1801) and others was being deduced.

The accurate medical delineation of specific syndromes in the 20th century progressed slowly after the pioneering efforts of Down in the 19th century (Beighton & Beighton, 1986; Penrose, 1949). The broad range of phenotypic expression of both genetic and teratogenic conditions contributed to the difficulties in this area. Such common and widespread syndromes as fetal alcohol and fragile X remained obscured until comparatively recently. Research on evolutionary issues, personality types, and the predisposition to psychiatric conditions all contributed to the difficulties in this work (Darwin, 1872/1969; Duchenne de Boulogne, 1862/1990; Kretschmer, 1936/1970). Paradoxically, the study of such group effects led to an increasing emphasis on the uniqueness of the individual: Francis Galton's quantitative investigation of fingerprints helped in the later delineation of many syndromes, and Sir Archibald Garrod's researches into alcaptonuria generated in 1909 the concept of inborn errors of metabolism (the "one gene–one enzyme" hypothesis).

The rediscovery and expansion of mendelian genetics in the early part of the 20th century (Bateson, 1909/1990) provided the needed scientific infrastructure but also opened the door to many abuses. Richard Dugdale (1841–1883) wrote *The Jukes: A Study of Crime, Pauperism, Disease, and Heredity* (1874), and Henry Herbert Goddard (1866–1957) wrote *The Kallikak Family: A Study in the Heredity of Feeblemindedness* (1912). Neither professional was a physician. At its inception, genetics was not viewed as a component of medical science, and the popularization of theories of the genetic determinism of mental defect came from nonphysicians. As with most social engineering, it was based on pseudoscience.

The books by Goddard and Dugdale tried to document that mental retardation was either an autosomal dominant or an autosomal recessive trait. They then argued that, if all persons with mental retardation in a single generation were prevented from reproducing, the disorder would be significantly decreased in the next generation and virtually eradicated within several generations. An international eugenics movement led to the passage of sterilization laws in the United States and euthanasia laws in Germany (Binding & Hoche, 1920/1975; Lifton, 1986). The extent to which euthanasia (direct or indirect) may have been carried out in the United States in this century remains unknown (Elks, 1993), but Gardner (1993) warned that pessimism and disillusionment may have been prevalent in institutional settings as early as the late 1850s, in the height of the "era of optimism." The history of mental retardation has few examples of linear progress, but appears to resemble more a complex tapestry with many interweaving and often conflicting strands.

Disorders of Higher Cortical Function

The 19th century had witnessed the identification of developmental disabilities whose presenting problem was delay—motor delay in the case of cerebral palsy and cognitive delay in the case of mental retardation. Identification of developmental disabilities whose presenting problem was dissociation between general ability or intelligence and the more specialized cognitive areas of language, learning, communication, and social interaction—disorders such as learning disabilities, communication disorders, and autism—came in the 20th century.

Late in the 19th century, select cases of a rare disorder referred to as congenital word blindness began to be reported (Hinshelwood, 1895, 1900; Morgan, 1896). The conceptualization of specific neurologically based deficits in reading ability (dyslexia) would need to wait the development of a psychology of reading (Huey, 1908/1968) as well as sufficient clarification of the novel quantification of intellectual capability, to allow any accurate understanding or diagnosis of such learning discrepancies or disabilities. Samuel Torrey Orton (1879–1948), after whom the Orton Society for the study of dyslexia was named, stressed the linkage between reading difficulties and speech and language disorders and interpreted all of these dysfunctions as neurologic in origin (1937, 1966; Critchley, 1970). Although there are several genetic markers for pure dyslexia, most reading deficits today are recognized as subtypes within the broader category of learning disabilities. It would not be until after the extensive study of head injuries in World War II by the Russian neurosurgeon Alexander Luria (1902–1977) that neuropsychology would begin to provide reasonably accurate brain localization for such isolated learning deficits (Luria, 1966). Gerstmann (1930) and Prechtl and Stemmer (1959) pioneered in the identification of specific neurocognitive and neurobehavioral syndromes; Rett syndrome and Smith-Magenis syndrome later would outline more definitively the future subspecialty area of behavioral genetics.

In a series of papers in *Lancet*, Sir George Frederick Still (1902) gave the first scientific description of a group of behavior disorder patterns in children—what later would be called attention-deficit/hyperactivity disorder. That occurrences of a similar pattern of behavior disorder were noted to follow an encephalitis epidemic shortly after World War I (Hohman, 1922) gave impetus to the interpretation of this syndrome as neurologically based. In an almost serendipitous discovery, benzedrine was noted to improve markedly many of these brain-damage–related behaviors in children (Bradley, 1937). In two large series of clinical research publications, the physician–psychologist Alfred Strauss (1897–1957) (Strauss & Kephart, 1955; Strauss & Lehtinen, 1947) and the educator William Cruickshank (1967) put forth the conceptualization of the child with brain injury as the model for special education; Cruickshank interpreted learning disabilities/language disorders and cerebral palsy as the two ends of a single continuum.

Hilda Knobloch and Benjamin Pasamanick (1959) suggested a continuum of reproductive casualty that allowed minimal cerebral damage to result from less than optimal pre- and perinatal care and that could present in infancy (Laufer & Denhoff, 1957). In 1967, Lenneberg presented a strong case for the biological foundation of language. Paul Wender (1971) first popularized the neurotransmitter imbalance theory and its correlative psychostimulant treatment for minimal brain dysfunction. Much of the earlier psychiatric literature that describes the controversial "moral insanity" or "moral imbecility" sounds very much like an attention deficit (similarly controversial) that has been superimposed on a wide variety of other conditions (Kraepelin, 1913/1985). It was not until 1943 that Leo Kanner first described the puzzling neurobehavioral syndrome of autism.

THE LESSONS OF HISTORY

The history of developmental disabilities documents medical leadership throughout the 19th century. The lack of effective medical therapies in all but a few disorders contributed to a rebellion by nonmedical professionals against medical dominance in the field. Physicians were targeted as arrogant, self-serving, and paternalistic. As the 20th century progressed, nonmedical professionals found themselves less and less able to scapegoat medicine as they fell into the same professional stereotype of arrogance, self-service, and paternalism (Blatt, 1987). A rebellion against the inadequacy of all professionals was led by parent groups that did not want theoretical promises of future cures but rather concrete solutions to practical, everyday problems. The current phase of the eternal rebellion against the hard fact of being human and worthwhile yet different has now struck at the parents themselves as being arrogant, self-serving, and paternalistic (Shapiro, 1993). Self-advocacy for persons with mental retardation now places them in an adversarial relationship with their own families. Such advocacy needs, of course, facilitators such as those used in facilitated communication and as are proposed in the equal rights for children movement. However, as Purdy (1992) queries, does respect for others always rule out paternalism?

The current disabilities rights movement is heavily rooted in the Whorf-Sapir theory of linguistic determinism (or linguistic relativism). This hypothesis states that language shapes reality. It is an old theory that is little accepted in linguistic circles; its conceptualization of language as determining rather than reflecting social reality is a type of dialectical materialism that was historically disproven—insofar as any theory can ever be so disproven—by the collapse of communism in Europe. The idea that such negative terms as *idiot, imbecile,* and *moron* determined how society valued people is rendered untenable in the presence of such facts as the deliberate creation of the term *moron* as a value-free and neutral label by Goddard in 1910.

Political and social activism not infrequently have a negative impact on science (Eyer, 1993; Fletcher, 1991). Bad science, poor science, corrupt science, no science—these all open the door to quackery and irrational belief systems (Holbrook, 1959) that, with their false hope and their wasting of limited resources, eventually damage people. History, including this last decade of the 20th century, is all too full of examples from which we refuse to learn. We try to write history as a linear progression, stepping from one great scientific discovery to the next social quantum leap, when in fact continuity and sameness are the most striking hallmarks of human endeavor. Other centuries were not exclusively barbarically cruel to children and persons with disabilities (Boswell, 1988; Pollock, 1983). Indeed, our own century has probably exceeded all others in the deliberate destruction and extermination of human life without value—and it has done so with the best of pseudoscientific and social need rationalizations (Lasch, 1977).

In the earlier half of the century, Doll (1953) advocated an emphasis on the social skill dimension in the assessment of outcome for special education. In the intervening time, little progress has been made to quantitate the measurement of such abilities. One of the major rationales for shifting from a cognitive to a social competence basis for the definition of mental retardation is the simple but tacitly ignored fact that all attempts to raise intelligence in persons with mental retardation and to prove the educability hypothesis have failed (Blatt, 1987; Spitz, 1986). If the "mantle of advocacy" is apparently to replace the objectivity of science (Spitz, 1986), those professionals committed to the application of science to the diagnosis and treatment of developmental disorders may need to redefine their terminology. Cognitive limitation and cognitive subtyping are, from a neurobiologic perspective, measurable if not fixed parameters necessary for the clear delineation of syndromes. For example, a geneticist working on associating marker chromosomes with cognitive functioning will need to classify patients by IQ score as a measure of severity, rather than by level of social supports needed for functioning in the community, because the latter would be much more variable.

Modern science has as its hallmark an emphasis on quantitative measurement; some may interpret this as a weakness or limitation, but it remains science's greatest and most productive strength. Physicians and scientists dealing with developmental disabilities are diagnosing static encephalopathies that include cognitive limitation, motor impairment, language and learning deficits, and neurobehavioral symptomatology. Such brain disorders are relatively permanent, although their manifestations may be alleviated by both educational and environmental interventions. To pursue its diagnostic, research and therapeutic goals successfully, pediatric developmental medicine must conceptualize developmental disabilities as organic impairments. That the diagnosis of such disabilities implies no devaluation of the human person goes without saying.

Taking the lead from a popular article by Gesell, Doll (1917) suggested the appropriateness of several different definitions of mental retardation according to the concerns of the different professional disciplines involved. Thus, varying with the diagnostic instruments used and the goals for diverse treatments, there might be separate definitions of mental retardation for the psychologist, the social worker, the educator, and the physician. Scientific medical progress would seem to warrant such a splitting in the present political climate.

REFERENCES

Accardo, P.J. (1980). Deformity and character: Dr. Little and the diagnosis of Richard III. *JAMA, 244.* 2746–2747.

Accardo, P.J. (1981). An early case report of muscular dystrophy: A footnote to the history of neuromuscular disorders. *Archives of Neurology, 38,* 144–146.

Accardo, P.J. (1982). Freud on diplegia: Commentary and translation. *American Journal of Diseases of Children, 136,* 452–456.

Accardo, P.J. (1989). William John Little (1810–1894) and cerebral palsy in the nineteenth century. *Journal of the History of Medicine and Allied Sciences, 44,* 56–71.

Accardo, P.J. (1992). *The medical almanac.* Totowa, NJ: Humana Press.

Alexander, F.G., & Selesnick, S.T. (1968). *The history of psychiatry.* New York: New American Library.

Allardyce, I. (1912). *Historical shrines of Spain.* Quebec: Franciscan Missionary Press.

Andry, N. (1743). *Orthopaedia: Or, the art of correcting and preventing deformities in children* (2 vols.). London: A. Millar. (Reprinted 1980, Birmingham, AL: Classics of Medicine Library)

Barbeau, A. (1981). History of movement disorders. In A. Barbeau (Ed.), *Disorders of movement* (pp. 1–28). Philadelphia: J.B. Lippincott.

Bateson, W. (1909). *Mendel's principles of heredity.* Cambridge, England: Cambridge University Press. (Reprinted 1990, Birmingham, AL: Classics of Medicine Library)

Beighton, P., & Beighton, G. (1986). *The man behind the syndrome.* New York: Springer-Verlag.

Binding, K., & Hoche, A. (1920). *Die Freigabe der Vernichtung lebensunwerten Lebens: Ihr Mass und ihre Form.* Leipzig: F. Meiner. (Translated 1975, *The release of the destruction of life devoid of value: It's measure and its form.* Santa Ana, CA: Life Quality)

Binet, A., & Simon, T. (1916). *The development of intelligence in children.* Baltimore: Williams & Wilkins. (Reprinted 1973, New York: Arno Press)

Blatt, B. (1987). *The conquest of mental retardation.* Austin, TX: PRO-ED.

Boswell, J. (1988). *The kindness of strangers: The abandonment of children in Western Europe from late antiquity to the renaissance.* New York: Pantheon Books.

Boyd, E. (1980). *Origins of the study of human growth.* Eugene: University of Oregon Health Sciences Center Foundation.

Bradley, C. (1937). The behavior of children receiving benzedrine. *American Journal of Psychiatry, 94,* 577–585.

Brown, G.W. (1976). Berkson fallacy revisited: Spurious conclusions from patient surveys. *American Journal of Diseases of Children, 130,* 56–60.

Cameron, H.C. (1958). Spasticity and the intellect: Dr. Little versus the obstetricians. *Cerebral Palsy Bulletin, 2,* 1–5.

Chase, A. (1980). *The legacy of Malthus: The social costs of the new scientific racism.* Urbana: University of Illinois Press.

Clarke, E., & O'Malley, C.D. (1968). *The human brain and spinal cord.* Berkeley: University of California Press.

Critchley, M. (1939). *The language of gesture.* London: Edward Arnold.

Critchley, M. (1949). *Sir William Gowers, 1845–1915.* London: William Heinemann Medical Books.

Critchley, M. (1970). *The dyslexic child.* Springfield, IL: Charles C Thomas.

Cruickshank, W.M. (1967). *The brain injured child in home, school and community.* Syracuse, NY: Syracuse University Press.

Darwin, C. (1872). *The expression of the emotions in man and animals.* London: John Murray. (Reprinted 1969, Bruxelles: Culture et Civilisation)

Denny-Brown, D. (1980). Historical aspects of the relation of spasticity to movement. In R.G. Feldman, R.R. Young, & W.P. Koella (Eds.), *Spasticity: Disordered motor control* (pp. 1–15). Chicago: Year Book Medical Publishers.

Doll, E.A. (1917) *Clinical studies in feeble-mindedness.* Boston: Richard G. Badger.

Doll, E.A. (1953). *Measurement of social competence.* Circle Pines, MN: American Guidance Service.

Doll, E.E. (1972). A historical survey of research and management of mental retardation in the United States. In E.P. Trapp & P. Himelstein (Eds.), *Readings on the exceptional child: Research and theory* (pp. 47–97). New York: Appleton-Century-Crofts.

Down, J.L. (1887). *On some of the mental affections of childhood and youth.* Classics in Developmental Medicine No. 5. Philadelphia: J.B. Lippincott. (Reprinted 1990)

Duchenne de Boulogne, G.-B. (1862). *The mechanism of human facial expression*. Paris: Jules Renouard. (Translated 1990, New York: Cambridge University Press)

Dugdale, R. (1874). *The Jukes: A study of crime, pauperism, disease, and heredity*. New York: Putnam.

Elks, M.A. (1993). The "lethal chamber": Further evidence for the euthanasia option. *Mental Retardation, 31,* 201–207.

Esquirol, E. (1845). *Mental maladies: A treatise on insanity* (E.K. Hunt, Trans.). Philadelphia: Lea and Blanchard. (Reprinted 1987, Birmingham, AL: Classics of Medicine Library)

Eyer, D.E. (1993). *Mother-infant bonding: A scientific fiction*. New Haven, CT: Yale University Press.

Fletcher, R. (1991). *Science, ideology and the media: The Cyril Burt scandal*. New Brunswick, NJ: Transaction Publishers.

Freud, S. (1968). *Infantile cerebral paralysis* (L.A. Russin, Trans.). Coral Gables, FL: University of Miami Press. (Original work published 1897)

Gardner, J.F. (1993). The era of optimism, 1850–1870: A preliminary reappraisal. *Mental Retardation, 31,* 89–95.

Garrison, F.H. (1923). History of pediatrics. In I.A. Abt (Ed.), *A system of pediatrics* (Vol. 1, pp. 1–130). Philadelphia: W.B. Saunders.

Gerstmann, J. (1930). Zur Symptomatologie der Hirnlasionen im Ubergangsgebiet der unteren Parietal- und mittleren Occipitalwindung. (Das Syndrom: Fingeragnosie, Rechts-Links-Storung, Agraphie, Akalkulie). *Nervenarzt, 3,* 691–695.

Gesell, A., & Amatruda, C.S. (1947). *Developmental diagnosis: Normal and abnormal child development: Clinical methods and pediatric applications*. New York: Paul B. Hoeber.

Gilson, E. (1955). *History of Christian philosophy in the middle ages*. New York: Random House.

Goddard, H.H. (1912). *The Kallikak family: A study in the heredity of feeblemindness*. New York: MacMillan.

Gordon, B.L. (1959). *Medieval and renaissance medicine*. New York: Philosophical Library.

Gould, G.M., & Pyle, W.L. (1896). *Anomalies and curiosities of medicine*. Philadelphia: W.B. Saunders. (Reprinted 1956, New York: Julian Press)

Gowers, W.R. (1893). *A manual of diseases of the nervous system* (2 vols.). (Reprinted 1970, Darien, CT: Hafner)

Gruner, O.C. (1930). *A treatise on the canon of medicine of Avicenna*. London: Luzac & Co. (Reprinted 1984, Birmingham, AL: Classics of Medicine Library)

Hinshelwood, J. (1895). Word-blindness and visual memory. *Lancet, 2,* 1564–1570.

Hinshelwood, J. (1900). *Letter-, word-, and mind-blindness*. London: H.K. Lewis.

Hohman, L.B. (1922). Post encephalitic behavior disorders in children. *Johns Hopkins Bulletin, 33,* 372–375.

Holbrook, S.H. (1959). *The golden age of quackery.* New York: Collier Books.

Holt, L.E. (1897). *The diseases of infancy and childhood*. New York: D. Appleton and Company. (Reprinted 1980, Birmingham, AL: Classics of Medicine Library)

Howell, M., & Ford, P. (1980). *The true history of the elephant man*. New York: Penguin Books.

Huey, E.B. (1908). *The psychology and pedagogy of reading*. New York: Macmillan. (Reprinted 1968, Cambridge, MA: MIT Press)

Ireland, W.W. (1877). *Idiocy and imbecility*. London: J. & A. Churchill.

Itard, J.M.-G. (1962). *The wild boy of Aveyron* (G. & M. Humphrey, Trans.). New York: Appleton-Century-Crofts. (Original work published 1801/1806)

Jones, W.H.S. (Trans.). (1923). *Hippocrates* (4 vols.). Cambridge, MA: Harvard University Press.

Kanner, L. (1943). Autistic disturbances of affective contact. *Nervous Child, 2,* 227–250.

Kanner, L. (1964). *A history of the care and study of the mentally retarded*. Springfield, IL: Charles C Thomas.

Knobloch, H., & Pasamanick, B. (1959). Syndrome of minimal cerebral damage in infancy. *JAMA, 170,* 1384–1387.

Kraepelin, E. (1913). *Lectures on clinical psychiatry*. New York: William Wood & Co. (Reprinted 1985, Birmingham, AL: Classics of Medicine Library)

Kraft, I. (1961). Edouard Seguin and 19th century moral treatment of idiots. *Bulletin of the History of Medicine, 35,* 393–418.

Kretschmer, E. (1970). *Physique and character: An investigation of the nature of constitution and the theory of temperament*. New York: Cooper Square Publishers. (Original work published 1936)

Lane, H. (1977). *The wild boy of Aveyron*. New York: Bantam.

Lasch, C. (1977). *Haven in a heartless world*. New York: Basic Books.

Laufer, M.J., & Denhoff, E. (1957). Hyperkinetic behavior syndrome in children. *Journal of Pediatrics, 50,* 463–473.

Lenneberg, E. (1967). *Biological foundations of language*. New York: John Wiley & Sons.

LeVay, D. (1990). *The history of orthopaedics*. Park Ridge, NJ: Parthenon Publishing Group.

Lifton, R.J. (1986). *The Nazi doctors: Medical killing and the psychology of genocide*. New York: Basic Books.

Little, W.J. (1853). *On the nature and treatment of the deformities of the human frame: Being a course of lectures delivered at the Royal Orthopaedic Hospital in 1843: With numerous notes and additions to the present time*. London: Longman Brown and Greene & Longmans. (Reprinted 1993, New York: Classics of Neurology and Neurosurgery)

Little, W.J. (1861–1862). On the influence of abnormal parturition, difficult labours, premature birth, and asphyxia-neonatorum, on the mental and physical condition of the child, especially in relation to deformities. *Transactions of the Obstetrical Society of London, 3,* 293–344.

Locke, J. (1959). *An essay concerning human understanding* (2 vols.). New York: Dover Publications. (Original work published 1690)

Luria, A.R. (1966). *Higher cortical functions in man.* New York: Basic Books.

Malson, L. (1972). *Wolf children and the problem of human nature.* New York: Monthly Review Press.

McGrew, R. (1985). *Encyclopedia of medical history.* London: Macmillan.

McHenry, L.C., Jr. (1969). *Garrison's history of neurology.* Springfield, IL: Charles C Thomas.

Mettler, C.C. (1947). *History of medicine.* Philadelphia: Blakiston.

Montessori, M. (1972). *The discovery of the child* (J. Costelloe, Trans.). New York: Ballantine Books.

Morgan, W.P. (1896). Congenital word blindness. *British Medical Journal, 2,* 1378.

Neuburger, M. (1981). *The historical development of experimental brain and spinal cord physiology before Flourens* (E. Clarke, Trans.). Baltimore: Johns Hopkins University Press. (Original work published 1897.)

O'Neill, Y.V. (1980). *Speech and speech disorders in western thought before 1600.* Westport, CT: Greenwood Press.

Orton, S.T. (1937). *Reading, writing and speech problems in children.* New York: W.W. Norton & Co.

Orton, S.T. (1966). *"Word-blindness" in school children and other papers on strephosymbolia.* Pomfret, CT: The Orton Society.

Osler, W. (1889). *The cerebral palsies of children.* Philadelphia: P. Blakiston, Son.

Owen, A.R.G. (1971). *Hysteria, hypnosis and healing: The work of J.-M. Charcot.* New York: Garrett Publications.

Paré, A. (1982). *On monsters and marvels* (J.L. Pallister, Trans.). Chicago: University of Chicago Press. (Original work published 1573)

Payne, W.H. (Trans.). (1892). *Rousseau's Emile or treatise on education.* New York: D. Appleton and Co.

Peiper, A. (1963). *Cerebral function in infancy and childhood.* New York: Consultants Bureau.

Penrose, L.S. (1949). *The biology of mental defect.* London: Sidgwick & Jackson.

Peterson, J. (1926). *Early conceptions and tests of intelligence.* World Book Company. (Reprinted 1969, Westport, CT: Greenwood Press)

Pinel, P. (1983). *A treatise on insanity.* (D.D. Davis, Trans.). Birmingham, AL: Classics of Medicine Library. (Original work published 1806)

Pollock, L.A. (1983). *Forgotten children: Parent-child relations from 1500 to 1900.* Cambridge, England: Cambridge University Press.

Prechtl, H.F.R., & Stemmer, C.J. (1959). Ein choreatiformes syndrom bei kindern. *Wiener Medizinische Wochenschrift, 19,* 1–9.

Purdy, L.M. (1992). *In their best interest? The case against equal rights for children.* Ithaca, NY: Cornell University Press.

Rademaker, G.G.J. (1931). *Das stehen.* Monograph in General Neurology and Psychiatry No. 59. Berlin: Julius Springer. (Translated 1980, *The physiology of standing: Postural reactions and equilibrium with special reference to the behavior of decerebellate animals.* Minneapolis: University of Minnesota Press)

Ray, I. (1838). *A treatise on the medical jurisprudence of insanity.* Boston: Charles C. Little and James Brown. (Reprinted 1987, Birmingham, AL: Classics of Medicine Library)

Rosen, M., Clark, G.R., & Kivitz, M.S. (Eds.). (1976). *The history of mental retardation: Collected papers* (2 vols.). Baltimore: University Park Press.

Ruhrah, J. (1925). *Pediatrics of the past.* New York: Paul B. Hoeber.

Ruhrah, J. (1932). *Pediatric biographies.* Baltimore: American Medical Association.

Scheerenberger, R.C. (1983). *A history of mental retardation.* Baltimore: Paul H. Brookes Publishing Co.

Scheerenberger, R.C. (1987). *A history of mental retardation: A quarter century of promise.* Baltimore: Paul H. Brookes Publishing Co.

Schleichkorn, J. (1987). *"The sometime physician": William John Little—Pioneer in treatment of cerebral palsy and orthopedic surgery.* Farmingdale, NJ: Jay Schleichkorn.

Seguin, E. (1866). *Idiocy and its treatment by the physiological method.* New York: William Wood & Co. (Reprinted 1971, New York: Augustus M. Kelley)

Shapiro, J.P. (1993). *No pity: People with disabilities forging a new civil rights movement.* New York: Times Books.

Spencer, W.G. (Trans.). (1938). *Celsus: De medicina* (3 vols.). Cambridge, MA: Harvard University Press.

Spitz, H.H. (1986). *The raising of intelligence: A selected history of attempts to raise retarded intelligence.* Hillsdale, NJ: Lawrence Erlbaum Associates.

Still, G.F. (1902). Some abnormal psychic conditions in children. *Lancet, 1,* 1008–1012, 1077–1082, 1163–1168.

Still, G.F. (1931). *The history of paediatrics.* Oxford, England: Oxford University Press. (Reprinted 1965, London: Dawsons of Pall Mall)

Strauss, A.A., & Kephart, N.C. (1955). *Psychopathology and education of the brain-injured child. Vol. II: Progress in theory and clinic.* New York: Grune & Stratton.

Strauss, A.A., & Lehtinen, L.E. (1947). *Psychopathology and education of the brain-injured child: Vol 1. Fundamentals and treatment of brain-injured children.* New York: Grune & Stratton.

Talbot, M.E. (1964). *Edouard Seguin: A study of an educational approach to the treatment of mentally defective children.* New York: Teachers College Press.

Tanner, J.M. (1981). *A history of the study of human growth.* Cambridge, England: Cambridge University Press.

Treves, F. (1923). *The elephant man and other reminiscences.* London: Cassell and Co. (Reprinted 1993, New York: Classics of Medicine Library)

Warkany, J. (1971). Teratology of the past. In J. Warkany (Ed.), *Congenital malformations, notes and comments* (pp. 6–20). Chicago: Year Book Medical Publishers.

Weir, N. (1990). *Otolaryngology: An illustrated history.* London: Butterworths.

Weiskrantz, L. (Ed.). (1988). *Thought without language.* Oxford, England: Clarendon Press.

Wender, P. (1971). *Minimal cerebral dysfunction in children.* New York: Wiley Interscience.

Wolf, T.H. (1973). *Alfred Binet.* Chicago: University of Chicago Press.

Wolfensberger, W. (1972). *Normalization: The principle of normalization in human services.* Toronto: National Institute on Mental Retardation.

PART I

THE CONTINUUM OF MOTOR DISORDERS AND DISORDERS OF HIGHER CORTICAL FUNCTION

Chapter 2

From Fetal Life to Developmental Disabilities

Claudine Amiel-Tison, M.D.

I am not a great curer, I know only a few songs.

a Ju/Wa healer from Namibia

There is increasing knowledge of the association between developmental disabilities on the one hand and less than optimal circumstances during fetal life and the intrapartum and/or immediate postnatal periods on the other hand. However, it has proved so difficult to collect truly prospective data in this field that perinatologists and developmental neurologists often have been discouraged and, as a result, many of the existing data sets are incomplete. For example, obstetricians and neonatologists only rarely have been able to obtain satisfactory data on the short-term, much less the long-term, outcomes of the populations in their care, and neuropediatricians have been unable to obtain the perinatal data that are essential if they are to understand the etiology of the disabilities they observe in their clinics. Moreover, for a variety of reasons that may not always be admitted, there remains some reluctance to establish a causal link between perinatal events and later developmental disabilities.

Although not ideal, a coherent picture can be obtained by amalgamating existing data pertaining to fetal life, infancy, and the school-age child, provided strict attention is paid to consistency of methodology and data recording. Methodologic consistency is particularly important in the assessment of perinatal risk and of neurologic signs in the neonatal period and later. From this type of analysis, it is clear that perinatal brain damage may cause the full spectrum of neuromotor impairment, from the trivial to the most severe (as discussed in Chapter 6, this volume). It is also clear that neuromotor

impairments often are associated with other developmental disabilities (as discussed in Chapter 6, this volume). For example, a large proportion of children who walk late (from 18 to 24 months) talk late (after 3 years) and often will struggle later in school on account of learning disabilities. Any improvement of our ability to predict later outcome from data obtained in the first 18 months of life (corrected age) will increase our confidence in using these early outcome measures as markers, along with mortality and neonatal morbidity, to assess advances in perinatal care.

In this chapter, I focus on methodology and trends rather than attempt to produce cumulative figures from published work, because the data rarely are completely compatible. Instead, I wish to share my experience gained from working in the maternity wards of Port-Royal-Baudelocque as the pediatrician member of a team caring for high-risk pregnancies. This position allowed me to collect my own prospective data, uninterrupted, from fetal life through infancy to childhood, and it also gave me the opportunity to participate in antenatal decision making with my obstetric colleagues. Thus, as a team we were able to use our own data as the basis for antenatal management and did not have to rely on the statistics of others, with all the uncertainties relating to the application of data from other times, other places, and other ethical attitudes.

PERINATAL DATA: THE OPTIMALITY CONCEPT

Prechtl introduced the optimality concept to perinatology (Prechtl, 1967, 1968), advocating that all perinatologists use it (Prechtl, 1980). He reported that common statistical methods such as correlations and factor analysis produced unsatisfactory findings that did not demonstrate properly the extent to which neonatal neurologic morbidity resulted from pre- and perinatal complications. Prechtl developed a new method for prospective collection of obstetric data:

> The lack of normative data and the difficulty of defining strict criteria hampered the usefulness of a normal-abnormal dichotomy in the case of many items. However, if then the emphasis was placed on finding the best possible condition rather than on normality, abnormality or pathology, many of the aforementioned problems disappeared. For a representative and comprehensive description of the pre- and perinatal condition of the mother, the fetus and the placenta, a list defining the criteria for the most favourable and optimal conditions could be drawn up. This was based on common clinical experience and on perinatal mortality data. Applying this concept, lists of obstetrical and newborn optimality criteria were designed. (1980, pp. 201–202)

Originally, Prechtl used a list of 42 items to define optimality. A point was awarded for each item meeting the defined optimality criteria, resulting in a maximum (good) score of 42. Prechtl identified the failure to achieve a perfect score as *nonoptimality*:

> The lower the total score in the individual case, the less optimal the course of pregnancy and/or delivery had been. As different weights were not given to the different items, the scores indicated quantitatively the numbers of items which had been found not to be optimal. It turned out empirically that most of the "important" items were associated with a simultaneous lack of optimality in many other items. This meant that the system was self-weighting. (1980, p. 202)

Prechtl concluded that the application of the optimality concept to describe pre- and perinatal conditions not only avoids the normal–abnormal dichotomy but has the advantages of an easily applicable, flexible system. Many researchers subsequently applied the optimality concept to their data, each having to adapt criteria to their routine clinical practice, to concurrent advances in obstetric management, and to the specific goals of their investigations (Amiel-Tison, Cabrol, & Shnider, 1994; Kyllerman & Hagberg, 1983; Michaelis, Dopfer, Gerbig,

Dopfer-Feller, & Rohr, 1979; Michaelis, Dopfer-Feller, Dopfer, Gerbig, & Rohr, 1979; Sonnander & Gustavson, 1987; Touwen et al., 1980). Moreover, this presentation of the data appears less threatening.

NEUROLOGIC SIGNS IN THE NEONATAL PERIOD

Typical Patterns of Cerebral Damage Caused by Circulatory Problems

The majority of cases of cerebral damage caused by circulatory problems fall into one of four categories—hypoxic-ischemic encephalopathy (HIE), periventricular leukomalacia (PVL), intraventricular hemorrhage (IVH), and cerebral arterial infarction—in which risk circumstances, anatomic findings, clinical signs, and prognosis are distinctive. An "identikit" of the four most common types of lesion is presented in Tables 1 through 4. This presentation is an admitted oversimplification; although any moderate or mild lesions of the same mechanism can occur, only the most severe damage is tabulated. For instance, for HIE (Table 1), mild and moderate cases can be recognized as well and in fact occur more frequently than the severe form. It is of primary importance to recognize them and to inform the obstetrician.

In these four categories, a diminution of cerebral blood flow—chronic, acute, or both—is always implied in the insult leading to cell damage. However, directly or indirectly, the maturative stage of the brain at the time of the hypoxic–ischemic insult will determine the type of lesion; that is, the gestational age is the most important factor to consider in order to understand the mechanisms involved (Feess-Higgins & Larroche, 1987; Levene & Lifford, 1995; Volpe, 1995).

Influence of Gestational Age
Direct Effects   By 23–24 weeks' gestation, the hemispheric cortex is not yet formed; an enormous mass of immature cells known as the germinal matrix is lying under the lateral ventricles. These immature cells will migrate in the following weeks toward the surface of the hemispheres. In the very preterm infant, the cerebral hemispheres are mainly represented by

Table 1. Severe hypoxic–ischemic encephalopathy (HIE)—clinical course and prediction for outcome

Risk situations
  Pre- and/or intrapartum, more often near-term, acute
  event, or superimposed on chronic hypoxia
	Hypoxic–ischemic episodes (cord compression,
	  abruptio placentae, fetal hemorrhage, maternal
	  circulatory failure)

Elective sites of cellular damage	**Massive cellular necrosis in cortical areas**
	  ± Subcortical leukomalacia
	  ± Basal ganglia, cerebellum, brain stem lesions

Acute clinical features	Low Apgar score **Major CNS depression** **Seizure activity** ± Brain stem signs
Investigations	**EEGs** confirm seizures, show severe interictal abnormalities Ultrasound poorly contributive (edema ± hemorrhage) **CT or MRI** may show early destructive aspects

Prediction of a poor outcome
  CP + MR + epilepsy; diagnosis established within
  the first 6 months
	Based on:
	  severe neurologic signs
	  persisting EEG abnormalities
	  slow cephalic growth
	  cerebral atrophy on imaging within the first month

Prediction of a favorable outcome
  No or mild impairment in various areas of brain
  function (more brain edema than cellular damage)
	Based on:
	  absence of brain stem signs
	  seizuring activity of short duration
	  moderate CNS depression (suck and swallow at
	    Day 7)
	  EEG: subnormal interictal activity
	  normal imaging by end of first month

Intermediate situations
  Uncertainties until school age
	Based on:
	  insufficient head growth
	  persisting hypertonicity in limbs
	  slow development of axial tone
	  independent walking after 18 months
	  abnormalities in behavior and contact

Note: CNS, central nervous system; CP, cerebral palsy; CT, computed tomography; EEG, electroencephalogram; MR, mental retardation; MRI, magnetic resonance imaging.

white matter, and the tissue is fragile and rich in water. Also by 23–24 weeks, the arterial network is irrigating primarily the germinal matrix; a few weeks later the white matter itself is more irrigated. As a consequence, up to 33–34 weeks' gestation, hemorrhages will occur in the germinal matrix and extend to the lateral ventricles. Ischemic cell damage will be located in the periventricular white matter and will be very severe. PVL will heal within a few weeks, leaving holes (porencephalic cysts) or atrophy (hydrocephaly ex vacuo). These lesions will partially or totally interrupt the descending motor pathways through the internal capsule, resulting in spastic cerebral palsy. Cortical damage may be associated, but usually only moderate impairment of cognitive functions will be observed.

After 34 weeks, with the cortex being formed, the arterial irrigation is displaced toward the cortical layers to fulfill the high meta-bolic demand. Therefore, the regions at risk for ischemic damage are the cortex, the subcortical white matter, or both. The more mature the fetus at the time of the insult, the more cortical will be the cell damage: Motor and sensory areas can be destroyed partially or totally, as can the wide associative areas. The resulting motor disability will be of the same type as in the preterm infant, but cognitive functions will be very defective as well in most of the cases. Because the brain tissue is more organized, the lesions will be much less visible than in a very preterm infant; therefore, normal imaging will not be as reassuring as in a preterm infant.

Indirect Effects The immaturity of every organ in the very preterm infant will result in various difficulties in adapting to extrauterine life. Respiratory distress syndrome (RDS) and its hemodynamic consequences are responsible for hypoxia, acidosis, and unstable blood flow with

Table 2. Periventricular leukomalacia (PVL)—clinical course and prediction for outcome

Risk situations
  Mainly in **preterm infants with RDS**
  but possible at any gestational age
	Postnatal (approximately 85% of cases), hemodynamic
	  failure caused by severe RDS in preterm infants or later
	  apneic spells with bradycardia
	Antenatal (approximately 15% of cases) in severe IUGR
	  Risk increased by materno-fetal bacterial infection

Elective sites of cellular damage	**Ischemic lesions in white matter**
	  internal capsule (periventricular border zones)
	  interrupting ascending and descending pathways

Neonatal clinical course	No specific neurologic signs in the neonatal period in very sick infants Poor visual pursuit, poor alertness
Investigations	**Ultrasound:** hyperechogenicity at the acute stage in the periventricular border zones **EEG:** positive rolandic spikes

Prediction of a poor outcome
  Severe CP + MR; spastic diplegia is most
  common outcome
	Based on:
	  abnormal ultrasound within the first month
	  cerebral atrophy in white matter
	  porencephalic cysts and/or gliosis
	  hydrocephaly ex vacuo

Prediction of a favorable outcome
  No or moderate motor impairment with typical or
  impaired cognitive function
	Based on:
	  normal ultrasound and normal clinical assessment at 40
	    weeks (corrected), including normal axial tone, normal
	    fix and track, alertness, and interaction

Intermediate situations
  Uncertainties until school age
	Based on:
	  suspicion of subtle PVL with normal ultrasound at
	    1 month but abnormal neurological findings since 40
	    weeks (corrected)

	Associated problems may be very misleading
	  in VLBW (muscle shortening–bony deformations;
	  poor nutrition; chronic lung disease)

Note: CP, cerebral palsy; EEG, electroencephalogram; IUGR, intrauterine growth retardation; MR, mental retardation; RDS, respiratory distress syndrome; VLBW, very low birth weight.

wide variations during the first days of life (Lou et al., 1979), all circumstances placing the infant at high risk for hemorrhage, cell damage, or both. This explains why there is a high correlation, before 34 weeks' gestation, between RDS and IVH.

Mechanical Difficulties During Labor In the preterm infant, in whom the skull is soft, molding and deformations can be extreme. The brain is therefore poorly protected and hemorrhages are frequent in the arachnoid or subdural space. This partly explains why cesarean section often seems to provide the safest birth for the very low birth weight (VLBW) infant (Ment et al., 1992).

In the term infant, the brain is better protected by a more resistant skull; however, cephalopelvic disproportion may contribute to mechanical difficulties at the high- or mid-pelvis level.

Role of Asphyxia

Perinatal Asphyxia Asphyxic factors during labor are more clearly defined in the term delivery. Prolapse of the cord, for instance, is one of the most typical causes of bradycardia and acute fetal asphyxia. Repeated decelerations with contractions, which may indicate some degree of fetal hypoxia, are less easy to interpret. When they occur, the situation as a whole (including the parity) is evaluated by the obstetrician according to the stage of cervical dilatation and descent. An emergency cesarean section may be indicated.

It is beyond the scope of this chapter to analyze the controversy surrounding electronic fetal monitoring (see Chapter 13, Volume I). There are different schemes of pattern interpretation, and most alterations of the fetal heart rate (FHR) do not indicate brain damage but rather indicate a risk situation. Therefore, these

Table 3. Intraventricular hemorrhage (IVH)—clinical course and prediction for outcome

Risk situations **Before 34 weeks'** gestation in infants ventilated for RDS **postnatal** event	Risk and severity increase when gestational age decreases Very high risk at 31 weeks and below Exceptional after 34 weeks
Elective site of hemorrhage	**Germinal matrix,** then spread to lateral ventricles, third and fourth ventricles, foramina of Magendie and Lushka, arachnoid space
Neonatal clinical course	In typical cases, **abrupt deterioration** in a ventilated preterm infant; coma ± seizures after a free interval of a few hours or days Often not contributive in a very sick infant
Investigations	**Ultrasound diagnosis & gradation:** Germinal matrix + mild IVH (stage I) IVH without distention (stage II) IVH with distention (stage III)
Prediction of a poor outcome Severe CP & MR; spastic diplegia is most common outcome	Based on: **associated PVL** plus risk of posthemorrhagic **hydrocephalus**
Prediction of a favorable outcome No or moderate motor impairment with typical or impaired cognitive function	Based on: **absence of PVL in grade I or II IVH** lateral ventricles of normal size complete resorption of blood within about 10 days
Intermediate situations Uncertainties until school age	Based on: suspicion of subtle PVL on clinical grounds

Note: CP, cerebral palsy; MR, mental retardation; PVL, periventricular leukomalacia; RDS, respiratory distress syndrome.

alterations do not correlate well with brain damage. Moreover, acute alterations of the FHR pattern during labor (prolonged decelerations or bradycardia) do not always imply abnormal labor because they can occur in a fetus already compromised before labor and therefore unable to cope with the stress of even a normal labor. Despite its limitations, electronic fetal monitoring is considered as having contributed to the improvement of perinatal outcome (Schiffrin, 1990).

Postnatal Asphyxia Postnatal asphyxia in the delivery room also must be considered. A low Apgar score at 1 minute of life indicates fetal compromise. If active resuscitation is started immediately, appropriate oxygenation and blood flow will be reestablished within a few minutes. In the absence or delay of such emergency care, the central nervous system depression, meconium aspiration, or both will be responsible for adding minutes of postnatal asphyxia to minutes of prenatal asphyxia. However, fast and efficient postnatal care does not guarantee a favorable outcome in every case because the brain damage may already exist at the time of birth. This explains why correlations are so poor between low Apgar score at 1 minute and outcome. Correlations are better between

outcome and the 5-minute Apgar score; the latter reflects the quality of postnatal care plus the neonate's capacity to establish vital functions, a capacity that is much higher when fetal distress has been short and has occurred in a previously healthy fetus.

The quality of immediate postnatal care is extremely important in the very preterm infant. Large variations of pO_2, pCO_2, and temperature are responsible for an instability in blood flow as a result of impaired autoregulation of cerebral blood flow that will increase the risk for IVH. In infants weighing less than 1,000 g, the risk is so high that the effects of prevention are difficult to demonstrate. In infants between 1,000 and 1,500 g, the incidence and severity of IVH will depend largely on an early stabilization of vital functions.

Outcome Several classifications of outcome have been proposed in the literature (Amiel-Tison, 1979; Levene, Grindulis, Sands, & Moore, 1986; Sarnat & Sarnat, 1976). For example, outcome is generally excellent in the mild degree of HIE. Sequelae can be observed with moderate HIE; the prediction of outcome in this grade is not very accurate because signs of brain edema and early signs of cell damage are difficult to separate. A normal electroen-

Table 4. Infarction of an arterial territory—clinical course and prediction for outcome

Risk situations Mainly **prenatal**, independent of gestational age	Multiple pregnancies Septicemia with **DIC** **No risk circumstances in most cases**
Elective sites of cellular damage	**Left middle cerebral artery** Other localizations are rare
Neonatal clinical course	**Status epilepticus** after a free interval, in the absence of risk factors for HIE Unilateral neurologic findings

Investigations	Ultrasound: poorly contributive
	Early CT scan (within first 3 days): large zone of low
	    density in the corresponding arterial territory; already
	    organized lesion = prenatal
	EEG: focal abnormalities with otherwise subnormal
	    tracing

Prediction of a poor outcome
    CP, MR, epilepsy
	Based on:
	    imaging at birth (extensive and hemorrhagic infarction)
	    severe clinical signs (coma and protracted seizures)
	    severe EEG findings (cortical involvement)

Prediction of a favorable outcome
    mild spastic hemiplegia with minimal lower limb
    impairment, moderate impairment of speech and
    cognitive abilities
	Based on:
	    limited area involved on CT scan
	    rapid clinical improvement
	    discrete EEG findings

Note: CP, cerebral palsy; CT, computed tomography; DIC, disseminated intravascular coagulation; EEG, electroencephalogram; HIE, hypoxic–ischemic encephalopathy; MR, mental retardation.

cephalogram (EEG) in an infant with moderate HIE is a good predictor of a normal outcome, whereas normal imaging studies are not.

The predictive value of investigations other than clinical (Hope, 1994) is beyond the scope of this discussion. As a rough indication, for example, imaging from transfontanelar echography within the first month of life has a very good correlation with outcome in preterm infants with PVL because the resulting lesions are very destructive before 33 weeks' gestation. Conversely, in term or near-term newborn infants, the EEG tracings gathered during the first week of life have a good correlation with outcome, whereas the imaging does not, because lesions are more cortical and less clearly destructive in more mature infants.

Conclusion   In many cases, both the causative factors and the neonatal picture will fit with one of the four typical patterns described here and therefore will allow a precise anatomic and clinical diagnosis to be made. In these cases, a follow-up program can be proposed in continuity with treatment provided during the neonatal period, with no resulting gap in services. Early intervention will be indicated according to the diagnosis and level of severity.

Less Typical Patterns of Cerebral Damage Caused by Circulatory Problems

In less typical cases, the nature and quantification of signs and their pattern of evolution often can orient the search for a possible etiology. Usually, when the hypoxic–ischemic insult is acute or subacute and is recent (most often concomitant with labor in the full-term infant), the signs of cerebral damage change demonstrably from one day to the next. A worsening often is observed within the first 3–4 days, probably as a result of brain edema; improvement occurs by the end of the first week, sometimes with complete recovery. Conversely, if the insult is chronic or more distant from birth, then the signs are usually quite stable during the first weeks.

Clues to Other Causes of Cerebral Damage: Malformations, Infections, or Toxic Disorders

Most gross cerebral malformations now are diagnosed during the second trimester of pregnancy by fetal ultrasound imaging; the diagnosis is easily suspected at birth by the shape of the skull and easily confirmed by neonatal imaging. However, in many cases, neurologic signs present since birth are linked with genetic problems, polymalformations with no precise diagnosis. The diagnosis can be even more difficult when the child received a low Apgar score at birth not as a result of any abnormalities in labor and delivery but because of the fragility of the malformed fetus. A complete physical evaluation may help to establish a diagnosis (see Chapter 15, Volume I).

There are many infectious causes of cerebral damage in the neonatal period; these are often obvious, as in the case of bacterial or viral infections (e.g., meningitis or meningoencephalitis). However, some cases of fetal infection, such as cytomegalovirus infection (Remington & Klein, 1990), are often underdiagnosed. The only clue may be the relative microcephaly, hyperexcitability, and poor visual interaction in a newborn who does not appear very sick at first. The search for cytomegalovirus virus must be performed in the neonatal period (see Chapter 8, Volume I).

Toxic problems during fetal life may present as unexpected surprises if the mother did not benefit from prenatal care and if she denies any drug addiction or alcohol intoxication (Chasnoff, 1991; see also Chapter 10, Volume I). In these cases, hyperexcitability appears as the most prominant symptom. Abnormalities are noted more often in visual fixation and orienting responses: Eye contact is brief, and "fix and track" responses to sound are very fragmented. These abnormalities are good clues to consider investigating possible maternal substance abuse.

The problem of identifying causes of cerebral damage other than circulatory is still out of our reach in many cases. For instance, we are just beginning to learn about cerebral dysgenesis (Sarnat, 1992), abnormalities of cellular migration that occur early in fetal life. Magnetic resonance imaging is identifying these cases in vivo (see Chapter 22, Volume I), and it appears that toxic or infectious factors might be partly responsible for these developmental errors.

"Normal Brain" in the Appropriate-for-Gestational-Age Full-Term Newborn Infant

The neurobehavioral competence of the full-term newborn infant is such that typical devel-

opment can be affirmed, however poor the condition at birth has been. A low Apgar score at 1 minute and a good Apgar score at 5 minutes is a common finding after a hypoxic insult of short duration in the second stage of delivery. Stabilization of vital functions with spontaneous correction of metabolic acidosis is observed within a few minutes or hours. The neurologic assessment can be performed at this time, but responses must be perfect to affirm that the brain is intact. The full-term newborn is in a transitional phase: The ascending myelinization of subcortical motor pathways is completed but the descending maturation of the corticospinal tract is only beginning, so higher control is not yet fully established (Sarnat, 1989). To be predictive of a typical outcome, including cognitive functions, the neurologic assessment must rely more on the emerging upper control than on the subcortical control (postural tone and primary reflexes). This emerging upper control is first detectable by three maneuvers: testing fixation and tracking; evaluating flexor versus extensor tone by the raise-to-sit maneuver; and evaluating the spontaneous movements of fingers, including abduction of the thumbs (Amiel-Tison et al., 1994; see also Chapter 16, Volume I). When this higher cortical control is demonstrable in an appropriate-for-gestational-age full-term newborn with a normal head circumference, the prediction of normalcy is highly accurate (Amiel-Tison, Dubé, Lévy, Maillard, & Shnider, 1988).

SHORT-TERM OUTCOME: THE FIRST 18 MONTHS OF LIFE

Except in very severe HIE with damage extending to the brain stem and early signs of decerebration, brain lesions of perinatal origin are located mainly in the cerebral hemispheres, cortex, and white matter. This explains why the resulting neuromotor impairment will be represented by spastic cerebral palsy of various degrees of severity and topography, and why all types of sensory loss or deficits in intellectual functions also can be observed, usually in association with the motor findings. Because the maturation of the motor pathways is very rapid in the first year of life, it is not surprising that looking for neuromotor impairment provides the most reliable clues.

Neuromotor
Impairment and Motor Disability

The neuromotor assessment must be performed in relation to the rapid maturation of the infant, in whom there is a striking development of cortical control superceding subcortical control. Relaxation is observed first in the upper limbs and later in the lower limbs, with physiologic hypotonia achieved by 9 months (Amiel-Tison & Grenier, 1986). During the same period, axial tone progresses from the head (allowing head control) to the back (allowing independent sitting) and to the lower limbs (allowing standing and independent walking). Simultaneously, the primitive reflexes and excessive postural reactions in extension disappear. Independent finger movements develop. The head growth velocity parallels the development of the hemispheres in the first 6 months and then proceeds more slowly.

However, if damage is present (e.g., motor cells in the cortex, subcortical or periventricular damage in motor pathways), various neuromotor findings will appear, with various levels of severity but reflecting deficits in the higher control of motor function:

Brain stem activity (excessive postural reactions, persistence of primitive reflexes) will not disappear in the first trimester.
Passive tone will remain as flexion in the limbs.
Passive axial tone will show more extension than flexion.
Signs of spasticity will appear during the second 6 months of life, mainly in the postural muscles (e.g., abnormal stretch reflex in the sural triceps).
Head growth will not progress normally.

According to the degree of severity and the course observed within the first year, a gradation can be defined:

1. In *severe damage*, the diagnosis of cerebral palsy is proposed by the end of the first year (or even sooner in very severe cases).
2. In *moderate damage*, an improvement is observed by the end of the first year; however, a few signs persist (Amiel-Tison & Stewart, 1994): imbalance in passive axial tone, a moderate (phasic) stretch reflex obtained by the fast dorsiflexion of the foot, and a squamous ridge revealing that head growth has not been optimal.
3. In *minor damage*, the signs observed in the first 6 months completely disappear by 8–10 months. However, these transient neuromotor findings may provide a clue to the involvement of other cerebral functions (Amiel-Tison, Dubé, Garel, & Jequier, 1983).

Any type of neuromotor impairment usually will result in some alterations of the pattern of motor acquisitions. The resulting functional disability, however, will be very variable in degree and timing, and therefore must be described separately as a functional consequence of the impairment. The use of the Clinical Adaptive Test (CAT) (see Chapter 20, Volume I) should allow the pediatrician to describe the child functionally with more precision (see also Chapters 17 and 21, Volume I).

Other Indicators

The prelinguistic stages of language development can be tested within the first year by the Clinical Linguistic and Auditory Milestones Scale (CLAMS) (Capute et al., 1986), evaluating, according to the mother's observations, the first steps of reception and expression (see Chapters 17 and 20, Volume I). Early deviation from normal language development will correlate well with later language testing in the second or third year of life.

Psychometric testing in the first 2 years of life is represented mainly by the Bayley Scales of Infant Development (Bayley, 1993). The predictive value of the recent restandardization remains to be determined (see Chapter 20, Volume I).

Predictive Value of Abnormalities

Neuromotor Impairment Except when the family environment is extremely abnormal, neuromotor development progresses in a manner that is relatively independent of socioeconomical factors. Therefore, in those cases in which extreme deprivation can be eliminated, neuromotor impairments in infancy, even if mild or transient, may be associated with later impairments in cognitive function and fine motor function. In the case of a very stimulating family environment, or if a very active intervention program is available, these deficits can be masked until 3–5 years of age. However, they will be revealed later by learning disabilities. A typical outcome remains possible for one third of children with transient motor signs (Amiel-Tison et al., 1983). Therefore, at the present time, one can consider that mild or moderate neuromotor findings represent a clue to later deficits, perhaps not on an individual basis but certainly on a statistical basis.

The short-term outcome based on neuromotor findings at 18 months of age can be used by obstetricians and neonatologists to assign infants to one of three categories:

1. *Clearly damage:* cerebral palsy, mental retardation, sensory deficit, hydrocephalus, and epilepsy represent the most common sequelae.

2. *Potentially at risk for cognitive dysfunction,* when mild or even transient neuromotor findings have been detected. Our knowledge is progressing very fast in this area as a result of increasing sophistication in the clinical approach and greater precision in the morphologic and functional exploration of the brain. This means that the diagnosis of various types of learning disabilities can be improved by recognizing their association with neurologic signs and primary disorder of vigilance, and attempting a localization of the mild lesions in the right or left hemisphere (Levy, Harper, & Weinberg, 1992; Weinberg & Brumback, 1992). As pointed out by Rapin (1982), although the school years are often very difficult for infants with mild neuromotor impairments, later, as adults, most of them will find their place in society. These consequences of perinatal difficulties cannot be considered too minor to take into consideration. For example, the high incidence of these problems cannot be ignored in the group of VLBW infants; only about 50% of these infants have expected cerebral function when tested at school age.

3. *At low risk for late deficit,* in the absence of neuromotor findings and with normal CAT/CLAMS results and head growth. In the cohort of preterm (less than 33 weeks) infants from the neonatal intensive care unit (NICU) of University College in London (Roth et al., 1994), neurologic impairment at 1 year was a highly significant independent predictor of outcome at 8 years ($p<.001$), whereas development quotient (DQ) at 1 year was not. Abnormal DQ only detected very severe damage. Among neurologic impairments, imbalance of axial passive tone and stretch reflexes in the sural triceps are common findings; these anomalies represent a good marker for continued follow-up cognitive testing.

Psychometric Tests Short-term outcome based on psychometric tests is discussed elsewhere in this book (see Chapter 20, Volume I). However, one particular warning seems important because many short-term follow-up studies are based on the Bayley scale without a control group and not on neuromotor findings: It has been shown recently (Gross, Slagle, D'Eugenio, & Mettelman, 1992), and it is known by experience, that the Bayley scores in control groups at 6, 15, and 24 months are nowadays not 100 but between 110 and 115. Consequently, classifying as "normal" the high-risk infant who obtains a score of 85 or higher (1 standard deviation [*SD*] below the mean), using the instrument norms only, will provide inappropriate reassurance in nearly half of the cohort, who in fact should be classified as having mild or moderate disability, defined by a score between 69 and 84 (between 1 and 2 SD below the mean). The McCarthy General Cognitive Scale (McCarthy, 1972) at 4 years will be disappointing in comparison. This is particularly important to estimate the long-term outcome in VLBW infants, who represent a group particularly at risk for learning disabilities. A meta-analysis of 80 recently published studies that evaluated the outcome of low birth weight (LBW) infants stressed the need for control groups (Aylward, Pfeiffer, Wright, & Verhulst, 1989).

Decision Making in Obstetrics and Neonatology

Obstetrics The obstetrician often has no choice but to accept premature labor. If there is a choice, however, then a few situations will be handled according to expectations about outcome.

In pregnancies delivered after spontaneous preterm labor or rupture of the membranes, the birth weight threshold at which obstetric efforts intended to delay delivery might potentially improve rates of neonatal morbidity and mortality has been decreasing with advances in perinatal care. In recent years in sophisticated NICUs, the birth weight threshold for neonatal mortality is 1,600 g (p <.001); for neonatal morbidity, the threshold is between 1,600 and 1,900 g (p <.008) (de Palma, Leveno, Kelly, Sherman, & Carmody, 1992). Every decision made in response to this crucial problem must be considered as *provisional* (varying constantly with the improvement of neonatal care, as recently stressed by Perlman et al., 1995) and *circumstancial* (varying according to countries and perinatal centers; Stewart & Pezzani-Goldsmith, 1994).

The problem of extreme low birth weight has been summarized by Hack and Fanaroff (1988). The tendency at the present time is to separate the 23- to 25-weeks group, with very high risk of sequelae, from the 26 weeks and up group, in which survival and outcome are better. The results of Allen, Donohue, and Dusman (1993) are in agreement with those of Hack et al. (1995) as well. The consensus among obstetricians is to begin to consider FHR monitoring and cesarean section at 26 weeks or 750 g birth weight, but rarely below (Amon, Shyken, & Sibai, 1992). The problem of the parallelism of survival and outcome has been studied by Hagberg and Hagberg (1989) for over 40 years. It seems clear that, in Sweden, a rupture of parallelism has been observed in extremely LBW survivors. This warning should be quoted exactly: In the period from 1979 to 1982, a "gain" of nearly 4,000 "healthy" infants (at least without cerebral palsy) was observed, compared to the period from 1967 to 1970.

The contemporary "cost" was nearly 300 cases of cerebral palsy, among whom a new category of extremely preterm infants with combinations of severe neuroimpairments (cerebral palsy, mental retardation, hydrocephalus, epilepsy and retinopathy) constitutes the most alarming signal. We think that as long as the survival of preterm infants

continues to increase and extends to ever lower gestational ages there will be yet more such damaged children. (Hagberg & Hagberg, 1989, p. 372)

However, these data, and therefore this pessimistic warning, are not universal. A Canadian regionally based study (Robertson, Hrynchyshynt, Etches, & Pain, 1992) does not show this increase in severe sequelae and proposes as an explanation for this difference a better regionalization of care in Canada.

The decision is different in stressed pregnancies because one must compromise between the risk of prematurity and the risk of fetal distress. Such a situation typically occurs in two not uncommon instances of fetal compromise: hypertension in pregnancy and multiple pregnancies. As long as fetal growth is progressing, even on a low percentile, and as long as FHR patterns show good variability, until the gestational age reaches 31 weeks, every day spent in utero will decrease the risk inherent to prematurity (i.e., RDS, IVH, and PVL). However, if the restriction of supplies becomes very severe, if the Doppler velocimetry shows changes in cerebral blood flow, and, above all, if the FHR variability becomes abnormal on the nonstress test, then the risk of fetal brain damage may be greater than the risk of postnatal complications resulting from immaturity. In fact, in many of these cases, adaptive phenomena are observed in the fetus during these stressed pregnancies (Amiel-Tison & Pettigrew, 1991): An acceleration of lung maturity of several weeks will decrease the risk for RDS, and an acceleration of brain stem maturity of several weeks will facilitate the adaptation to extrauterine life. However, in multiple pregnancies, a decision for early extraction, often favorable for the small fetus, may be poorly tolerated by the other(s). At 34 weeks or later, the risk of lung and brain immaturity is so much lower that any sign of fetal distress makes cesarean section advisable.

Anxiety about these decisions is obviously the consequence of uncertainty (Fischer & Stevenson, 1987). The physician would like to provide intensive care support to only those neonates with a reasonable chance of survival without disabilities, but often we simply do not know enough to decide with certainty.

Neonatology Neonatologists have little choice but to do their best in the delivery room to establish and maintain vital functions in a very preterm newborn or in a full-term infant after severe anoxia, as long as a few heartbeats or gasps were present at birth. After a few days or weeks, they can be faced with an infant with a very destructive encephalopathy (or white matter damage in a preterm or grey matter damage in a full-term infant), at a time when vital functions are maintained spontaneously. A very gloomy outcome is predictable, and withdrawal of care must be discussed (Richards, 1989). The "do not resuscitate" label is one possible step; in any case, decision making about such very sick infants cannot be avoided.

The historic approach, as pointed out by Knobloch, Malone, Ellison, Stevens, and Zdeb (1982), allowed us to anticipate that the good results obtained in infants above 1,000 g birth weight will extend to infants weighing less than 1,000 g:

> Improvements in prenatal, obstetric, and neonatal care appear to be doing for the 751- to 1,000-g group now what the then high level care in 1952 did for the 1,000- to 1,500-g group, when mortality decreased but only half of those were normal. (p. 285)

However, at the moment it seems we have reached a limit around 750 g—not a technical limitation, but one produced by extreme immaturity. These issues also must be discussed in the group of 500- to 750-g newborn infants (Young & Stevenson, 1990). In this VLBW group, the "ethics of uncertainty" must be analyzed (Rhoden, 1986); three ethical strategies are in use:

1. Treat all such infants vigorously, until we know better (the attitude adopted in most of the perinatal centers in the United States).
2. Withhold treatment when the prognosis is uncertain or grim—the "statistical prognosis strategy" advocated in Sweden.
3. Start treatment for all, and reevaluate regularly on the basis of clinical prognostic indications—the "individualized prognostic strategy," an attitude in between the two extremes above that has been adopted in several European countries, including the

United Kingdom, France, and Holland (Sauer, 1992).

Pitfalls and Prejudices in Interpreting the Data

Oversimplification A reductionist attitude, "cerebral palsy (CP) or not CP," often prevails in many follow-up studies concerning the outcome of surviving VLBW infants. Such a classification could be satisfactory if a careful and comprehensive gradation of the neurologic impairment were defined and universally accepted. Grading according to functional consequences usually underestimates both the incidence (moderate and mild impairments are overlooked as long as the child walks by 18 months) and the severity of the motor disability (secondary musculoskeletal deformations increase during the life span). Although apparently satisfactory for epidemiologists, "CP or not CP" does not adequately describe the outcome of perinatal care. Developmental pediatricians will have to improve the analytic part of their work in order to offer epidemiologists more satisfactory data, really reflecting the trends observed. At the present time, the use of CP as a marker to monitor the quality of perinatal care therefore seems misleading; it is consequently not surprising that the results published generate useless controversies.

The Family Environment Premature and LBW infants are known to be at greater risk for developmental disabilities than appropriate-for-gestational-age full-term newborns. The quality of the home environment of a LBW infant predicts developmental outcome better than any single biologic risk factor. This was shown by the British National Child Development Study (Davie, Butler, & Goldstein, 1972): The percentage of "educational backwardness" is much higher in the fifth-born full-term child of a "manual" family than in the first-born preterm child in a "nonmanual" family. This effect of home environment is shown by the transactional model presented by Sameroff and Chandler (1975), but it has been used to minimize the weight of perinatal brain damage for the sake of an ideological demonstration. Used in very large studies with insufficient perinatal data, this approach weights sociocultural factors more heavily than organic damage. In contrast, in small cohorts with careful neurologic and psychometric measurements, it often is not possible to split such a small number of infants into various sociocultural categories. This design limitation contributes to ignoring sociocultural factors and favoring the organic lesional aspect. Both attitudes are extremist in a way; unfortunately, "medium-size" studies that could avoid both pitfalls are infrequent. To minimize these difficulties, the identification of specific clinical signs as markers for perinatal brain damage, as described above, appears necessary (Amiel-Tison & Stewart, 1989, 1990).

CONCLUSIONS

The results of perinatal care in the 1990s have been discussed here according to both remarkable achievements and painful uncertainties. In fact, these uncertainties are not restricted to the most extreme preterm infants but include every case in which very severe brain damage becomes obvious within the first days of life of a newborn infant. The emphasis is on both pain and cost. "One thing is certain: when resources become scarce, are perceived to be scarce, or are relatively scarce, concerns about distributive justice increase in intensity until the point is reached when they can no longer be ignored" (Young & Stevenson, 1990, p. 551). We cannot forget that perinatologists must operate with the consent and support of the communities they serve.

Another point also must be raised when discussing distributive justice concerning standardized perinatal care in the 1990s: The quality of care is very unevenly distributed in many countries. This is a political problem that nations must face. Moreover, the lay public is informed sooner and sooner about the advances of care and dazzling technical achievements but is less informed about failures and physiologic limits. As a consequence, the expectation in the lay public is still far beyond reality concerning the outcome of survivors from the NICU.

REFERENCES

Allen, M.C., Donohue, P.K., & Dusman, A.E. (1993). The limit of viability—Neonatal outcome of infants born at 22 to 25 weeks gestation. *New England Journal of Medicine, 329,* 1597–1601.

Amiel-Tison, C. (1979). Birth injury as a cause of brain dysfunction in fullterm newborns. In R. Korobkin & C. Guilleminault (Eds.), *Advances in perinatal neurology* (pp. 57–83). New York: Spectrum.

Amiel-Tison, C., Cabrol, D., & Shnider, S. (1994). The safety of fullterm birth. In C. Amiel-Tison & A. Stewart (Eds.), *The newborn infant: One brain for life* (pp. 93–147). Paris: Inserm.

Amiel-Tison, C., Dubé, R., Garel, M., & Jequier, J.C. (1983). Outcome at age five years of fullterm infant with transient neurologic abnormalities in the first year of life. In L. Stern, H. Bard, & B. Friis-Hansen (Eds.), *Intensive care of the newborn IV* (pp. 247–258). New York: Masson.

Amiel-Tison, C., Dubé, R., Lévy, A., Maillard, F., & Shnider, S.M. (1988). Early prediction for a normal outcome based on a normal neurobehavioral assessment in the fullterm newborn. In *XIth European Congress of Perinatal Medicine* (Abstr. CIC, p. 70). Rome: Ed. Internazionali.

Amiel-Tison, C., & Grenier, A. (1986). *Neurological assessment during the first year of life.* New York: Oxford University Press.

Amiel-Tison, C., & Pettigrew, A. (1991). Adaptive changes in the developing brain during intrauterine stress. *Brain and Development, 13,* 67–76.

Amiel-Tison, C., & Stewart, A. (1989). Follow up studies during the first five years of life: A pervasive assessment of neurological function. *Archives of Disease in Childhood, 64,* 496–502.

Amiel-Tison, C., & Stewart, A. (1990). *Neuromotor assessment during the first years of life* [videotape]. London: UCL Images, University College London.

Amiel-Tison, C., & Stewart, A. (1994). Apparently normal survivors: Neuromotor and cognitive function as they grow older. In C. Amiel-Tison & A. Stewart (Eds.), *The newborn infant: One brain for life* (pp. 227–237). Paris: Inserm.

Amon, E., Shyken, J.M., & Sibai, B.M. (1992). How small is too small and how early is too early? A survey of American obstetricians specializing in high-risk pregnancies. *American Journal of Perinatology, 9,* 17–21.

Aylward, G.P., Pfeiffer, S.I., Wright, A., & Verhulst, S. (1989). Outcome studies of low birth weight infants published in the last decade: A metaanalysis. *Journal of Pediatrics, 115,* 515–520.

Bayley, N. (1993). *Bayley Scales of Infant Development—Second edition manual.* San Antonio, TX: Psychological Corporation.

Capute, A.J., Palmer, F.B., Shapiro, B.K., Wachtel, R.C., Schmidt, S., & Ross, A. (1986). Clinical Linguistic and Auditory Milestone Scale: Prediction of cognition in infancy. *Developmental Medicine and Child Neurology, 28,* 762–771.

Chasnoff, I.J. (1991). Chemical dependency and pregnancy. *Clinics in Perinatology, 18.*

Davie, R., Butler, N., & Goldstein, H. (1972). *From birth to seven: The second report of the National Child Development Study (1958 cohort)* (p. 167). London: Longman and National Children's Bureau.

de Palma, R.J., Leveno, K.J., Kelly, M.A., Sherman, M.L., & Carmody, T.J. (1992). Birth weight threshold for postponing preterm birth. *American Journal of Obstetrics and Gynecology, 167,* 1145–1149.

Feess-Higgins, A., & Larroche, J.C. (1987). *Development of the human foetal brain, an anatomical atlas.* Paris: Masson.

Fischer, A.F., & Stevenson, D.K. (1987). Consequences of uncertainty: An empirical approach to medical decision making in neonatal intensive care. *Journal of the American Medical Association, 258,* 1929–1931.

Gross, S.J., Slagle, T.A., D'Eugenio, D.B., & Mettelman, B.B. (1992). Impact of a matched term control group on interpretation of developmental performance in preterm infants. *Pediatrics, 90,* 681–687.

Hack, M., & Fanaroff, A. (1988). How small is too small? Considerations in evaluating the outcome of the tiny infant. *Clinics in Perinatology, 15,* 773–788.

Hack, M., Wright, L.L., Shankaran, S., Tyson, J.E., Horbar, J.D., Baver, C.R., & Younes, N. (1995). Very-low-birth-weight outcomes of the National Institute of Child Health and Human Development Neonatal Network, November 1989 to October 1990. *American Journal of Obstetrics and Gynecology, 172,* 457–464.

Hagberg, B., & Hagberg, G. (1989). The changing panorama of infantile hydrocephalus and cerebral palsy over forty years: A Swedish survey. *Brain and Development, 11,* 368–373.

Hope, P. (1994). The role of imaging and technology. In C. Amiel-Tison & A. Stewart (Eds.), *The newborn infant: One brain for life* (pp. 199–212). Paris: Inserm.

Knobloch, H., Malone, A., Ellison, P., Stevens, F., & Zdeb, M. (1982). Considerations in evaluating changes in outcome for infants weighing less than 1,501 grams. *Pediatrics, 69,* 285–295.

Kyllerman, M., & Hagberg, G. (1983). Reduced optimality in pre- and perinatal conditions in a Swedish newborn population. *Neuropediatrics, 14,* 37–42.

Levene, M.I., Grindulis, H., Sands, C., & Moore, J.R. (1986). Comparison of two methods of predicting outcome in perinatal asphyxia. *Lancet, 1,* 67–69.

Levene, M.I., & Lifford, R.J. (1995). *Fetal and neonatal neurology and neurosurgery* (2nd ed.). London: Churchill Livingstone.

Levy, H.B., Harper, C.R., & Weinberg, W.A. (1992). A practical approach to children failing in school. *Pediatric Clinics of North America, 39,* 895–928.

Lou, H.C., Lassen, N.A., Tweed, W.A., Johnson, G., Jones, M., & Palahniuk, R.J. (1979). Pressure passive cerebral blood flow and breakdown of the blood-brain barrier in experimental fetal asphyxia. *Acta Paediatrica Scandinavica, 68,* 57–63.

McCarthy, D.A. (1972). *Manual for the McCarthy Scales of Children's Abilities.* New York: Psychological Corporation.

Ment, L.R., Oh, W., Philip, A.G.S., Ehrenkranz, R.A., Duncan, C.C., Allan, W., Taylor, K.J.W., Schneider, K., Katz, K.H., & Makuch, R.W. (1992). Risk factors for early intraventricular hemorrhage in low birthweight infants. *Journal of Pediatrics, 121,* 776–783.

Michaelis, R., Dopfer, R., Gerbig, W., Dopfer-Feller, P., & Rohr, M. (1979). I- Die Erfassung obstetrischer und postnataler Risikofaktoren durch eine Liste optimaler Bedingungen. *Monatsschrift Kinderheilkunde, 127,* 149–155.

Michaelis, R., Dopfer-Feller, P., Dopfer, R., Gerbig, W., & Rohr, M. (1979). II- Die Verteilung obstetrischer und postnataler Risikofaktoren bei 400 zufällig ausgewählten Neugeborenen. *Monatsschrift Kinderheilkunde, 127,* 196–200.

Perlman, M., Claris, D., Hao, Y., Pandit, P., Whyter, H., Chipman, M., & Liu, P. (1995). Secular changes in the outcomes to eighteen to twenty-four months of age of extremely low birth weight infants, with adjustments for changes in risk factors and severity of illness. *Journal of Pediatrics, 126,* 75–87.

Prechtl, H.F.R. (1967). Neurological sequelae of prenatal and perinatal complications. *British Medical Journal, 4,* 763–767.

Prechtl, H.F.R. (1968). Neurological findings in newborn infants after pre- and para natal complications. In J.H.P. Jonxis, H.K.A. Visser, & J.A. Troelstra (Eds.), *Aspects of prematurity and dysmaturity* (Nutritia Symposium) (pp. 303–321). Leiden, Holland: Stenfert-Kroese.

Prechtl, H.F.R. (1980). The optimality concept. *Early Human Development, 4,* 201–205.

Rapin, I. (1982). *Children with brain dysfunction* (p. 211). New York: Raven Press.

Remington, J.S., & Klein, J.O. (1990). *Infectious diseases of the fetus and newborn infant* (3rd ed.). Philadelphia: W.B. Saunders.

Rhoden, N.K. (1986). Treating Baby Doe: The ethics of uncertainty. *Hastings Center Report, 16,* 34–42.

Richards, M.P.M. (1989). Reflections on the withdrawal of treatment from newborn infants. *Early Human Development, 18,* 263–272.

Robertson, C.M.T., Hrynchyshynt, G.J., Etches, P.C., & Pain, K.S. (1992). Population-based study of the incidence, complexity, and severity of neurologic disability among survivors weighing 500 through 1250 grams at birth: A comparison of two birth cohorts. *Pediatrics, 90,* 750–755.

Roth, S.C., Baudin, J., Pezzani-Goldsmith, M., Townsend, J., Reynolds, E.O.R., & Stewart, A.L. (1994). *Relation between neurodevelopmental status of very preterm infants at one and eight years. Developmental Medicine and Child Neurology, 36,* 1049–1062.

Sameroff, A.J., & Chandler, M.J. (1975). Reproductive risk and the continuum of care-taking casualty. In F.D. Horowitz, M. Hetherington, S. Scarr-Salapater, et al. (Eds.), *Review of child development research* (Vol. 4, pp. 187–244). Chicago: University of Chicago.

Sarnat, H.B. (1989). Do the corticospinal and corticobulbar tracts mediate functions in the human newborn? *Canadian Journal of Neurological Sciences, 16,* 157–160.

Sarnat, H.B. (1992). *Cerebral dysgenesis: Embryology and clinical expression.* New York: Oxford University Press.

Sarnat, H.B., & Sarnat, M.S. (1976). Neonatal encephalopathy following fetal distress: A clinical and electroencephalographic study. *Archives of Neurology, 33,* 697–705.

Sauer, P.J.J. (1992). Ethical decisions in neonatal intensive care units: The Dutch experience. *Pediatrics, 90,* 729–732.

Schiffrin, B.S. (1990). *Exercises in fetal monitoring.* Saint Louis: C.V. Mosby.

Sonnander, K., & Gustavson, K.H. (1987). Reduced optimality as an indicator of developmental status at 18 months and school achievement at 8 years. *Neuropediatrics, 18,* 131–137.

Stewart, A., & Pezzani-Goldsmith, M. (1994). Longterm outcome of extremely low birthweight infants. In C. Amiel-Tison & A. Stewart (Eds.), *The newborn infant: One brain for life* (pp. 151–166). Paris: Inserm.

Touwen, B.C.L., Huisjes, H.J., Jurgens van der Zee, A.D., Bierman van Eendenburg, M.E.C., Smrkovsky, M., & Olinga, A.A. (1980). Obstetrical condition and neonatal neurological morbidity: An analysis with the help of the optimality concept. *Early Human Development, 4,* 207–228.

Volpe, J. (1995). *Neurology of the newborn* (3rd ed.). Philadelphia: W.B. Saunders.

Weinberg, W.A., & Brumback, R.A. (1992). The myth of attention deficit-hyperactivity disorder: Symptoms resulting from multiple causes. *Journal of Child Neurology, 7,* 431–461.

Young, E.W.D., & Stevenson, D.K. (1990). Limiting treatment for extremely premature, low-birthweight infants (500 to 750 g). *American Journal of Diseases of Children, 144,* 549–552.

Chapter 3

Preterm Development

Marilee C. Allen, M.D.

We may think of the cycle of human life as a series of events which run a course and which fill the long interval between conception and death. The events occur in a single dimension of time; but they are manifested in various facets: anatomical, physiological, psychological. In spite of the bewildering diversity of these manifestations, the cycle is unitary and continuous. It has a beginning and an end.

The life cycle is essentially a growth cycle . . . So closely are time and growth linked together that, whenever we think of a degree of maturity, we also think of age. To understand the maturity of a growing organism, we must know how old it is. And the younger the organism, the more exactly we must know its chronological age. For the younger the organism, the more rapidly it develops—and the more rapidly it grows old. (Gesell & Amatruda, 1945, p. 12)

Development is a dynamic process that implies change over time, and human development is characterized by a continuum from fertilized ovum to morula, blastocyst, embryo, fetus, newborn, infant, toddler, child, adolescent, and adult (Gesell & Amatruda, 1945; Illingworth, 1972; Saint-Anne Dargassies, 1977).

What may be normal at one stage of development may be very abnormal at another stage. For example, the characteristics of the normal neurodevelopmental examination of the full-term newborn infant (e.g., hyperreflexia, flexor hypertonia, pathologic and primitive reflexes, poorly coordinated voluntary movements) are signs of cerebral palsy in a 2-year-old. Knowledge of the sequence of normal development allows the patterns of abnormal development to be identified.

The embryo and fetus are relatively inaccessible, so, in the past, knowledge of development prior to term was limited to observations of a few viable preterm infants and of nonviable aborted fetuses and of (Gesell & Amatruda,

1945; Hooker, 1952; Hooker & Hare, 1954; Humphrey, 1964, 1969; R.J. Robinson, 1966; Saint-Anne Dargassies, 1977). Improvements in obstetric and neonatal intensive care have lowered the limit of viability to 23–24 weeks' gestation, and thus have allowed close observation of much more immature viable premature infants (Allen & Capute, 1986a, 1986b, 1990). In addition, real-time ultrasound technology has improved so that it is now possible to observe not just fetal anatomy and gross fetal body movements but finer movements, such as eye movements, hand and finger movements, and fetal breathing movements (Birnholz, Stephens, & Faria, 1978; deVries, Visser, & Prechtl, 1982; Ianniruberto & Tajani, 1981). These movements, together with observations of fetal heart rate (FHR) patterns, are useful in descriptions of fetal behavior and fetal behavioral states, and someday may be useful in identifying abnormal fetuses prior to delivery (deVries, 1987; Nijhuis, Martin, & Prechtl, 1984).

Understanding the sequence of normal development prior to term allows the identification of patterns of abnormal development. The goal of this chapter is to discuss what is currently known about the development of muscle tone, reflexes, and behavior in the fetus and the premature infant.

THE EMBRYO

Embryologists date fetuses from the time of fertilization, which occurs approximately 12–15 days after the onset of the last menstrual period (Finnstrom, 1972; Saito et al., 1972). This is the true gestational age, as calculated from the time of fertilization. Most clinicians do not know the time of conception for a given fetus. The only date available is the day of onset of the last menstrual period (LMP). Clinicians, then, tend to date pregnancies from the LMP, which adds approximately 2 weeks onto the true gestational age. Although this age is more precisely a menstrual age, common clinical usage refers to it as the gestational age of the fetus.

Streeter (1942, 1948) described a series of developing external and internal features of the embryo, characterized as Horizons I–XXIII, to describe the maturation of embryos from fertilization to Day 47 (England, 1983). The first 3 days (Horizons I–III) are characterized by cell division, from the single-cell fertilized oocyte to the morula, which implants in the uterine wall during Days 4–7 (Horizon IV) (England, 1983; Streeter, 1942, 1948). During Days 7–12 (Horizon V), the blastocyst (a hollow sphere) develops, embedding deeply into the uterine wall and developing exocelomic and amniotic cavities. The branching of the chorionic villi and development of the yolk sac and the primitive streak characterize Horizons VI–VIII (Days 13–19). The ectoderm neural plate is the first rudiment of the nervous system and develops into neural folds that rise and form the neural tube. On Days 20–23 (Horizons IX and X), the embryo elongates, the somites form, and the cephalic and caudal ends can be distinguished. It is at this point (true gestational age 2–3 weeks, clinical gestational age 4–5 weeks) that a urinary pregnancy test first becomes positive, but the symptoms of pregnancy (e.g., nausea, breast tenderness, lassitude) may not generate recognition of pregnancy for several more weeks. Using vaginal (or transvaginal) ultrasound, a gestational sac also may be detected at this time (Goldstein, Snyder, Watson, & Danon, 1988; Timor-Tritsch, Farine, & Rosen, 1988).

At 24–27 days (Horizons XI and XII), the neural groove closes, the primary brain vesicles and the optic vesicles form, the limb buds appear, the two heart tubes fuse in the midline and begin to contract, and the primordia of the liver, pancreas, lungs, thyroid gland, and mesonephric tubules appear (England, 1983). On Days 27–29 (Horizon XIII), the embryo is flexed in a "C" shape, the four branchial arches are present, and the arm and leg buds are easily seen. At this point (true gestational age 4 weeks, clinical gestational age 6 weeks), abdominal ultrasound can detect the gestational sac, and endovaginal ultrasound can detect a fetal heartbeat

(Jouppila & Piiroinen, 1975; Timor-Tritsch et al., 1988).

During the next week (4–5 weeks' true gestational age, Horizons XIV–XVII), the primary bronchi of the lungs develop, the limb buds elongate and differentiate (i.e., shoulder, elbow, hand and thigh, leg, foot), the intestinal loops and gut mesentery develop, the midgut herniates into the umbilical cord, the external auditory meatus forms, the peripheral nerves grow in the limb buds and trunk, and the right and left sides of the heart differentiate (England, 1983). By true gestational age week 4, the main divisions of the central nervous system (i.e., forebrain, midbrain, hindbrain, and spinal cord) are formed; by week 5, both the forebrain and hindbrain further divide and differentiate. During true gestational age weeks 5–6 (Horizons XVIII–XX), the eyelids and retina form, the external and inner ear form, the secondary bronchi of the lungs branch, the renal pelvis branches to form calyces, and the embryo's trunk elongates and straightens. At clinical gestational age 8 weeks, ultrasound can detect the embryo within the sac and can differentiate it from a blighted ovum.

True gestational age weeks 6–8 (Horizons XXI–XXIII) are characterized by further differentiation of the hands, fingers, feet, toes, eyelids, external ears, nose, and mouth (England, 1983). The choroid plexuses of the lateral third and fourth ventricles form and secrete cerebrospinal fluid. The eyes move from the sides of the head to the front of the face. The spinal cord and peripheral nerves have spread throughout the length of the embryo by 8 weeks (true gestational age). At this point (clinical gestational age 10 weeks), fetal heartbeats and movements can be detected reliably by abdominal and endovaginal ultrasound (Birnholz et al., 1978; deVries, 1987; deVries et al., 1982; Ianniruberto & Tajani, 1981; Timor-Tritsch et al., 1988).

It is clear that anatomic development of the embryo proceeds at a very rapid pace: Much development has occurred before the pregnancy can be detected, and most of the major organ systems are formed by 8 weeks' true gestational age (10 weeks' clinical gestational age). It is only at the end of this period that the signs (i.e., nausea, breast tenderness, lassitude) and symptoms (uterine fullness, cervical changes) of pregnancy generally appear and ultrasound can detect movement and heartbeats of the embryo. Most of the major organ systems are formed before the pregnancy is diagnosed.

THE FETUS

Structure

The fetus continues to grow rapidly throughout the remainder of the pregnancy, especially during weeks 11–22. (Clinical gestational age is used exclusively for the remainder of the chapter.) The body proportions change and the organs and tissues continue to differentiate. At 11 weeks, the head is almost half the size of the fetus. The body length doubles by the 14th week, and the head grows more slowly. The head is one third the body size at 5 months and one quarter at term (40 weeks' gestation). By 12 weeks, the fetus's body is so curved that sonographic measurements of its length are inaccurate.

By 14 weeks' gestation, the midgut returns to the enlarged abdominal cavity, the eyelids fuse, the fingernails appear, and the genitalia become fully differentiated. Vernix caseosa is secreted to cover and protect the skin from amniotic fluid, lanugo (fine hair) covers the body, brown fat has begun to form, and the spinal cord begins to myelinate by weeks 25–27. The eyelids and eyebrows are well developed, and, for the most part, the fetus looks like the full-term newborn (except for its size and lack of subcutaneous tissue). The fetus continues to grow, deposit fat, develop nails, and lose its lanugo. By 37–40 weeks, the brain is formed and myelination begins.

Clinical Assessment

Pregnancies traditionally have been monitored clinically by following uterine growth, recognizing fetal heartbeats by stethoscope, and questioning mothers about fetal activity (Johnson, Walker, & Niebyl, 1986). Uterine growth is followed by measuring fundal height (the length from the symphysis pubis to the tip of the uterus). From the 18th to the 36th week of pregnancy, the fundal height (in centimeters) roughly corresponds with the week of pregnancy. The fetal heartbeat generally can be heard by fetoscope at 19–20 weeks, or by Doppler at 12–14 weeks. Mothers generally can detect their infants' movements (i.e., quickening) at 17–20 weeks.

Fetal activity, as recorded by the mother, has been used as a measure of fetal well-being during pregnancy. Because a sudden decrease or cessation of fetal activity may be a sign of imminent fetal death, any report of this warrants a careful evaluation of mother and infant (Sadovsky & Yaffe, 1973). The amount of perceived fetal movement increases during early pregnancy, then decreases during the last 1–2 months (Sadovsky, Laufer, & Allen, 1979). Mothers have been able to distinguish among different types of fetal movements (e.g., rolling, ripples, kicks, hiccups) and have noted that they vary in frequency and strength with gestational age.

Sonographic Assessment

Although the primary use of ultrasound has been to confirm gestational age and assess fetal growth, its use has now been expanded to include assessment of congenital anomalies and fetal well-being. Fetal heart rate patterns, breathing movements, body movements, behavioral states, and responses to stimuli (e.g., vibroacoustic stimuli) have been used to evaluate fetal well-being.

Ultrasound measurements of fetal crown–rump length correlate highly (± 3–5 days) with gestational age between 6 and 12 weeks, but beyond 12–14 weeks they are less accurate because the fetus curves too much (H.P. Robinson & Fleming, 1975). The biparietal diameter of the fetus has a linear relationship with gestational age from 12 to 40 weeks but is most accurate at 12–17 weeks (Kurtz et al., 1980). Errors in later gestation can be due to variability in head growth (e.g., intrauterine growth retardation). To improve accuracy, many physicians use serial measurements and add measurements of femur length and chest diameter.

Improvements in ultrasound technology have enhanced efforts to diagnose congenital anomalies prenatally. A list of anomalies that can be diagnosed prenatally would be long and rapidly outdated. Before discussions are made regarding a plan of action (i.e., termination of pregnancy, intervention), it is important to confirm the diagnosis by repeat ultrasounds read by experienced sonographers.

Electronic or ultrasonic monitoring of FHR patterns has been used to detect early signs of fetal distress. Abnormal FHR patterns include persistent tachycardia or bradycardia, variable or late FHR decelerations, loss of beat-to-beat variability, and loss of baseline variation. It is important to recognize normal variations in FHR patterns. Fetal heart rate reactivity can be influenced by maternal medications, maternal emotional state, and uterine contractions (Goodlin & Schmidt, 1972). Light or vibroacoustic stimulation can accelerate FHR, sometimes producing a prolonged tachycardia (Jensen, 1984; Peleg & Goldman, 1980; Read & Miller, 1977; Thomas et al., 1989).

Ultrasound can detect fetal movements as early as 6–8 weeks (Birnholz et al., 1978; deVries, 1987; deVries et al., 1982; deVries, Visser, & Prechtl, 1984; Ianniruberto & Tajani, 1981). The earliest movements are described as smooth vermicular or just discernible movements at 6–8 weeks; by 8 weeks, rapid generalized movements characterized by twitches or startles are noted. Fetal movements become more differentiated with age and include general body movements; isolated arm, leg, or head movements; hiccups; jaw opening; and hand-to-face movements. Fetal breathing movements can be appreciated at 10–14 weeks, and their frequency increases with gestational age (deVries, 1987; deVries et al., 1982, 1984; Fox, Inglis, & Steinbrecher, 1979; Ianniruberto & Tajani, 1981). Although diurnal variations in fetal movement are not noted at 13 weeks' gestation, significant diurnal variations can be observed in fetal breathing movements, fetal movements, FHR, and FHR variation at 20–40 weeks (deVries, 1987; Roberts, Little, Cooper, & Campbell, 1979).

The rich and varied repertoire of fetal movements and their specific and recognizable patterns of evolution have encouraged investigators to evaluate the quality of fetal movements in pregnancies complicated by pathologic fetal or maternal conditions. Anencephalic fetuses demonstrate very abnormal fetal movements even in the first half of pregnancy: Movements are forceful, jerky, and of large amplitude and

occur only in burst–pause patterns (deVries, 1987). Growth-retarded fetuses have been described as having decreased fetal breathing and body movements, especially after late FHR decelerations (Bekedam & Visser, 1985; Ianniruberto & Tajani, 1981). Decreased fetal movements have been observed in fetuses with threatened abortion, severe preeclampsia, severe Rh isoimmunization, and maternal diabetes during an episode of hypoglycemia (Ianniruberto & Tajani, 1981). Fetuses with meningomyeloceles or hydrocephalus have been noted to have relatively immobile extended lower extremities with scissoring (Ianniruberto & Tajani, 1981).

Fetal body movements, eye movements, and heart rate patterns are used to classify fetal behavioral states, from 1F (quiescence) to 4F (vigorous, continual activity) (Nijhuis, Prechtl, Martin, & Bots, 1982; Nijhuis et al., 1984). From 36 weeks on, the fetus demonstrates well-organized behavioral states in which there is concordance among those three parameters for at least 3 minutes at a time. These behavioral states correspond to the behavioral states seen in neonates. As in preterm infants, fetuses below 36 weeks' gestational age demonstrate cycles of activity and rest, regular and irregular respirations, and presence or absence of eye movements, but some think that these cycles seldom overlap for a long enough period to demonstrate well-organized behavioral states (Nijhuis et al., 1982, 1984; Prechtl, Fargel, Weinmann, & Bakker, 1979). External environmental stimuli (e.g., vibroacoustic stimulation) can change fetal behavioral states and therefore fetal movement, fetal breathing, and FHR patterns (Birhnolz & Benacerraf, 1983; Goodlin & Schmidt, 1972; Read & Miller, 1977; Thomas et al., 1989). When assessing any fetal movement or fetal responsiveness to stimuli, it is important to determine and take into account the fetal behavioral state.

Ultrasound has proved to be the most useful and promising method of assessing the fetus. However, its use in identifying congenital anomalies, fetal distress, and abnormalities of the fetal central nervous system is still being explored and defined. It is important to continue to observe and describe normal patterns of fetal development and to assess the significance of variations from these patterns. Variation from normal may represent pathology or may be a physiologic adaptation to an unusual or stressful environment. Extreme caution must be exercised in interpreting and acting on these findings because we have only begun to learn the signs the fetus sends us.

Nonviable Aborted Fetuses

Several researchers have studied the movement and responses of nonviable aborted fetuses of various gestational ages in the minutes to hours prior to their deaths (Gesell & Amatruda, 1945; Hooker, 1952; Hooker & Hare, 1954; Humphrey, 1964, 1969; Saint-Anne Dargassies, 1977). Hooker (1952; Hooker & Hare, 1954) demonstrated reflex activity in a human embryo at 7.5 weeks' gestational age. Prior to that, human fetal muscle contraction occurred only in response to electrical stimulation. The first cutaneous sensory nerve to be functional is the trigeminal nerve: Stroking the lip with a hair causes contralateral flexion of the neck and upper trunk at 7.5 weeks. Until 10 weeks, the perioral area is the only area sensitive to cutaneous stimuli. Hooker found that the extent and character of fetal responses to exteroceptive cutaneous stimuli were so specific at each age up to 11 weeks that they could be used to date an embryo. Beyond 11 weeks, increasing individual variability in responses of fetuses of the same age was noted.

The earliest reaction to perioral stimulation is generalized avoidance-type body movement (contralateral neck and trunk movement at 7.5 weeks) (Hooker, 1952; Hooker & Hare, 1954; Humphrey, 1964, 1969). By 9.5 weeks, the movement involves more of the body (upper extremities, trunk, pelvis). At 8.5 weeks, ipsilateral movements (lateral head and trunk flexion, rump rotation toward the side of the stimulus) are seen in response to perioral stimulation as well. A more localized reaction (contralateral rotation of the face without trunk movement) appears by 14 weeks. The earliest localized reaction noted in the human fetus is a squint movement in response to stroking the upper eyelid. By 14 weeks, localized reflexes predominate and the entire surface of the body is sensitive to stimulation. Avoidance movements predominate early, and movements toward a stimulus (generally related to feeding) evolve somewhat later.

The earliest coordinated reflexes are related to feeding (Hooker, 1952; Hooker & Hare, 1954; Humphrey, 1964). Mouth opening is observed by 9.5 weeks, and ipsilateral head rotation with perioral stimulation (possibly a precursor of the rooting reflex) by 11.5 weeks. Momentary lip closure and swallowing with lip stimulation is noted by 12.5 weeks, with a more sustained response appearing by 14 weeks. Components of the Babkin and palmomental reflexes can be elicited by 13 weeks. Tongue movements are noted at 14 weeks, the gag reflex at 18 weeks, and protrusion of the lips and pursing of the lips by 20–22 weeks. Sucking begins at approximately 20–24 weeks.

The grasp reflexes are also seen very early. By 10.5 weeks, the fetus closes its fingers when its palm is stroked; by 11.5 weeks, the toes plantar flex in response to stimulation of the sole (Hooker, 1952; Humphrey, 1964). Spontaneous finger movements appear by 13.5 weeks. By 14 weeks, finger closure is more complete, and by 18 weeks a weak but true grasp reflex appears. By 12.5–13.5 weeks, stimulation of the sole often is followed by dorsiflexion of the toes (the Babinski reflex), and from then on the two reflexes (lower extremity grasp and Babinski) compete.

Much has been learned about early reflexes and responses from detailed observations of nonviable aborted fetuses. However, observations of this type are limited by factors that affect the overall status of the fetus: progressive anoxia, maternal anesthetics, trauma from manipulation when delivered, and cold stress (Hooker, 1952).

THE PREMATURE INFANT

Observations of viable preterm infants by Gesell and Amatruda (1945) and by Saint-Anne Dargassies (1977) have provided data on the development of tone and reflexes prior to term. Since the 1960s and 1970s, improvements in technology and monitoring in obstetrics and neonatology have allowed for more detailed observations of larger populations of relatively healthy preterm infants (Allen & Capute, 1986a, 1986b, 1990; Dubowitz, Dubowitz, Morante, & Verghote, 1980; Fawer & Dubowitz, 1982; Morante, Dubowitz, Levene, & Dubowitz, 1982).

As Saint-Anne Dargassies has emphasized, development prior to term proceeds in an orderly manner, according to postmenstrual age (PMA). Postmenstrual age is defined as the infant's clinical gestational age plus the infant's chronologic age at the time of the examination. Thus, a 4-week-old infant born at 28 weeks' gestation has a postmenstrual age of 32 weeks. "Postconceptional age" is used synonymously with postmenstrual age, but is somewhat of a misnomer because the gestational age used is that determined by the obstetrician and is calculated from the mother's LMP. The mother's LMP or the obstetrician's best estimate (from early examinations, sonograms, or both) is preferable to postnatal assessments of gestational age (e.g., Ballard, Dubowitz, lens vessels) in extremely premature infants. Postnatal assessments of gestational age have a tendency to overestimate gestational age assessed by LMP or sonogram by 2–3 weeks in preterm infants below 32–34 weeks' gestation (Constantine et al., 1987; Sanders et al., 1989; Spinnato, Sibai, Shaver, & Anderson, 1984).

The evolution of tone and reflexes in the preterm infant proceeds in an orderly, sequential manner from birth to term, in accordance with PMA. Two patterns—a caudocephalad pattern (lower to upper extremity) and a centripetal pattern (distal to proximal)—guide the development of tone and reflexes prior to term. Although most infants follow the normal pattern and sequence of development, there can be considerable individual variability in the timetable. As Illingworth has emphasized, "The sequence of development is the same in all children, but the rate of development varies from child to child" (1972, p. 137). In addition to normal individual variability, prenatal stress may accelerate neurologic maturity in some preterm infants (Amiel-Tison, 1980; Gould, Gluck, & Kulovich, 1977).

Development of preterm infants from birth to term is described here with respect to extremity tone, axial tone, deep tendon reflexes, patho-

logic reflexes, primitive reflexes, oromotor responses, auditory responses, visual responses, and behavior. Although the focus is on normal patterns and timetables, common deviations from these patterns and their significance also are discussed.

Extremity Tone

Although preterm infants are primarily hypotonic, they tend to demonstrate greater flexor tone immediately after birth because of the flexed posture in utero (Saint-Anne Dargassies, 1977). They generally assume a more hypotonic posture within 12–72 hours after delivery. Preterm infants below 28–30 weeks' PMA are generally quite hypotonic but may assume a semiflexed posture spontaneously (Allen & Capute, 1990). The development of flexor tone is manifest first in posture, then in maneuvers that reflect passive tone (e.g., heel-to-ear maneuver, popliteal angle) and in measures of active tone (e.g., recoil).

Flexor tone develops in a caudocephalad manner prior to term. Mild flexor tone appears in the lower extremities as early as 29 weeks' PMA as measured by popliteal angle or heel-to-ear maneuver (Allen & Capute, 1990). Subjective assessment of flexor tone and assessment of flexor tone by recoil maneuver (Amiel-Tison, 1968; Saint-Anne Dargassies, 1977; Thomas, Chesni, & Saint-Anne Dargassies, 1960) can detect mild flexor tone in the lower extremities by 31 weeks' PMA and in the upper extremity by 34 weeks (Allen & Capute, 1990). Flexor tone becomes stronger with increasing PMA and peaks at term (with flexor hypertonia in both upper and lower extremities and fisting). After term, the flexor tone is lost (or becomes more balanced with extensor tone), also in a caudocephalad manner. By 1–2 months past term, the infant generally has more recoil in the upper than in the lower extremities. By 3–4 months past term, extremity tone is equal and no longer flexor, and the infant is unfisted most of the time.

Axial Tone

Mild hip adductor tone can be appreciated by 31–33 weeks' PMA, and becomes stronger by 35–37 weeks' PMA (Allen & Capute, 1990).

Some degree of frog-legged posture is common in preterm infants until hip adductor tone becomes strong enough to overcome gravity, generally by 36–37 weeks. The normal prone posture of a full-term infant is with flexion of all extremities and the buttocks up in the air as a result of strong hip adductor and flexor tone (Illingworth, 1972; Saint-Anne Dargassies, 1977).

Preterm infants prior to 35 weeks' PMA demonstrate shoulder hypotonia, with both anterior scarf sign (Amiel-Tison, 1968; Thomas et al., 1960; Saint-Anne Dargassies, 1977) and posterior scarf sign (i.e., elbows touch in back) and with slip through at the shoulders. The posterior scarf sign generally is lost first (by 37–38 weeks' PMA), followed by the anterior scarf and slip through (by 38–39 weeks' PMA) (Allen & Capute, 1990). Although the majority of premature infants at term (38–40 weeks' PMA) no longer demonstrate either the anterior or posterior scarf signs, up to 30% may still demonstrate slip through at the shoulders.

Truncal hypotonia can be appreciated in preterm infants by holding them in ventral suspension and measuring the curve of the back (Thomas et al., 1960; Illingworth, 1972; Saint-Anne Dargassies, 1977). Trunk tone progressively improves with increasing PMA, and by term (40 weeks' PMA) the infant should be able briefly to achieve a horizontal position (Allen & Capute, 1990; Saint-Anne Dargassies, 1977).

The earliest sign of neck flexor tone may appear as early as 33 weeks' PMA (Allen & Capute, 1990). However, neck flexor tone takes longer to mature than any other aspect of tone. Nuchal tone can be measured best by pulling the infant to a sitting position from supine and observing the position of the head with respect to the body (Amiel-Tison, 1968, 1974). For extremely preterm infants, the forward movement of the head is passive and dominated by the pull of gravity, with very little modulation of the forward movement. With increasing PMA, the preterm infant develops better flexor tone and first is able to modulate the forward movement (so that the head no longer flops forward so dramatically) and then (by 37 weeks' PMA) can actively flex the head forward even against gravity (Allen & Capute, 1990). Most term infants have a head lag on pull to sit from supine, and, by 2–3 months from term, the infant can flex the neck actively so that the head remains in line with the body on pull to sit. Although the pull-to-sit maneuver is a good way of assessing nuchal tone, it frequently is stressful in extremely preterm and hypotonic infants. It should never be used to assess nuchal tone in infants with Down syndrome or other conditions that carry an increased risk of atlanto-occipital instability. Gently lifting the infant 1–2 cm off the bed by the shoulders can demonstrate marked nuchal hypotonia in extremely immature or hypotonic infants.

Development of neck flexor tone prior to term is balanced against the development of neck extensor tone. However, in some infants, neck extensor tone predominates, signifying abnormal development. One way to appreciate neck extensor hypertonia is by observing the infant's posture in supine (Amiel-Tison, 1974; Amiel-Tison, Korobkin, & Esque-Vaucouloux, 1977). The term infant should have no visible space behind the neck: Increased space behind the neck suggests neck extensor hypertonia. Neck extensor hypertonia can cause such marked neck and trunk extension that the infant is not able to lie in supine, but rather maintains a lateral decubitus posture. Preterm infants are frequently so dolichocephalic (i.e., they have long narrow heads with prominent occiputs) that they have increased space behind the neck. However, their spines are generally supple enough that the shoulders are flat to the bed. Neck extensor hypertonia is suggested by increased space behind the shoulders in preterm infants.

Neck extensor hypertonia also can be evaluated by the pull-to-sit maneuver and rocking in sitting (Amiel-Tison, 1974; Amiel-Tison et al., 1977). Infants with neck extensor hypertonia have head lag on pull to sit, and, when the body moves forward, the head does not move forward with gravity but holds back, and is very slow to flop forward onto the chest. When the infant is rocked in sitting, the neck tends to remain extended, even against gravity.

The infant with pronounced neck extensor hypertonia also may manifest the tonic labyrinthine reflex, characterized by shoulder retraction and lower extremity extension with neck extension, and shoulder protraction and lower extremity flexion with neck flexion. When extreme, neck extensor hypertonia can precipitate shoulder retraction and trunk and lower extremity extension (opisthotonus). This posture makes positioning and holding the infant very difficult, can lead to the development of contractures, and may interfere with the later development of voluntary motor activity (e.g., rolling, midline hand regard transfer).

Neck extensor hypertonia has been associated with later cerebral palsy in term infants (Nelson & Ellenberg, 1979). In preterm infants, neck extensor hypertonia may be related to prolonged intubation, tracheostomy, or the maintenance of an open airway in infants with chronic lung disease. However, its relationship to central nervous system damage cannot be ignored in these infants. Attempts must be made to position the infant correctly (with head midline, shoulders protracted, and lower extremities flexed and adducted) whenever possible and to follow the child's neurodevelopmental status very carefully.

Head righting is the earliest postural reaction to evolve and can be demonstrated prior to term in preterm infants. The infant is placed in a supported sitting position and gently tilted to the side. A more mature infant or adult would right his or her head by laterally flexing it. The premature infant's earliest response is to rotate the head laterally away from the tilt. This response should be present by term.

Mild extremity or axial hypotonia or both at a given PMA may reflect merely individual variability or health factors (e.g., improper nutrition, chronic lung disease). Development of normal lateral head righting can be reassuring in the infant with mild hypotonia. However, moderate to severe hypotonia (at least 3–4 weeks behind) is worrisome, and the child should be followed very carefully. As the hypotonic infant matures, he or she may develop maladaptive postures (e.g., fixation in a frog-legged posture) and even contractures (e.g., tensa fascia lata contractures) that may interfere with further voluntary motor development. Attention to the infant's handling and positioning may help to circumvent these difficulties.

Deep Tendon and Pathologic Reflexes

Extremely preterm infants are initially hyporeflexic. They develop deep tendon reflexes in a caudocephalad pattern: These reflexes generally can be elicited consistently at 30 weeks' PMA in the lower extremities and at 33 weeks' PMA in the upper extremities (Allen & Capute, 1990). Most premature infants develop hyperreflexia and frequently demonstrate unsustained clonus at the ankles, knees, or both by term. Sustained clonus is rare and somewhat worrisome.

The vast majority of preterm infants demonstrate many of the pathologic reflexes (i.e., Babinski, Chaddock's sign, mass reflex, and crossed adduction) by term. The more distal pathologic reflexes (e.g., Babinski, Chaddock's) can be elicited as early as 29 weeks' PMA, and the more proximal pathologic reflexes can be elicited at 33–34 weeks' PMA (Allen & Capute, 1990). The only worrisome finding with respect to the pathologic reflexes is the presence of asymmetric reflexes.

As with the evolution of tone, the evolution of the deep tendon and pathologic reflexes demonstrates the caudocephalad and centripetal patterns of development.

Primitive Reflexes

The primitive reflexes are stereotyped, complex, automatic movement patterns that are present at birth in full-term infants and, with central nervous system maturation, become more difficult to elicit during the first year of life when voluntary activity is emerging (Capute, Accardo, Vining, Rubenstein, & Harryman, 1978; Capute et al., 1982, 1984). The primitive reflexes actually emerge prior to term: They are initially incomplete and weak, and progressively become stronger, more complete, and easier to elicit with increasing PMA (Allen & Capute, 1986b, 1989; Robinson, 1966; Saint-Anne Dargassies, 1977).

A weak grasp reflex was elicited at 10–14 weeks in nonviable aborted fetuses (Hooker, 1952). A more sustained finger grasp could be elicited by 20 weeks in nonviable aborted fetuses and by 25 weeks' PMA in viable premature infants (Allen & Capute, 1990; Hooker,

1952; Humphrey, 1964, 1969). By 36 weeks' PMA, upward traction when eliciting the upper extremity grasp reflex will elicit flexion at the elbows (Allen & Capute, 1986b, 1990; R.J. Robinson, 1966; Saint-Anne Dargassies, 1977). Approximately 40% of preterm infants at term can be lifted off the bed with their upper extremity grasp reflex, in comparison to 60% of full-term newborns (Allen & Capute, 1986b; Saint-Anne Dargassies, 1977).

The Moro, Galant, and asymmetric tonic neck reflexes have been noted in nonviable aborted fetuses in a weak and incomplete form at 20–25 weeks' gestation (Gesell & Amatruda, 1945; Hooker, 1952; Saint-Anne Dargassies, 1977). In a study of graded primitive reflexes in viable extremely premature infants studied weekly from 25 weeks' PMA to term, all three reflexes emerged at 25–30 weeks' PMA; became stronger, more complete, and easier to elicit with increasing PMA; and were universally present by term (Allen & Capute, 1986b).

The initial flexor component of lower extremity placing emerges early (27–32 weeks' PMA), but the complete placing reflex, with flexion followed by extension, is not consistently present until 35–36 weeks' PMA (Allen & Capute, 1986b). This reflex is described as universally present in full-term newborns (Paine, 1960; Saint-Anne Dargassies, 1977). The newborn positive support and stepping can be seen as early as 27–28 weeks' PMA, but is not a frequent response until 35–36 weeks' PMA (Allen & Capute, 1986a). As in full-term newborns, both the newborn positive support and stepping responses are variable and may be absent in normal premature infants at term (Allen & Capute, 1986b; Capute et al., 1984; Paine et al., 1964; Saint-Anne Dargassies, 1977).

The tonic labyrinthine and symmetric tonic neck reflex also emerge at approximately 30 weeks' PMA in normal premature infants (Allen, 1987). The expression of one frequently interferes with the expression of the other, and neither is universally present at term.

The pattern of development of primitive reflexes reflects the pattern of development of tone (Allen & Capute, 1990). The flexion response of lower extremity placing emerges as lower extremity flexor tone emerges (31–33 weeks' PMA). Elbow flexion with upward traction (a component of the upper extremity grasp) and good upper extremity flexion with the Moro reflex emerge at 35–36 weeks' PMA, when upper extremity flexor tone emerges. Consistent posture changes with the asymmetric tonic neck reflex emerge first in the lower, then in the upper extremities. With the upper extremity grasp reflex, strong finger flexion can be elicited more than 5 weeks before elbow flexion. Thus, primitive reflexes also emerge in both a caudocephalad and a centripetal manner.

Preterm infants who demonstrate deviations from this pattern of development of primitive reflexes should be viewed as suspect, as should infants with primitive reflexes that are absent (or too weak) or obligatory. Primitive reflexes also can be used to evaluate symmetry.

Oromotor Responses

The earliest coordinated behavior a fetus demonstrates is related to sucking. The premature infant can suck at 24–25 weeks' PMA (and frequently is observed sucking on an endotracheal tube) and demonstrates a weak rooting response by 28 weeks' PMA (Saint-Anne Dargassies, 1977). However, coordination of the suck and swallow is not reliably present until 32–34 weeks' PMA, and preterm infants may not efficiently nipple feed until 34–36 weeks' PMA. The sucking rate and number of sucks increase with PMA.

The newborn's pattern of sucking, with rhythmic up-and-down movement of the jaw and protraction/retraction stripping action of the tongue, actually is called "suckling" because a more mature sucking pattern generally develops later (at 6–8 months) (Morris, 1978). The mature suck is characterized by less jaw movement, more independent up-and-down movement of the tongue, and a tighter seal with the lips, thus creating more negative pressure within the oral cavity. The full-term infant generally demonstrates a strong, well-coordinated suckle pattern, may still demonstrate a loose seal with the lips, and has a well-developed four-cardinal-point rooting reflex.

A number of neurologic and medical complications can contribute to difficulty feeding. The child with chronic lung disease may have a neurologically normal pattern of sucking but may be unable to sustain it because of exercise intolerance. The nipple can easily be removed from the mouth of an infant with a weak suck caused by generalized illness. The child with an inefficient suck may have excessive up-and-down movement of the jaws. Some infants may not develop a consistent rhythm of sucking. The premature infant may have difficulty coordinating the suck and swallow, and may have periods of apnea, bradycardia, and/or coughing and gagging with feedings. This should improve with time and be rare by term.

Tongue thrust and tonic bite, if consistently present, are generally signs of central nervous system damage. Tongue thrust is the forceful protrusion of the tongue beyond the lips, with the tongue appearing thick and bunched. Tongue thrust interferes with inserting the nipple and initiating the normal feeding pattern. The tonic bite is a strong closure of the jaws when the gums are stimulated, with difficulty opening the jaws once the bite is elicited. It is always worrisome and greatly interferes with feeding the infant.

An occupational, physical, or speech-language therapist who is experienced in feeding abnormalities of infants and children may be helpful in analyzing the feeding difficulty and developing intervention techniques designed to enhance feeding ability. These techniques include proper positioning of the infant to optimize tone as much as possible (e.g., inhibit extensor tone) and methods of introducing the nipple and supporting the jaw.

Auditory Responses

By 24–32 weeks' gestation, the fetus in utero responds to auditory or vibroacoustic stimulation with movement or heart rate acceleration (Birnholz & Benacerraf, 1983; Jensen, 1984). Preterm infants at the limit of viability (23–26 weeks' PMA) demonstrate change in heart or respiratory rate in response to a bell and auditory brain stem responses (to 70-dB stimuli) (Allen & Capute, 1986a; Starr, Amile, Martin, & Sanders, 1977). By 28–30 weeks' PMA, the alerting response (i.e., movement in response to a bell) and auditory brain stem responses can be obtained reliably (Allen & Capute, 1986a; Despland & Galambos, 1980; Fawer & Dubowitz, 1982). Using auditory brain stem responses, an auditory threshold of 30 dB has been reported in preterm infants (Despland & Galambos, 1980).

It is difficult to distinguish between habituation (i.e., the mechanism by which the central nervous system blocks out repetitive, distracting, and meaningless stimuli) and fatigue of the central nervous system. Nevertheless, apparent habituation to repetitive auditory stimuli has been demonstrated both in fetuses and in preterm infants (by 30–31 weeks' PMA) (Allen & Capute, 1986a).

A number of tools have been used to assess hearing in preterm and newborn infants. The crib-o-gram records infant movement in response to a loud (90-dB) stimulus, but, because of high false-positive and false-negative rates and its inability to detect anything less than a bilateral profound hearing loss, it is no longer used. Auditory brainstem responses (ABRs) can be detected early (at 23–26 weeks' PMA), and can be obtained reliably by 28 weeks' PMA. However, the pattern matures with increasing PMA: The threshold falls, latency decreases, and the amplitude of the waveform increases (Despland & Galambos, 1980; Fawer & Dubowitz, 1982; Starr et al., 1977). Both unilateral and bilateral hearing impairment can be detected, and stimuli as low as 30 dB can be used (although immaturity and background noise in a neonatal intensive care unit may contribute to a high false-positive rate at this level). Use of ABRs has been increasingly cost-effective but continues to demonstrate a high rate of false positives (Duara, Suter, Bessard, & Gutberlet, 1986). Transient evoked otoacoustic emissions (TEOE) is a newer methodology that is widely used to evaluate hearing in neonates in Europe, with increasing use throughout the United States (Kemp & Ryan, 1993). Most neonatal intensive care units screen their infants using one of these techniques and bring back those infants with abnormal responses for more definitive audiologic evaluation at 3–6 months from term.

Visual Responses

Preterm infants reliably blink in response to bright light as early as 25–26 weeks' PMA (Allen & Capute, 1986a; R.J. Robinson, 1966). Pupillary constriction in response to bright light can be elicited by 29–31 weeks' PMA, and the preterm infant turns his or her head toward diffuse light by 32–36 weeks' PMA (Robinson, 1966). The preterm infant is able to fixate visually, begins to demonstrate optokinetic nystagmus with an optokinetic nystagmus drum, and can differentiate between different visual patterns at 30–32 weeks' PMA (Allen & Capute, 1986b; Dubowitz et al., 1980; Hack, Mostow, & Miranda, 1976; Hack, Muszynski, & Miranda, 1981; Morante et al., 1982). These abilities all mature with increasing PMA and are universally present at term. The literature is divided as to whether preterm infants at term do as well as, the same as, or better than full-term infants on measures of visual attention, orientation, and discrimination (Allen & Capute, 1986a; Dubowitz et al., 1980; Ferrari, Grosoli, Fontana, & Cavazzuti, 1983; Kurtzberg et al., 1979; Morante et al., 1982; Palmer, Dubowitz, Verghote, & Dubowitz, 1982; van Hof-van Duin & Mohn, 1984).

Visual acuity in preterm infants at term and in full-term newborns is estimated to range from 10/150 to 20/16,000 (Hack, 1983). The full-term newborn should be able to fixate and follow (i.e., track) an object briefly. Both preterm and full-term infants have a fixed focal length of 19 cm (8–9 inches), and any object held closer or farther from their eyes will be more blurry. The ability to follow an object with the eyes and then to include head movement improves over the next 2–3 months. The ability to blink in response to a threatening gesture is not present in preterm infants prior to term or in newborns but generally can be elicited by 2–4 months past term (Allen & Capute, 1989; van Hof-van Duin & Mohn, 1984).

Behavior

Movements of both the fetus and the preterm infant increase in frequency and become smoother, more isolated, more integrated, and more sustained with increasing gestational age (Birnholz et al., 1978; Prechtl et al., 1979; Saint-Anne Dargassies, 1977). Startles and jerky movements involving the whole body are present by 24 weeks' PMA. By 28 weeks' PMA, the premature infant's movements are slow and global, with some isolated extremity movements (e.g., leg flexion and extension). The full-term infant demonstrates fewer movements (because flexor tone is increased), but the movements demonstrate greater control, strength, and integration. After term, the infants become more adept at integrating controlled flexion and extension, thereby demonstrating movement that is more voluntary.

Preterm and full-term infants demonstrate a continuum of states of alertness and arousal. For simplicity in describing an infant's behavior, we differentiate this continuum into specific stages or states (Hack, 1983; Wolff, 1959). A normal range of states includes quiet sleep or deep sleep, active sleep or light sleep, drowsiness, quiet alert, agitated, and intense crying. The infant's state affects his or her behavior, response to stimuli, muscle tone, posture, expression of primitive reflexes, deep tendon reflexes, and voluntary movements. Assessment of each of these parameters must be viewed in terms of the state the child is in at the time. For example, an infant may be more hypertonic and hyperreflexic when crying than when asleep.

It is important to note a given infant's range of states and transition from state to state. Most infants are capable of all states and move smoothly from one to another. Some irritable infants are capable of all states and move smoothly from one to another. Other irritable infants go immediately from sleep to crying and spend little or no time in the quiet alert state. Some lethargic infants are either asleep or drowsy and do not achieve higher states. Comatose infants appear to be in a sleep state and are poorly responsive to external stimuli.

The infant's state of alertness can be influenced by environmental stimuli, physiologic needs, position, temperature, drugs, asphyxia or coma, metabolic abnormalities, and jaundice (Hack, 1983). Swaddling, soothing touch and voice, rhythmic sounds, rocking, and encouraging sucking are environmental stimuli that can induce lower states. Rubbing, stroking, tickling, painful stimuli, interesting visual stimuli, and variations in sound can induce higher states. The hungry infant is generally more active, and the infant who recently was fed tends to sleep. The infant tends to be more active in the supine position, and tends to sleep in the prone position. A lower environmental temperature increases activity and higher temperature reduces activity.

The infant's state influences a number of physiologic functions (Hack, 1983). The infant's heart rate and respirations are slow and regular in quiet sleep. During active sleep and awake states, heart rate and respirations are faster and more irregular. Infants may have periodic breathing and apnea during active sleep. Oxygen consumption is lowest during quiet sleep and highest when the infant is crying. The infant has lower blood oxygen levels during active sleep than during quiet sleep. Blood pressure is lowest in quiet sleep, variable during active sleep, and highest when awake and crying. In terms of endocrine function, there is higher cortisol secretion when the infant is awake.

The time spent in various states varies with age. Fetuses in utero demonstrate a circadian rhythm to their body movements and fetal breathing movements (Roberts et al., 1979). Preterm infants have very short periods (seconds) of alertness by 30 weeks' PMA, with increasing duration with gestational age (Saint-Anne Dargassies, 1977). Prior to 36 weeks' PMA, cycles of rest and activity, regular and irregular respirations, and eye movements may alternate independently, and they may not coincide to produce consistent behavioral states in the infant (or fetus) until 36 weeks' PMA (Nijhuis et al., 1984; Prechtl et al., 1979).

It takes the full-term newborn infant 4–5 days to establish a regular sleep–wake cycle following birth (which disrupts the cycle). Sleep cycles are short in preterm infants and increase with age, with a gradual increase in the amount of time spent in quiet sleep over time spent in active sleep (Hack, 1983; Michaelis, Parmalee, Stern, & Haber, 1972).

In assessing and working with infants, it is important to be aware of their states of alertness. These states influence the infant's behavior and neurodevelopmental examination. Time spent in the various states varies with age, and various internal and external stimuli influence the transition from state to state.

COMPARISON OF PREMATURE AND FULL-TERM INFANTS

With respect to tone, reflexes, and behavior, preterm and full-term newborns are more similar than different (Saint-Anne Dargassies, 1977). However, the differences that do exist are worth noting: Although preterm infants at term demonstrate flexor hypertonia, their flexor tone is generally not quite as hypertonic as that of full-term newborns (Kurtzberg et al., 1979; Palmer et al., 1982; Saint-Anne Dargassies, 1977). Preterm infants at term demonstrate more lower extremity and trunk extensor tone than full-term newborns (Palmer et al., 1982). Except for preterm infants demonstrating a stronger positive support (probably as a result of more lower extremity extensor tone), the patterns of pathologic and primitive reflexes in preterm infants at term and full-term newborns are more similar than different (Allen & Capute, 1986a; Capute et al., 1984). Many preterm infants demonstrate asymmetries on examination, and these do not generally relate to abnormalities on cranial ultrasound (unless there is a severe Grade IV intraparenchymal hemorrhage) (Hinderliter, Allen, Nussbaum, & Jones, 1989; Howard, Parmalee, Kopp, & Littman, 1976).

Auditory abilities and visual acuity are similar in preterm infants at term and full-term newborns (Allen & Capute, 1990; van Hof-van, Duin & Mohn, 1984). There is, however, some controversy as to whether preterm infants at term do better or worse than full-term newborns on tests of visual orientation, pattern preferences, visual evoked responses, and state transition (Dubowitz et al., 1980; Ferrari et al., 1983; Howard et al., 1976; Kurtzberg et al., 1979; Michaelis et al., 1972; Palmer et al., 1982).

It is not clear whether these differences between preterm infants at term and full-term newborns are due to subtle abnormalities of the central nervous system, medical conditions (e.g., mild pulmonary disease, nutritional status), or a different (extrauterine versus intrauterine) environment, or to a combination of factors.

Because of the specific problems of preterm birth and the large number of variables affecting the preterm infant we consider it impossible to characterize the preterm infant as more or less neurologically mature than the full-term but rather as different in several important respects. (Palmer et al., 1982, p. 188)

After term, development continues to proceed in an orderly manner. There continues to be some controversy over whether chronologic age or age corrected for degree of prematurity (the term age equivalent, or adjusted age) is the valid measurement scale for premature infants. It may be important to try to answer this question separately for each stream of development, because one stream may be more or less affected by the extrauterine environment. Motor development appears to proceed according to age corrected for degree of prematurity (i.e., term age equivalent) (Allen & Alexander, 1990; Palisano, 1986). Although most psychologists correct for degree of prematurity up to age 1 or 2 when assessing cognitive abilities in premature infants, many continue to be concerned that this practice "overcorrects" and fails to identify abnormal preterm infants (Barrera, Rosenbaum, & Cunningham, 1987; Hunt & Rhodes, 1977; Miller, Dubowitz, & Palmer, 1984; Siegel, 1983). It also may be important to separate language from problem-solving abilities. Some early data suggest that, beyond 9 months, chronologic age is the best measurement scale for language abilities (Belcher, Allen, Gittelsohn, & Capute, 1988).

Clearly, further research must be done because this issue is of both theoretical and great practical concern. As more preterm infants born at 23–28 weeks' gestational age survive, this 3- to 4-month difference can make a difference in determining that a 6- to 12-month-old preterm infant is developing normally or has mental retardation, and will make a difference as to whether or not that infant is referred for early intervention services.

SIGNIFICANCE OF ABNORMALITIES ON EXAMINATION

Significant abnormalities on neonatal neurodevelopmental examination have been associated with later developmental disability in full-term newborns, in asphyxiated newborns, and in high-risk preterm infants (Allen & Capute, 1989; Bierman-van Eedenburg, Jurgens-van der Zee, Olinga, Huisjes, & Touwen, 1981; Brown, Purvis, Forfar, & Cockburn, 1974; DeSouza & Richards, 1978; Donovan, Coues, & Paine, 1962; Dubowitz et al., 1984; Nelson & Ellenberg, 1979; Parmalee et al., 1970; see also Chapter 16, Volume I). The more abnormalities on examination, the higher risk of neurologic disability (Allen & Capute, 1989; Brown et al., 1974). The neonatal exam appears to be better able to predict cerebral palsy and other neurologic impairments than mental retardation: There are few (if any) good indicators of cognition in neonates.

Sensitivity and specificity rates are good (70%–90%) for the ability of the neonatal exam to predict later neuromotor outcome (Allen & Capute, 1989; Dubowitz et al., 1980). A normal neonatal neurodevelopmental examination is reassuring because the vast majority of preterm and full-term infants with normal exams do well: Negative predictive values range from 90% to 97% (Allen & Capute, 1989; Bierman-van Eendenberg at al., 1981; Donovan et al., 1962; Dubowitz et al., 1980). However, most studies note a relatively poor positive predictive value (16%–64%). This is due to the generally low incidence of neuromotor abnormalities in the populations studied (up to 26%) and the impressive potential for recovery that the newborn exhibits.

The neonatal neurodevelopmental examination, then, cannot be used to diagnose developmental disability in the newborn because of the high rate of false positives. It can be used, however, to select a group of newborns (preterm or full-term infants) who are at high risk of developing developmental disabilities. This strategy would allow for more efficient utilization of follow-up and early intervention services. All high-risk infants, however, should be followed for cognitive deficits and academic and behavior problems through school age.

CONCLUSIONS

The embryo, fetus, and newborn represent the earliest stages in the continuum of human development. Their development proceeds in an orderly manner along a timetable determined by postmenstrual (or postconceptional) age. Knowledge of normal patterns of development allows identification of abnormal development.

In most cases, the major organ systems have formed before a pregnancy is diagnosed. The most rapid growth and structural development occurs by 22 weeks' gestation. Ultrasound has improved accessibility of the fetus and can be used to date a pregnancy accurately; follow fetal growth; diagnose congenital anomalies prenatally; and assess fetal well-being by evaluating fetal heart rate, movements, behavioral states, and responses.

Earlier observations of fetal muscle tone and reflexes were made in nonviable aborted fetuses and in a few viable preterm infants born beyond 28–30 weeks' gestation. Improvements in obstetrics and neonatology have allowed detailed sequential observations of the development of tone and reflexes in extremely preterm infants, from 25 weeks' postmenstrual age to term. Extremity and axial tone and deep tendon, pathologic, and primitive reflexes all emerge prior to term in a caudocephalad (lower to upper extremity) and a centripetal (distal to proximal) manner. Deep tendon, pathologic, and primitive reflexes become stronger, easier to elicit, and more complete with increasing postmenstrual age. Auditory and visual responses can be elicited at birth in preterm infants and become more mature by term. With a few exceptions, the preterm infant at term is more similar to than different from the full-term newborn.

What is normal at one point in time can be very abnormal at another point in time. Although there may be some individual variability in rate, most infants follow a normal pattern of development. Deviations from these patterns and marked variation from the normal timetable are worrisome. Some findings (e.g., neck extensor hypertonia, persistent extremity extensor tone, sustained clonus, tonic bite) can be viewed as abnormal at any point in development. Although a normal neonatal neurodevelopmental examination is reassuring, an abnormal neonatal examination cannot be used for definitive diagnosis of developmental disability. However, the examination can be used to select infants at high risk for developmental disability so that they can be followed carefully during infancy and childhood.

In conclusion, much development of the major organ systems, muscle tone, reflexes, auditory responses, visual responses, and regulation of behavior occurs prior to term in the fetus and preterm infant. Understanding the normal sequences and timetables allows us both to identify abnormal development and to recognize reassuringly normal development when it occurs.

REFERENCES

Allen, M.C. (1987). The symmetric tonic neck reflex (STNR) as a normal finding in premature infants prior to term. *Pediatric Research, 21,* 208A.

Allen, M.C., & Alexander, G.R. (1990). Gross motor milestones in very preterm infants: Correction for degree of prematurity. *Journal of Pediatrics, 116,* 955–959.

Allen, M.C., & Capute, A.J. (1986a). Assessment of early auditory and visual abilities of extremely premature infants. *Developmental Medicine and Child Neurology, 28,* 458–466.

Allen, M.C., & Capute, A.J. (1986b). The evolution of primitive reflexes in extremely premature infants. *Pediatric Research, 20,* 1284–1289.

Allen, M.C., & Capute, A.J. (1989). Neonatal neurodevelopmental examination as a predictor of neuromotor outcome in premature infants. *Pediatrics, 83,* 498–506.

Allen, M.C., & Capute, A.J. (1990). Tone and reflex development before term. *Pediatrics Supplement, 85,* 393–399.

Amiel-Tison, C. (1968). Neurological evaluation of the maturity of newborn infants. *Archives of Disease in Childhood, 43,* 89–93.

Amiel-Tison, C. (1974). Neurologic evaluation of the small neonate: The importance of head straightening reactions. In L. Gluck (Ed.), *Modern perinatal medicine* (pp. 347–357). Chicago: Year Book Medical Publishers.

Amiel-Tison, C. (1980). Possible acceleration of neurological maturation following high-risk pregnancy. *American Journal of Obstetrics and Gynecology, 138,* 303–306.

Amiel-Tison, C., Korobkin, R., & Esque-Vaucouloux, M. (1977). Neck extensor hypertonia: A clinical sign of insult to the central nervous system of the newborn. *Early Human Development, 1,* 181–190.

Barrera, M.E., Rosenbaum, R.L., & Cunningham, C.E. (1987). Corrected and uncorrected Bayley scores: Longitudinal developmental patterns in low and high birth weight preterm infants. *Infant Behavior and Development, 10,* 337–346.

Bekedam, D.J., & Visser, G.H.A. (1985). Effect of hypoxemic events on breathing, body movements, and heart rate variation: A study in growth retarded human fetuses. *American Journal of Obstetrics and Gynecology, 153,* 52–56.

Belcher, H.M.E., Allen, M.C., Gittelsohn, A.M., & Capute, A.J. (1988). Longitudinal language assessment of preterm infants: Full versus partial correction for prematurity. *Pediatric Research, 23,* 441A.

Bierman-van Eedenberg, M.E.C., Jurgens-van der Zee, A.D., Olinga, A.A., Huisjes, H.H., & Touwen, B.C.L. (1981). Predictive value of neonatal neurological examination: A follow-up study at 18 months. *Developmental Medicine and Child Neurology, 23,* 296–305.

Birnholz, J.C., & Benacerraf, B.R. (1983). The development of human fetal hearing. *Science, 222,* 516–518.

Birnholz, J.C., Stephens, J.C., & Faria, M. (1978). Fetal movement patterns: A possible means of defining neurologic developmental milestones in utero. *American Journal of Roentgenology, 130,* 537–540.

Brown, J.K., Purvis, R.J., Forfar, J.O., & Cockburn, F. (1974). Neurological aspects of perinatal asphyxia. *Developmental Medicine and Child Neurology, 16,* 567–580.

Capute, A.J., Accardo, P.J., Vining, P.G., Rubenstein, J.E., & Harryman, S. (1978). *Primitive reflex profile.* Baltimore: University Park Press.

Capute, A.J., Palmer, F.B., Shapiro, B.K., Wachtel, R.C., Ross, A., & Accardo, A.J. (1984). Primitive reflex profile: A quantification of primitive reflexes in infancy. *Developmental Medicine and Child Neurology, 26,* 375–383.

Capute, A.J., Shapiro, B.K., Accardo, P.J., Wachtel, R.C., Ross, A., & Palmer, F.B. (1982). Motor functions: Associated primitive reflex profiles. *Developmental Medicine and Child Neurology, 24,* 662–669.

Constantine, N.A., Kraemer, H.C., Kendall-Tackett, K.A., Bennett, F.C., Tyson, J.E., & Gross, R.T. (1987). Use of physical and neurological observations in assessment of gestational age in low birth weight infants. *Journal of Pediatrics, 110,* 921–928.

DeSouza, S.W., & Richards, B. (1978). Neurological sequelae in newborn babies after perinatal asphyxia. *Archives of Disease in Childhood, 53,* 564–569.

Despland, P., & Galambos, R. (1980). The auditory brainstem response (ABR) is a useful diagnostic tool in the intensive care nursery. *Pediatric Research, 14,* 154–158.

deVries, J.I.P. (1987). *Development of specific patterns in the human fetus.* Groningen, The Netherlands: Drukkerij Van Denderen B.V.

deVries, J.I.P., Visser, G.H.A., & Prechtl, H.F.R. (1982). The emergence of fetal behavior. I. Quantitative aspects. *Early Human Development, 7,* 301–322.

deVries, J.I.P., Visser, G.H.A., & Prechtl, H.F.R. (1984). Fetal motility in the first half of pregnancy. In H.F.R. Prechtl (Ed.), *Continuity of neural functions* (Clinics in Developmental Medicine No. 94) (pp. 46–64). Philadelphia: J.B. Lippincott.

Donovan, D.E., Coues, P., & Paine, R.S. (1962). The prognostic implications of neurologic abnormalities in the neonatal period. *Neurology, 12,* 910–914.

Duara, S., Suter, C.M., Bessard, K.K., & Gutberlet, R.L. (1986). Neonatal screening with auditory brainstem responses: Results of follow-up audiometry and risk evaluation. *Journal of Pediatrics, 108,* 276–281.

Dubowitz, L.M.S., Dubowitz, V., Morante, A., & Verghote, M. (1980). Visual function in the preterm and full-term newborn infant. *Developmental Medicine and Child Neurology, 22,* 465–475.

Dubowitz, L.M.S., Dubowitz, V., Palmer, P.G., Miller, G., Fawer, C., & Levene, M.I. (1984). Correlation of neurologic assessment in the preterm newborn infant with outcome at 1 year. *Journal of Pediatrics, 105,* 452–456.

England, M.A. (1983). *Color atlas of life before birth: Normal fetal development.* Chicago: Year Book Medical Publishers.

Fawer, C., & Dubowitz, L.M.S. (1982). Auditory brainstem response in neurologically normal preterm and full-term newborn infants. *Neuropediatrics, 13,* 200–206.

Ferrari, F., Grosoli, M.V., Fontana, G., & Cavazutti, G.B. (1983). Neurobehavioral comparison of low-risk preterm and full-term infants at term conceptional age. *Developmental Medicine and Child Neurology, 25,* 450–458.

Finnstrom, O. (1972). Studies on maturity in newborn infants. *Acta Paediatrica Scandinavica, 61,* 33–41.

Fox, H.E., Inglis, J., & Steinbrecher, M. (1979). Fetal breathing movements in uncomplicated pregnancies. *American Journal of Obstetrics and Gynecology, 134,* 544–546.

Gesell, A.L., & Amatruda, C.S. (Eds.). (1945). *The embryology of behavior.* New York: Harper & Brothers.

Goldstein, S.R., Snyder, J.R., Watson, C., & Danon, M. (1988). Very early pregnancy detection with endovaginal ultrasound. *Obstetrics and Gynecology, 72,* 200–204.

Goodlin, R.C., & Schmidt, W. (1972). Human fetal arousal levels as indicated by heart rate recordings.

American Journal of Obstetrics and Gynecology, 114, 613–621.

Gould, J.B., Gluck, L., & Kulovich, M.V. (1977). The relationship between accelerated pulmonary maturity and accelerated neurological maturity in certain chronically stressed pregnancies. *American Journal of Obstetrics and Gynecology, 127,* 181–186.

Hack, M. (1983). The sensorimotor development of the preterm infant. In A.A. Fanaroff, R.J. Martin, & I.R. Merkatz (Eds.), *Neonatal-perinatal medicine* (pp. 328–346). St. Louis: C.V. Mosby.

Hack, M., Mostow, A., & Miranda, S.B. (1976). Development of attention in preterm infants. *Pediatrics, 58,* 669–674.

Hack, M., Muszynski, S.Y., & Miranda, S.B. (1981). State of awakeness during visual fixation in preterm infants. *Pediatrics, 68,* 87–92.

Hinderliter, S.A., Allen, M.C., Nussbaum, A., & Jones, M.D., Jr. (1989). Does asymmetry of intraventricular hemorrhage (IVH) predict neurologic asymmetry in premature infants? *Pediatric Research, 25,* 254A.

Hooker, D. (1952). *The perinatal origin of behavior.* New York: Hafner Publishing Company.

Hooker, D., & Hare, C. (1954). Early human fetal behavior with a preliminary note on double simultaneous fetal stimulation. *Research Publications—Association for Research in Nervous and Mental Disease, 33,* 98–113.

Howard, J., Parmalee, A.H., Jr., Kopp, C.B., & Littman, B. (1976). A neurologic comparison of preterm and full-term infants at term conceptional age. *Journal of Pediatrics, 88,* 995–1002.

Humphrey, T. (1964). Some correlations between the appearance of human fetal reflexes and the development of the nervous system. *Progress in Brain Research, 4,* 93–135.

Humphrey, T. (1969). Postnatal repetition of human prenatal activity sequences with some suggestions of their neuroanatomical basis. In R.J. Robinson (Ed.), *Brain and early behavior: Development of the fetus and infant* (pp. 43–84). New York: Academic Press.

Hunt, J.V., & Rhodes, L. (1977). Mental development of preterm infants during the first year. *Child Development, 48,* 204–210.

Ianniruberto, A., & Tajani, E. (1981). Ultrasonographic study of fetal movements. *Seminars in Perinatology, 5,* 175–181.

Illingworth, R.S. (Ed.). (1972). *The development of the infant and young child.* Baltimore: Williams & Wilkins.

Jensen, O.H. (1984). Fetal heart rate response to controlled sound stimuli during the third trimester of normal pregnancy. *Acta Obstetrica et Gynaecologica Scandinavica, 63,* 193–197.

Johnson, T.R.B., Walker, M.A., & Niebyl, J.R. (1986). Prenatal care. In S.G. Gabbe, J.R. Niebyl, & J.L. Simpson (Eds.), *Obstetrics: Normal and problem pregnancies* (pp. 159–182). New York: Churchill Livingstone.

Jouppila, P., & Piiroinen, O. (1975). Ultrasonic diagnosis of fetal life in early pregnancy. *Obstetrics and Gynecology, 46,* 616–620.

Kemp, D.T., & Ryan, S. (1993). The use of transient evoked otoacoustic emissions in neonatal hearing screening programs. *Seminars in Hearing, 14,* 30–44.

Kurtz, A.B., Wapner, R.J., Kurtz, R.J., Dershaw, D.D., Rubin, C.S., Cole-Beuglet, C., & Goldberg, B.B. (1980). Analysis of bi-parietal diameter as an accurate indicator of gestational age. *Journal of Clinical Ultrasound, 8,* 319–326.

Kurtzberg, D., Vaughan, H.G., Jr., Daum, C., Grelong, B.A., Albin, S., & Rotkin, L. (1979). Neurobehavioral performance of low-birthweight infants at 40 weeks conceptional age: Comparison with normal full-term infants. *Developmental Medicine and Child Neurology, 21,* 590–607.

Michaelis, R., Parmelee, A.H., Stern, E., & Haber, A. (1972). Activity states in premature and term infants. *Developmental Psychobiology, 6,* 209–215.

Miller, G., Dubowitz, L.M.S., & Palmer, P. (1984). Follow-up of pre-term infants: Is correction of the developmental quotient for prematurity helpful? *Early Human Development, 9,* 137–144.

Morante, A., Dubowitz, L.M.S., Levene, M., & Dubowitz, V. (1982). Development of visual function in normal and neurologically abnormal preterm and full-term infants. *Developmental Medicine and Child Neurology, 24,* 771–784.

Morris, S.E. (1978). Oral-motor development: Normal and abnormal. In J.M. Wilson (Ed.), *Oral-motor function and dysfunction in children* (pp. 114–206). Chapel Hill, NC: University of North Carolina, Department of Medical Allied Health Professions, Division of Physical Therapy.

Nelson, K.B., & Ellenberg, J.H. (1979). Neonatal signs as predictors of cerebral palsy. *Pediatrics, 64,* 225–232.

Nijhuis, J.C., Martin, C.B., Jr., & Prechtl, H.F.R. (1984). Behavioral states of the human fetus. *Clinics in Developmental Medicine, 94,* 65–78.

Nijhuis, J.G., Prechtl, H.F.R., Martin, C.B., Jr., & Bots, R.S.G.M. (1982). Are there behavioral states in the human fetus? *Early Human Development, 6,* 177–195.

Paine, R.S. (1960). Neurologic examination of infants and children. *Pediatric Clinics of North America, 7,* 471–510.

Paine, R.S., Brazelton, J.B., Donovan, D.E., Drorbaugh, J.E., Hubbell, J.P., Jr., & Sears, E.M. (1964). Evolution of postural reflexes in normal infants and in the presence of chronic brain syndromes. *Neurology, 14,* 1036–1048.

Palisano, R.J. (1986). Use of chronological and adjusted ages to compare motor development of healthy preterm and fullterm infants. *Develop-*

mental Medicine and Child Neurology, 28, 180–187.

Palmer, P.G., Dubowitz, L.M.S., Verghote, M., & Dubowitz, V. (1982). Neurological and neurobehavioral differences between preterm infants at term and full-term newborns. *Neuropediatrics, 13,* 183–189.

Parmalee, A.H., Jr., Minkowski, A., Saint-Anne Dargassies, S., Dreyfuss-Brisac, C., Leziae, I., Berges, J., Cheruin, G., & Stern, E. (1970). Neurological evaluation of the premature infant. *Biology of the Neonate, 15,* 65–78.

Peleg, D., & Goldman, J.A. (1980). Fetal heart rate acceleration in response to light stimulation as a clinical measure of fetal well-being: A preliminary report. *Journal of Perinatal Medicine, 8,* 38–41.

Prechtl, H.F.R., Fargel, N.W., Weinmann, H.M., & Bakker, H.H. (1979). Postures, motility, respiration of low-risk pre-term infants. *Developmental Medicine and Child Neurology, 21,* 3–27.

Read, J.A., & Miller, F.C. (1977). Fetal heart rate acceleration in response to acoustic stimulation as a measure of fetal well-being. *American Journal of Obstetrics and Gynecology, 129,* 512–517.

Roberts, A.B., Little, D., Cooper, D., & Campbell, S. (1979). Normal patterns of fetal activity in the third trimester. *British Journal of Obstetrics and Gynaecology, 86,* 4–9.

Robinson, H.P., & Fleming, J.E.E. (1975). A critical evaluation of sonar "crown-rump length" measurements. *British Journal of Obstetrics and Gynaecology, 82,* 702–710.

Robinson, R.J. (1966). Assessment of gestational age by neurological examination. *Archives of Disease in Childhood, 41,* 437–447.

Sadovsky, E., Laufer, N., & Allen, J.W. (1979). The incidence of different types of fetal movements during pregnancy. *British Journal of Obstetrics and Gynaecology, 86,* 10–14.

Sadovsky, E., & Yaffe, H. (1973). Daily fetal movement recording and fetal prognosis. *Obstetrics and Gynecology, 41,* 845–850.

Saint-Anne Dargassies, S. (1977). *Neurological development of the full-term and premature neonate.* New York: Excerpta Medica.

Saito, M., Yazawa, K., Hashiguchi, A., Kumasaka, T., Nisha, N., & Kato, K. (1972). Time of ovulation and prolonged pregnancy. *American Journal of Obstetrics and Gynecology, 112,* 31–38.

Sanders, M.R., Allen, M.C., Graeber, J.E., Alexander, G.R., Yankovich, J., Johnson, J.B.R., & Repka, M.X. (1989). Gestational age assessment in premature infants less than 1500 grams. *Pediatric Research, 25,* 262A.

Siegel, L.S. (1983). Correction for prematurity and its consequences for the assessment of the very low birth weight infant. *Child Development, 54,* 1176–1188.

Spinnato, J.A., Sibai, B.M., Shaver, D.C., & Anderson, G.D. (1984). Inaccuracy of Dubowitz gestational age in low birth weight infants. *Obstetrics and Gynecology, 63,* 491–495.

Starr, A., Amile, R.N., Martin, W.H., & Sanders, S. (1977). Development of auditory function in newborn infants revealed by auditory brainstem potentials. *Pediatrics, 60,* 831–839.

Streeter, G.L. (1942). Developmental horizons in human embryos. Description of age group XI, 13–20 somites and age group XII, 21–29 somites. (Carnegie Institution of Washington Publication No. 541.) *Contributions to Embryology, 30,* 211–254.

Streeter, G.L. (1948). Developmental horizons in human embryos. Description of age groups XV, XVI, XVII, and XVIII. (Carnegie Institution of Washington Publication No. 575). *Contributions to Embryology, 32,* 133–203.

Thomas, A., Chesni, Y., & Saint-Anne Dargassies, S. (1960). *The neurological examination of the infant.* (Little Club Clinics in Developmental Medicine, No. 1). London: Spastic Society Medical Education and Information Unit in association with William Heinemann Medical Books.

Thomas, R.L., Johnson, T.R.B., Besinger, R.E., Rafkin, D., Treanor, C., & Strobino, D. (1989). Preterm and term fetal cardiac and movement responses to vibratory acoustic stimulation. *American Journal of Obstetrics and Gynecology, 161,* 141–145.

Timor-Tritsch, I.E., Farine, D., & Rosen, M.G. (1988). A close look at early embryonic development with the high frequency vaginal transducer. *American Journal of Obstetrics and Gynecology, 159,* 676–681.

Touwen, B.C.L. (1984). Primitive reflexes— conceptional or semantic problem? *Clinics in Developmental Medicine, 94,* 115–125.

van Hof-van Duin, J., & Mohn, G. (1984). Vision in the preterm infant. *Clinics in Developmental Medicine, 94,* 93–114.

Walters, C.E. (1964). Reliability and comparison of four types of fetal activity and of total activity. *Child Development, 35,* 1249–1256.

Wolff, P.H. (1959). Observations on newborn infants. *Psychosomatic Medicine, 121,* 110.

Chapter 4

Mental Retardation and Learning Disorders

A Neuropathologic Differentiation

Walter E. Kaufmann, M.D.

Cognitive disorders affecting infants and children have been classified according to different criteria, most commonly based on the type and severity of deficient skills (Kinsbourne, 1980). Two large groups of deficits can be recognized: those affecting global cognitive development (e.g., mental retardation) and specific disorders, usually less severe, that involve predominantly only one sphere of cognition (e.g., dyslexia), known as learning disabilities.

A second dimension of analysis of developmental cognitive disorders is the temporal one. There are conditions associated with a progressive loss of cognitive skills, which display a wide range of cognitive function, including levels comparable to mental retardation, and are categorized as dementias (Kaufmann, 1992; Rapin, 1989). Typical examples of this group are metabolic disorders affecting either gray or white matter, such as neuronal ceroid lipofuscinosis and leukodystrophies (Dyken & Krawlecki, 1983; Naidu & Moser, 1990; Rapin, 1989).

By contrast, most of the developmental cognitive disorders are more or less stable. This category includes both classic mental retardation and learning disabilities. Moreover, several developmental conditions, such as neurofibromatosis type 1 (NF 1) and tuberous sclerosis, can present the whole spectrum of cognitive impairment from learning disability to severe mental retardation (Berg, 1991; B.H. Cohen, 1991). Finally, underachievement of intellectual functions usually is accompanied by de-

viant behavior that could be either a constant and primary feature, as in autism, or a secondary adaptive phenomenon (Kinsbourne, 1980). This extremely simplified overview underscores the complexity and importance of understanding the neurobiologic bases of developmental cognitive disorders as a necessary step to improve their diagnosis and treatment. This chapter attempts to characterize and differentiate developmental cognitive disorders from an anatomic perspective, with special emphasis on the neuropathology of mental retardation and learning disabilities.

NEUROANATOMY OF DEVELOPMENTAL COGNITIVE DISORDERS

Neuropathology traditionally has provided key information for a clearer neurobiologic understanding of many neurologic diseases (Hornykiewicz, 1963). However, by reviewing the available neuropathologic literature, it becomes evident that there is no systematic approach to the neuroanatomic bases of disorders affecting the development of intellectual function. Textbooks on neuropathology usually classify brain disorders according to categories that combine etiology, pathogenesis, and morphology (Adams & Duchen, 1992). For example, perinatal brain damage that leads to cognitive impairment usually is classified under perinatal or hypoxic–ischemic categories. This etiologic/pathogenic/morphologic classification

This chapter was supported by National Institutes of Health Grant No. HD 01046, an Epilepsy Foundation of America Research Award, and a Merck Clinician Scientist Award.

of mental impairment has some use in clinical management of mental retardation (Jones, 1988; Smith & Simons, 1975); however, there is poor correlation between a particular etiology and its neurobehavioral outcome (Kinsbourne, 1980). Consequently, a mechanistic or pathogenic approach makes it extremely difficult to characterize the neurobiologic or common morphologic features subjacent to developmental cognitive impairment. In spite of this, neuropathologic studies on mental retardation (Huttenlocher, 1991) and dyslexia (Galaburda, Sherman, Rosen, & Kaufmann, 1987) have emphasized the consistent involvement of the cerebral cortex in these disorders. Furthermore, the introduction of advanced neuroimaging, more specifically magnetic resonance imaging (MRI) morphometry, has expanded our neuroanatomic knowledge of mental retardation (Gabrielli et al., 1990; Reiss et al., 1993); dyslexia (Rumsey et al., 1986); and other related cognitive disorders such as developmental dysphasia (Jernigan, Hesselink, Sowell, & Tallal, 1991), attention-deficit/hyperactivity disorder (ADHD) (Hynd, Semrud-Clikeman, Lorys, Novey, & Eliopulos, 1990), and Tourette syndrome (Singer et al., 1993). These radiologic investigations again have confirmed the critical role of developmental cortical anomalies in developmental cognitive disorders.

NEUROPATHOLOGY OF MENTAL RETARDATION

Of all the developmental cognitive syndromes affecting the pediatric age group, mental retardation is unquestionably the most comprehensibly studied, although still not fully understood. Currently, few unifying hypotheses that can explain the mental and behavioral abnormalities in the majority of cases of mental retardation are available. I begin my exposition by presenting data pertinent to mental retardation, emphasizing the general principles that also can be applied to other developmental cognitive disabilities.

From both clinical and anatomic viewpoints, mental retardation is a heterogeneous condition (Smith & Simons, 1975). There are individuals with mild cognitive impairment who show a sustained developmental profile slightly below standards. These cases mainly relate to socioenvironmental factors (Drillien, 1968; Drillien, Jameson, & Wilkinson, 1966; Dobbing & Smart, 1974; Riessman, 1962), and milder forms of chromosopathies and metabolic disorders (Jones, 1988), and sometimes are associated with minor brain malformations (Blomquist, Gustavson, & Holmgren, 1981). On the other end of the spectrum, one finds individuals with minimal intellectual capabilities who exhibit a developmental delay compatible with psychomotor "stagnation" rather than retardation. In this group, a higher frequency of genetic disorders (mainly chromosopathies) and major brain malformations is found (Gustavson, Hagberg, Hagberg, & Sars, 1977a, 1977b). The etiologic differentiation between mild and severe mental retardation can be exemplified by the distinct proportion of prenatal (23% and 55%, respectively) and perinatal (18% and 15%–20%, respectively) etiologies (Hagberg & Kyllerman, 1983).

Anatomically, both ends of the spectrum, which can be seen in entities such as Down syndrome, could be characterized by unremarkable and grossly abnormal brains, respectively. Major brain malformations (e.g., agyria/lissencephaly spectrum, pachygyria) (Aicardi, 1991; Goertchen, 1975) almost invariably are associated with severe mental disabilities and frequently are accompanied by anomalies in other organs (Jones, 1988). These conditions show greatly deviated macroscopic parameters of the central nervous system (CNS)—for example, brain weight, brain shape, and gray/white matter ratio. Nevertheless, the most severely abnormal structures are the cerebral cortex and subjacent white matter (Barth, 1987; Sarnat, 1987). By contrast, no clearly abnormal brain morphology and a high frequency of cases (40%–50%) without an identified cause are characteristic of mild mental retardation (Blomquist et al., 1981). Yet, the pathologic observations in severe forms of mental retardation have clinical implications if one considers that microcephaly constitutes one of the best predictors of mental retardation (Dolk, 1991). However, the lack of direct evidence of brain pathology, by standard clinical and imaging techniques

(Jones, 1988), has been an obstacle to explaining the significant proportion of severe mental retardation (15%–20%) (Benassi et al., 1990; Gustavson et al., 1977b) without an etiology, to adopting prophylactic measures in many instances, and to determining a prognosis as well.

Standard neuropathology, including microscopic evaluations, was considered an alternative approach to clarify these issues. Nevertheless, pathologic studies are scarce and not particularly informative in terms of disclosing an etiology or pattern of abnormalities in a large proportion of mental retardation cases (Crome & Stern, 1972; Freytag & Lindenberg, 1967). This is especially true of mental retardation that is not associated with particular syndromes, usually termed *unclassified* (Jellinger, 1972). Negative pathologic findings in mental retardation raise two related questions: What is the cause of most of the mild to moderate cases, and what is the common substrate of the wide spectrum known as mental deficiency? Fortunately, a combination of more sophisticated morphologic techniques, along with quantitative imaging studies, is beginning to answer these clinical dilemmas.

SYNAPTIC CIRCUITRY AND MENTAL RETARDATION

Cytoarchitectonic techniques have helped to delineate better the large group of brain malformations commonly labeled *neuronal migration disorders* (NMDs), which are associated with mental retardation (Barth, 1987). These abnormalities are diffuse and more severely involve the neocortex, and are characterized by a combination of anomalous neuronal density, laminar organization, heterotopic tissue, and aberrant cytodifferentiation (Friede, 1989; Warkany, Lemire, & Cohen, 1981). Milder forms of NMDs (microdysgeneses) that are not detected grossly, and that include heterotopias and cortical dysplasias, are seen at a higher frequency in persons with mental retardation when compared to other neurologic disorders (Rorke, 1994). By contrast, in individuals without macro- or microscopic malformations, such as most of those with an unclassified etiology, only morphometric techniques have showed cytoarchitectonic anomalies as aberrant distribution and orientation of small pyramidal neurons that are involved in local circuitry (Logdberg & Brun, 1993). Cytoarchitectonic findings such as microdysgenesis frequently are characterized poorly and are reported as minor anomalies in routine diagnoses. To understand the significance of these cytoarchitectonic abnormalities, it is important to consider that discrete areas of NMD also are seen in small numbers in neurologically normal subjects (Kaufmann & Galaburda, 1989). Therefore, microdysgeneses would be functionally significant only when they cover large or critical areas, or both, of the cortex and hippocampus. Cytoarchitectonic abnormalities imply disarrangements of brain circuitry in terms of spatial relationships between neurons; for instance, they can reflect aberrant numbers of a particular cell population or anomalous laminar and columnar orientation of a neuronal type. In addition, they indirectly show abnormal neuronal processes, particularly those arising from the neuronal soma (dendrites). All these parameters have pathophysiologic implications to the extent that they evidence aberrant morphology of the basic neural unit: the synapse. In this regard, the introduction of more sophisticated histologic techniques, principally Golgi impregnations that reveal, in detail, neuronal processes and therefore the synaptic surface, has been the single most important advance in approaching the neurobiology and neuropathology of mental retardation.

The staining by Golgi methods of autopsy and biopsy samples from individuals with mental retardation is the consequence of the reintroduction, in the 1970s, of these techniques in experimental neuroanatomy. Studies of normal cortical structure and development (Greenough, 1984; Petit, LeBoutillier, Gregorio, & Libstug, 1988) and animal models relevant to mental retardation (Hohmann, Kwiterovich, Oster-Granite, & Coyle, 1991; Nigam & Labar, 1979) and learning disabilities (Adaro, Fernández, & Kaufmann, 1986) have provided an important base and stimulus for extension of these methods to human developmental disorders. Although many technical issues, such as fixation, postmortem interval, and selection of appropriate controls (Buell, 1982; Huttenlocher, 1991; Williams, Ferrante, & Caviness, 1978), have brought into question the results of many investigations, there are general conclusions to be made.

There are dendritic anomalies in a wide variety of mental retardation–related conditions (Jagadha & Becker, 1989) (Table 1). Four groups of brains from individuals with mental retardation have been studied in a more systematic way: those with unclassified mental retardation, chromosopathies, malformations (NMDs), and metabolic disorders. The findings in unclassified mental retardation are prototypic in the neocortex and hippocampus: decreased dendritic arborizations (apical and basilar branches) and sparse dendritic spines (Huttenlocher, 1970, 1974; Purpura, 1974, 1975). Moreover, qualitative changes of dendritic spines, characterized

by long and thin processes, suggest a developmental arrest at early stages of dendritic spine formation (Purpura, 1974). These dendritic spine anomalies, termed *dysgenesis*, have been studied extensively in chromosomal disorders by Marin-Padilla (1972, 1974, 1976), and, although not specific to these forms of mental retardation, they seem to be characteristic of each chromosomal syndrome. These investigations have included Down syndrome (Fábregues & Ferrer, 1983; Marin-Padilla, 1976; Suetsugu & Mehraein, 1980; Takashima, Becker, Armstrong, & Chan, 1981), perhaps the most extensively studied form of mental retardation (Barth, 1987). In this syndrome, quantitation of dendritic branches has suggested that anomalies are present in an age-dependent pattern, with infants and older individuals showing definitive abnormalities while fetuses and neonates show

Table 1. Cerebrocortical pathology in mental retardation

Disease/condition	Abnormality
Diffuse NMDs (lissencephaly, pachygyria)	Abnormal neuronal density
	Anomalous lamination
	Distorted neuronal orientation
	Abnormal neuronal location
	Aberrant cell typology
	Anomalous neuronal size and shape
	Major dendritic aberration
	Reduced dendritic spines
Focal NMDs (polymicrogyria, heterotopias)	Abnormal neuronal location
	Anomalous lamination
	Abnormal neuronal density
	Distorted neuronal orientation
	Aberrant cell typology
	Minor dendritic aberration
Down syndrome	Abnormal neuronal location
	Anomalous neuronal density
	Reduced dendritic tree
	Aberrant dendritic spines
	Decreased spine density
	Aberrant perisomatic processes
	Reduced synaptic density
	Increased synaptic density
	Immature synapses
Rett syndrome	Increased neuronal density
	Reduced neuronal size
	Decreased dendritic tree
Unclassified mental retardation	Reduced dendritic tree
	Aberrant dendrites and spines
	Decreased spine density

Note: NMD, neuronal migration disorder.

rather normal dendritic trees (Becker, Armstrong, & Chan, 1986; Jagadha & Becker, 1989).

Dendritic shaft and spine abnormalities are important in understanding mental retardation for several reasons. First, they also are seen in disorders affecting cerebrocortical lamination focally (e.g., polymicrogyria) (Richman, Stewart, & Caviness, 1974; Williams, Ferrante, & Caviness, 1976) or diffusely (e.g., lissencephaly or agyria/pachygyria) (Ferrer, 1984; Ferrer & Fernández-Alvarez, 1977; Jagadha & Becker, 1989; Robain & Deonna, 1983; Stewart, Richman, & Caviness, 1975; Williams, Ferrante, & Caviness, 1975). These malformations correspond to the category of NMDs even though four-layered polymicrogyria would most likely be the result of postmigrational necrosis (Barth, 1987; Humphreys, Rosen, Press, Sherman, & Galaburda, 1991). Based on correlations of cytoarchitectonics with dendritic patterns by Golgi impregnations in NMDs, we can draw several conclusions. First, dendritic anomalies are more subtle signs of neuronal pathology, often overlooked in regions with minor laminar disturbances, such as those adjacent to conspicuous lesions. In fact, Golgi studies of cortical tubers in tuberous sclerosis have underscored the anomalous architecture of the cortex in this syndrome (Ferrer, Fábregues, Coll, Ribalta, & Rives, 1984). Consequently, brains of individuals with mental retardation that show only dendritic aberrations would represent the opposite end to gross malformations in the spectrum of cerebrocortical anomalies associated with these disorders. Second, most of these studies point to a decrease in dendritic length, which represents a decrease in overall postsynaptic surface. It is intuitive to associate this feature with hypofunction of the cerebral cortex, a presumed cause of cognitive impairment. Third, there are qualitative and quantitative changes involving dendritic spines in typical cases of mental retardation. This is the more generalized and direct evidence of synapse pathology in mental retardation, considering that dendritic spines are excrescences that represent postsynaptic sites for axodendritic synapses. Hence, not only decreased available synaptic sites but also aberrant ones would underlie cortical dysfunction in mental retardation. Fourth, the introduction of immunocytochemical techniques to the study of developmental disorders has confirmed the value of Golgi data in assessing neuronal differentiation and synaptic components (Takashima, Chan, Becker, & Kuruta, 1991) and promises to expand the spectrum of tools to assess neuropathologic changes in mental retardation. Finally, data from well-characterized models of mental retardation and learning disabilities (Adaro et al., 1986; Hohmann et al., 1991; Nigam & Labar, 1979) have shown results similar to the pathology of mental retardation and proved the feasibility of these methods in evaluating dynamics of developmental processes and their functional implications.

Is the reduction and distortion in the cortical postsynaptic surface a hallmark of mental retardation? Despite the consistency of Golgi impregnation findings in mental retardation, several troublesome issues remain. Long postmortem interval and agonal changes (Buell, 1982; Williams et al., 1978), as well as confounding variables, mainly the presence of cardiac malformations in chromosopathies (Huttenlocher, 1991), are factors that preclude considering dendritic changes as specifics of mental retardation. In this regard, discrepancies among investigations could be the consequence of technical variables or methodology of assessment (qualitative vs. quantitative) (Huttenlocher, 1974; Williams, Ferrante, & Caviness, 1979; Williams, Hauser, Purpura, DeLong, & Swisher, 1980). Furthermore, in several metabolic disorders affecting primarily the cerebral cortex, there are dendritic abnormalities similar to those seen in typical mental retardation (Bauman & Kemper, 1982; Della Giustina, Goffinet, & Landrieu, 1981; Takashima, Chan, Becker, Houdu, & Suzuki, 1991). Nevertheless, the fundamental defect in these disorders—that is, the accumulation of storage material in neuronal somata and proximal dendrites and axons (Friede, 1989)—leads to a somewhat different Golgi pattern. The anomalies are more pronounced in axons, especially in the proximal segments, which are markedly distended (Braak, Braak, & Goebel, 1983; Goldman, Katz, & Rapin, 1981; Paula-Barbosa et al., 1981; Purpura, 1978; Purpura & Suzuki, 1976; Takashima, Becker, Chan, & Augustin, 1985;

Williams, Lott, & Ferrante, 1977). Therefore, dendritic aberrations in classic storage disorders such as gangliosidoses and neuronal ceroid lipofuscinosis affect predominantly axons (the presynaptic domain) and include anomalous spatial configurations of cortical neurons (Purpura & Suzuki, 1976).

Are these findings an indication that, in mental retardation there are also presynaptic disturbances? Not necessarily; although the cognitive profile of children with storage disorders may resemble that of classic mental retardation, these metabolic conditions are not stable but rather progressive (Dyken & Krawlecki, 1983). The clinical picture at a particular stage can be comparable with mild mental retardation and, at a later time point, with severe mental retardation. In fact, there are Golgi data showing progression of dendritic pathology in a case of gangliosidosis (Jagadha & Becker, 1989). It is possible to conclude that metabolic–degenerative disorders show qualitative and quantitative alterations of dendritic and axonal morphology that correlate with cognitive impairment as in mental retardation; however, these are dynamic changes and share with mental retardation their diffuse and severe magnitude. The pathogenesis of these abnormalities in metabolic disease is usually postnatal when the basic cytoarchitecture of the cortex is already established, and they can be considered as secondary processes. By contrast, in mental retardation, an earlier disturbance of corticogenesis is suspected, probably dating to the beginning of neuronal differentiation.

An extremely interesting situation is represented by autistic syndromes, a group of heterogeneous disorders that have been correlated with a variety of neuroanatomic anomalies (Lotspeich & Ciaranello, 1993; Williams et al., 1980). Mental retardation is a frequent manifestation in autistic individuals and, of particular interest, is the condition known as Rett syndrome. This entity affects almost exclusively girls, with a progressive course during early childhood that resembles a degenerative disorder. Nevertheless, by late childhood and adolescence, neurologic deficit, including cognitive dysfunction, stabilizes as in typical cases of mental retardation (Hagberg, 1989). Pathologi-

cally, cytoarchitectonic analyses demonstrate an increased cell packing density, particularly marked in the neocortex and hippocampus. These changes reflect a reduced dendritic tree, probably caused by developmental arrest, as has been corroborated by preliminary Golgi studies (Armstrong, 1992). These reports have shown no age dependency of these anomalies, as expected from clinical observations. Hence, reduced dendritic trees seem to be an indicator of cognitive impairment and not of evolution of developmental anomalies in this form of mental retardation. This is not surprising if one considers that a decrease in dendritic arborizations also has been demonstrated in most neurodegenerative disorders associated with aging, such as Alzheimer's disease (Catalá, Ferrer, Galofré, & Fábregues, 1988; Jagadha & Becker, 1989; Kaufmann, 1992). Therefore, it is necessary to analyze Golgi studies in mental retardation in the context of, and complementing, other sophisticated morphologic techniques in order to discern their specificity and pathophysiologic role.

It is still unknown whether dendritic tree reductions in most mental retardation–related conditions represent a true developmental arrest, as it has been demonstrated in Rett syndrome by morphometry showing decreased neuronal body surfaces (Armstrong, 1992). Therefore, more comprehensive qualitative and morphometric examinations, using Golgi and other techniques, that cover a wider spectrum of cases of mental retardation are essential. This approach has been successful in other conditions such as Huntington disease and human immunodeficiency virus encephalopathy, where it has resolved long-term dilemmas by disclosing a primary cortical involvement accompanied by peculiar plastic (compensatory) responses (Kaufmann, 1992; Sotrel, Williams, Kaufmann, & Myers, 1993). Likewise, more electron microscopic studies, which have been circumscribed almost exclusively to Down syndrome, directly examining synapses would help to clarify contradictory information. There are reports of both decreased (Wisniewski, Laure-Kamionowska, Connell, & Wisniewski, 1985) and increased (Cragg, 1975) synaptic density as well as of arrest in synaptic development (Petit,

LeBoutillier, Alfano, & Becker, 1984). Finally, neuropathologic studies in mental retardation present another difficulty in their interpretation. A few studies, which have compared individuals with mild to those with severe mental retardation, have found dendritic anomalies only in the most profoundly affected individuals (Huttenlocher, 1974; Williams et al., 1980). A bias toward severe forms of neurologic disease is not unusual because of the wider availability of specimens for neuropathology. Nevertheless, the experience in conditions such as dyslexia (Galaburda, Sherman, Rosen, Aboitiz, & Geschwind, 1985) has shown that at least some features found in severe cases (e.g., symmetry in the planum temporale) are also detected by MRI in vivo in more typical individuals (Hynd et al., 1990). Therefore, careful quantitation of Golgi staining combined with immunocytochemistry or other advanced methods most likely would be revealing even in milder cases of mental retardation.

CEREBROCORTICAL DEVELOPMENT AND MENTAL RETARDATION

As stated in the two previous sections, there are two relatively consistent types of anatomic abnormalities associated with mental retardation: malformations of the cerebral cortex and related structures and dendritic/synaptic anomalies in otherwise well-formed brains (Table 1). Although NMDs are seen almost invariably in severe mental retardation, dendritic pathology can be seen in milder forms. How can we explain this wide range of anomalies in severe mental retardation? A better understanding of the basic processes of cerebrocortical development and the techniques employed in their study can be helpful. The traditional view of CNS developmental abnormalities correlates phenotype with a fundamental developmental process. Thus, it is possible to categorize anomalies in a few groups: induction disorders (e.g., anencephaly); proliferation and migration anomalies, or NMDs (e.g., lissencephaly); and cytodifferentiation abnormalities (e.g., failure in myelination or dendritic growth) (Gabriel, 1974). Recently, it has become evident that this simple approach is accurate only in general terms. For instance,

in most NMDs, including those relatively minor types, there is also a disorder of neuronal differentiation and programmed cell death (Rorke, 1994). The consequence of this multiple process anomaly is that the fine architecture of the cerebral cortex is distorted substantially not only by deficient synaptic structures but also by "extra" and aberrant neuronal circuitry. At this time, there is no technology available to distinguish, functionally, a neuron with normal morphology that is part of a minor aberrant circuit from one appropriately connected. Indeed, Golgi impregnations have revealed normal dendritic trees in neurons that clearly are situated abnormally (Williams et al., 1975). It is likely that normal dendritic staining in mild mental retardation (Huttenlocher, 1974) and other conditions (Williams et al., 1979, 1980) represents the limitations of Golgi methods in detecting aberrant synaptic relationships when dendritic patterns are otherwise normal.

Regressive events such as cell death and synapse elimination play a critical role in shaping normal brain wiring. Failure of neuronal death in the cerebral cortex could have significant cognitive and behavioral consequences, and it has been suggested in conditions such as schizophrenia (Akbarian et al., 1993); its role in mental retardation is unknown. Disturbances in synapse pruning might be present in mental retardation, as implied by growth-arrested dendritic spines in chromosopathies and unclassified mental retardation (Marin-Padilla, 1972; Purpura, 1974). Consequently, a subtle but diffuse involvement of neuronal architecture and circuitry of the cerebral cortex eventually can lead to cognitive impairment similar to that produced by a major cortical malformation. The role of subcortical nuclei in mental retardation is still unknown. In severe NMDs, anomalies of the basal ganglia and thalamus are not unusual (Barth, 1987). Even in the absence of malformations, as in Rett and Down syndromes, macroscopic (Reiss et al., 1993) and histologic (Armstrong, 1992; Casanova, Walker, Whitehouse, & Price, 1985) anomalies in basal ganglia, substantia nigra, and basal forebrain strongly support the involvement of pathways from and to the cortex. Moreover, the clear association between perinatal pathology, which usually involves subcortical nuclei and connections to the cortex (Friede, 1989), and mental retardation in a significant proportion of cases (Chaney, Givens, Watkins, & Eyman, 1986; Hagberg & Kyllerman, 1983) emphasizes a subcortical role in the pathogenesis of mental retardation. A schematic representation of the relationship between abnormal anatomic circuitry and mental retardation is provided in Figure 1.

NEUROPATHOLOGY OF LEARNING DISABILITIES

Our limited knowledge about neurobiologic bases of developmental cognitive disorders is even more evident in the field of learning disabilities. Neuropathologic studies have been infrequent because of the difficulty in identifying cases for postmortem examination and because surgical specimens have been available only oc-

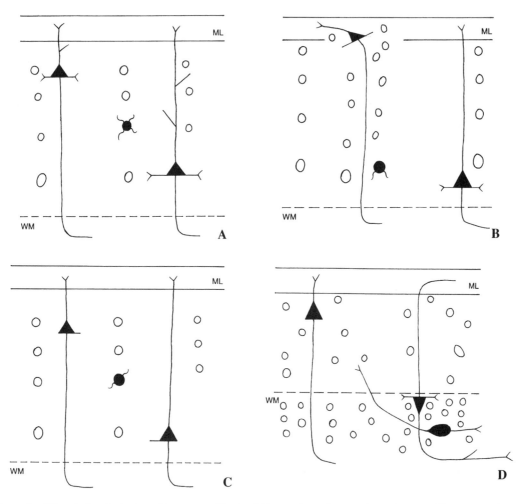

Figure 1. Disrupted cortical cytoarchitecture, and its dendritic correlates, in mental retardation and learning disabilities. *A*, Normal. All six neocortical layers are well defined, and pyramidal and nonpyramidal neurons display rich apical and basilar dendritic trees. *B*, Learning disability. Microdysgenetic cortex, as seen in dyslexia and NF 1. There are ectopic neurons in layer I and laminar disarrangement beneath this abnormality (cortical dysplasia). Dendritic anomalies are focal in nature. *C*, Mild mental retardation. Cortical laminar organization is relatively well preserved; however, moderate reduction in dendritic arborizations is widespread. *D*, Severe mental retardation. Typical cortical disorganization seen in generalized NMD. Neuronal density, typology, orientation, and differentiation are affected. There are major qualitative and quantitative changes in dendritic arborizations. Other cases of severe mental retardation, without malformations, show only dendritic anomalies. (ML, molecular layer, cortical surface; WM, white matter; NMD, neuronal migration disorder.)

casionally for more sophisticated methods such as Golgi impregnations and immunocytochemistry. Of all learning disorders, the best characterized is developmental dyslexia (Duanne, 1989). In this situation, neuropathology not only has provided specific information regarding affected areas of the brain, but also has allowed for the development of a research program on neurobiologic bases that extends from animal models to clinical evaluations (Galaburda, 1991). Neurofibromatosis type 1 and ADHD, without association to dyslexia, are two other learning disabilities to be considered in more detail in this analysis.

Developmental Dyslexia

Developmental dyslexia is associated with several consistent and characteristic anatomic anomalies. First, there is a deviation from the usual pattern of asymmetry of the planum temporale, which is larger on the left side (Galaburda, 1991, 1993; Galaburda et al., 1985, 1987). The planum temporale corresponds to a triangular region of associative neocortex located immediately behind the primary auditory cortex. Dyslexic individuals exhibit a symmetric planum, which seems more similar to the standard larger left side. Magnetic resonance imaging studies have confirmed plana symmetry (Rumsey et al., 1986); however, the direction of this deviation is still a controversial issue (Galaburda, 1993; Hynd et al., 1990). Radiologic studies have detected other anomalies in hemispheric symmetry involving the right frontal, insular, right parietal opercular, and right occipital cortices (Galaburda, 1993). These changes have not yet been demonstrated in pathologic specimens and require further confirmation. A second neuropathologic feature in dyslexic brains is the presence of multiple foci of microdysgenesis in the frontal and temporal lobes. These developmental anomalies are distributed mainly in the left perisylvian region (Galaburda et al., 1985, 1987), although multiple lesions are still found on the right and ventral aspects of the cortex (Humphreys, Kaufmann, & Galaburda, 1990).

The specificity of these two types of anatomic anomalies in dyslexia is underscored by MRI investigations in children with language and learning impairment, who were not selected on the basis of reading disability. These children also demonstrated deviation of normal asymmetry in the posterior perisylvian region (Jernigan et al., 1991). Also, MRI comparisons of individuals with dyslexia with normal and ADHD subjects corroborated the consistent association of dyslexia and planum temporale symmetry (Hynd et al., 1990). Furthermore, a preliminary neuropathologic investigation of a case of developmental dysphasia, a language disorder that usually precedes dyslexia, demonstrated microdysgenetic lesions, consistent in cortical dysplasia or laminar disorganization, in the medial (insular) left temporal cortex in association with symmetry of the planum temporale (M. Cohen, Campbell, & Yaghmai, 1989). From these studies and others evaluating cortical function (Rumsey et al., 1992), we can conclude that anomalous development of the left perisylvian and posterior temporal cortex seems to be a consistent anatomic substrate for developmental language deficits, such as those seen in dysphasia and dyslexia. Figure 1 shows a representation of microdysgenetic cortex in learning disability and its dendritic correlates.

Nevertheless, the cerebral cortex is not the only brain structure involved in dyslexia. More subtle anomalies have been found in subcortical nuclei in dyslexic subjects. Cytoarchitectonic/morphometric analyses of both lateral and medial geniculate nuclei show a shift in neuronal size toward smaller cells (Galaburda & Livingstone, 1993; Galaburda, Menard, & Rosen, 1994). These two centers, which are the thalamic-specific nuclei for the visual and auditory pathways, respectively, are essential in the processing of these sensory modalities. Reduction in neuronal size is correlated with decreased speed of neural transmission; therefore, information carried by these affected thalamic nuclei would arrive with delay to the respective cortical regions. In the case of the visual pathway, it is the magnocellular division of the lateral geniculate that displays these anomalies. The magnocellular system, which is segregated from the parvocellular pathway from the retina to the visual cortex, is responsible for processing fast, low-contrast visual stimuli. As expected, children with dyslexia have difficulties in the perception of these stimuli (Galaburda, 1993). Moreover, a study of visual evoked potentials confirmed that perception of magnocellular-mediated and not parvocellular-dependent stimuli (slow, color selective, contrast sensitive) is slowed in people with dyslexia (Livingstone, Rosen, Drislane, & Galaburda, 1991). Similarly, people with dyslexia show impairment in fast auditory processing that may correlate with less well-defined changes in the auditory thalamus (Galaburda, 1993; Galaburda et al., 1994). In summary, in dyslexia there are anatomic abnormalities that involve different levels of the central neural pathways of at least two critical sensory modalities: vision and audition. These features suggest that the substrate of this learning disability is a combination of inappropriate cortical input and altered cortical processing by defective cortical organization.

Are these findings in dyslexia a model of the neuroanatomic substrate for specific cognitive deficits/learning disabilities in general? Because of the limited information available on other developmental learning disabilities, we do not have a definitive answer to this question. However, there are some sparse experimental, radiologic, and pathologic data on other types of learning disability that tend to support, as in dyslexia, a corticosubcortical defect.

Neurofibromatosis Type 1

Neurofibromatosis type 1 (NF 1) is a genetic disorder that long has been associated with a variety of developmental cognitive disorders, including mental retardation and learning disabilities (Berg, 1991; Riccardi, 1981). Although most of the neuropathologic literature on NF 1 has focused on tumors, several studies have demonstrated the presence of multiple NMDs (pachygyria, polymicrogyria, cortical dysplasias, neuronal heterotopias in deep white matter, glial nodules) involving mainly the cerebral cortex (Lott & Richardson, 1981; Rosman & Pearce, 1968; Rubinstein, 1986). In one of the few comprehensive analyses on the subject to date, Rosman and Pearce (1968) showed a positive correlation between the extent of the cortical microdysgenesis and the cognitive impairment in terms of IQ. They found fewer lesions in intellectually normal subjects with

NF 1, but more than in normal subjects without NF 1. Limited characterization of the subjects in neuropsychological terms, lack of precise topographic data, and application of only conventional pathologic methods impair generalization of these results. Furthermore, a large number of NF 1 cases do not exhibit the global and severe cognitive involvement reported in the mentioned study. In fact, learning disability in the form of visuospatial or visuomotor impairment, without significant language or reading difficulties (Eliason, 1986) or left shift in the normal range of IQ (Eldridge et al., 1989), which occurs in 30%–45% of children with NF 1, seems to be the predominant type of cognitive disorder in NF 1 (Riccardi, 1981).

The recognition of this specific learning disability occurred at a moment when great interest and controversy were originated by descriptions of a high frequency of bright abnormal images on MRI present only in children with NF 1. These prolonged T_2-weighted images are located subcortically mainly in the deep cerebral white matter, basal ganglia (globus pallidus), brain stem, and cerebellum (white matter) (Duffner, Cohen, Seidel, & Shucard, 1989; Dunn & Ross, 1989; Goldstein, Curless, Post, & Quencer, 1989; see also Chapter 22, Volume I). Their incidence in the pediatric NF 1 population ranges from 43% to 79% (Aoki et al., 1989; Duffner et al., 1989; Dunn & Ross, 1989), similar to the proportion of children with NF 1 who are affected by mental retardation or learning disabilities. Several questions arose about these MRI abnormalities. First, what is their nature? It was speculated that they corresponded to hamartomas or microdysgeneses (Dunn & Ross, 1989). Only one preliminary study has correlated MRI with histology, and it showed that these abnormalities are areas of atypical glial infiltrate and perivascular gliosis with microcalcifications, dysmyelination, and spongy degeneration of the white matter in the pallidum and midbrain (Zimmerman et al., 1992). This study, on two pediatric NF 1 cases, must be expanded to cover a wider age spectrum.

A second issue related to these subcortical abnormalities deals with their temporal dimension: Are they a transient phenomenon because of their rare occurrence in patients older than 20 years (Aoki et al., 1989)? The limited prospective information indicates that these lesions tend to decrease over time, but they do not disappear by 16 years (Sevick et al., 1992). Based on the pathologic data, it is difficult to understand how glial changes of an astrocytic proliferation type can be reversible. It is more likely that anomalies in extracellular fluid composition and myelin biochemistry could generate aberrant MRI images that can return to normal after brain maturation is finished.

Finally, the third critical question regarding these MRI anomalies concerns their functional significance. Lack of correlation between MRI lesions and neurologic manifestations initially was reported (Duffner et al., 1989; Dunn & Ross, 1989). Nevertheless, a later larger scale study has shown a negative correlation between MRI abnormalities and several neuropsychological parameters, including IQ, language scores, and visuomotor integration and coordination (North et al., 1994). Indeed, according to the authors, MRI abnormalities divide pediatric NF 1 into two clearly distinct groups in terms of cognitive development.

In conclusion, a combination of cortical and subcortical, perhaps transient, abnormalities underlies mental retardation and learning disabilities as seen in NF 1. It is not clear whether specific pathways connecting the cortex with subcortical nuclei are critical in NF 1 learning disability, as in dyslexia, but this is a likely possibility. In this regard, the association of visuomotor impairment and MRI anomalies in the basal ganglia and related structures support a distinct corticosubcortical model. Contrasting the left cortex/thalamic pattern seen in dyslexia, NF 1 would show a right cortex/basal ganglia–deficient axis. At this point, only clinical data indicate right hemisphere pathology in NF 1 learning disability (B.H. Cohen, 1991), as well as the nature of subcortical lesions, which is an issue that deserves further neuropathologic study.

Attention-Deficit/Hyperactivity Disorder

Attention-deficit/hyperactivity disorder is one of the most prevalent forms of learning disability. Unfortunately, there are no direct neuropathologic data on this disorder because of the difficulties in premortem characterization of

this condition. Nevertheless, analyses of both subjects with selective developmental language impairment and dyslexics with ADHD are informative regarding the likely neurobiologic bases of ADHD. (For more comprehensive reviews on the subject, see Kaufmann [1993] and Zametkin & Rapoport [1987].) Comparative analyses of brain symmetry, using MRI scans, in subjects with dyslexia and subjects with ADHD have demonstrated that, whereas symmetry of the planum temporale is a feature associated with dyslexia, a rather symmetric prefrontal region is common to both dyslexia and ADHD. Specifically, the two groups show smaller right anterior width measurements in comparison with controls, who show an asymmetry in favor of the right side (Hynd et al., 1990). These results are intriguing if one considers that the brains of people with dyslexia exhibit multiple dysgenetic lesions in the dorsolateral and orbital frontal cortex, particularly on the right side (Humphreys et al., 1990). These abnormalities have not clearly implicated a cognitive substrate in dyslexia and might contribute to attentional deficits, at least in this population. As mentioned above, in general terms, a left temporal developmental anomaly would be a base for selective language disorders, and an aberrant formation of the right anterior frontal cortex would predispose for attentional disturbances. Frontal cortex dysfunction in ADHD is also supported by a variety of functional studies, including evaluations of blood flow (Lou, Henriksen, & Bruhn, 1984), glucose utilization (Zametkin et al., 1990), and cognition/behavior (Benson, 1991). These investigations not only have confirmed a frontal cortex abnormality, particularly on the right side, but also indicate an involvement of subcortical regions such as the striatum (more on the right) and the midbrain (Lou et al., 1989; Lou, Henriksen, Bruhn, Borner, & Nielsen, 1989).

A combined cortical/subcortical anomaly in ADHD has been suggested by numerous animal studies of normal and abnormal attention (Colby, 1991; Heilman, Voeller, & Nadeau, 1991). Although anatomic data on subcortical anomalies are not available in humans, experimental investigations have provided valuable information that must be evaluated in postmortem material. Several discrete subcortical regions, mainly components of dopaminergic pathways (e.g., ventral tegmental area) have been implicated in hyperactivity and deficient attention in adult animals (Kaufmann, 1993). Based on these results, and clinical studies demonstrating abnormal dopamine metabolism in ADHD (Shaywitz, Cohen, & Bowers, 1977), a murine neonatal model of decreased dopamine with hyperactivity was generated (Shaywitz, Yager, & Klopper, 1976). From these and other reports, it was established that disruptions of mesocortical dopaminergic systems play a critical role in the most salient manifestations of ADHD (Clark, Geffen, & Geffen, 1987; Miller, Heffner, Kotake, & Seiden, 1981). Future directions in the neuropathology of ADHD require the evaluation of these brain regions and other monoaminergic systems, as pointed out by clinical observations (Zametkin & Rapoport, 1987). Striatal lesions also are correlated to hyperactivity, as well as to some of the cognitive manifestations (e.g., motor impersistence) of ADHD (Kaufmann, 1993). Moreover, studies on neurobiology of normal attentional processes have emphasized their distributed nature, involving not only multiple cortical regions (Mesulam, 1981) but also nuclei in the brain stem, diencephalon, and basal ganglia (Colby, 1991). Finally, experimental data on primates emphasize the role of frontal cortex dysfunction in virtually all the signs associated with ADHD (Kaufmann, 1993).

Tourette Syndrome and Tuberous Sclerosis

There are two other learning disability syndromes that are not so well characterized as dyslexia or NF 1, but can provide an insight to the neurobiology of learning disabilities in general. Tourette syndrome is a movement disorder condition characterized by motor and vocal tics. Although intelligence is normal, there is an increased incidence of ADHD and learning difficulties (B.H. Cohen, 1991). Neuropsychological data indicate that Tourette syndrome learning disability is similar to NF 1 learning disability in its visuomotor/visuospatial impairment profile (Matthews, 1988). Interestingly, it long has been recognized that there is an increase in dopamine activity in Tourette syn-

drome, considering that drugs that reduce dopamine production or block its receptors alleviate symptomatology (B.H. Cohen, 1991). Recently, the nature of the biochemical defect has been pinpointed to a deficiency in dopamine reuptake in the striatum (Singer, Hahn, & Moran, 1991). This involvement of the basal ganglia is not surprising, given the fact that the most prominent symptom in Tourette syndrome is a movement disorder. Moreover, MRI volumetric analyses have shown a deviation from the normal pattern of asymmetry of the putamen, normally left sided, with increased incidence of right-sided asymmetry. Tourette syndrome cases with ADHD typically had this putamenal right-sided asymmetry, and also a significant reduction in left globus pallidus volume when compared with Tourette syndrome cases without ADHD and controls (Singer et al., 1993). Cortical pathology has not been described in Tourette syndrome; however, it cannot be excluded until comprehensive studies are performed. These findings in Tourette syndrome emphasize the association of developmental anomalies of the basal ganglia with learning disabilities, particularly of the nonverbal type.

Tuberous sclerosis is a neurocutaneous syndrome also associated with mental retardation and learning disabilities in a high proportion (Berg, 1991). Tubers, the characteristic lesions in this syndrome, usually are located in the cortex, but they can be found in the basal ganglia, where they are smaller. They are more or less circumscribed lesions characterized by large and bizarre cells with glial and neuronal features. Similar abnormal cells are seen in the two other typical subventricular or subependymal lesions, subventricular nodules and giant cell tumors. Golgi impregnations have clarified that, at least on morphologic grounds, the tubers are composed of astrocytes and small neurons. These neurons are primitive in appearance, stellate or pyramidal, with short dendrites and a few aberrant spines and an anomalous dendritic orientation that forms neuronoglial contacts (Ferrer et al., 1984; Machado-Salas, 1984). Cytoarchitectonic evaluations demonstrate a lack of laminar organization in the region of the tubers (Ferrer et al., 1984), and Golgi preparations reveal reduced dendritic trees in adjacent and, to a lesser extent, in distant cortices (Huttenlocher & Heydemann, 1984). These findings stress the multifocal nature of the distortion of circuitry in the cerebral cortex with tuberous sclerosis. Although no correlations between magnitude of cortical involvement by tubers and cognitive profile have been made (Huttenlocher, 1991), difficulties in detection of small tubers, particularly beneath the cortex, may prevent this assessment. It is likely that large numbers of lesions underlie mental retardation and a few cortical and subcortical tubers are present in patients with learning disabilities and cognitively typical patients.

Summary

In learning disability syndromes, there is variable neuroanatomic involvement of the cerebral cortex and subcortical nuclei. A pattern of left hemisphere–thalamus anomaly emerges in verbal learning disabilities, such as dyslexia. In contrast, nonverbal learning disabilities, such as NF 1 and Tourette syndrome, seem to have right cortical–basal ganglia disturbances. Frontal cortex–striatum-midbrain axis anomalies would predispose to attentional and motor inhibition deficits. In this regard, the direct role of the basal ganglia in cognitive processes should not be underestimated (Alexander, DeLong, & Strick, 1986). With respect to the pathogenesis of learning disability abnormalities, it is clear that they represent disorders of brain formation: NMD in dyslexia, NF 1, and Tourette syndrome and cytodifferentiation in tuberous sclerosis. ADHD-related pathology is still unclear in origin. Animal studies have pointed to genetic factors in NMDs associated with learning disabilities (Galaburda, 1991); however, perinatal damage—including prematurity, which involves the subcortical white matter (Gordon, 1991; Towbin, 1971), cortex, hippocampus, basal ganglia, and brain stem (Fuller, Guthrie, & Alvord, 1983)—has been associated consistently with learning disabilities. New etiologies of learning disability are emerging; prenatal exposure to drugs of abuse, such as cocaine, is one of them. Learning disabilities in the form of ADHD have been reported preliminarily in these children (Dow-Edwards, 1991; Volpe, 1992). Only one neuropathologic study, in infants, is available. Kaufmann and Cuello (1991) found increased neuronal density in subcortical white matter and retarded neuronal cytodifferentiation in the neocortex. Mild cytoarchitectonic disarrangements that resemble these human abnormalities also have been described in a rodent model of prenatal exposure to cocaine (Gressens, Kosofsky, & Evrard, 1992). More clinical and pathologic data are necessary to clarify whether or not prenatal drug exposure also is associated with corticosubcortical anomalies.

GENES, ENVIRONMENT, AND DEVELOPMENTAL COGNITIVE DISORDERS

In order to develop solid programs in prevention and treatment of mental retardation and learning disabilities, it is important to recognize factors involved in the predisposition to and genesis of developmental anomalies underlying these disorders. Traditional views of developmental conditions differentiate two distinct categories: genetic and environmental variables. In the first group, major alterations in quantity (e.g., Down syndrome) or quality (e.g., phenylketonuria) of genetic material would lead to an aberrant structural phenotype associated with mental retardation, learning disabilities, or both. The second category corresponds to factors whose presence or deficiency disturbs an otherwise normal genetic program (e.g., connatal infection, perinatal hypoxic–ischemic damage, postnatal malnutrition) (Dobbing & Smart, 1974; Jones, 1988; Kinsbourne, 1980). This simple categorization, although valid in very general terms, overlooks the complex interaction of gene expression and the environment occurring during brain development, as disclosed by advances in developmental neuroscience.

Brain development is characterized by an organized and stereotypic sequence of events—neural induction, proliferation, migration, and cytodifferentiation—that occur in a precise temporospatial sequence (Gabriel, 1974; McConnell, 1988). It has been postulated that these processes reflect also precise sequences of gene activation (Rorke, 1994). Some of the critical regulatory genes (e.g., homeogenes) have been identified in early stages of embryonic formation, such as during hindbrain segmentation (Keynes & Lumsden, 1990). Since the late 1980s and early 1990s, gene expression in cognitively relevant areas during histogenesis has been reported. Multiple regulatory genes, including transcription factors (TFs), are expressed in the prenatal cortex, hippocampus, and basal ganglia in extremely complex patterns (Bulfone et al., 1993; He et al., 1989). Nevertheless, the precise role of these master genes in mammalian development is unknown and has been inferred from studies in invertebrates and in simpler systems, such as neural cells in culture. These investigations have demonstrated that growth factors, membrane potential changes, and neurotransmitters activate distinct gene programs (Bartel, Sheng, Lau, & Greenberg, 1989; Greenberg, Ziff, & Greene, 1986). Transcription factors, proteins that induce the expression of specific or target genes, are the best understood of these molecules (Sheng & Greenberg, 1990). Members of the *Fos* and *Jun* TF families (Smeyne, Curran, & Morgan, 1992) and zinc finger TFs (Kaufmann, Yamagata, Andreasson, & Worley, 1994; Worley et al., 1990; Yamagata, Kaufmann, et al., 1994) are expressed at relatively high levels during critical stages of cerebrocortical development. These regulatory genes are important for understanding normal and aberrant cortical formation for several reasons. First, these TFs clearly are involved in programs of cell growth and differentiation (Nathans et al., 1991). Second, they are involved in long-term, or "plastic," changes in neural structures (Kaufmann et al., 1994; Montarolo et al., 1986). These synaptically dependent long-term changes share many features with cytodifferentiation of neural structures occurring during cerebrocortical development (Worley et al., 1990). In addition, TFs are induced by physiologic neural stimuli (Hunt, Pini, & Evan, 1987; Sheng & Greenberg, 1990) and seem to participate in complex activity-dependent changes in adult cerebral cortex (Chaudhuri & Cynader, 1993; Yamagata, Kaufmann, et al., 1994).

Cellular interactions play a critical role in "decision making" during brain development (McConnell, 1988). In addition to the well-known radial glial–neuroblast interaction, which allows the migration of the future cortical neuron to the right place (Gabriel, 1974), intercellular communication of the synaptic type or mediated by neurotransmitters is present from early stages of cerebrocortical development. Neuroblasts are electrically coupled in the germinal matrix (Lo Turco & Kriegstein, 1991) (the ventricular proliferation zone), are regulated in their migration by neurotransmitter receptor activity (Komuro & Rakic, 1993), and express these receptors shortly after their arrival at the cortex in formation (Blanton & Kriegstein, 1992). Moreover, postnatal neural activity-dependent modulation of neuronal maturation has been demonstrated clearly in experimental animals (Greenough, 1984; Kaufmann et al., 1994; Kleinschmidt, Bear, & Singer, 1987; Worley et al., 1990). These cellular interactions, synaptic or not, would constitute the microenvironment that triggers the expression of regulatory or effector genes essential for that particular phase of neural development. In other words, despite the existence of a genetic blueprint, cortical development can be modulated at every critical step by local factors. Indeed, the precise patterns of connectivity of many regions, including the cortex, are determined by neural activity (Goodman & Shatz, 1993). Therefore, NMDs and dendritic anomalies, already mentioned in the neuropathology of mental retardation and learning disabilities, can be explained in terms of an aberrant, local signal-gene induction process (Kaufmann et al., 1994; Rorke, 1994). The best characterized of these intercellular factors is the activation of a particular type of glutamate receptor, the so-called *N*-methyl-D-aspartate (NMDA). This receptor is involved, for instance, in cerebellar cortex neuronal migration (Komuro & Rakic, 1993) and visual cortex organization (ocular dominance patterns) (Kleinschmidt et al., 1987). Changes in NMDA activity by pharmacologic agents modulate regulatory gene expression, particularly of TFs (Kaufmann et al., 1994; Worley et al., 1990).

The search for other neural activity-induced genes is very active (Nedivi, Hevroni, Naot, Israeli, & Citri, 1993) given their importance in brain physiology and development. Of particular interest are reports of activity-dependent genes expressed at very early stages of cortical development (e.g., neuronal migration), when TFs modulated by activity are virtually not expressed (Kaufmann et al., 1994; Yamagata, Kaufmann, et al., 1994). One of these novel regulatory genes, termed *rheb*, is also modulated by growth factors and NMDA-dependent activity. *rheb* encodes a *Ras*-related protein, and belongs, as does this oncogene, to the large category of G proteins. Intriguing is the fact that two conditions leading to mental retardation and learning disabilities, Miller-Dieker lissencephaly (Reiner et al., 1993) and NF 1 learning disability (Xu et al., 1990), are linked to G protein–like genes. Consequently, the neural manifestations of these two syndromes could be the result not only of general disturbances in development but also of specific alterations in brain formation.

Finally, the identification of nonregulatory-type activity-dependent genes (Qian, Gilbert, Colicos, Kandel, & Kuhl, 1993) has opened the possibility of a more direct influence of neural activity on brain physiology and development. *COX-2* is one of these genes, with high expression during the critical period of postnatal cortical development (Kaufmann et al., 1994; Yamagata, Andreasson, Kaufmann, Barnes, & Worley, 1993), similar to zinc finger TFs (Worley et al., 1990; Kaufmann et al., 1994; Yamagata, Kaufmann, et al., 1994). *COX-2* encodes the inducible form of cyclooxygenase, the enzyme that catalyzes the first step in prostaglandin synthesis. In the brain, prostaglandins are involved in modulation of synaptic activity and have direct actions in areas such as the hypothalamus. Their role in cortical function is unknown; however, *COX-2* is expressed predominantly in cognitive-related regions and is regulated by NMDA-dependent activity in developing and adult cortex (Yamagata et al., 1993). In conclusion, a better understanding of the specific role of genes expressed during cortical development, and their regulation by growth factors, neurotransmitters, and TFs, provides the opportunity for designing new strategies in prevention and amelioration of brain pathology associated with mental retardation and learning disabilities. Furthermore, the iden-

tification and characterization of these neural activity-dependent genes will help to develop improved histochemical markers for the study of these conditions.

CONCLUSIONS: COMPARATIVE NEUROPATHOLOGY OF MENTAL RETARDATION AND LEARNING DISABILITIES

It can be concluded that different, but not exclusive, neuroanatomic bases underlie mental retardation and learning disabilities. The latter show a consistent and characteristic combination of cortical and subcortical anomalies. In most learning disabilities, there is focal involvement of specific cortical regions (left perisylvian in dyslexia, prefrontal in ADHD, and perhaps right hemisphere in NF 1) while the rest of the cerebral cortex seems to be normal. These cortical areas, at least in dyslexia and ADHD, clearly are linked to the specific deficits of the particular learning disability. The left perisylvian cortex, which corresponds to the classic language areas of Broca and Wernicke, displays dysgenetic lesions and contributes to an anomalous planum temporale in dyslexia (Galaburda, 1993). Similarly, in ADHD, the prefrontal cortex, which has been implicated in attentional and executive skills (Fuster, 1989), shows functional abnormalities that seem to be more severe on the right. Nevertheless, the most characteristic neuropathologic feature of learning disabilities is the additional involvement of specific subcortical nuclei. In the case of dyslexia, thalamic nuclei that are part of sensory pathways are affected, causing an impairment in processing fast modalities of visual and auditory information. In NF 1 and tuberous sclerosis, at least the globus pallidus, which is the output nucleus for the basal ganglia, would be anomalous, leading to disturbed visuomotor integration. Finally, in ADHD, the striatum and other brain stem monoaminergic nuclei seem to be dysfunctional, causing disruption of circuits involved in attention and motor inhibition.

In mental retardation, the unifying feature is a disturbance in synaptic relationships or circuitry, or both, affecting the cerebral cortex. Abnormal architecture of cortical regions, aberrant synaptic surfaces, or both occur in a generalized manner, leading probably to dysfunction in multimodal processing and integration. Although in mental retardation there is no clear selective cortical involvement or subcortical pathology in most instances, features common to learning disabilities should not be excluded. In fact, several NMDs affect preferentially some cortical areas; for instance, in polymicrogyria the perisylvian distribution is quite characteristic. In addition, subcortical heterotopias and other abnormalities are common in generalized NMD (Aicardi, 1991; Barth, 1987). Given the extent of the cortical pathology, it is not surprising that subcortical abnormalities have been greatly overlooked in mental retardation. A

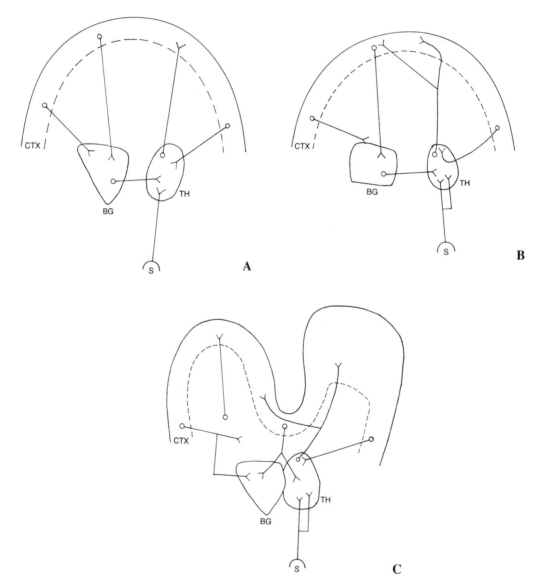

Figure 2. Postulated patterns of involvement of corticosubcortical circuits in mental retardation and learning disabilities. *A,* Normal relationships between neocortex (CTX), basal ganglia (BG), and thalamus (TH). (S, sensory pathway.) *B,* In learning disability, there are selective abnormalities in connections between cortex and basal ganglia or cortex and thalamus. *C,* In severe mental retardation associated with malformations, major cytoarchitectonic disruptions originate aberrant corticosubcortical pathways. In addition, primary developmental abnormalities of basal ganglia and thalamus can contribute to these anomalous relationships.

schematic diagram of the postulated differential neuropathology of mental retardation and learning disabilities is represented in Figure 2.

In conclusion, aberrant synaptic arrangements of developmental origin that compromise brain regions critical for cognition are the neuroanatomic/neurobiologic bases of developmental cognitive disorders. Specific circuits in learning disabilities, and a more generalized disturbance in connectivity in mental retardation, are beginning to be characterized. An increased understanding of gene–environment interaction during brain development, especially of neural activity-dependent genes, may provide new approaches for prevention, diagnosis, and treatment of developmental cognitive disorders.

REFERENCES

Adams, J.H., & Duchen, L.W. (Eds.). (1992). *Greenfield's neuropathology.* New York: John Wiley & Sons.

Adaro, L., Fernández, V., & Kaufmann, W. (1986). Effects of nutritional-environmental interactions upon body weight, body size and development of cortical pyramids. *Nutrition Reports International, 33,* 1013–1020.

Aicardi, J. (1991). The agyria-pachygyria complex: A spectrum of cortical malformations. *Brain and Development, 13,* 1–8.

Akbarian, S., Bunney, W.E., Jr., Potkin, S.G., Wigal, S.B., Hagman, J.O., Sandman, C.A., & Jones, E.G. (1993). Altered distribution of nicotinamideadenine dinucleotide phosphate-diaphorase cells in frontal lobe of schizophrenics implies disturbances of cortical development. *Archives of General Psychiatry, 50,* 169–177.

Alexander, G.E., DeLong, M.R., & Strick, P.L. (1986). Parallel organization of functionally segregated circuits linking basal ganglia and cortex. *Annual Review of Neuroscience, 9,* 357–381.

Aoki, S., Barkovich, A.J., Edwards, M.S.B., Koch, T., Berg, B., & Lempert, T. (1989). Neurofibromatosis types 1 and 2: Cranial MRI findings. *Radiology, 172,* 527–534.

Armstrong, D.D. (1992). The neuropathology of the Rett syndrome. *Brain and Development, 14*(Suppl.), 89–98.

Bartel, D.P., Sheng, M., Lau, L.F., & Greenberg, M.E. (1989). Growth factors and membrane depolarization activate distinct program of early response gene expression: Dissociation of *fos* and *jun* induction. *Genes and Development, 3,* 304–313.

Barth, P.G. (1987). Disorders of neuronal migration. *Canadian Journal of Neurological Sciences, 14,* 1–16.

Bauman, M.L., & Kemper, T.L. (1982). Morphologic and histoanatomic observations of the brain in untreated phenylketonuria. *Acta Neuropathologica, 58,* 55–63.

Becker, L.E., Armstrong, D.L., & Chan, F. (1986). Dendritic atrophy in children with Down's syndrome. *Annals of Neurology, 20,* 520–526.

Benassi, G., Guarino, M., Cammarata, S., Cristoni, P., Fantini, M.P., Ancona, A., Manfredini, M., & D'Alessandro, R. (1990). An epidemiological study on severe mental retardation among school children in Bologna, Italy. *Developmental Medicine and Child Neurology, 32,* 895–901.

Benson, F.D. (1991). The role of frontal dysfunction in attention deficit hyperactivity disorder. *Journal of Child Neurology, 6*(Suppl.), 9–12.

Berg, B.O. (1991). Current concepts of neurocutaneous disorders. *Brain and Development, 13,* 9–20.

Blanton, M.G., & Kriegstein, A.R. (1992). Properties of amino acid neurotransmitter receptors of embryonic cortical neurons when activated by exogenous and endogenous agonists. *Journal of Neurophysiology, 67,* 1185–2000.

Blomquist, H.K., Gustavson, K.H., & Holmgren, G. (1981). Mild mental retardation in children in a northern Swedish county. *Journal of Mental Deficiency Research, 25,* 169–186.

Braak, H., Braak, E., & Goebel, H.H. (1983). Isocortical pathology in type C Niemann-Pick disease: A combined Golgi pigmentoarchitectonic study. *Journal of Neuropathology and Experimental Neurology, 42,* 671–687.

Buell, S.J. (1982). Golgi-Cox and rapid Golgi methods as applied to autopsied human brain tissue: Widely disparate results. *Journal of Neuropathology and Experimental Neurology, 41,* 500–507.

Bulfone, A., Puelles, L., Porteus, M.H., Frohman, M.A., Martin, G.R., & Rubenstein, J.L.R. (1993). Spatially restricted expression of *Dlx-1, Dlx-2 (Tes-1), Gbx-2,* and *Wnt-3* in the embryonic day 12.5 mouse forebrain defines potential transverse and longitudinal segmental boundaries. *Journal of Neuroscience, 13,* 3155–3172.

Casanova, M.F., Walker, L.C., Whitehouse, P.J., & Price, D.L. (1985). Abnormalities of the nucleus basalis in Down's syndrome. *Annals of Neurology, 18,* 310–313.

Catalá, I., Ferrer, I., Galofré, E., & Fábregues, I. (1988). Decreased numbers of dendritic spines on cortical pyramidal neurons in dementia: A quantitative Golgi study on biopsy samples. *Human Neurobiology, 6*, 255–259.

Chaney, R.H., Givens, C.A., Watkins, G.P., & Eyman, R.K. (1986). Birth injury as the cause of mental retardation. *Obstetrics and Gynecology, 67*, 771–775.

Chaudhuri, A., & Cynader, M.S. (1993). Activity-dependent expression of the transcription factor Zif268 reveals ocular dominance columns in monkey visual cortex. *Brain Research, 605*, 349–353.

Clark, C.R., Geffen, G.M., & Geffen, L.B. (1987). Cathecolamines and attention. I. Animal and clinical studies. *Neuroscience and Biobehavioral Research, 11*, 341–352.

Cohen, B.H. (1991). Neurologic causes of learning disabilities. *Seminars in Neurology, 11*, 7–13.

Cohen, M., Campbell, R., & Yaghmai, F. (1989). Neuropathological abnormalities in developmental dysphasia. *Annals of Neurology, 25*, 567–570.

Colby, C.L. (1991). The neuroanatomy and neurophysiology of attention. *Journal of Child Neurology, 6*(Suppl.), 90–118.

Cragg, B.G. (1975). The density of synapses and neurons in normal, mentally defective and aging human brains. *Brain, 98*, 81–90.

Crome, L., & Stern, J. (1972). *Pathology of mental retardation*. Edinburgh: Churchill Livingstone.

Della Giustina, E., Goffinet, A.M., & Landrieu, P. (1981). A Golgi study of the brain malformation in Zellweger's cerebro-hepato-renal disease. *Acta Neuropathologica, 55*, 23–28.

Dobbing, J., & Smart J.L. (1974). Vulnerability of developing brain and behaviour. *British Medical Bulletin, 30*, 164–168.

Dolk, H. (1991). The predictive value of microcephaly during the first year of life for mental retardation at seven years. *Developmental Medicine and Child Neurology, 33*, 974–983.

Dow-Edwards, D.L. (1991). Cocaine effects on fetal development: A comparison of clinical and animal research findings. *Neurotoxicology and Teratology, 163*, 1535–1542.

Drillien, C.M. (1968). Studies in mental handicap. II. Some obstetric factors of possible aetiological significance. *Archives of Disease in Childhood, 43*, 283–294.

Drillien, C.M., Jameson, S., & Wilkinson, E.M. (1966). Studies in mental handicap. I. Prevalence and distribution by clinical type and severity of defect. *Archives of Disease in Childhood, 41*, 528–538.

Duanne, D.D. (1989). Neurobiological correlates of learning disorders. *Journal of the American Academy of Child and Adolescent Psychiatry, 28*, 314–318.

Duffner, P.K., Cohen, M.E., Seidel, F.G., & Shucard, D.W. (1989). The significance of MRI abnormalities in children with neurofibromatosis. *Neurology, 39*, 373–378.

Dunn, D.W., & Ross, K.L. (1989). MRI evaluation of learning difficulties and incoordination in neurofibromatosis type 1. *Neurofibromatosis, 2*, 1–5.

Dyken, P., & Krawlecki, N. (1983). Neurodegenerative diseases of infancy and childhood. *Annals of Neurology, 13*, 351–364.

Eldridge, R., Denckla, M.B., Bien, E., Myers, S., Kaiser-Kupfer, M.I., Pikus, A., Schlesinger, S.L., Parry, D.M., Dambrosia, J.M., Zasloff, M.A., & Mulvihill, J.J. (1989). Neurofibromatosis type 1 (von Recklinghausen's disease): Neurologic and cognitive assessment with sibling controls. *American Journal of Diseases of Children, 143*, 833–837.

Eliason, M.J. (1986). Neurofibromatosis: Implications for learning and behavior. *Developmental and Behavioral Pediatrics, 7*, 175–179.

Fábregues, I., & Ferrer, I. (1983). Abnormal perisomatic structures in nonpyramidal neurons in the cerebral cortex in Down's syndrome. *Neuropathology and Applied Neurobiology, 9*, 165–170.

Ferrer, I. (1984). A Golgi analysis of unlayered polymicrogyria. *Acta Neuropathologica, 65*, 69–76.

Ferrer, I., Fábregues, I., Coll, J., Ribalta, T., & Rives, A. (1984). Tuberous sclerosis: A Golgi study of cortical tuber. *Clinical Neuropathology, 3*, 47–51.

Ferrer, I., & Fernández-Alvarez, E. (1977). Lisencefalia. Agiria. Un estudio con el método de Golgi. *Journal of Neurological Sciences, 34*, 109–120.

Freytag, E., & Lindenberg, R. (1967). Neuropathologic findings in patients of a hospital for the mentally deficient: A survey of 359 cases. *Johns Hopkins Medical Journal, 121*, 379–392.

Friede, R.L. (1989). *Developmental neuropathology*. Berlin: Springer-Verlag.

Fuller, P.W., Guthrie, R.D., & Alvord, E.C., Jr. (1983). A proposed neuropathologic basis for learning disabilities in children born prematurely. *Developmental Medicine and Child Neurology, 25*, 214–231.

Fuster, J.M. (1989). *The prefrontal cortex*. New York: Raven Press.

Gabriel, R.S. (1974). Malformations of the central nervous system. In J.H. Menkes (Ed.), *Textbook of child neurology* (pp. 161–237). Phildelphia: Lea & Febiger.

Gabrielli, O., Salvolini, U., Coppa, G.V., Catassi, C., Rossi, R., Manca, A., Lanza, R., & Giorgi, P.L. (1990). Magnetic resonance imaging in the malformative syndromes with mental retardation. *Pediatric Radiology, 21*, 16–19.

Galaburda, A.M. (1991). Neuropathologic correlates of learning disabilities. *Seminars in Neurology, 11*, 20–27.

Galaburda, A.M. (1993). Neurology of developmental dyslexia. *Current Opinion in Neurobiology, 3*, 237–242.

Galaburda, A.M., & Livingstone, M. (1993). Evidence for a magnocellular defect in developmental dyslexia. *Annals of the New York Academy of Sciences, 682*, 70–82.

Galaburda, A.M., Menard, M.T., & Rosen, G.D. (1994). Evidence for aberrant auditory anatomy in developmental dyslexia. *Proceedings of the Na-*

tional Academy of Sciences of the United States of America, 91, 8010–8013.

Galaburda, A.M., Sherman, G.F., Rosen, G.D., Aboitiz, F., & Geschwind, N. (1985). Developmental dyslexia: Four consecutive patients with cortical anomalies. Annals of Neurology, 18, 222–233.

Galaburda, A.M., Sherman, G.F., Rosen, G.D., & Kaufmann, W.E. (1987). Neuropathologic findings and neurodevelopmental hypothesis in dyslexia [Abstract]. Neuroscience, 22(Suppl.), 2017W.

Goertchen, R. (1975). On pathology of the diffuse pachygyria. Zentralblatt fur Allgemeine Pathologie und Pathologische Anatomie, 119, 3–14.

Goldman, F., Katz, D., & Rapin, I. (1981). Chronic G_{M1} gangliosidosis presenting as dystonia. I. Clinical and pathological features. Annals of Neurology, 9, 465–475.

Goldstein, S.M., Curless, R.G., Post, J.D., & Quencer, R.M. (1989). A new sign of neurofibromatosis on magnetic resonance imaging in children. Archives of Neurology, 46, 1222–1224.

Goodman, C.S., & Shatz, C.J. (1993). Developmental mechanisms that generate precise patterns of neuronal connectivity. Cell/Neuron, 72(10, Suppl.), 77–98.

Gordon, N. (1991). Specific learning disorders: The possible role of brain damage. Brain Development, 13, 143–147.

Greenberg, M.E., Ziff, E.B., & Greene, L.A. (1986). Stimulation of neuronal acetylcholine receptor induces rapid gene transcription. Science, 234, 80–83.

Greenough, W.T. (1984). Structural correlates of information storage in the mammalian brain: A review and hypothesis. Trends in Neuroscience, 7, 229–233.

Gressens, P., Kosofsky, B., & Evrard, P. (1992). Cocaine-induced disturbances of corticogenesis in the developing murine brain. Neuroscience Letters, 140, 113–116.

Gustavson, K.H., Hagberg, B., Hagberg, G., & Sars, K. (1977a). Severe mental retardation in a Swedish county. I. Epidemiology, gestational age, birth weight and associated CNS handicaps in children born 1959–1970. Acta Paediatrica Scandinavica, 66, 373–379.

Gustavson, K.H., Hagberg, B., Hagberg, G., & Sars, K. (1977b). Severe mental retardation in a Swedish county. II. Etiologic and pathogenetic aspects of children born 1959–1970. Neuropadiatrie, 8, 293–304.

Hagberg, B.A. (1989). Rett syndrome: Clinical peculiarities, diagnostic approach, and possible course. Pediatric Neurology, 5, 75–83.

Hagberg, B., & Kyllerman, M. (1983). Epidemiology of mental retardation—a Swedish survey. Brain and Development, 5, 441–449.

He, X., Treacy, M.N., Simmons, D.M., Ingraham, H.A., Swanson, L.W., & Rosenfeld, M.G. (1989).

Expression of a large family of POU-domain regulatory genes in mammalian brain development. Nature, 340, 35–41.

Heilman, K.M., Voeller, K.K.S., & Nadeau, S.E. (1991). A possible pathophysiologic substrate of attention deficit hyperactivity disorder. Journal of Child Neurology, 6(Suppl.), 76–81.

Hohmann, C.F., Kwiterovich, K.K., Oster-Granite, M.L., & Coyle, J.T. (1991). Newborn basal forebrain lesions disrupt cortical cytodifferentiation as visualized by rapid Golgi staining. Cerebral Cortex, 1, 143–157.

Hornykiewicz, O. (1963). Die topische Lokalisation und das Verhalten von Noradrenalin und Dopamin (3-hydroxytyramin) in der Sustantia Nigra des normalen und Parkinson kranken Menschen. Wiener Klinische Wochenschrift, 75, 309–312.

Humphreys, P., Kaufmann, W.E., & Galaburda, A.M. (1990). Developmental dyslexia in women: Neuropathological findings in three cases. Annals of Neurology, 28, 727–738.

Humphreys, P., Rosen, G.D., Press, D.M., Sherman, G.F., & Galaburda, A.M. (1991). Freezing lesions of the developing rat brain. I. A model for cerebrocortical microgyria. Journal of Neuropathology and Experimental Neurology, 50, 145–160.

Hunt, S.P., Pini, A., & Evan, G. (1987). Induction of c-fos-like-protein in spinal cord neurons following sensory stimulation. Nature, 328, 632–634.

Huttenlocher, P.R. (1970). Dendritic development and mental defect. Neurology, 20, 381.

Huttenlocher, P.R. (1974). Dendritic development in neocortex of children with mental defect and infantile spasms. Neurology, 24, 203–210.

Huttenlocher, P.R. (1991). Dendritic and synaptic pathology in mental retardation. Pediatric Neurology, 7, 79–85.

Huttenlocher, P.R., & Heydemann, P.T. (1984). Fine structure of cortical tubers in tuberous sclerosis: A Golgi study. Annals of Neurology, 16, 595–602.

Hynd, G.W., Semrud-Clikeman, M., Lorys, A.R., Novey, E.S., & Eliopulos, D. (1990). Brain morphology in developmental dyslexia and attention deficit disorder. Archives of Neurology, 47, 919–926.

Jagadha, V., & Becker, L. (1989). Dendritic pathology: An overview of Golgi studies in man. Canadian Journal of Neurological Sciences, 16, 41–50.

Jellinger, K. (1972). Neuropathological features of unclassified mental retardation. In J.B. Cavanagh (Ed.), The brain in unclassified mental retardation (pp. 293–306). London: Churchill Livingstone.

Jernigan, T.L., Hesselink, J.R., Sowell, E., & Tallal, P.A. (1991). Cerebral structure on magnetic resonance imaging in language- and learning-impaired children. Archives of Neurology, 48, 539–545.

Jones, K.L. (1988). Smith's recognizable patterns of human malformation. Philadelphia: W.B. Saunders.

Kaufmann, W.E. (1992). Editorial: Cerebrocortical changes in AIDS. Laboratory Investigation, 66, 261–264.

Kaufmann, W.E. (1993). Experimental and clinical models of attention deficit disorder hyperactivity syndrome. In A.J. Capute, P.J. Accardo, & B.K. Shapiro (Eds.), *The spectrum of developmental disabilities: Learning disability spectrum—ADD, ADHD and learning disabilities* (pp. 17–36). Baltimore: York Press.

Kaufmann, W.E., & Cuello, N. (1991). Prenatal exposure to cocaine in humans [Abstract]. *Teratology, 43*, 486.

Kaufmann, W.E., & Galaburda, A.M. (1989). Cerebrocortical microdysgenesis in neurologically normal subjects: A histopathologic study. *Neurology, 39*, 238–244.

Kaufmann, W.E., Yamagata, K., Andreasson, K.I., & Worley, P.F. (1994). Rapid response genes as markers of cellular signaling during cortical histogenesis: Their potential in understanding mental retardation. *International Journal of Developmental Neuroscience, 12*, 263–271.

Keynes, R., & Lumsden, A. (1990). Segmentation and the origin of regional diversity in the vertebrate central nervous system. *Neuron, 2*, 1–9.

Kinsbourne, M. (1980). Disorders of mental development. In J.H. Menkes (Ed.), *Textbook of child neurology* (pp. 636–666). Phildelphia: Lea & Febiger.

Kleinschmidt, A., Bear, M.F., & Singer, W. (1987). Blockade of "NMDA" receptors disrupts experience-dependent plasticity of kitten striate cortex. *Science, 238*, 355–358.

Komuro, H., & Rakic, P. (1993). Modulation of neuronal migration by NMDA receptors. *Science, 260*, 95–97.

Livingstone, M.S., Rosen, G.D., Drislane, F.W., & Galaburda, A.M. (1991). Physiological and anatomical evidence for a magnocellular defect in developmental dyslexia. *Proceedings of the National Academy of Sciences of the United States of America, 88*, 7943–7947.

Logdberg, B., & Brun, A. (1993). Prefrontal neocortical disturbances in mental retardation. *Journal of Intellectual Disability Research, 37*, 459–468.

Lotspeich, L.J., & Ciaranello, R.D. (1993). The neurobiology and genetics of infantile autism. *International Review of Neurobiology, 35*, 87–129.

Lott, I.T., & Richardson, E.P., Jr. (1981). Neuropathological findings and the biology of neurofibromatosis. *Advances in Neurology, 29*, 23–32.

Lo Turco, J.J., & Kriegstein, A.R. (1991). Clusters of coupled neuroblasts in embryonic neocortex. *Science, 252*, 563–566.

Lou, H.C., Henriksen, L., & Bruhn, P. (1984). Focal cerebral hypoperfusion in children with dysphasia and/or attention deficit disorder. *Archives of Neurology, 41*, 825–829.

Lou, H.C., Henriksen, L., Bruhn, P., Borner, H., & Nielsen, J.B. (1989). Striatal dysfunction in attention deficit disorder. *Archives of Neurology, 465*, 48–52.

Machado-Salas, J. (1984). Abnormal dendritic patterns and aberrant spine development in Bourneville's disease—a Golgi survey. *Clinical Neuropathology, 3*, 52–58.

Marin-Padilla, M. (1972). Structural abnormalities of the cerebral cortex in human chromosomal aberrations: A Golgi study. *Brain Research, 44*, 625–629.

Marin-Padilla, M. (1974). Structural organization of the cerebral cortex (motor area) in human chromosomal aberrations: A Golgi study. I. D_1 (13-15) trisomy, Patau syndrome. *Brain Research, 66*, 373–391.

Marin-Padilla, M. (1976). Pyramidal cell abnormalities in the motor cortex of a child with Down's syndrome: A Golgi study. *Journal of Comparative Neurology, 167*, 63–82.

Matthews, W.S. (1988). Attention deficits and learning disabilities in children with Tourette's syndrome. *Pediatric Annals, 17*, 410–416.

McConnell, S.K. (1988). Development and decision-making in the mammalian cerebral cortex. *Brain Research Reviews, 13*, 1–23.

Miller, F.E., Heffner, T.G., Kotake, C., & Seiden, L.S. (1981). Magnitude and duration of hyperactivity following neonatal 6-hydroxydopamine is related to the extent of dopamine depletion. *Brain Research, 229*, 123–132.

Montarolo, P.G., Goelet, P., Catellucci, V.F., Morgan, J., Kandel, E.R., & Schacher, S. (1986). A critical period for macromolecular synthesis in long-term heterosynaptic facilitation in aplysia. *Science, 234*, 1249–1254.

Naidu, S., & Moser, H.W. (1990). Peroxisomal disorders. *Neurologic Clinics, 8*, 507–528.

Nathans, D., Christy, B.A., DuBois, R., Lanahan, A., Sanders, L.K., & Nakabeppu, Y. (1991). Transcription factors induced by growth-signaling agents. In J. Brugge, T. Curran, E. Harlow, & I. McCormick (Eds.), *Origins of human cancer: A comprehensive review* (pp. 353–364). New York: Cold Spring Harbor Laboratory Press.

Nedivi, E., Hevroni, D., Naot, D., Israeli, D., & Citri, Y. (1993). Numerous candidate plasticity-related genes revealed by differential cDNA cloning. *Nature, 363*, 718–722.

Nigam, M.P., & Labar, D.R. (1979). The effect of hyperphenylalaninemia on size and density of synapses in rat neocortex. *Brain Research, 179*, 195–198.

North, K., Joy, P., Yuille, D., Cocks, N., Mobbs, E., Hutchins, P., McHugh, K., & de Silva, M. (1994). Specific learning disability in children with neurofibromatosis type 1: Significance of MRI abnormalities. *Neurology, 44*, 878–883.

Paula-Barbosa, M.M., Tavares, M.A., Silva, C.A., Pereira, S., Hogg, E., & Patrick, A.D. (1981). Axodendritic abnormalities in a case of juvenile neuronal disease. *Journal of Submicroscopic Cytology and Pathology, 13*, 657–665.

Petit, T.L., LeBoutillier, J.C., Alfano, D.P., & Becker, L.E. (1984). Synaptic development in the human fetus: A morphometric analysis of normal and Down's syndrome neocortex. *Experimental Neurology, 83*, 13–23.

Petit, T.L., LeBoutillier, J.C., Gregorio, A., & Libstug, H. (1988). The pattern of dendritic development in the cerebral cortex of the rat. *Developmental Brain Research, 41*, 209–219.

Purpura, D.P. (1974). Dendritic spine "dysgenesis" and mental retardation. *Science, 186*, 1126–1128.

Purpura, D.P. (1975). Dendritic differentiation in human cerebral cortex: Normal and aberrant developmental patterns. *Advances in Neurology, 12*, 91–116.

Purpura, D.P. (1978). Ectopic dendritic growth in mature pyramidal neurones in human ganglioside storage disease. *Nature, 276*, 520–521.

Purpura, D.P., & Suzuki, K. (1976). Distortion of neuronal geometry and formation of aberrant synapses in neuronal storage disease. *Brain Research, 116*, 1–21.

Qian, Z., Gilbert, M.E., Colicos, M.A., Kandel, E.R., & Kuhl, D. (1993). Tissue-plasminogen activator is induced as an immediate-early gene during seizure, kindling and long-term potentiation. *Nature, 361*, 453–457.

Rapin, I. (1989). Cerebral degenerations of childhood: Differential diagnosis. In L.P. Rowland (Ed.), *Merritt's textbook of neurology* (pp. 568–576). Philadelphia: Lea & Febiger.

Reiner, O., Carrozo, R., Shen, Y., Wehnert, M., Faustinella, F., Dobyns, W.B., Caskey, C.T., & Ledbetter, D.H. (1993). Isolation of a Miller-Dieker lissencephaly gene containing G protein b-subunit-like repeats. *Nature, 364*, 717–721.

Reiss, A.L., Faruque, F., Naidu, S., Abrams, M., Beaty, T., Bryan, R.N., & Moser, H. (1993). Neuroanatomy of Rett syndrome: A volumetric imaging study. *Annals of Neurology, 34*, 227–234.

Riccardi, V.M. (1981). von Recklinghausen neurofibromatosis. *New England Journal of Medicine, 305*, 1617–1626.

Richman, D.P., Stewart, R.M., & Caviness, V.S., Jr. (1974). Cerebral microgyria in a 27-week fetus: An architectonic and topographic analysis. *Journal of Neuropathology and Experimental Neurology, 33*, 374–384.

Riessman, F. (1962). *The culturally deprived child.* New York: Harper & Row.

Robain, O., & Deonna, T. (1983). Pachygyria and congenital nephrosis disorder of migration and neuronal orientation. *Acta Neuropathologica, 60*, 137–141.

Rorke, L.B. (1994). A perspective: The role of disordered genetic control of neurogenesis in the pathogenesis of migration disorders. *Journal of Neuropathology and Experimental Neurology, 53*, 105–117.

Rosman, N.P., & Pearce, J. (1968). The brain in multiple neurofibromatosis (von Recklinghausen's disease): A suggested neuropathological basis for the associated mental defect. *Brain, 90*, 829–837.

Rubinstein, L.J. (1986). The malformative central nervous system lesions in the central and peripheral forms of neurofibromatosis: A neuropathological study of 22 cases. *Annals of the New York Academy of Sciences, 486*, 14–29.

Rumsey, J.M., Andreason, P., Zametkin, A.J., Aquino, T., King, A.C., Hamburger, S.D., Pikus, A., Rapoport, J.L., & Cohen, R.M. (1992). Failure to activate the left temporoparietal cortex in dyslexia: An oxygen 15 positron emission tomographic study. *Archives of Neurology, 49*, 734–739.

Rumsey, J.M., Dorwart, R., Vermess, M., Denckla, M.B., Kruesi, M.J.P., & Rapoport, J.L. (1986). Magnetic resonance imaging of brain anatomy in severe developmental dyslexia. *Archives of Neurology, 43*, 1045–1046.

Sarnat, H.B. (1987). Disturbances of late neuronal migrations in the perinatal period. *American Journal of Diseases of Children, 141*, 969–980.

Sevick, R.J., Barkovich, A.J., Edwards, M.S.B., Koch, T., Berg, B., & Lempert, T. (1992). Evolution of white matter lesions in neurofibromatosis type 1. *American Journal of Radiology, 159*, 171–175.

Shaywitz, B.A., Cohen, D.J., & Bowers, M.B. (1977). CSF monoamine metabolites in children with minimal brain dysfunction: Evidence for alteration of brain dopamine. *Journal of Pediatrics, 90*, 67–71.

Shaywitz, B.A., Yager, R.D., & Klopper, J.H. (1976). Selective brain dopamine depletion in developing rats: An experimental model of minimal brain dysfunction. *Science, 191*, 305–308.

Sheng, M., & Greenberg, M.E. (1990). The regulation and function of Fos and other immediate early genes in the nervous system. *Neuron, 4*, 477–485.

Singer, H.S., Hahn, I.H., & Moran, T.H. (1991). Abnormal dopamine uptake sites in postmortem striatum from patients with Tourette's syndrome. *Annals of Neurology, 30*, 558–562.

Singer, H.S., Reiss, A.L., Brown, J.E., Aylward, E.H., Shih, B., Chee, E., Harris, E.L., Reader, M.J., Chase, G.A., Bryan, R.N., & Denckla, M.B. (1993). Volumetric MRI changes in basal ganglia of children with Tourette's syndrome. *Neurology, 43*, 950–956.

Smeyne, R.J., Curran, T., & Morgan, J.I. (1992). Temporal and spatial expression of a *fos-lacZ* transgene in the developing nervous system. *Molecular Brain Research, 16*, 158–162.

Smith, D.W., & Simons, F.E. (1975). Rational diagnostic evaluation of the child with mental deficiency. *American Journal of Diseases of Children 129*, 1285–1290.

Sotrel, A., Williams, R.S., Kaufmann, W.E., & Myers, R.H. (1993). Evidence for neuronal degeneration and dendritic plasticity in cortical pyramidal neurons of Huntington's disease (HD): A quantitative Golgi study. *Neurology, 43*, 2088–2096.

Stewart, R.M., Richman, D.P., & Caviness, V.S., Jr. (1975). Lissencephaly and pachygyria: An architectonic and topographic analysis. *Acta Neuropathologica, 31*, 1–12.

Suetsugu, M., & Mehraein, P. (1980). Spine distribution along the apical dendrites of the pyramidal neurons in Down's syndrome: A quantitative Golgi study. *Acta Neuropathologica, 50*, 207–210.

Takashima, S., Becker, L.E., Armstrong, D.L., & Chan, F. (1981). Abnormal neuronal development in the visual cortex of the human fetus and infant with Down's syndrome. A quantitative and qualitative Golgi study. *Brain Research, 225*, 1–21.

Takashima, S., Becker, L.E., Chan, F.-W., & Augustin, R. (1985). Golgi and computer morphometric analysis of cortical dendrites in metabolic storage disease. *Experimental Neurology, 88*, 652–672.

Takashima, S., Chan, F., Becker, L., Houdu, S., & Suzuki, Y. (1991). Cortical cytoarchitectural and immunohistochemical studies on Zellweger syndrome. *Brain & Development, 13*, 158–162.

Takashima, S., Chan, F., Becker, L., & Kuruta, H. (1991). Aberrant neuronal development in hemimegalencephaly: Immunohistochemical and Golgi studies. *Pediatric Neurology, 7*, 275–280.

Towbin, A. (1971). Organic causes of minimal brain dysfunction: Perinatal origin of minimal cerebral lesions. *JAMA, 217*, 1207–1214.

Volpe, J.J. (1992). Effect of cocaine use on the fetus. *New England Journal of Medicine, 327*, 399–407.

Warkany, J., Lemire, R.J., & Cohen, M.M., Jr. (1981). *Mental retardation and congenital malformations of the central nervous system.* Chicago: Year Book Medical Publishers.

Williams, R.S., Ferrante, R.J., & Caviness, V.S., Jr. (1975). Neocortical organization in human cerebral malformations: A Golgi study [Abstract]. *Society for Neuroscience Abstracts, 1*, 776.

Williams, R.S., Ferrante, R.J., & Caviness, V.S., Jr. (1976). The cellular pathology of microgyria: A Golgi analysis. *Acta Neuropathologica, 36*, 269–283.

Williams, R.S., Ferrante, R.J., & Caviness, V.S. (1978). The Golgi rapid method in clinical neuropathology: The morphologic consequences of suboptimal fixation. *Journal of Neuropathology and Experimental Neurology, 37*, 13–33.

Williams, R.S., Ferrante, R.J., & Caviness, V.S., Jr. (1979). The isolated human cortex: A Golgi analysis of Krabbe's disease. *Archives of Neurology, 36*, 134–139.

Williams, R.S., Hauser, S.L., Purpura, D.P., DeLong, G.R., & Swisher, C.N. (1980). Autism and mental retardation: Neuropathologic studies performed in four retarded persons with autistic behavior. *Archives of Neurology, 37*, 749–753.

Williams, R.S., Lott, I.T., & Ferrante, R.J. (1977). The cellular pathology of neuronal ceroid-lipofuscinosis: A Golgi-electronmicroscopic study. *Archives of Neurology, 34*, 298–305.

Wisniewski, K.E., Laure-Kamionowska, M., Connell, F., & Wisniewski, H.M. (1985). Quantitative determination of synaptic density and their morphology during the postnatal brain development in visual cortex of Down syndrome brain [Abstract]. *Journal of Neuropathology and Experimental Neurology, 44*, 342.

Worley, P.F., Cole, A.J., Murphy, T.H., Christy, B.A., Nakabeppu, Y., & Baraban, J.M. (1990) Synaptic regulation of immediate-early genes in brain. *Cold Spring Harbor Symposia on Quantitative Biology, 55*, 213–223.

Xu, G., O'Connell, P., Viskochil, D., Cawthon, R., Robertson, M., Culver, M., Dunn, D., Stevens, J., Gesteland, R., White, R., & Weiss, R. (1990). The neurofibromatosis type 1 gene encodes a protein related to GAP. *Cell, 63*, 851–859.

Yamagata, K., Andreasson, K.I., Kaufmann, W.E., Barnes, C.A., & Worley, P.F. (1993). Expression of a mitogen-inducible cyclooxygenase in brain neurons: Regulation by synaptic activity and glucocorticoids. *Neuron, 11*, 371–386.

Yamagata, K., Kaufmann, W.E., Lanahan, A., Papapavlou, M., Barnes, C.A., Andreasson, K.I., & Worley, P.F. (1994). *Egr3/Pilot*, a zinc-finger transcription factor, is rapidly regulated by activity in brain neurons and colocalizes with *Egr1/zif268*. *Learning and Memory, 1*, 140–152.

Yamagata, K., Sanders, L.K., Kaufmann, W.E., Yee, W., Barnes, C.A., Nathans, D., & Worley, P.F. (1994). *Rheb*, a growth factor- and synaptic activity-regulated gene, encodes a novel Ras-related protein. *Journal of Biological Chemistry, 269*, 16333–16339.

Zametkin, A.J., Nordahl, T., Gross, M., King, C., Semple, W.E., Rumsey, J., Hamburger, S., & Cohen, R.M. (1990). Cerebral glucose metabolism in adults with hyperactivity of childhood onset. *New England Journal of Medicine, 323*, 1361–1366.

Zametkin, A.J., & Rapoport, J.L. (1987). Neurobiology of attention deficit disorder with hyperactivity: Where have we come in 50 years? *Journal of the American Academy of Child and Adolescent Psychiatry, 26*, 676–686.

Zimmerman, R.A., Yachnis, A.T., Rorke, L.B., Rebsamen, S.L., Bilaniuk, L.T., & Zackai, E. (1992). Pathology of findings of high signal intensity findings in neurofibromatosis type 1 [Abstract]. *Radiology, 186*, 123.

PART II
CEREBRAL PALSY

Chapter 5

Epidemiology and Etiology of Cerebral Palsy

Karin B. Nelson, M.D.

Individuals with cerebral palsy (CP), except those with the mildest degrees of this disorder, experience life-limiting problems. As compared with children with asthma, epilepsy, blindness, or deafness, it is those with CP for whom normal activities of childhood are most limited (Newacheck & Taylor, 1992). It is estimated that more than 100,000 persons less than 18 years old in the United States manifest CP (Kuban & Leviton, 1994) and that about 5,000 children with moderate or severe congenital CP are added to the population of the United States each year (Cummins, Nelson, Grether, & Velie, 1993). With good care, most persons with CP, even those with serious involvement, now survive into adult life (Evans, Evans, & Alberman, 1990). Provision of that care is demanding: Feeding, bathing, and administration of medications requires about 24 hours per week (Barabas, Matthews, & Zumoff, 1992). The economic cost per year in the United States for care of persons with CP is about $5 billion (Kuban & Leviton, 1994).

There is obviously much reason for efforts to prevent CP. If we are to improve our preventive capability, we will require a better understanding of the causes of CP than has yet been achieved.

DEFINITION

Cerebral palsy is an umbrella term for a group of chronic neurologic disorders manifested by abnormal control of movement, beginning early in life, and not due to underlying progressive disease. Obviously such a categorization does not define a single disease; the term is analogous with the category *mental retardation*, which groups individuals according to another important limitation, cognitive disability. A chief purpose for such categorizations according to significant disabilities is to provide a grouping of affected persons according to their similar needs for medical, educational, and social services. Another reason is that such a categorization can be used in studies of etiology to explore for common associated factors. For example, persons with CP are more likely than those unaffected to have been born low in birth weight, and that knowledge can be a basis for further explorations of associated factors that may improve understanding of causal pathways to motor disability of differing types.

In the field of mental retardation, the last decades have seen a good deal of progress in recognizing etiologic subgroups: There are genetic disorders such as Down and fragile X syndromes, toxic syndromes such as fetal alcohol syndrome, metabolic disorders such as phenylketonuria and its variants, and so on. Recognition of these specific substituent disorders in mental retardation has opened new possibilities for counseling and intervention. In the field of CP, we are at a much earlier stage in the recognition of pathogenetically specific subsyndromes, but the basic task is comparable with that in mental retardation: We must learn to identify specific entities, learn their biologic substrates, and—we hope—progress to better strategies for management and prevention.

Although the defining disability in CP is motor, persons with CP often experience other disabilities related to their underlying brain abnormalities. More than half of persons with CP

---

have mental retardation, a third or more experience epilepsy, and about a fifth have disorders of vision or hearing (Evans, Elliot, Alberman, & Evans, 1985). The more severe the motor disorder, the greater the likelihood of additional impairments. Severe spastic quadriplegia is the type of CP most likely to be accompanied by other neurologic and sensory disorders.

EPIDEMIOLOGY

Variations in definition and severity, different methods and ages of ascertainment, and exclusions complicate the comparison of prevalence estimates from different sources and in different time periods. Some abnormalities of movement and posture are not apparent early in life, and mild spasticity in very young children tends to improve with age. Despite this variability in methods, studies in a number of developed countries indicate a CP prevalence of 1.2–2.5 per 1,000 children of early school age. In industrialized countries, approximately 12%–20% of persons with CP acquired their disability after the first month of life (Kuban & Leviton, 1994).

Cerebral palsy is somewhat more common in boys and more common in black than in white children (Cummins et al., 1993; Murphy, Yeargin-Allsopp, Decoufle, & Drews, 1993), the latter apparently related to the greater frequency of low birth weight in blacks. In one study, infants born to women 40 years old or older more often had CP, especially if those mothers were high in parity. Children born to teenage mothers or fathers (even if the mothers were members of the next older age group) were also at somewhat higher risk for CP (Cummins et al., 1993). Neither early initiation of prenatal care nor delivery in a hospital with a neonatal intensive care unit was related to lower risk of CP in that large majority of babies born weighing more than 1,500 g (Cummins et al., 1993).

In the 1970s, there was a good deal of optimism that, as obstetrics improved, CP largely would disappear. Obstetrics did indeed improve, and markedly so as measured by the drop in deaths and injuries to mothers and to babies. Unfortunately, the hoped-for decrease in the frequency of CP has not materialized (Mutch, Al-

berman, Hagberg, Kodama, & Perat, 1992). In a meta-analysis of 85 cohorts, the CP rate in survivors born weighing less than 1,500 g has remained fairly stable from the mid-1960s to the present (Escobar, Littenberg, & Petitti, 1991). Several population-based studies, however, have noted increases in the CP rate among infants under 1,500 g, a group in which survival has greatly improved.

It has been estimated that, in the United States, the childhood prevalence of CP has risen about 20% between 1960 and 1986 (Bushan, Paneth, & Kiely, 1993). The improved survival rate of very low birth weight infants, which has allowed many babies who would have died in earlier times to become healthy citizens, has also increased the number of persons with disabilities.

Mortality has decreased among babies of normal birth weight as well, and CP prevalence has not dropped among them; in some populations it has risen (e.g., Hagberg, Hagberg, & Olow, 1993). There is some suggestion that the combination of CP and severe mental retardation may be more frequent than heretofore (Nicholson & Alberman, 1992; Stanley, 1994).

Thus as obstetric and neonatal care have improved greatly, the occurrence of CP has not declined. Cerebral palsy is not a good outcome by which to measure the quality of medical care.

ETIOLOGY

Until the 1970s and 1980s, many people thought that CP arose chiefly through calamities during the process of birth. The more recent literature, using appropriate controls, avoiding known sources of bias, and evaluating the contributions of risk factors present before labor began, has led to some change in that perception: "Cerebral palsy in children born at term most often appears to reflect phenomena that precede the onset of labor" (Kuban & Leviton, 1994, p. 193), whereas CP arising in preterm children more often may include both prenatal and perinatal factors (see Chapter 13, Volume I).

The number of methodologically appropriate studies of the etiology of CP is still not large. To date, the major risk factors identified for CP have been low birth weight and birth asphyxia.

Low Birth Weight

Freud asked whether prematurely born infants have a higher risk of abnormality because of their premature birth or are born prematurely because of some intrinsic abnormality of the child or pregnancy; there is still no clear-cut answer to his question. Factors that contribute to preterm birth have been reviewed recently (Berkowitz & Papiernik, 1993; Lumley, 1993).

During a period in which survival of low birth weight infants has improved, the prevention of preterm birth has not yet been successful (Alexander, Weiss, Hulsey, & Papiernik, 1991), and the rate of neurologic morbidity among infants of very low birth weight has not decreased (Cooke, 1993). The net result is that the CP arising in low birth weight infants has become a large minority of all CP cases. Babies born weighing less than 1,500 g constituted 0.68% of survivors but contributed 28% of cases of CP (Cummins et al., 1993). Survivors with birth weights below 1,000 g, a group among which few survived in the past, contributed 8.7% of CP cases in singletons. Overall, almost half of CP cases arose in infants under 2,500 g.

Although low birth weight is especially associated with spastic diplegia, the form of bilateral spastic CP affecting legs more prominently than arms and hands, tiny babies may have any form of CP, and diplegia may occur in term infants.

Low birth weight and low gestational age are independent predictors of CP; thus both preterm birth and poor growth for duration of gestation are probably related to risk of neurologic morbidity. Mildly or moderately premature infants who are small for their gestational ages may be at special risk (Blair & Stanley, 1990; Nelson & Ellenberg, 1985b). Unfortunately, problems in determination of gestational age, an imperfect procedure in general, may be especially serious in very low birth weight infants (DiPietro & Allen, 1991). Estimation of gestational age also may present special problems in relation to CP because aberrant menstrual cycles are more common in mothers of children with CP (Nelson & Ellenberg, 1985a; Torfs, van den Berg, Oechsli, & Cummins, 1990), and tone and head size may be atypical for gestational age in infants who are neurologically abnormal.

The causes of poor intrauterine growth may themselves be important in outcome. Viral infection, congenital malformations, chromosomal anomalies, and certain maternal illnesses can be causes of abnormal growth and of brain dysfunction after birth.

Low birth weight of a previous child born to the same mother is an important predictor of low birth weight in the current pregnancy. Other factors that contribute to the likelihood of low birth weight, and can be associated with risk of CP even in big babies, are congenital malformations, inflammations of the placenta, and twinning or higher order multiple births.

Evidence of maldevelopment of the brain or other organ systems is more common in children with CP (Blair & Stanley, 1993; Nelson & Ellenberg, 1985a). There is an association of malformations with low birth weight, and low birthweight infants with congenital malformations are at increased risk of CP (Nelson & Ellenberg, 1985b).

Inflammation of the placenta is a risk factor for CP in babies of all birth weights (Nelson & Ellenberg, 1985a) but is especially common in infants born prematurely; evidence of inflammation is present in 50%–80% of very premature births (Steer, 1991). Infection can trigger a cascade of cell biologic processes, mediated by the release of endogenous cytokines (Gibbs, Romero, Hillier, Eschenbach, & Sweet, 1992). Some of these agents have potential effects on development of neurons and glia within the brain (Leviton, 1993).

Multiple births now contribute about 10% of CP, and, in multiple births, low birth weight is relatively frequent (Grether, Nelson, & Cummins, 1993). The rate of CP in twins is higher than in singletons, and in triplets is higher still (Petterson, Nelson, Watson, & Stanley, 1993).

If one twin dies, the risk of CP in the surviving twin is more than 100 times higher than the risk in a singleton (Grether et al., 1993). Brain pathology in the surviving twin is most often multicystic encephalomalacia, and often there are also defects in other organs, with renal cortical defects or horseshoe kidney, intestinal atresia, terminal limb defects, or other manifestations of *the vascular disruption sequence* (Scheller & Nelson, 1992). A major hypothesis as to etiology of the brain pathology in the surviving twin is related to linked circulations in the placenta in monozygotic twin pairs: When one twin dies, the other is thought to exsanguinate into the pressure sink and, before pressure relationships can stabilize, may suffer irreparable harm. The risk of CP in unlike-sex twin pairs, all of whom are dizygous, is not lower than in like-sex pairs, however, so it is likely that vascular anastomoses in the placenta are not the only pathogenetic mechanism in the CP in the surviving co-twin.

The disappearance during pregnancy of one member of a twin pair whose earlier existence was visualized by ultrasound examination during the pregnancy or by placental examination at the time of delivery is not infrequent. Some otherwise unexplained cases of CP may arise by this mechanism. A large study relating early ultrasound examinations to outcome would be required to test this possibility.

Twinning and tripletting have increased strikingly in the United States and in other developed countries, probably related in major part to the use of assistive reproductive technologies. The short-term costs and stresses related to this increase in multiple births have been discussed in both the medical and the lay press. It seems likely that the increase in multiple gestations also will lead to an increase in long-term neurologic morbidity.

In preterm babies, neuroimaging findings thought to represent necroses of white matter have shown reasonable reliability and good sensitivity and predictive power for later CP (Kuban & Leviton, 1994). In infants of very low birth weight, imaging procedures—usually cranial ultrasonography, which is safe and cost-effective—by the time of nursery discharge can permit recognition of infants at especially high risk for CP.

It appears likely, based on current incomplete evidence, that both prenatal and perinatal factors may contribute to neurologic morbidity in infants of very low birth weight.

Birth Asphyxia

The term *birth asphyxia* has been used with a wide variety of meanings and with so little validation that the American College of Obstetri-

cians and Gynecologists (1991) has concluded that the term is imprecise and should not be used. Furthermore,

> Evidence associating cerebral palsy with measures of birth asphyxia is difficult to interpret as we have such poor measures of birth asphyxia.. . . Abnormal fetal heart rate traces are notorious in terms of interobserver variation, do not predict long term neurologic handicap well.. . . Other measures such as presence of meconium, cord blood pH, Apgar scores and time to first breath all suffer from similar problems of, "what are they really measuring?" (Stanley, 1994, pp. 5–6)

Acute obstetric catastrophes occur occasionally, with a prolapsed, pulseless cord or massive abruption of the placenta, for example. The infant in such cases may be born in a neurologically depressed state, may experience evidence of encephalopathy in the first days of life, and may experience early neonatal convulsions. Such infants may go on to experience lifelong neurologic morbidity. The great misfortune of such occurrences brands such a history on the memory of all who are in contact with it. It does not follow logically, however, that every neurologically depressed infant has his or her symptoms for a similar reason, nor that the natural history of the condition will necessarily be the same when the initiating pathogenetic events are different. We have seen uncritical application of the word *asphyxiated* to any infant with a low Apgar score, despite evidence that a wide variety of factors can produce a lowered Apgar score. For example, chorionitis was associated, in babies both over and under 2,500 g, with a marked increase in 5-minute Apgar scores of 5 or less (Nelson & Ellenberg, 1984, Table 1).

The topic of birth asphyxia and its relationship to CP has recently been reviewed (Nelson & Emery, 1993). Medical evidence using such indicators as are currently available indicates that interference with oxygen supply to the fetus during birth must be severe and prolonged and accompanied by abnormality of blood flow as well as of oxygen saturation, if it is to be associated with increased risk of long-term neurologic abnormality. Many or most infants who experience that degree of abnormality do not survive it. Surprisingly, most infants who do survive even major asphyxial stress are later clinically normal. Unless the fetus cannot muster an anaerobic response for some reason, meaningful interruption of oxygen supply during birth will result in metabolic acidemia. The presence of low pH is therefore an important marker of intrapartum asphyxia. However, pH must be extremely low—below 7.00—to be associated with significant increase in risk (Goldaber, Gilstrap, Leveno, Dax, & McIntire, 1991). Even in the presence of such marked acidosis, surviving term babies without additional problems are usually normal (Goodwin, Belai, Hernandez, Durand, & Paul, 1992). An important additional point is that a substantial share of infants who have low Apgar scores or low pH, or both and who survive and are abnormal have congenital malformations or other characteristics suggestive of increased vulnerability or other determinants of poor outcome.

Spastic quadriplegia, especially if accompanied by movement disorder, is the form of CP most often linked with serious birth asphyxia, but other etiologies can produce a similar clinical picture. A recent study of children with moderate or severe spastic quadriplegia found boys to be overrepresented among this group. Most of these children had multiple disabilities. An intrapartum cause was considered possible in almost a quarter of these children, but half of that number were either very small for gestational age or had experienced only "comparatively minor intrapartum insult" (Stanley, Blair, Hockey, Petterson, & Watson, 1993, p. 199). The authors concluded that half of those whose onset might have been intrapartum had evidence of compromise before labor began.

It is clearly possible for irreversible, and even for preventable, neurologic injury to occur during birth, but the percentage of children with CP who were normal before labor began and were injured irreversibly during birth is thought, on the basis of current evidence, to be a small part of the total. Even more troubling is the fact that there is so little to assist the birth attendant to recognize the fetus in real danger during labor, at a time when clinical decisions must be made. It was hoped at one time that the widespread introduction of electronic fetal monitoring of the heart rate during labor would lead to a decrease in CP, but despite the increased rate of surgical delivery, that decrease has not been achieved.

In an infant who displays signs of neurologic dysfunction in the first minutes after birth, with hypotonia, reflex unresponsiveness, and respiratory depression, a low Apgar score is assigned. An infant who manifests such signs in the days after birth, sometimes accompanied by seizures, is often given a diagnosis of *hypoxic–ischemic encephalopathy* (HIE). That diagnosis is often one of exclusion, given if cultures are not positive and if major malformations or metabolic defects are not apparent. However, ascertainment of these conditions is distinctly insensitive, so "HIE" or "birth asphyxia" is often a clinical diagnosis made by default, without much clear-cut positive supporting evidence. Neuroimaging or blood flow study evidence of ischemia does not help in identifying the fundamental pathogenetic processes, because ischemia is a potential late feature of a wide variety of different basic problems. More objective and descriptive clinical investigations of neurologically depressed infants, and fewer unsupported assumptions, would better serve individual patients and the progress of the field.

Other Factors

Physical trauma at birth is probably an uncommon factor underlying long-term neurologic disability in developed countries today. Babies weighing 4,000–4,500 g, once a group vulnerable to birth injury, had the lowest rate of CP of any birth weight group in a recent American study (Cummins et al., 1993).

In one case series, abnormalities of neuronal migration were observed by magnetic resonance imaging in nearly one third of persons with CP (Truwit, Barkovich, Koch, & Ferriero, 1992). The presence of other evidence of maldevelopment, in the brain or elsewhere, already has been commented on as more frequent in persons with CP than in others.

Athetoid CP has become less frequent as better approaches to rH sensitization and neonatal hyperbilirubinemia have been developed. Congenital infection with certain viral agents, such as rubella and cytomegalovirus, can lead to CP, and toxoplasmosis is another potentially causative agent. In utero abnormalities of thyroid hormone levels and exposure to methyl mercury or exogenous thyroid hormone and es-

trogen have been implicated, as has been exposure to benzyl alcohol in the newborn period
(Benda, Hiller, & Reynolds, 1986). Some of
these and other factors have been associated
with increased risk of CP (Table 1). Some of
these are directly related to potential causes of
brain abnormality; others, such as maternal age
and high parity, may be markers for some other
factor not directly identified.

In developing countries, it is likely that infection, maternal anemia and hemorrhage, neona-
tal-hypothermia, and obstetric trauma are con-
tributors to motor disability.

CONCLUSIONS

There still has not been a great deal of research
into the etiology of CP and very little that has
pressed to understand the factors that predict
CP. If better preventive strategies are to be developed, a good deal more clinical research is
still needed. Furthermore, there is great need to
relate clinical research about CP to rapidly increasing knowledge in the basic developmental
neurosciences that is likely, in future, to help us

Table 1. Risk factors for cerebral palsy based on epidemiologic studies

Recognizable at time of first prenatal visit
Mother
  Thyroid disorder[a]
  Menstrual cycle > 36 days[a]
  Previous pregnancy loss or neonatal deaths[a]
  Mental retardation
  Seizure disorder
Prior-born child
  < 2,000 g[a]
  Motor deficit
  Mental retardation or sensory deficit

In current pregnancy
  Polyhydramnios[a]
  Treatment with thyroid hormone[a] and/or estrogen,
    progesterone
  Congenital malformations[a]
  Multiple gestation[a]
  Maternal seizure disorder
  Severe late proteinuria, hypertension
  Bleeding in third trimester

[a] Factor noted in more than a single study.

to understand—and, it is hoped, to prevent—
many of the problems that now confront our patients and their families.

REFERENCES

Alexander, G.R., Weiss, J., Hulsey, T.C., & Papiernik, E. (1991). Preterm birth prevention: An
   evaluation of programs in the United States. *Birth,
   18*, 160–169.
Barabas, G., Matthews, W., & Zumoff, P. (1992).
   Care-load for children and young adults with severe cerebral palsy. *Developmental Medicine and
   Child Neurology, 34*, 979–984.
Benda, G.I., Hiller, J.L., & Reynolds, J.W. (1986).
   Benzyl alcohol toxicity: Impact on neurologic
   handicaps among surviving very low birth weight
   infants. *Pediatrics, 77*, 507–512.
Berkowitz, G.S., & Papiernik, E. (1993). Epidemiology of preterm birth. *Epidemiologic Reviews, 15*,
   414–442.
Blair, E., & Stanley, S.J. (1990). Intrauterine growth
   and spastic cerebral palsy. I. The association with
   birth weight for gestational age. *American Journal
   of Obstetrics and Gynecology, 162*, 229–237.
Blair, E., & Stanley, F. (1993). When can cerebral palsy
   be prevented? The generation of causal hypotheses
   by multivariate analysis of a case-control study. *Pae-
   diatric and Perinatal Epidemiology, 7*, 272–301.
Bushan, V., Paneth, N., & Kiely, J.L. (1993). Impact
   of improved survival of very low birth weight in-

fants on recent secular trends in the prevalence of
   cerebral palsy. *Pediatrics, 91*, 1094–1100.
Cooke, R.W.I. (1993). Annual audit of three year out-
   come in very low birthweight infants. *Archives of
   Disease in Childhood, 69*, 295–298.
Cummins, S.K., Nelson, K.B., Grether, J.K., & Velie,
   E.M. (1993). Cerebral palsy in four northern Cali-
   fornia counties, births 1983 through 1985. *Journal
   of Pediatrics, 123*, 230–237.
DiPietro, J.A., & Allen, M.C. (1991). Estimation of
   gestational age: Implications for developmental
   research. *Child Development, 62*, 1184–1199.
Escobar, G.J., Littenberg, B., & Petitti, D.B. (1991).
   Outcome among surviving very low birthweight
   infants: A meta-analysis. *Archives of Disease in
   Childhood, 66*, 204–211.
Evans, P., Elliot, M., Alberman, E., & Evans, S.
   (1985). Prevalence and disabilities in 4- to 8-year-
   olds with cerebral palsy. *Archives of Disease in
   Childhood, 60*, 940–945.
Evans, P.M., Evans, S.J.W., & Alberman, E. (1990).
   Cerebral palsy: Why we must plan for survival.
   Archives of Disease in Childhood, 65, 1329–1333.
Gibbs, R.S., Romero, R., Hillier, S.L., Eschenbach,
   D.A., & Sweet, R.L. (1992). A review of premature

birth and subclinical infection. *American Journal of Obstetrics and Gynecology, 166,* 1515–1528.

Goldaber, K.G., Gilstrap, L.E., III, Leveno, K.J., Dax, J.S., & McIntire, D.D. (1991). Pathologic fetal acidemia. *Obstetrics and Gynecology, 78,* 1103–1107.

Goodwin, T.M., Belai, I., Hernandez, P., Durand, M., & Paul, R.H. (1992). Asphyxial complications in the term newborn with severe umbilical acidemia. *American Journal of Obstetrics and Gynecology, 162,* 1506–1512.

Grether, J.K., Nelson, K.B., & Cummins, S.K. (1993). Twinning and cerebral palsy: Experience in four northern California counties, births 1983 through 1985. *Pediatrics, 92,* 854–858.

Hagberg, B., Hagberg, G., & Olow, I. (1993). The changing panorama of cerebral palsy in Sweden. VI. Prevalence and origin during the birth year period 1983–1986. *Acta Paediatrica Scandinavica, 82,* 287–293.

Kuban, K.C.K., & Leviton, A. (1994). Cerebral palsy. *New England Journal of Medicine, 330,* 188–195.

Leviton, A. (1993). Preterm birth and cerebral palsy: Is tumor necrosis factor the missing link? *Developmental Medicine and Child Neurology, 35,* 553–558.

Lumley, J. (1993). The epidemiology of preterm birth. *Bailliere's Clinical Obstetrics and Gynaecology, 7,* 477–498.

Murphy, C.C., Yeargin-Allsopp, M., Decoufle, P., & Drews, C.D. (1993). Prevalence of cerebral palsy among ten-year-old children in metropolitan Atlanta, 1985 through 1987. *Journal of Pediatrics, 123,* S13–S19.

Mutch, L., Alberman, A., Hagberg, B., Kodama, K., & Perat, M.L. (1992). Cerebral palsy epidemiology: Where are we now and where are we going? *Developmental Medicine and Child Neurology, 34,* 547–555.

Nelson, K.B., & Ellenberg, J.H. (1984). Obstetric complications as risk factors for cerebral palsy or seizure disorders. *Journal of the American Medical Association, 251,* 1843–1848.

Nelson, K.B., & Ellenberg, J.H. (1985a). Antecedents of cerebral palsy. I. Univariate analysis of risks. *American Journal of Diseases of Children, 139,* 1031–1038.

Nelson, K.B., & Ellenberg, J.H. (1985b). Predictors of low and very low birthweight and the relation of these to cerebral palsy. *Journal of the American Medical Association, 254,* 1473–1479.

Nelson, K.B., & Emery, E.S., III. (1993). Birth asphyxia and the neonatal brain: What do we know and when do we know it? *Clinics in Perinatology, 20,* 327–344.

Newacheck, P.W., & Taylor, W.R. (1992). Childhood chronic illness: Prevalence, severity and impact. *American Journal of Public Health, 82,* 364–371.

Nicholson, A., & Alberman, E. (1992). Cerebral palsy—An increasing contributor to severe mental retardation? *Archives of Disease in Childhood, 67,* 1050–1055.

Petterson, B., Nelson, K.B., Watson, L., & Stanley, F. (1993). Twins, triplets, and cerebral palsy in births in Western Australia in the 1980s. *British Medical Journal, 307,* 1239–1243.

Scheller, J.M., & Nelson, K.B. (1992). Twinning and neurologic morbidity. *American Journal of Diseases of Children, 146,* 1110–1113.

Stanley, F.J. (1994). Cerebral palsy trends: Implications for perinatal care. *Acta Obstetrica et Gynecological Scandinavica, 73,* 5–9.

Stanley, F.J., Blair, E., Hockey, A., Petterson, B., & Watson, L. (1993). Spastic quadriplegia in Western Australia: A genetic and epidemiological study. I. Case population and perinatal risk factors. *Developmental Medicine and Child Neurology, 35,* 191–201.

Steer, P.J. (1991). Premature labour. *Archives of Disease in Children, 66,* 1167–1170.

Torfs, C.P., van den Berg, B.J., Oechsli, F.W., & Cummins, S. (1990). Prenatal and perinatal factors in the etiology of cerebral palsy. *Journal of Pediatrics, 116,* 615–619.

Truwit, C.L., Barkovich, A.J., Koch, T.K., & Ferriero, D.M. (1992). Cerebral palsy: MR findings in 40 patients. *American Journal of Neuroradiology, 13,* 67–78.

Chapter 6

Cerebral Palsy

The Spectrum of Motor Dysfunction

Arnold J. Capute, M.D., M.P.H., and Pasquale J. Accardo, M.D.

Cerebral palsy refers to a group of brain damage syndromes in which a static and nonprogressive cerebral lesion produces significant motor delay, abnormal neuromotor findings, onset during the developmental period, and other central nervous system deficits in the areas of cognition and neurobehavior. The severity of cerebral palsy is determined by the degree of motor impairment rather than the associated neurologic signs that are used to classify the (sub)type. There remains the possibility of a striking dissociation between the abnormal neuromotor findings on physical examination and the motor delay; the former tend to exhibit greater fluctuation over time. The neuromotor impairment in cerebral palsy is often of such severity as to require orthopedic surveillance for optimal management.

For the classic forms of cerebral palsy, this degree of motor delay usually equates with a motor developmental quotient (MDQ) of less than 50, where the MDQ is the motor age divided by the chronologic age times 100 (Capute & Shapiro, 1985). Although the cerebral lesion remains static and nonprogressive, the peripheral neuromotor signs change with brain maturation. For example, hypotonia evolves into spasticity or rigidity; choreoathetosis often is transformed into dystonia (Figure 1), and contractures develop later. Despite such changes in the clinical presentation over time, the general overall trend is for motor function to improve with age. In the presence of otherwise unexplained regression or loss of motor skills, active neurologic disease should be ruled out.

The cerebral insult or injury that causes cerebral palsy occurs during early brain development, where "early" is variously defined as prenatal (congenital central nervous system malformation), perinatal (intraventricular and intracerebral hemorrhages, brain asphyxia associated with difficult delivery, and respiratory disorders associated with prematurity), and postnatal (trauma, infectious and toxic agents), with age cutoffs such as 3 years (when brain growth achieves approximately three quarters of adult size), 5 years, 8 years (end of cerebral plasticity), and 16 years (in line with the upper limit of the developmental period for the onset of mental retardation). A major change in thinking over the past two decades has been the marked reduction in the role assigned to obstetric risk factors in the etiology of cerebral palsy (Nelson, 1988). Thus, one might say that an "unusual brain" gives rise to an unusual gestational period, labor, and delivery, making one think twice before placing blame on obstetric care. A prenatal etiology can be suspected in the presence of multiple minor malformations (Coorssen, Msall, & Duffy, 1991).

Although some studies have suggested the possibility of an overall decline in the occurrence of cerebral palsy with improvements in prenatal care and neonatal intensive care technologies for at-risk infants, the prevailing impression is one of a fairly consistent prevalence of cerebral palsy at school age of 2 per 1,000 live births, with 10% of these cases being of postnatal origin. Increased, decreased, or static prevalence rates as an effect of salvaging extremely low birth weight premature infants continue to be debated. Although the overall prevalence for cerebral palsy has probably not changed significantly in the past half century,

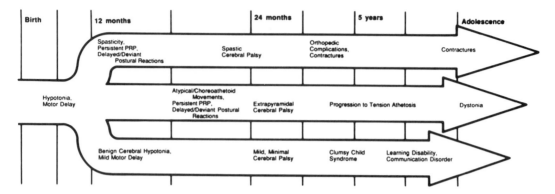

Figure 1. Evolution of motor disorders. As the brain matures, the peripheral neuromotor signs of cerebral palsy change. (PRP, primitive reflex profile.)

the relative contribution of specific subtypes has altered dramatically. Before the introduction of exchange transfusion a quarter of a century ago, the majority of cases of choreoathetosis were secondary to bilirubin encephalopathy (kernicterus). These children often displayed relatively typical cognitive abilities along with their severe motor impairment. After the virtual eradication of this subtype through preventive measures, the majority of children today with choreoathetoid cerebral palsy have diffuse asphyxial brain damage not uncommonly resulting in severe to profound mental retardation.

Epidemiologic studies of cerebral palsy are plagued by two problems. First, clinically used definitions and terminology remain inconsistent, confusing, and subjective (Blair & Stanley, 1985). Thus, whereas some clinicians report mixed cerebral palsy as a common diagnosis, other studies omit the category altogether. Second, the understanding of cerebral palsy as an "all-or-none" phenomenon ignores the more prevalent but less severe motor involvement that many children exhibit as a result of brain insult or injury. The cerebral palsy that is "a disorder of movement and posture that occurs during the developmental period of brain growth" (Bax, 1964, p. 295) must allow for the full spectrum of motor dysfunction with subclinical types (Capute, Shapiro, & Palmer, 1981). These subclinical types—*mild* and *minimal* cerebral palsy—are markers for the same associated deficits that in classic cerebral palsy can be more devastating and disabling than the motor disability itself.

ASSOCIATED DEFICITS

The associated deficits found in cerebral palsy reflect a continuum of central nervous system dysfunction. They include

1. Mental retardation (60% of cases, with the remainder at high risk for lowered intelligence, learning disability, or other cognitive impairment even though global intelligence may be within the normal range)
2. Hearing (deafness in 6%–16% of cases) and visual disturbances, especially in the choreoathetoid type
3. Strabismus (50% of cases, with an increased incidence of refractive errors)
4. Sensory impairment, especially in hemiplegia (thought to be due to parietal lobe involvement)
5. Seizures (20%–30% of cases, of which 70% are the spastic type and 20% are the athetoid type)
6. Emotional problems, especially during the adolescent years

Seizures in patients with cerebral palsy tend to have a poorer prognosis with regard to the discontinuation of anticonvulsant medication (Aksu, 1990). Poor physical growth can reflect a variety of etiologic factors, including feeding and swallowing problems, endocrine dysfunction, constipation, and a more nonspecific general debility (Stallings, Charney, Davies, & Cronk, 1993). The following physiologic and topographic classifications can provide clues to the presence of such associated deficits.

PHYSIOLOGIC CLASSIFICATION

Cerebral palsy is divided into two main physiologic groups, the *pyramidal* (a term somewhat inexactly used to refer to cases in which spasticity is prominent) and the *extrapyramidal* types (Table 1). The latter term is often used interchangeably with choreoathetoid cerebral palsy because this is the most common subtype in this category.

Spasticity is a clinical sign manifested by an increased resistance of a limb to externally imposed joint extension. The spastic types of cerebral palsy have neuromotor findings that are consistent and persistent: Neurologic abnormalities remain during quiet periods and sleep and do not vary much during the active state or when degrees of emotional stress or irritability are present. In contrast, in the extrapyramidal type there is marked variability in tone during relaxation and sleep and especially during wakefulness when stressful situations arise. This is one reason for performing serial neurodevelopmental examinations prior to rendering a physiologic diagnosis. The examiner may on one occasion see a sleepy or relaxed child who exhibits mild hyperreflexia and mild tone changes. If, at another time, the infant is alert and active, stressed, or agitated, a different constellation of neuromotor signs and tone changes—hyperreflexia and rigidity—will be

present. This variability can be extremely confusing to professionals unfamiliar with cerebral palsy. Because of the more consistent hypertonicity, the spastic child is more prone to early development contractures and other orthopedic deformities. Such contractures can be seen later in individuals with choreoathetoid cerebral palsy, particularly when they have used a wheelchair for years. In these latter cases, the positional types of contractures are more typical, mainly hip and knee flexion contractures, with or without scoliosis.

Probably all cases of cerebral palsy have some degree of mixed findings, and at times it can be difficult to find the proper diagnostic terminology. It is important to note that, in a child with significant extrapyramidal findings and atypical (other than hip and knee flexion) contractures, one should look for underlying extrapyramidal findings that may diagnose a mixed cerebral palsy. There are no generally accepted criteria for the diagnosis of mixed cerebral palsy; it is a pragmatic and heuristic clinical classification that helps explain confusing findings and predicts a different pattern of associated deficits.

Several important factors must be considered regarding tone. Spastic hypertonus is elicited by rapidly increasing the resistance of muscles by passive movement at a joint. The classical descriptor of spasticity is the "clasp knife" resis-

Table 1. Physiologic classification of cerebral palsy

Characteristic	Spastic/pyramidal	Extrapyramidal/choreoathetoid
Neurodevelopmental findings	Persistent, consistent	Variable
Contractures	Common, nonpositional	Uncommon; usually positional especially with prolonged seating in wheelchair
Increased tone	Clasp knife	Lead pipe (candle wax), putty like
Primitive reflexes	Common and pronounced, early	More common, more pronounced, and more prolonged
Deep tendon reflexes	1–4 +; sustained ankle clonus	1–3 +; ankle clonus unsustained
Pathologic reflexes	Babinski, Chaddock, Gordon, Oppenheim	Elicited as part of foot positioning seen with choreoathetosis; spontaneous extensor plantar responses
Oromotor findings	Pseudobulbar palsy; "flat facies"	Athetotic facial movements, "hung-up grimace," pseudobulbar palsy
Seizures	Common (especially in hemiplegia)	Less common
Growth delay	Less severe	More severe

tance that is followed by a sudden "give." This can be compared to the opening or closing of a penknife. Extrapyramidal hypertonicity, in contrast, is represented by increased tone persisting throughout repeated flexion and extension of an extremity. It is often described as "lead pipe" or "candle wax" rigidity. However, combinations or alternations of both these tone patterns in the same patient are not uncommon, especially when the cerebral insult is extensive. Thus, in a child with severe motor involvement, a more "clasp knife" quality may prevail at one examination, and the presence of "lead pipe" rigidity at a later examination then may suggest a mixed picture.

It is important to note that a sudden stretching of the tendon will accentuate spasticity, whereas slow, evenly applied pressure is needed to elicit the extrapyramidal component. "Cogwheel" rigidity (a series of "catches") is an unusual finding in children with cerebral palsy, usually occurring during the preadolescent years but sometimes occurring following a traumatic brain insult. This clinical observation applies also to ballismus, the sudden involuntary thrusting out of an extremity. Primitive reflexes are more exaggerated and persist longer in the extrapyramidal types of cerebral palsy.

The deep tendon reflexes are not very helpful in differentiating the physiologic types of cerebral palsy. Although deep tendon reflexes are usually more brisk in the spastic type, one must look to other neurologic findings for differential diagnosis. Sustained ankle clonus (ankle clonus that persists during that period of time the Achilles tendon remains on stretch) does point to spasticity. However, unsustained ankle clonus (only several beats elicited during stretch) can be found in the extrapyramidal type as well. In eliciting ankle clonus, it is important to have the Achilles tendon in the proper anatomic position so that it can be kept stretched for a sufficient period of time. Although an extensor plantar response that is positive or upgoing (Babinski sign) can be a physiologic response in the first 2 years of life, it is usually a very prominent finding in the spastic type of cerebral palsy. In the extrapyramidal type of cerebral palsy, a spontaneous extensor plantar response is often choreoathetoid postur-

ing and can be confused with the more traditional Babinski sign. In observing the infant or child with choreoathetoid manifestations, it is important to compare the degree to which the extensor plantar response is present when the child is not being stimulated to the degree of response when the sign is elicited by stroking the lateral border of the sole of the foot. If this response is more exaggerated during the former situation, the presence of a true Babinski sign should be questioned. However, if lateral stroking elicits a greater degree of extensor response, a true Babinski sign should be recorded. One should also note the presence of asymmetry with this response. (In eliciting the Babinski response, one should not cross the hallucal area because this will elicit the plantar flexor response and confuse the interpretation. Other means of eliciting the extensor plantar response, such as stimulating the area around the external malleolus, can also be used.)

Oromotor findings can be useful in differentiating the type of cerebral palsy present. With choreoathetosis, one can observe a "hung-up" smile and "adderlike" tongue movements (tongue thrusts), which are not found in the spastic type. However, both types of cerebral palsy can exhibit suprabulbar palsy, as manifested by a flat or expressionless facies (Blasco, Allaire, & Consortium on Drooling, 1992).

In addition to the choreoathetoid type, other less frequent forms of extrapyramidal cerebral palsy can be diagnosed. The cerebellar or ataxic form can be difficult to delineate and frequently is confused with choreoathetosis. The presence of truncal titubation along with such pathognomonic manifestations as dysmetria (past pointing) and dysdiadochokinesia, with or without the characteristic cerebellar eye movements, can help in the differential diagnosis. Cerebellar manifestations often require further investigation to rule out a degenerative disorder such as the Louis-Bar syndrome (ataxia-telangiectasia), Friedreich's ataxia, Refsum's disease, Hartnup disease, or Marinesco-Sjogren syndrome.

Rigidity is another form of extrapyramidal cerebral palsy that manifests either a decorticate (tonic labyrinthine reflex) or decerebrate posturing that diminishes with sleep or decreased stress. In the tension athetoid subtype, the infant assumes a rigid posture on stimulation and exhibits choreoathetoid movements on relaxation. This subtype progresses into the rigid or dystonic type at a later age, with a course similar to that of bilirubin encephalopathy. Bilirubin encephalopathy is characterized by a tetrad of findings: 1) choreoathetosis in 100% of cases; 2) vertical gaze palsy (usually supraversion—the child cannot look up) in 90% of cases but diminishing or disappearing by adolescence; 3) dental enamel dysplasia in 80% of cases, usually with green staining of the teeth; and 4) neurosensory hearing loss, usually coupled with central auditory imperception, in 50% of cases (Perlstein, 1961). Bilirubin encephalopathy exhibits a predictable physiologic course, with initial extensor spells (1–2 months) progressing to hypotonia (1–5 years), then choreoathetosis (usually before 5 years), and finally dystonia (during adolescence). The pure tremor type of cerebral palsy is extremely rare. Further subclassification of the extrapyramidal group is not very useful clinically.

Seizures, orthopedic complications, and contractures are all more prevalent in the spastic type. Children with extrapyramidal cerebral palsy and average intelligence exhibit a higher incidence of emotional disorders. Both groups of children with cerebral palsy exhibit poor growth. This tends to be more severe with extrapyramidal disorders, but appears to be amenable to nutritional enhancement (Shapiro, Green, Krick, Allen, & Capute, 1986).

TOPOGRAPHIC CLASSIFICATION

Extrapyramidal cerebral palsy has four-limb involvement, with the upper extremities typically being functionally more involved than the lower extremities. This precludes further useful topographic breakdown. (It is important to realize that upper extremity function is essential for vocational rehabilitation.) One occasionally sees children with choreoathetoid or dystonic hemiplegia, but, prior to considering them as atypical presentations of cerebral palsy, an intracerebral lesion should be ruled out and a diagnosis of mixed cerebral palsy considered. Therefore, for all practical purposes, topographic classification is restricted to the spastic group (Table 2).

The most common spastic presentation is hemiplegia. It is also the single most common type of cerebral palsy in general. Findings are lateralized to one side, with the homolateral upper extremity more involved than the lower. Although the incidence of seizures is high (approaching 70%), cognitive abilities are usually spared. These individuals function well in society and typically do not consider themselves significantly physically incapacitated (O'Malley & Griffith, 1977).

Neuroradiologic studies of the brains of people with cerebral palsy typically reveal a wide variety of abnormalities that do not necessarily reflect the topography, physiology, or severity of the clinical picture. Candy, Hoon, Capute, and Bryan (1993) reported that over three quarters of persons with cerebral palsy demonstrated abnormal brain findings on magnetic resonance imaging (see also Chapter 22, Volume I). Hemiplegia at least usually displays more significant involvement of the contralateral motor strip region. Wiklund and Uvebrant (1991) were able to show that brain maldevelopment and cortical and subcortical atrophy were associated with arm-dominant hemiplegia, more severe hemiplegia, decreased IQ, and an increased risk of seizures; more normal computerized tomogra-

Table 2. Topographic types of cerebral palsy

Type	Pattern of involvement
Hemiplegia	Homolateral arm and leg; arm more functionally impaired than leg
Diplegia	All four extremities; legs more involved than arms, which are relatively spared
Quadriplegia	All four extremities; some asymmetry, but all severely impaired with lower extremities more involved than upper
Double hemiplegia	All four extremities; both upper extremities more involved than both lower extremities
Monoplegia	One extremity, usually upper; probably reflects a mild hemiplegia or a birth palsy
Triplegia	One upper extremity and both lower extremities; probably reflects a variation of a quadriplegia or the combination of a diplegia with a hemiplegia

phy scans were associated with milder clinical presentations of leg-dominated hemiplegia.

The diplegic type has involvement of all four limbs, with the minimally impaired upper extremities maintaining good functional abilities. The lower extremities are more severely involved, with some degree of asymmetry being common. Whereas children with hemiplegia usually develop handedness before 12 months of age, children with diplegia usually do not develop handedness until well after 24 months, even when their diplegia is asymmetrical. The quadriplegic type is more severe than the diplegic type: All four limbs are significantly involved, with considerable compromise of both upper and lower extremity function. These children usually have severe mental retardation and often have seizures as well. Inverse to the quadriplegic type is bilateral (or "double") hemiplegia, in which the upper extremities are more involved than the lower extremities. These children usually have severe mental retardation and seizures, but the latter at a lower rate than that observed in children with quadriplegia. Triplegia can be considered a variant of quadriplegia. The rare monoplegic subtype is a remnant of hemiplegia when an upper extremity is involved and of diplegia when a lower extremity is involved.

With regard to the clinical value of the above classifications, several points should be made. The physiologic typing and the topographic localization serve primarily as indicators of associated deficits (Table 3), although they can also suggest an etiology (Table 4). With regard to topography, the more extensive the limb involvement (with regard to both number and degree), the greater the incidence of associated deficits. If the upper extremities are significantly involved, vocational rehabilitation may be a serious problem.

The diagnosis of hemiplegia, for example, suggests the need for further investigation, as 25% of these patients will have homonymous hemianopsia, and 50% will have sensory impairments involving stereognosis, two-point discrimination, and position sense. These sensory impairments are more likely to be present if growth arrest (present in 50%) is evident. Hemiparesis has the highest incidence of

Table 3. Deficits associated with various types of cerebral palsy

Type of cerebral palsy	Associated deficits
Spastic hemiplegia	Epilepsy, hemianopsia, cortical sensory deficit (including visual field cut), growth arrest
Spastic diplegia	Strabismus
Spastic quadriplegia	Epilepsy, mental retardation, strabismus, dysarthria
Choreoathetosis	Mental retardation, auditory impairment, dysarthria

seizures in cerebral palsy. Unilateral hemiplegia is quite compatible with typical cognition, whereas bilateral hemiplegia is usually associated with significant mental retardation.

AUTOMATED RESPONSES AND EARLY DIAGNOSIS

It is essential to supplement traditional neurologic findings with neurodevelopmental ones to yield an accurate motor assessment. The neurodevelopmental assessment will require evaluation of two groups of automated responses as markers for motor dysfunction. The first group includes those early infant automated responses (*primitive reflexes*) that appear during the late gestational period and are present at birth but suppressed by higher cortical function before 6 months of age. These automated responses have been quantified and closely studied with regard to time of appearance and suppression (Blasco, 1994; Capute, 1979; Capute, Accardo, Vining, Rubenstein, & Harryman, 1978; Capute et al., 1984).

This group of responses remains a useful screening tool to aid in the early detection of motor problems (see Chapter 16, Volume I). The suppression of these primitive reflexes by 6

Table 4. Etiologic factors in cerebral palsy

Type of cerebral palsy	Etiology
Spastic diplegia	Prematurity
Choreoathetosis	Bilirubin encephalopathy, severe asphyxia
Spastic hemiplegia	Postnatal brain damage
Spastic diplegia	Hydrocephalus
Ataxia	Hydrocephalus

months of age is followed by the appearance of a second group of "late" infant *postural reactions*, which include both righting and equilibrium responses. Reactions from this latter group are especially prominent just prior to the appearance of motor milestones, and thus can be quite useful in evaluating readiness for and predicting motor function, such as rolling over, sitting (with support, alone, with pivoting), creeping, and crawling (Figure 2). The appendix at the end of this chapter presents illustrations of various primitive reflexes and postural reactions, as well as information on elicitation and grading.

Primitive Infant Reflexes

The *Moro reflex* is elicited by slapping the mattress or by lifting the child from the supine position and letting the head fall back onto a padded surface. The infant responds by extension of the upper extremities, followed by abduction and then adduction, along with semiflexion of the elbows, wrists, and fingers, with the first and second fin-

gers assuming a "C" posture (see Figure 4 in the appendix at the end of this chapter). Some examiners prefer placing the infant on the flexor surface of the forearm with the head supported in the palm of the hand and then letting the head suddenly drop to produce nuchal extension followed by the typical Moro pattern. The absence of a Moro reflex may indicate the presence of either a hemiplegia or a brachial palsy. It also correlates fairly well with global central nervous system integrity by its absence (abnormal in the first several months of life) or by being present to a significant degree (abnormal after 6 months of age).

The *Galant reflex* is supposed to indicate truncal instability. This response is elicited by stimulating the paravertebral area with the thumbnail or a tracing wheel, moving caudad from the lower thoracic to the sacral region. Truncal incurvature is elicited, with flexion of hips on the ipsilateral side (see Figure 5 in the appendix). The clinical value of this isolated response remains questionable.

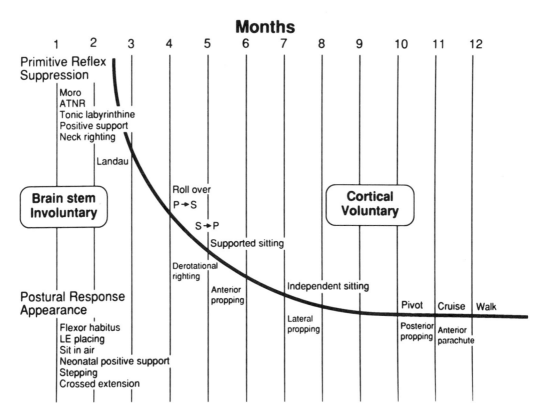

Figure 2. Evolution of motor development in infancy. (ATNR, asymmetrical tonic neck reflex; LE, lower extremity; P → S, prone to supine; S → P, supine to prone.)

The *asymmetrical tonic neck reflex* pattern is also referred to as the "fencer" position. Turning the head laterally elicits extension of the upper and lower extremities on the chin side and flexion of the limbs on the occiput side (see Figure 6 in the appendix). If this response is present to an obligatory degree, then the infant with cerebral palsy is at high risk for having occipital hip subluxation/dislocation and scoliosis. Because of the persistence of the tonal pattern of this reflex, it is essential for infants and young children to have their heads in a neutral or midline position to equalize limb tone throughout the neurologic examination for at least the first year of life. In the past this response sometimes was misinterpreted as indicating maternal rejection.

The *symmetrical tonic neck reflex* contradicts the tone and movement changes present in other early infantile automated responses. It is not present at birth, first appears at about 20 weeks of age, and is present to only a slight degree in a fairly small number of infants. Clinical experience shows that, when this response is present to a significant degree or for a longer period of time, it may indicate significant extrapyramidal involvement. This response has been described as the "cat" reflex because neck extension induces upper extremity extension with lower extremity flexion, as when a cat is about to jump up; neck flexion produces flexion of the upper extremities and extension of lower extremities, as when a cat is crouching to drink (see Figure 7 in the appendix). The time course for its true suppression remains unclear. However, as long as head movements control or strongly influence lower extremity positioning, reciprocal lower extremity movements will be inhibited. Thus, all traces of this reflex should be gone by 8 months, the time at which creeping and crawling begin to appear.

The *positive support reaction* represents a graded series of responses useful for determining lower extremity integrity, especially when evaluated in conjunction with reflex patterns such as stepping and the "downward parachute." The evolution of this response reflects the transition of reflex motor development from the neonatal stage, in which the infant "sits in air" when held in vertical suspension, to a state of momentary extension of the lower extremities that is elicited by hallucal stimulation, and on to the stage of reflex standing. The neonatal phase is present between birth and 2 months of age, after which time hallucal stimulation results in brief body support by lower extremity extension (see Figure 8 in the appendix). This mature reaction probably represents a transition into a righting response. It can be reinforced by nuchal extension that increases the lower extremity tone via the tonic labyrinthine response. (Earlier in development, nuchal extension facilitates a weak stepping response.)

The *tonic labyrinthine response* (physiologic decorticate posturing) is elicited by nuchal extension and flexion. Neck extension produces shoulder retraction with secondary flexion of the upper extremities and extension of the lower extremities, a pattern sometimes referred to as the "surrender" posture. Neck flexion produces shoulder protraction and lower extremity flexion (see Figure 9 in the appendix). Clinically, this response resembles decorticate posturing. Decerebrate posturing (shoulder retraction with extension and internal rotation of the upper extremities) is never seen in normal premature infants or neonates and, if present, indicates a pathologic state with an ominous prognosis for devastating cerebral involvement. This tonic labyrinthine reflex in prone, a total body flexor response, is probably responsible for the flexor habitus or fetal position that is evident in the early months of life and that persists until 3 months of age. Prior to this time, one can describe the automated responses as exhibiting a lessening or an increase of the predominant flexor tone. Whereas the primitive reflexes must be suppressed or be integrated prior to the development of specific motor functions, the postural reactions (equilibrium and righting responses) must evolve.

Equilibrium and Righting Postural Reactions

Three early postural reactions are closely associated with rolling over: 1) the *head-righting reaction*, present soon after birth; 2) the *Landau reaction*, present in 50% of 2-month-olds and 100% of 3-month-olds; and 3) the *derotative righting reactions* ("head-on-body" and "body-on-body"), present by 4 months of age. Although the majority of early infantile automated responses are not contiguous with postural reactions, there are exceptions that are valuable in determining the infant's motor developmental phase with regard to rolling over.

At birth, the infant has a head-righting reaction manifested by the ability to lift the head from the table while in the prone position. This should not be confused with the neck-righting response present in the newborn and elicited with the infant in the supine position by turning the head approximately 45 degrees to either side to produce a loglike roll of the body. Both these primitive head/neck reactions are suppressed with the evolution of the voluntary head-righting reaction into vertebral righting (Landau reaction) and later axial (centrifugal) extension (the derotative righting response noted just prior to rolling over at 4–5 months of age). The Landau reaction is elicited with the infant held in horizontal suspension when voluntary neck extension stimulates first vertebral extension and then lower extremity extension. The derotative righting reaction can be performed in two ways. Head-on-body is elicited when, with the infant in the supine position, turning the head laterally produces a derotative response—a spiral uncoiling—that progresses from the neck to the shoulders, hips, and lower extremities; body-on-body is elicited when, with the infant in the supine position, crisscrossing the lower extremities results in a derotative roll progressing from the lower extremities to the hips, trunk, shoulder, and neck (see Figure 10 in the appendix).

In order for these automated responses to be correlated with later motor function, it is essential that the examiner view them in a sequential fashion. The initial phase of rolling over is head righting (anterior nuchal righting), with its progression to the vertebral column (Landau reaction), and then spreading in a segmental manner (derotative righting). Thus, these three phases—head righting, Landau reaction, and derotative righting—must be present for rolling over to occur in a physiologic manner. One may thus consider this progression as Stages I, II, and III of prerolling. If all three stages are not present, the infant will not roll in a normal fashion. If sequentialness is absent, the examiner should determine which stage the infant has reached. (A similar analysis may also be applied to the positive support reflex, with Stage I being "sitting in air," Stage II having transient lower extremity extension, and Stage III presenting the most mature response or postural righting. These would then represent the three stages of prestanding.)

In addition to recording the sequentiality of the primitive responses and their integration with the postural reactions, the quality of these responses can also be diagnostically interpreted. For example, a child with diplegia in the hypertonic phase will have significant lower extremity extensor tone. This will influence the head-on-body derotative righting reaction to exhibit a log roll quality in the lower extremities but a derotative quality in the upper extremities. The opposite pattern can be seen in children with choreoathetosis because the upper extremities usually are more involved. In the positive support response, a diplegic infant will exhibit an obligatory response, with the increased lower extremity extensor tone being expressed clinically as toe walking with or without scissoring, and with the persistence of an evident stepping response. Delay and deviancy of the other automated responses are also important, and include the absence of the lower and upper extremity placing reactions; the neonatal "sitting in air" in vertical suspension or the stepping reaction remaining past 4–5 months; and the downward parachute (normally present at 6 months) appearing late (hypotonic phase) or early (hypertonic phase).

SPECTRUM OF MINOR MOTOR DYSFUNCTION

The classic types of major motor dysfunction comprising cerebral palsy have been described. However, the motor spectrum is not an all-or-none phenomenon, as it includes milder subclinical forms that are not given clinical prominence because orthopedic monitoring and therapy are not required (Capute et al., 1981). Society does not typically place a high premium on motor abilities unless athletic prowess is a goal. The classic forms of cerebral palsy exhibit MDQs of less than 50 (Capute & Shapiro, 1985). The subclinical form of cerebral palsy known as *mild motor disorder* is characterized by both delay and deviance, with an overall MDQ of between 50 and 70. By history, the infant may not roll over before 8 months, come to sit before 16 months, cruise before 16 months, and walk before 18 months. In addition to this delay, deviancy is exhibited, with early (at 1–2 months) rolling over from prone to supine as a result of an exaggerated tonic labyrinthine reaction, coming to standing rather than sitting when pulled from prone as a result of increased tone in the lower extremities, and either a prolonged "sitting-in-air" posture (if in the hypotonic state) or a misleadingly "mature" strong positive support response (if in the hypertonic phase). These infants will remain at high risk for either preschool or school-age learning problems. When this motor picture is discussed with the parents, the term "cerebral palsy" should not be used, just as, when counseling in the cognitive area, one would not equate borderline or low-average functioning with mental retardation.

When this continuum of motor dysfunction presents as motor deviancy without delay, a *minimal* type is noted in which the motor milestones appear on time, with a MDQ above 70. Motor deviancy without delay characterizes this minimal cerebral palsy. In counseling, mild motor delay is mentioned rather than cerebral palsy because of the connotations of the latter term. Both these subclinical forms—the mild and the minimal—are manifested early in life by having early infantile automated responses present to a significant degree and persisting for a longer period of time, followed by poorly developed righting and equilibrium reactions that usually are noted in children with minor neuromotor problems.

The importance of the *motor spectrum* concept is that both of these forms indicate an increased risk for preschool and school-age learning problems with minor neurologic dysfunction. Clinically, these children's subtle and "soft" neuromotor findings represent the residual of their earlier mild or minimal cerebral palsy patterns. The persistence of deviant righting and equilibrium reactions is noted by the child having problems maintaining balance. This is usually accompanied by atypical upper extremity posturing on various gait tests. Also noted are asymmetrical, increased, or decreased deep tendon reflexes; poorly executed alternat-ing movements of the forearms and finger apposition; and late development of handedness. Depending on the presence and degree of functional impairment, such children may also be described as clumsy or apraxic. Further physiologic and topographic classification of these minor motor types yields three main subclinical syndromes. In the *choreiform syndrome*, the child exhibits choreoathetoid movements with the eyes closed, along with hand drifting, spooning, and intentional tremor (Prechtl & Stemmer, 1962). The *diplegic syndrome* is characterized by persistent toe walking, increased tendon reflexes in the lower extremities, a knock-kneed gait, and late handedness. The *hemiplegic syndrome* is manifested by asymmetrical findings on the Fog walk, the tandem walk, deep tendon reflexes, finger apposition, and rapid alternating movements of the upper extremity.

These subclinical types are highlighted to stress the existence of this extended spectrum and its clinical implications (see Chapter 13, this volume). This spectrum must be appreciated by those managing preschool and school-age children with learning problems. Although these findings are insignificant in isolation, they represent an integral part of the three-dimensional view of the developmental disabilities triangle (Figure 3). If the motor side of the triangle is involved, one should look for associated cognitive deficits as well as neurobehavioral abnormalities. Appreciation of the motor spectrum mandates that pediatricians as well as orthopedic surgeons question parents of infants and children having motor delay or deviancy with regard to their overall developmental status. When one developmental stream is involved, the other streams should be investigated as well.

DIAGNOSTIC CLUES

The following clinical observations and hypothetical associations can help in the early diagnosis of cerebral palsy:

1.   Because of the age-related appearance of motor milestones, the rate of motor development can be precisely monitored by converting it into a MDQ.

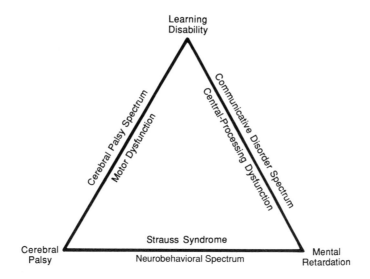

Figure 3. Developmental disabilities triangle.

2. Familiarity with the orderly sequence of motor milestone appearance will highlight any deviancy that occurs.

3. The quality of motor activity also should be noted. For example, "scooting" or "bunny hopping" is observed in diplegia (related to good upper extremity function). Infants with hypotonic diplegia come to sit in a reversed tailor, or "W," rather than in a circle or long-legged sitting position. Classic diplegias also exhibit a characteristic rolling-over "mermaid" pattern, retaining the primitive log roll (neck righting) of early infancy that typically is suppressed by 4 months of age.

4. All infants with cerebral palsy pass through an initial hypotonic phase. Significant spasticity present at birth indicates that the hypotonia occurred during intrauterine life.

5. During the first 6 months of life, many neurologic findings that are abnormal in adults are physiologic (e.g., ankle clonus, brisk reflexes, extensor plantar responses, palmomental reflex).

6. Observation of the infant or child with a motor problem frequently is omitted. Cerebral palsy is a disorder of movement and posture, and observation of spontaneous activity can be helpful clinically even when it is not diagnostic.

7. All cerebral palsy patients are mixed in type to some degree; guidelines must be developed for distinguishing these subtypes and relating them to cerebral topography.

8. All cerebral palsy is asymmetrical to some degree.

9. Adderlike movements (tongue thrusts) of the tongue or choreiform oromotor movements indicate a significant degree of choreoathetosis.

10. If a symmetrical tonic neck reflex is prominent, choreoathetosis should be sought.

11. If the upper extremities are significantly involved, oromotor dysfunction should be sought, and vice versa.

12. If the examiner is in doubt about the degree of extrapyramidal involvement, the infant should be examined when asleep because quietness accentuates the hypotonia.

13. The examination of deep tendon reflexes is not clinically helpful and actually can be confusing, particularly if they are symmetrical.

14. If one developmental stream (motor) is involved, another stream is likely to be involved as well (language, problem solving).

15. The "cross" evaluation should be used in motor dysfunction; each of the four extremities should be individually evaluated neurodevelopmentally for functional and physiologic manifestations, which then yield a topographic diagnosis.

MANAGEMENT

Because cerebral palsy reflects a static encephalopathy, reversibility is unobtainable and therapy must focus on either surgical intervention to circumvent the cerebral lesion or medical/ nonsurgical management of the limbs. These strategies and their implementations vary with the expertise and orientation of the various subspecialties involved in care. For example, orthopedic surgery monitors the motor development and intervenes periodically to prevent or correct deformities or to maintain or enhance motor abilities (Bleck, 1987). Lower extremity surgery includes such procedures as adductor tenotomy with or without obturator neurectomy for hip subluxation, femoral osteotomy for femoral anteversion, and arthrodesis for joint stabilization. Muscle transfers are also performed. Lower extremity involvement appears to benefit more from surgery, mainly because of the larger and fewer muscles and joints required for effective gross movement. Only a limited number of surgical procedures are available for upper extremity functional enhancement, because fine motor improvement is much more difficult to obtain. One of the newer procedures is rhizotomy, in which the posterior branches of the spinal nerves producing spasticity are severed. This operation alleviates spasticity and can provide more balanced muscle tone and better function in the involved limbs. In addition, intrathecal Baclofen and Botulin-A toxin studies are being pursued to determine efficacy.

Stereotactic brain surgery has been abandoned because of concern that such operations might impair speech and language. With improved techniques to isolate the target areas to be "destroyed," thalamic surgical measures will probably be rejuvenated.

Short leg braces, long leg braces with and without pelvic bands, crutches, various types of canes, and other orthotic devices are used in comprehensive care programs. In addition to the goals centered on the preventive aspects of orthopedic complications and function enhancement, they can also be used to determine potential effectiveness of surgery.

Within the medical armamentarium, one must not neglect the various medications that are available to alter muscle tone to prevent deformities and improve function. Dantrolene, diazepam, and baclofen (Albright, Cervi, & Singletary, 1991; Young & Delwaid, 1981) also can alleviate the flexor spasm that commonly follows surgical procedures of the hip, but the use of these drugs as well as other research pharmacologic agents must be carefully titrated against a child's total clinical picture (Armstrong, 1992).

The most common form of physical therapy employed in the United States is neurodevelopmental treatment, based on the concept that normal postural control against gravity is significantly compromised by cerebral damage. The Bobaths were pioneers in the development of this form of therapy, in which the early infantile tonic reflexes are analyzed along with the postural (righting and equilibrium) reflexes for synthesis of primary motor patterns. Passive positioning is introduced to inhibit the impact of primitive reflexes and to reduce the hypertonus. Postural reactions are simultaneously facilitated to give the child the experience of normal movements. Parents are taught to execute the various positioning maneuvers at home. The effectiveness of this therapeutic modality is still under debate (Law et al., 1991; Palmer et al., 1988).

Another therapy is sensory integration, based on an assumed failure of integration of tactile and proprioceptive inputs from the trunk and extremities that precludes proper vestibular function. This form of therapy was previously used with children with learning disabilities. Other interventions include the Rood method, in which various stimuli such as cold and heat reduce the hypertonus by simultaneously stimulating contraction of the antagonistic muscles. The Doman-Delacato approach stemmed from Temple Faye's interpretation of the evolution of crawling, with ontogeny recapitulating phylogeny. This therapy uses "patterning" (passive positioning and exercise) to imitate the evolutionary process of crawling from that exhibited by fish, amphibians, reptiles, primates, and humans. This form of therapy places serious demands on the family to carry out a home program. Conductive education (the Peto system) has not fared well in controlled outcome studies (Bairstow, Cochrane, & Hur, 1993).

Although these interventions have not been subjected to proper scientific scrutiny, they are used in the total management program (see Chapter 33, Volume I). Currently, the optimal form of management for the motor involvement of cerebral palsy appears to be a combination of home physical therapy input and continuing orthopedic surveillance to determine the necessity and timing of indicated surgical intervention. Drug therapy should be used sparingly when indicated.

CONCLUSIONS

Cerebral palsy represents a collection of complex and distinct motor disorders that exhibit sufficient family resemblance to be grouped together. It remains the most common cause of significant motor delay in childhood. "Floppy" infants will most commonly be diagnosed as having cerebral palsy or benign cerebral hypotonia, and only rarely will qualify for a diagnosis of congenital myopathy. The diagnosis of cerebral palsy is especially difficult early in infancy and requires a careful assessment of motor milestones, classic neurologic findings, motor deviance as reflected in a pattern of primitive postural and equilibrium responses, and a spectrum of associated central nervous system deficits. Therapeutic modalities include physical therapy, orthotic devices, orthopedic surgery, and drugs. The complex clinical evolution of each case makes accurate judgment of the efficacy of interventions very difficult.

REFERENCES

Aksu, F. (1990). Nature and prognosis of seizures in patients with cerebral palsy. *Developmental Medicine and Child Neurology, 32*, 661–668.

Albright, A.L., Cervi, A., & Singletary, J. (1991). Intrathecal baclofen for spasticity in cerebral palsy. *JAMA, 265*, 1418–1422.

Armstrong, R.W. (1992). Intrathecal baclofen and spasticity: What do we know and what do we need to know? *Developmental Medicine and Child Neurology, 34*, 739–745.

Bairstow, P., Cochrane, R., & Hur, J. (1993). *Evaluation of conductive education for children with cerebral palsy: Final reports (Parts I and II)*. London: Her Majesty's Stationery Office.

Bax, M.C.O. (1964). Terminology and classification of cerebral palsy. *Developmental Medicine and Child Neurology, 6*, 295–297.

Blair, E., & Stanley, F. (1985). Interobserver agreement in the classification of cerebral palsy. *Developmental Medicine and Child Neurology, 27*, 615–622.

Blasco, P.A. (1994). Primitive reflexes: Their contribution to the early detection of cerebral palsy. *Clinical Pediatrics, 33*, 388–397.

Blasco, P.A., Allaire, J.H., & Consortium on Drooling. (1992). Drooling in the developmentally disabled: Management practices and recommendations. *Developmental Medicine and Child Neurology, 34*, 849–862.

Bleck, E. (1987). *Orthopaedic management in cerebral palsy* (Clinics in Developmental Medicine, No. 99/100). Oxford: Blackwell Scientific Publications.

Candy, E.J., Hoon, A.H., Capute, A.J., & Bryan, R.N. (1993). MRI in motor delay: Important adjunct to classification in cerebral palsy. *Pediatric Neurology, 9*, 421–429.

Capute, A.J. (1979). Identifying cerebral palsy in infancy through study of primitive reflex profiles. *Pediatric Annals, 8*, 589–595.

Capute, A.J., Accardo, P.J., Vining, E.P.G., Rubenstein, J.E., & Harryman, S. (1978). *Primitive reflex profile*. (Monographs in developmental pediatrics, Vol. 1.) Baltimore: University Park Press.

Capute, A.J., Palmer, F.B., Shapiro, B.K., Wachtel, R.C., Ross, A., & Accardo, P.J. (1984). Primitive reflex profile: A quantitation of primitive reflexes in infancy. *Developmental Medicine and Child Neurology, 25*, 375–383.

Capute, A.J., & Shapiro, B.K. (1985). The motor quotient: A method for early detection of motor delay. *American Journal of Diseases of Children, 139*, 940–942.

Capute, A.J., Shapiro, B.K., & Palmer, F.B. (1981). Spectrum of developmental disabilities: Continuum of motor dysfunction. *Orthopedic Clinics of North America, 12*, 3–22.

Coorssen, E.A., Msall, M.E., & Duffy, L.C. (1991). Multiple minor malformations as a marker for prenatal etiology of cerebral palsy. *Developmental Medicine and Child Neurology, 33*, 730–736.

Law, M., Cadman, D., Rosenbaum, P., Walter, S., Russell, D., & DeMatteo, C. (1991). Neurodevelopmental therapy and upper extremity inhibitive casting for children with cerebral palsy. *Developmental Medicine and Child Neurology, 33*, 379–387.

Nelson, K.B. (1988) What proportion of cerebral palsy is related to birth asphyxia? *Journal of Pediatrics, 112*, 572–574.

O'Malley, P.J., & Griffith, J.F. (1977). Perceptuomotor dysfunction in the child with hemiplegia. *Developmental Medicine and Child Neurology, 19*, 172–178.

Palmer, F.B., Shapiro, B.Y., Wachtel, R.C., et al. (1988). The effects of physical therapy on cerebral palsy: A controlled trial in infants with gastric diplegia. *New England Journal of Medicine, 318,* 803–808.

Perlstein, M.A. (1961). *Kernicterus and its importance in cerebral palsy.* Springfield, IL: Charles C Thomas.

Prechtl, H.F.R., & Stemmer, C.J. (1962). The choreiform syndrome in children. *Developmental Medicine and Child Neurology, 4,* 119–127.

Shapiro, B.K., Green, P., Krick, J., Allen, D., & Capute, A.J. (1986). Growth of severely impaired children: Neurological versus nutritional factors. *Developmental Medicine and Child Neurology, 28,* 729–733.

Stallings, V.A., Charney, E.B., Davies, J.C., & Cronk, C.E. (1993). Nutritional status and growth of children with diplegic or hemiplegic cerebral palsy. *Developmental Medicine and Child Neurology, 35,* 997–1006.

Wiklund, L.-M., & Uvebrant, P. (1991). Hemiplegic cerebral palsy: Correlation between CT morphology and clinical findings. *Developmental Medicine and Child Neurology, 33,* 512–523.

Young, R.R., & Delwaid, P.J. (1981). Drug therapy: Spasticity. *New England Journal of Medicine, 304,* 28–33; 96–99.

Automated Responses in Infant Screening for Cerebral Palsy

Moro Reflex

Description   On sudden extension of the head, there is rapid, symmetrical abduction and upward movement of the arms. The hands open and there is gradual adduction and flexion of the arms in a clasping position; a similar but milder pattern or movement may be observed in the lower extremities.

Technique   The child is lifted in supine and the head is allowed to drop back suddenly from about 3 cm off a padded surface (Figure 4).

Grading

0   Absent. (If the response is flexion, the Moro is absent.)

1+   Minimal arm extension and abduction. Momentary extension of the fingers followed by some finger flexion may be observed.

2+   Arm extension/abduction immediately followed by arm adduction or wrist flexion.

3+   In addition to a 2+ response, the back arches (with minimal opisthotonus), or full (180-degree) extension of the lower extremities is observed.

4+   Obligatory neck extension, shoulder retraction, and back arching produce a picture of marked opisthotonus; finger splaying also is observed.

Galant Reflex

Description   On being stroked on the back along the paravertebral area, the child arches his or her trunk with concavity toward the stimulated side.

Technique   The child is tested in prone suspension. The back is stroked with a dressmaker's tracing wheel paravertebrally (approximately 2 cm from the midline) from about T5 to the sacrum (Figure 5). (A Wardenburg Sensory Testing Wheel may be used, but this tends to yield somewhat higher scores.) Lateral movement of the trunk is noted. This is repeated five times in succession on each side with the head in a flexed or neutral position. Testing may need to be repeated with a varying rate and pressure

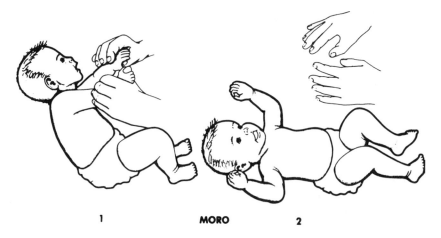

1   **MORO**   2

Figure 4.   Moro reflex.

From Capute, A.J., Accardo, P.J., Vining, E.P.G., Rubenstein, J.E., & Harryman, S. (1978). *Primitive reflex profile. Monographs in developmental pediatrics, Vol. 1.* Baltimore: University Park Press; reprinted by permission of the authors.

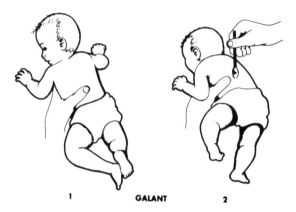

Figure 5. Galant reflex.

of stimulus after allowing the trunk to return to the midline.

Grading

0   Absent.
1+   Very mild and inconsistent truncal incurvature; more felt than seen.
2+   Persistent truncal incurvature less than 45 degrees.
3+   Exaggerated truncal incurvature with hips swinging laterally to 45 degrees or more.
4+   Persistent hip elevation.

Asymmetrical Tonic Neck Reflex (ATNR)

Description   When the child is in supine, he or she may be seen to lie with the head turned to one side, with extension of the extremities on that side (chin side) and flexion of the contralateral extremities (occiput side). This also may be noted in sitting; it often is described as the "fencer" position.

Technique   The child is placed in supine and observed for active head turning and subsequent extremity movement. The head then is turned passively (through 180 degrees) alternately to each side for 5 seconds (Figure 6). This is repeated five times on each side. If no movement is noted, the head turning is repeated and changes in tone are observed. Consistent tone changes must be felt in at least two extremities for the reflex to be scored as present.

Grading

0   Absent.
1+   With passive head rotation, there is no visible response but increased extensor tone

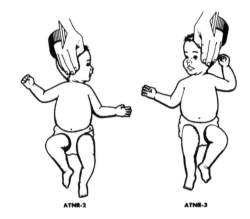

Figure 6. Asymmetrical tonic neck reflex.

is noted in extremities on chin side or increased flexor tone on occiput side. (Active movement may elicit visible response.)

2+   With passive movement of the head, visible extension of extremities on chin side or flexion on occiput side is noted. (In some babies, the visible component will be limited to flexion/extension of the fingers.)

3+   Passive head movement produces full (180-degree), if transient, extension in the extremities on the chin side or more than full (90-degree) flexion of extremities on the occiput side. (The upper extremities of some babies with a positive tonic labyrinthine reflex will start from a position of flexion, and therefore only slight visible movement will cause them to be scored 3+.)

4+ Obligatory (more than 30-second) extension of extremities on chin side or flexion of extremities on occiput side.

Symmetrical Tonic Neck Reflex (STNR)

Description On extending the head in midline, the arms extend and the legs flex; flexion of the head has the opposite effect—the arms flex and the legs extend.

Technique Active neck extension/flexion is sought through visual stimulus or command. Movement and tone change in the extremities are assessed. The neck is then passively extended and flexed; this is repeated five times for extension and flexion. In the newborn infant, upper extremity changes are best noted in prone suspension. In older infants, upper and lower extremity changes are best assessed in a supported sitting position (i.e., on the mother's lap) (Figure 7). (Because tone changes and movement in single extremities can be caused by overlap with either the tonic labyrinthine or Landau reflex, scoring is limited to patients demonstrating the reflex with consistent [3 of 5] and appropriate tone changes in at least one upper and one lower extremity.)

Grading

0   Absent.

1+ No visible response with passive neck extension, but increased extensor tone is noted in upper extremities and increased flexor tone in lower extremities; the reverse is noted with neck flexion. (Active head movement may elicit transient visible responses.)

2+ With passive neck extension, there is visible extension of the upper extremities or flexion of the lower extremities; the reverse is noted with neck flexion.

3+ Movement (as in 2+) is noted with full (180-degree) extension or more than full (90-degree) flexion of at least one extremity.

4+ With head manipulation, an obligatory (more than 30-second) reflex posture (as in 3+) is observed.

Positive Support Reaction (PSR)

Description On stimulation of the hallucal area, co-contraction of opposing muscle groups occurs so as to fix the joints of the lower extremities in a position capable of supporting weight.

Technique The child is suspended around the trunk below the axillae with the head in a neutral or midline flexed position and bounced five times on the balls of the feet. The balls of the feet then are brought in contact with the floor and the child held in a vertical position to assess the degree of supporting response (Figure 8).

Grading

0   Absent; child goes into flexion and does not support his or her weight.

1+ The child supports his or her weight momentarily (between 1 and 30 seconds).

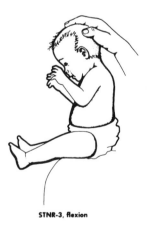
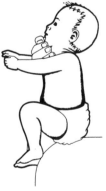

STNR-3, flexion   STNR-3, extension

Figure 7. Symmetrical tonic neck reflex.

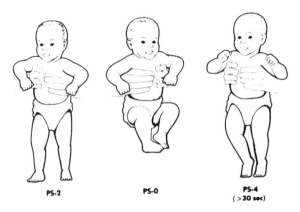

PS-2   PS-0   PS-4
                          (>30 sec)

Figure 8. Positive support reaction.

2+ The child is able to support his or her weight for longer than 30 seconds, with a quick (less than 5-second) movement from plantar flexion to dorsiflexion (i.e., the heel makes contact with the examining surface).

3+ There is delayed movement from plantar flexion to dorsiflexion; the child remains in the equinus position longer than 5 seconds but less than 30 seconds.

4+ The child remains (longer than 30 seconds) in an equinus position. (The child is unable to move out of this position without circumducting the legs.)

Tonic Labyrinthine Response

Description The position of the extremity changes with respect to the position of the head in space (orientation of labyrinths). With the neck extended 45 degrees, the limbs extend; with the neck flexed 45 degrees, the limbs flex (Figure 9).

Technique

Tonic Labyrinthine in Supine (TLS) In a supine position, support is placed between the shoulders so that the head is extended 45 degrees. Position and tone of the extremities (especially the shoulders) are assessed. Active neck flexion and grasp in the midline are sought

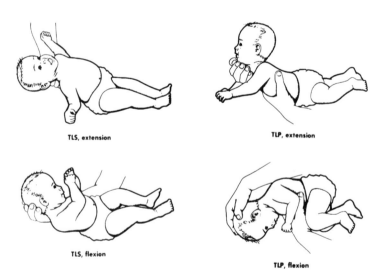

TLS, extension   TLP, extension

TLS, flexion

TLP, flexion

Figure 9. Tonic labyrinthine response: *Left,* in supine; *right,* in prone.

through visual stimulus or command. If active neck flexion beyond the midposition with grasp in the midline is not noted, the head then is flexed passively 45 degrees with the back still supported, and midline grasp again is sought.

Grading

0   Absent. (This may be seen in the "floppy" infant.)

1+   Increased extensor tone is felt in the neck, shoulders, trunk, or lower extremities, but shoulder retraction and extremity extension are not observed. (Neck flexion may be accompanied by some nonreflex protraction of the shoulders, with the hands approaching the midline.)

2+   With the head in extension, there is visible shoulder retraction. Trunk or leg extension (less than 180 degrees) may be noted; neck flexion results in shoulder protraction within 5 seconds and the disappearance of extensor posture.

3+   Response as in 2+ but with head flexion; shoulder retraction or full (180-degree) extension of lower extremities persists (5 to 30 seconds).

4+   With head flexion, shoulder retraction or full lower extremity extension persists (for more than 30 seconds).

Tonic Labyrinthine in Prone (TLP)   The child is held in prone suspension; the head is extended 45 degrees below the horizontal. Changes of posture and tone of extremities (especially the shoulders) are evaluated. Consistent tone changes must be present in at least one upper and one lower extremity for the reflex to be scored as present.

Grading

0   Absent.

1+   With head flexion, an increase in flexor tone is noted in the extremities.

2+   With head flexion, visible protraction of the shoulders or flexion of the lower extremities is noted.

3+   With the head flexed, the shoulders are protracted with the upper extremities under the trunk, or hips or knees flexed more than 90 degrees.

4+   With head flexion, the upper extremities remain protracted under the trunk or the lower extremities remain fully (greater than 90 degrees) flexed for greater than 30 seconds.

Derotative Righting Reaction

Description   The body turns to untwist itself in a segmental (derotational) fashion when rotation is applied along the body axis.

Technique   The child is placed in a supine position.

Segmental Rotation, Head on Body (SR-HB)   Initially, the head is flexed to approximately 45 degrees and slowly rotated in order to turn the shoulders; body rotation then is observed (Figure 10A). The head is manipulated with one hand on the side of the face near the chin and the other on the occiput. When the child is rolled to the right, the examiner's left hand is the face hand and the examiner's right hand is the occiput hand; when the child is rolled to the left, the positions of the examiner's hands are reversed.

Segmental Rotation, Body on Body (SR-BB)   One leg, flexed at the hip and knee, is held below the knee and, with that leg, the child is rotated to turn the pelvis toward the midline; body rotation then is observed (Figure 10B).

Grading

0   Body does not follow when head and shoulders are turned 30 degrees past midline; head and shoulders do not follow when hips are turned 30 degrees past midline (this is observed in "floppy" infants).

1+   The child does not roll over until the midline is surpassed by 30 degrees; performed in a derotational fashion.

2+   Before having the shoulders or hips reach the midline, the child completes the maneuver in a derotational (segmental) fashion; that is, movement occurs in a proximal-to-distal fashion when the head is turned (HB) and in a distal-to-proximal fashion when the pelvis is turned (BB).

3+   The body turns in a nonderotational manner; that is, rotating head on body, lower extremities rotate before upper; when ro-

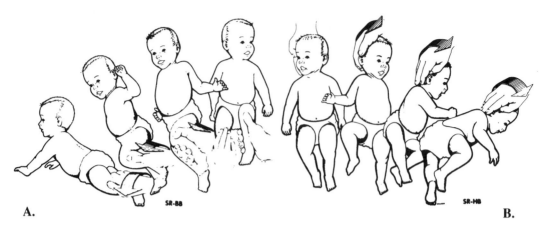

Figure 10.   Derotative righting reaction: *A*, head on body; *B*, body on body.

tating body on body, head and upper extremities rotate before lower extremities.

4+   The body follows repetitively in a "log-rolling" manner: When rotating head on body, the upper and lower extremities turn simultaneously; when rotating body on body, the head and upper extremities turn simultaneously. (As long as the hip and shoulder movements are simultaneous, the child does not need to complete the maneuver.)

Chapter 7

Orthopedic Intervention in Cerebral Palsy

Peter A. Blasco, M.D.

Among the surgical subspecialists involved in the care of children with cerebral palsy, the pediatric orthopedist is the most notable. This chapter is an attempt to describe the patient with cerebral palsy as seen through the eyes of the orthopedist, but it is written from the developmental pediatrician's point of view. The intent is to provide a primer in orthopedic evaluation and management for the developmental specialist and for the general pediatrician or family practitioner interested in the care of children with developmental disabilities. As an assist, terminology that is largely unique to orthopedics has been summarized in a glossary at the end of the chapter.

CLINICAL ASSESSMENT

Many view clinical orthopedics as a matter of simple logic—if a tendon is contracted, it is cut and lengthened. However, the mechanics of movement are much too complicated to allow for this simplistic view. Most muscles of ambulation are *two-joint* muscles. If you alter a tendon (or a bone), usually two joints are directly influenced and often a third is impacted by the domino effect. Gage (1991) viewed all the muscles and joints of ambulation as a system in balance, and each must be accounted for clinically when contemplating intervention, even for an apparently isolated abnormality.

The orthopedic clinical evaluation is based primarily on 1) a detailed visual and hands-on inspection of joint mobility and alignment, and 2) the subjective and sometimes objective analysis of the mechanical characteristics of posture and gait. Motor developmental milestones are accorded appropriate attention, but the cognitive aspects of development are addressed less completely. The neurologic examination, focusing on strength, tone, reflexes, and coordination, is thorough but less rigorous than that performed by the child neurologist or developmental pediatrician.

Subtypes of cerebral palsy are classified based on the extremities involved (e.g., hemiplegic, diplegic) and on the predominant movement disorder or tone pattern. The orthopedist will be very exact in describing which limbs are involved but tends to be less precise in diagnosing the exact nature of the underlying neurologic substrate. The orthopedic emphasis is on intervention (therapy, bracing, equipment, and surgery), and etiology most often receives little attention unless there is concern that an acute or a progressive process is occurring. In every respect, the orthopedic clinical approach to diagnosis complements information generated by professionals from other disciplines, especially the developmental pediatrician and the physical therapist. The expertise in the mechanics of movement is unique to the orthopedist and can rarely be provided by another discipline. Hence it comes as no surprise that especially close working relationships often develop between the pediatric orthopedist, the pediatric physical therapist, and the developmental pediatrician.

This chapter was written with expert advice generously provided by orthopedic colleagues Michael D. Sussman, M.D., John E. Lonstein, M.D., Tom F. Novachek, M.D., James R. Gage, M.D., Deborah S. Quanbeck, M.D., and Steven E. Koop, M.D.

Examination of Gait

The evaluation of station and gait is primarily done by visual inspection of body alignment, joint movement, and functional movement patterns. Objective measures of gait have recently become available through the use of the gait laboratory and gait analysis, both of which are addressed briefly later.

Station is defined as the position or posture assumed in standing (or sitting). Human stance is assessed from anterior, lateral, and posterior viewpoints with the subject standing erect. It is also valuable to view the individual from behind while he or she is bending forward (Figure 1). *Gait*, of course, refers to walking. Typically, the infant begins to walk without support around 1 year of age. He or she steps with a wide base and relative flexion of the hips and knees, holds the arms in abduction and the el-

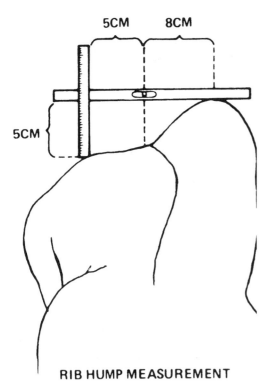

RIB HUMP MEASUREMENT

Figure 1.   Posterior view of trunk in a person with scoliosis. With the patient bent over, the hump associated with scoliosis becomes quite striking. (From Bleck, E.E. [1987]. *Orthopedic management in cerebral palsy* [Clinics in Developmental Medicine, No. 99/100, p. 31]. London: MacKeith Press; reprinted by permission.)

bows in flexion, and moves in a staccato manner. The width of the base diminishes gradually, movements become smoother, reciprocal arm swing appears, step length and walking velocity both increase, and an adult pattern of walking emerges by about 3 years of age. The 3-year-old's typical gait pattern shows a vigorous walk, reciprocal arm swing, well-developed heel strike, and smooth movements, all of which differ only slightly from those of an adult. By age 7, the child's gait is indistinguishable from that of an adult. *Step length*—defined as the distance covered in one step—obviously is related to leg length but also depends on muscle tone and range of joint motion. *Stride length* is the distance covered in two steps (i.e., one complete *gait cycle*). The *base* of the gait, measured as the perpendicular distance between the heels, is normally 5–10 cm, although it can be narrower.

Gait is assessed in progress, rather than beginning from a stationary position (Gage, 1991; Sutherland, 1984) (Figure 2). With the trunk slightly forward because of forward progression, the normal gait cycle begins with *heel strike* (better referred to as *initial contact*), whereby the leading foot first makes contact with the floor. It proceeds through *stance phase,* then *swing phase,* and then ends with heel strike of the same foot. Stance phase represents 60% of the gait cycle and swing phase 40%. Single-limb stance phase begins just after heel strike, when the ankle is flexed at a 90-degree angle (referred to as neutral), the knee is nearly fully extended, and the hip is flexed about 40 degrees. The ankle plantar flexes to get the foot flat on the floor as the body mass progresses forward over the stance-phase foot. In midstance, the foot is still flat on the floor, but the ankle is slightly dorsiflexed and the knee is slightly flexed as well. As the body continues forward, the foot remains flat and the ankle goes into increasing dorsiflexion while the knee progressively extends. As the contralateral foot makes initial floor contact (heel strike), the double-limb phase of stance begins. The stance foot rocks forward (i.e., the heel comes up from the floor) and prepares for *toe-off* as weight is transferred to the contralateral leg. Just before leaving the ground (toe-off, also called *terminal contact*) to enter swing phase, the ankle is plan-

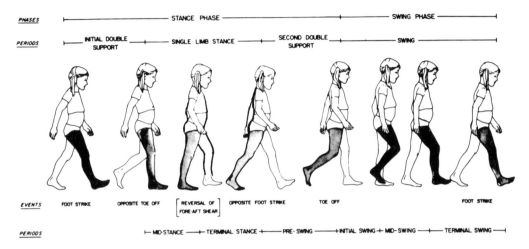

Figure 2. Normal gait cycle of a 7-year-old child. (From Sutherland, D.H. [1984]. *Gait disorders in childhood and adolescence,* p. 11. Baltimore: Williams & Wilkins; reprinted by permission.)

tar flexed 10–15 degrees and the knee is flexed 35 degrees.

Swing phase is separated into three periods: initial swing, midswing, and terminal swing. During initial swing, the knee and ankle must flex in order for the foot to clear the ground. This is followed by full extension of the knee as the leg swings through to terminal swing. Swing phase ends with heel strike, completing one gait cycle. Velocity during gait is not constant but varies slightly, speeding up through swing phase and slowing during stance phase.

As gait proceeds, the head moves up and down in a low sinusoidal curve. If one marks the center of gravity, located at about midpelvis, it describes essentially the same curve. The pelvis makes very little lateral rotational movement during gait. The more bobbing (up-and-down) movement that is created, the less efficient the gait becomes, leading to increased oxygen consumption.

In lower extremity spasticity, the typical pattern is one of a tendency toward flexion and adduction at the hip, flexion at the knee, plantar flexion (*equinus*) at the foot, and internal rotation of the entire lower extremity. This pattern produces a gait with increased bobbing of the pelvis, anterior pelvic tilt with lumbar hyperlordosis, increased side-to-side sway, decreased step length (because the knee and hip are restricted in extending), a wide base, abrupt changes in velocity, and a tendency to stay on the toes and therefore strike on the toe or forefoot rather than on the heel. This "natural" dynamic of the spastic limb produces extreme forces on the foot. Over time, instability of the subtalar joint frequently leads to collapse of the foot into a *valgus* position. In spastic diplegia, this usually occurs bilaterally. In hemiplegia, there tends to be little spastic hip adduction, more involvement in terms of knee and hip flexion, and an equinus foot. Eventually a heel cord contracture often develops.

Ataxic and choreoathetoid gaits have their own unique characteristics, which are both more complex and more variable than those of the spastic syndromes. The major features are a wide base and excessive body sway in ataxia and variable postural stability with erratic, jerky extremity movements in the choreoathetosis. The hallmark of these patterns is nonreproducibility on gait analysis.

Gait Analysis

The objective description of normal gait and gait disorders involves a thorough knowledge of force plate values, movement measurements, and electromyography. These measurements provide the foundation for kinematic description of movement (its geometry) and kinetic analysis of gait (the underlying forces). In children with cerebral palsy, there is an exceedingly complex interplay of tone abnormality, contracture, bone deformity, weakness, and multiple-joint dynamics that lead to gait aberrations. With the advent of gait analysis technology, objective criteria can begin to play a more prominent role in analyzing problems of locomotion in order to make rational decisions about surgery, orthotics, drugs, and physical therapy. Experienced clinicians appreciate that the decision not to treat is of equal if not more value than the decision to treat. In addition, gait analysis information allows the clinician to make objective comparisons before and after treatment to better understand the efficacy of his or her therapeutic maneuvers.

The sophisticated gait analysis laboratory requires a biotelemetry system consisting of three major subsystems: optical, electronic, and computer. The *optical system* requires motion picture recording with two or more cameras for true three-dimensional measurement. The subject to be studied is prepared with attached surface markers—sticks or light reflectors—placed at various critical points, especially joints. In addition, a digital time display is linked with the video.

The *electronic system* consists of force plate and electromyography (EMG) components. The force plate is a foot pressure sensor that is mounted in the floor. It measures forces in three planes: vertical, fore-and-aft, and medial–lateral. Muscle group electrical activity is monitored with surface electrodes for large muscle groups (e.g., hip adductors). Deeper muscles and isolated muscles cannot be monitored without the use of internal (i.e., needle) electrodes. These fine-wire intramuscular electrodes have limited use for clinical evaluations, especially in children. In addition, a sensor, called a *foot switch*, may be placed on each heel to indicate the instant of heel strike. Battery-operated radio transmitter units are used to relay these electrical pressure and EMG signals to a computer.

A *computer system* performs all calculations from the data gathered and presents them in either graphic or tabular form. It also creates a permanent record for storage on digital tape.

There are five major determinants of mature gait: duration of single-limb stance, walking velocity (i.e., the average distance traveled per second), cadence (i.e., the number of steps per minute), step length, and the ratio of pelvic span to ankle spread. Mean values for gait events in a group of normal 7-year-olds are shown in Figure 3.

Energy is required to walk, and the measurement of oxygen consumption during gait is the ultimate test of the cost of walking in terms of energy expenditure (Gage, 1991).

Passive Examination

Leg length should be measured with the patient supine using a tape measure. Measurement is from the anterior superior iliac spine to the medial malleolus. If the patient has a flexion contracture of the knee joint, the measurement should follow the contour of the leg itself. It can be divided into two measurements that are added in order to get an actual measurement of the limb length. *Orthoroentgenograms*, which are basically long-distance radiographs designed to measure bone length accurately require the patient to stand and are little used with people with cerebral palsy. *Scanograms* are most frequently used to measure bone length radiographically, particularly in hemiplegic children, and involve shooting a series of films that focus on a long ruler adjacent to the limb being examined.

Passive range of motion is intended to be a maximum (but not painful) measure and therefore requires that the patient be maximally relaxed. Obviously, this is not always possible in the awake infant and younger child. Hip range of motion is defined in terms of abduction and adduction. Hip abduction may be described in terms of the angle of the femurs when both are abducted or in terms of each femur individually as the angle of the abducted hip with a vertical plane. The latter method is preferable in order to identify and clearly document any asymmetry. Observations are made both with the hips flexed at 90 degrees and with them extended. The full range in the flexed position is normally 80–90 degrees on each side. With the legs extended, the normal range is 45–50 degrees on each side. Hip flexion contracture is common and can be measured in two ways, using either the Thomas test with the patient in supine (which is easier to accomplish) or the more accurate but more difficult method of Staheli (1977) with the patient in prone (Figure 4). With the patient in prone and the hips flush with the end of the table, the examiner places one hand on the posterior supe-

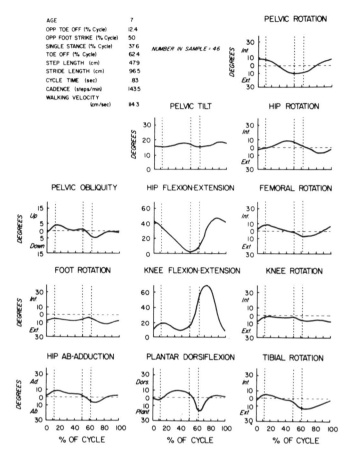

Figure 3. Mean values for gait events in a group of normal 7-year-old children. The column in the upper left-hand corner presents numerical data on events related to time and distance during walking. The graphs describe specific joint angles and their changes during the gait cycle. The first hashed vertical line represents initial toe-off, the second heel strike, and the third contralateral toe-off. (From Sutherland, D.H. [1984]. *Gait disorders in childhood and adolescence*, p. 22. Baltimore: Williams & Wilkins; reprinted by permission.)

rior iliac spines while the other hand brings the lower limb slowly into extension. The point at which the examiner feels the pelvis begin to rotate forward is the point of deformity. Limitation of extension can be produced by a tight iliopsoas, a tight rectus femoris, or a tight tensor fascia lata (or its tendon, the iliotibial band). The normal range of hip extension is 0–20 degrees except in newborns, who have physiologic flexion contractures usually in the neighborhood of −25 degrees.

Internal (medial) and external (lateral) hip rotation are measured with the patient in prone and the knees flexed to 90 degrees (Figure 5). The pelvis must be firmly stabilized to prevent hip rotation caused by lateral rolling of the pelvis. These values change substantially during childhood. Internal rotation is least in infants

and increases with age, reaching values of 20–60 degrees in adolescence. External rotation in infants averages 70 degrees and declines in adolescence to a range of 25–65 degrees.

During any of these examinations, further flexion of the knee (or abduction of the hip) done in a rapid manner can detect tightness (either spasticity or a contracture) in the quadriceps (or adductor) muscle groups. Knee flexor tightness in the hamstrings can be reliably measured with the patient supine. With the leg lying flat, the knee should extend fully to 0 degrees. The upper leg is then raised to flex the hip at 90 degrees, and the lower leg is gradually extended to its limit. Normal extension in the adult decreases to about 10–20 degrees shy of a straight line, and this quantity is referred to as the *popliteal angle*. (This is not actually the angle

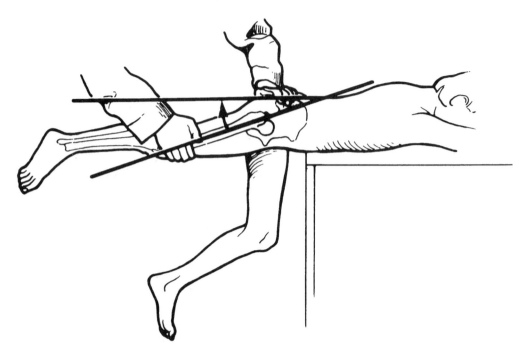

Figure 4.   Staheli's test for hip flexion contracture. The angle subtended by the femur and the horizontal plane represents the angle of hip *extension*. Therefore, angles above the horizontal are positive and those below are negative. (From Bleck, E.E. [1987]. *Orthopedic management in cerebral palsy.* [Clinics in Developmental Medicine, No. 99/100, p. 50]. London: MacKeith Press; reprinted by permission.)

of the popliteal space but rather the complement to it.) Newborns demonstrate physiologic knee flexion contractures, with a popliteal angle range of 20–40 degrees. This decreases to 0 degrees by 9–10 months of age (Reade, Hom, Hallum, & Lopopolo, 1984). At the same time, the position of the patella should be noted in relation to its normal location in the patellofemoral groove. Flexion contracture within the knee joint itself can be distinguished to some extent from hamstring contracture by simply observing the knee in relaxed extension flat on the table (i.e., with the hip extended). If firm pressure on the anterior aspect of the knee joint fails to extend the knee completely, a contracture of the joint itself is likely present. In the presence of a severe hamstring contracture, it would be practically impossible to identify additional contracture within the joint capsule.

Lower leg deformities generally are described in terms of tibial–fibular torsion and foot rotation. If the tibia is twisted inward (*internal tibial torsion*), the feet turn in. If the femurs are turned inward (*femoral anteversion*), the feet and the knees as well turn in. Precise measurements of tibial–fibular torsion are difficult and time con-

suming, but good approximations are easy and quick. Bleck (1987) recommended observing the patient sitting comfortably with knees flexed over the edge of the table (Figure 6). The angle from an imaginary line through the malleoli that intersects the plane of the table edge estimates the amount of tibial rotation (or torsion), which is normally in a range of 0–45 degrees (external). The thigh–foot angle is a close approximation of the same thing and is also easily measured. With the patient in prone and the knee flexed at 90 degrees, an imaginary line is drawn bisecting the thigh (femur) through the heel and another is drawn bisecting the plantar aspect of the foot. The intersection of these lines represents a slightly narrower angle than the one obtained by the previously described method, and the normal range is from −3 to +20 degrees. The foot must be at rest when carrying out either of these measurements. (For details, see Bleck, 1987, and Staheli, 1985.)

A foot that is positioned with the plane of the toes pointing down (i.e., with more than a 90-degree angle) is in *equinus*, and with the plane of the toes pointing up is in *calcaneus*. When the *hindfoot* (commonly called the heel)

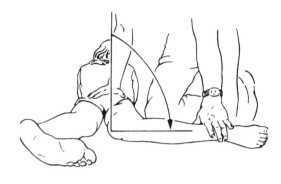

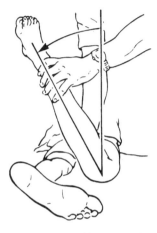

Figure 5. Measurement of hip internal rotation (top) and external rotation (bottom). (From Bleck, E.E. [1987]. *Orthopedic management in cerebral palsy* [Clinics in Developmental Medicine, No. 99/100, p. 50]. London: MacKeith Press; reprinted by permission.)

rolls in, it is called *varus*. When it rolls out, the foot appears to collapse medially, referred to as *valgus*. Varus is due to overpull of the tibialis posterior or tibialis anterior muscles. It is to be distinguished from *in-toeing*, which is due to rotation of the foot inward but with the heel still aligned flat on the floor. If these positions can be passively corrected, they are referred to as *dynamic*. If not, they are *fixed*. Equinus can also occur starting from the point of the midfoot, termed a *cavus deformity*. This excessive forefoot equinus is usually a fixed deformity and is also referred to as a *high arch*. Dorsiflexion of the ankle is measured with the foot held in slight inversion in order to lock the subtalar joint. It is important to check passive dorsiflexion with the knee both flexed and extended in order to distinguish soleus from gastrocnemius

contracture (the Silfverskiold test). With the knee flexed at 90 degrees, the gastrocnemius is relaxed, so any equinus deformity is due to contracture of the soleus. If deformity appears or worsens (i.e., there is *less* dorsiflexion possible) when the knee is extended, then the gastrocnemius is the main site of contracture or both muscles are implicated.

Toe deformities come in the form of flexion contractures and *hallux valgus*, an abduction deformity of the great toe. The former are common in individuals without cerebral palsy. In persons with cerebral palsy, they rarely cause a clinical problem in childhood. Hallux valgus, however, is associated with valgus foot deformity and can lead to significant pain at the first metatarsophalangeal joint in children with cerebral palsy.

Much of the passive orthopedic examination must be done on a floor mat or on a large examining table. Appreciating the ranges of normal and the subtle variations that depend on age and sex in typical children—let alone in children with various types of neuromuscular, connective tissue, or skeletal abnormalities—clearly depends on extensive clinical experience. This highlights the unique contribution of an experienced orthopedist to the interdisciplinary team.

COMMON CLINICAL CONDITIONS

The following are some commonly encountered conditions and minor deformities that may appear in isolation or may be associated with encephalopathy. In the latter circumstance, they may be more likely to require surgical intervention.

1. *Metatarsus adductus* is a term denoting adduction of the forefoot (i.e., curvature in a medial direction). In congenital metatarsus adductus, in contrast to congenital clubfoot, the heel is not in varus and there is no fixed equinus. In children with spastic cerebral palsy, spastic metatarsus adductus consists of forefoot adduction. It is a late-developing phenomenon and appears to be due to spasticity of the intrinsic muscles of the foot. Although initially dynamic, it tends to evolve into a fixed deformity (Bleck, 1987).

2. Congenital *clubfoot deformities* (*talipes equinovarus* and others) consist of varying de-

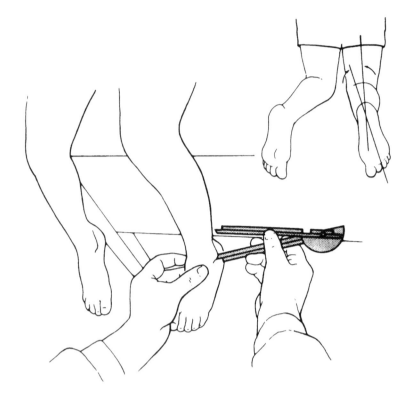

Figure 6. Measurement of tibial–fibular torsion. *Left,* A goniometer is used to measure the angle of the transmalleolar line and the vertical plane of the tibia (represented by the table edge). *Right,* The thigh–foot angle is determined from imaginary lines bisecting each. (From Bleck, E.E. [1987]. *Orthopedic management in cerebral palsy* [Clinics in Developmental Medicine, No. 99/100, p. 55]. London: MacKeith Press; reprinted by permission.)

grees of fixed foot deformity, equinovarus being the most common. Neither congenital nor acquired clubfeet are seen more commonly among children with cerebral palsy than in children without disabilities.

3. *Excessive tibial torsion* occurs more frequently in the presence of neurologic impairment. Surgical correction is rarely needed except in children with cerebral palsy or other neuromuscular disorders. Although internal tibial torsion may appear quite dramatic in the typical child, it will almost always self-correct by 3 years of age. Self-correction may occur in children with cerebral palsy as well.

4. *Excessive femoral anteversion* develops in almost all cases of spastic cerebral palsy. It can be thought of as maintenance of the fetal (newborn) angle rather than the creation of a new deformity. Femoral anteversion can be measured by radiography but is just as well monitored clinically. The femur has a normal angle of anteversion, so the abnormal circum-

stance should be called *increased* femoral anteversion. As with tibial torsion, even dramatic femoral anteversion in the child without disabilities almost always resolves spontaneously.

5. *Genu varum* and *genu valgum* are commonly referred to as "bow legs" and "knock knees," respectively. They rarely require surgery and are not seen more frequently in children with cerebral palsy than in children without disabilities. Genu varum is physiologic in the newborn, with the angle of the femur and tibia averaging +17 degrees. This progresses to a maximum valgus angle of −10 degrees at 3 years of age, then returns to the stable adult range of 0–10 degrees by 6 or 7 years of age (Salenius & Vankka, 1975). This is to be distinguished from Blount's disease, which is a pathologic entity consisting of progressive varus deformity of the proximal tibia (therefore *tibia* vara) and which does require surgical intervention.

6. *Congenital hip dysplasia and dislocation* has recently been renamed *developmental dys-*

plasia of the hip (DDH) to better reflect the evolving nature of the disorder. The hip is not really dysplastic at birth but becomes so in susceptible individuals. When unilateral, DDH is much more likely to be left sided than right sided. Bilateral involvement is present about one third of the time, and DDH is six times more common in girls than in boys. Almost all cases are considered idiopathic and occur in isolation. If coincidentally present in an infant with cerebral palsy, DDH is greatly aggravated by the presence of spasticity after birth. Acquired hip dislocations secondary to spasticity are addressed in the following section.

TREATMENT

General Considerations

The orthopedic surgeon's conceptual approach to treatment is no different from that of the developmental pediatrician. Ideally, all members of the interdisciplinary team approach the patient within the same general framework, which defines the elements of treatment as

1. Prerequisite data: accurate diagnosis of
   • Primary disability
   • Associated problems
2. Treatment modalities
   • Hands-on therapy
   • Orthoses
   • Adaptive and assistive equipment
   • Medical treatments
   • Surgery

Accurate diagnosis, including some appreciation for severity and for associated problems, is the essential first step toward understanding the patient's problems, both actual and potential, current and future. Treatment follows from this and begins with hands-on therapy interventions that may have immediate impact or are at least worth a trial for some period of time. Adaptive equipment (such as a seat insert), orthoses, and numerous other assistive devices (such as canes or an augmentative communication system) are provided as adjuncts.

At one time it was mistakenly believed that cumbersome metal and leather braces could "fully control" the limbs of children with cere-

bral palsy, allowing them to develop walking skills naturally without acquiring deformities. (These were the so-called Phelps braces, named for Winthrop Phelps, an orthopedist who pioneered many treatment approaches for children with cerebral palsy.) Orthotic devices are currently used to prevent deformity (i.e., through control of spasticity), to improve function (i.e., maintaining foot position in stance or swing), and occasionally to impose partial postoperative immobilization. They are now made primarily of lightweight plastic and are attached by means of Velcro straps. The AFO (ankle-foot orthosis) is particularly useful because it can control all motions of the foot and ankle: equinus, varus, and valgus. It is also convenient because it can be worn over a sock in an ordinary shoe. The primary indications for AFO use are spastic equinus or hypotonia, and AFO construction has a number of variations to suit specific purposes (Gage, 1991). Knee hyperextension (*genu recurvatum*) sometimes can be managed with a rigid AFO molded to keep the foot in a few degrees of dorsiflexion, thereby mechanically driving the knee toward more flexion (Rosenthal, Deutsch, Miller, Schumann, & Hall, 1975). As another example, after hamstring lengthening and posterior capsulectomy of the knee joint, the KAFO (knee-ankle-foot orthosis) can be employed to control excessive flexion for a variable length of time until the patient regains quadriceps strength and competence during gait (Bleck, 1987). Orthoses seem to have little benefit for choreoathetoid patients. They may be somewhat useful to help maintain a stable, plantar-grade foot position. The smaller shoe insert–type orthoses—heel cups or UCBLs (named for the original brand, University of California Biomechanics Laboratory)—have limited utility, although some advocate their use to stabilize the valgus hindfoot.

Medication management consists primarily of drug treatment intended specifically to diminish spasticity or lessen extraneous movements. The list of medications to choose from is very long, but the likelihood of gaining substantial clinical benefit (beyond modest tone reduction) is rather small. Diazepam is the drug most commonly employed and can reduce spastic as well as extrapyramidal hypertonus.

With all drug options, however, the balance between benefits and side effects is often quite narrow, and predicting whether a given drug will help or make matters worse is almost impossible. The use of baclofen intrathecally to relieve spasticity is a new treatment with some promise that is currently under investigation (Albright, Cervi, & Singletary, 1991; Armstrong, 1992). The extent of its benefits and associated risks is yet to be clearly defined. General pediatric care for associated medical problems (such as seizures) and intercurrent acute problems to which these children are more susceptible is an important element of the overall management plan.

Surgical intervention is not a last resort, but an adjunct to other modalities of treatment. Surgery should be judiciously applied when the need becomes apparent. The general goals of surgery are to maximize function, minimize deformity, and keep interventions to a minimum. The first goal of surgery is to diminish muscle imbalance. This is accomplished by weakening muscles and decreasing spasticity (tendon lengthening and tendon release procedures) and by altering the direction of muscle force (specific muscle transfer procedures). Most muscle procedures are muscle shortening procedures, whereby muscle origins or tendons are released or the tendons are lengthened. This weakens the muscle by reducing the resting length (Figure 7) and diminishes tension on the muscle spindle and tendon organs, thereby reducing spasticity (Inman, Ralston, & Todd, 1981). The second goal is to prevent bony and soft tissue deformity. Where deformity has developed already, correcting bony deformity and releasing soft tissue contracture become necessary. Most bony procedures involve realignment/angulation changes in order to achieve better position and better mechanical advantage. The resulting bone realignment and joint stabilization lead once again back to maximal function.

The reasons for pursuing these operative procedures are several. Simple mechanical disadvantage may be the main factor impeding developmental progress. Pain may be a significant immediate or predictable future problem that can be eliminated. Ease of management and reduction of general care are potential benefits even in those situations in which independent function is unlikely. Improved positioning with assistive devices can benefit the patient both in functional ways and in minimizing the long-term development or progression of deformity. Cosmesis, although almost never a primary indication for limb surgery, is almost always an associated benefit (e.g., improved functional gait). The ultimate long-term goal is to avoid the pain and superimposed disability associated with later degenerative arthritis as a result of chronic and often unappreciated joint trauma.

The timing of surgery is determined primarily by functional need. Age of the patient, although a major consideration for spine surgery, is generally a secondary factor in limb surgery. There is often a necessary degree of uncertainty about the exact nature or the exact extent of any procedures to be performed in the operating room. This is because the surgeon has the unique opportunity to supplement his or her routine clinical examination and the gait analysis data with an examination under anesthesia. Occasionally, the findings will dictate a slightly different plan than what was anticipated.

Bleck (1987) wrote cogently about preoperative management of the child and family. He maintained that the orthopedic surgeon who is conscientious and cautious in terms of preoperative analysis, selection of surgical procedure, surgical technique, and good follow-up care, and who clearly defines the aims of surgery, can expect an 80%–90% "good result." Promoting a trusting relationship is the fundamental basis for minimizing physiologic and psychological discomfort surrounding the surgical procedure. To foster this attitude, sufficient time should be allowed for the physical therapist and patient to become acquainted, and a close working relationship should exist between therapist and surgeon.

In the treatment of cerebral palsy, more objective measures of outcome of orthopedic surgery should lead to better decisions in the selection of the surgical procedure. This concept extends to other modalities (e.g., physical therapy, drugs, orthotics) as well. Gait analysis provides the technology to meet this need.

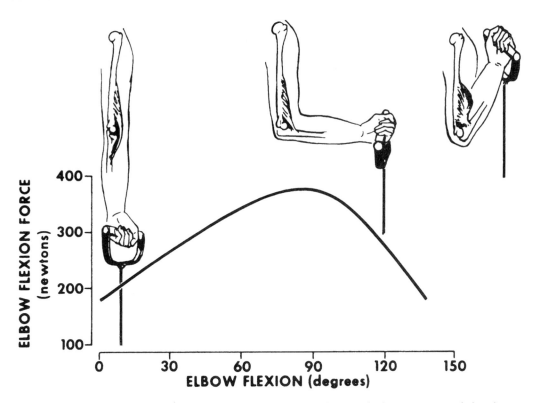

Figure 7. Muscle force graph. Maximal force is plotted against elbow flexion, which represents muscle length. Muscle strength is greatest at midlength and diminishes as the muscle is lengthened or shortened (as occurs with tendon release surgery). This is analogous to the Starling curve for myocardial contractility. (From Inman, V.T., Ralston, J.H., & Todd, F. [1981]. *Human walking*, p. 96. Baltimore: Williams & Wilkins; reprinted by permission.)

Specific Surgical Procedures

Procedures About the Ankle and Foot Ankle and foot problems represent the most common deformities in patients with cerebral palsy. In order to function as an adjustable base of support for standing, the foot must be flat and stable. Therefore, fixed deformity in a position that is functional rarely needs surgery. The other role of the foot is as a sensory device to provide proprioceptive feedback information, especially during dynamic movement.

The most common ankle deformity is equinus, which may be aligned straight but most commonly is associated with medial (varus) or lateral (valgus) deviation of the foot. Any equinus deformity destabilizes the base of support and probably reduces or alters sensory input as well. This in turn will increase tone through the "fixing" reaction that accompanies disequilibrium. Equinovarus usually does not need surgery because it can often be controlled by

AFO use. If spasticity interferes with gait without a fixed deformity (*dynamic* equinovarus), gastrocnemius recession is considered. When a fixed contracture occurs, Achilles tendon lengthening or fascial lengthening of the gastrocnemius are the two principal surgical choices (Rose, DeLuca, Davis, Ounpuu, & Gage, 1993). The major caution is to avoid overlengthening, which results in a crouched gait. This is all too common a mistake, and more children have had a worse outcome from having their heel cords injudiciously lengthened than from any other orthopedic procedure.

Postoperative management consists of short leg casting for 5 weeks, rapid resumption of ambulation, and long-term protection with night splints (AFOs). The AFOs may reduce recurrence rates, which are reported as between 5% and 20% in various series. It may be, however, that as many as another 5%–20% are lengthened inappropriately.

Varus deformity in children with spastic cerebral palsy is due to imbalance of the two muscles governing medial and lateral ankle movement. The peroneal on the lateral side is overpowered as a result of overpull of the tibialis posterior or anterior medially. There are three surgical options:

1. Posterior tibial tendon lengthening with immediate ambulation in short leg casts for 3 weeks.

2. Split posterior tibial tendon transfer, which requires long leg casting. The tendon is split in half and the lateral segment is detached from its insertion on the navicular and reattached laterally to the tendon of the peroneus brevis muscle. Hence the spastic tibialis posterior muscle basically balances itself. Weight bearing soon after surgery is acceptable. If there is a fixed bony deformity present, calcaneal wedge osteotomy for varus, combined with posterior tibial and sometimes Achilles tendon lengthening, is required.

3. Split anterior tibial tendon transfer (SPLATT) whereby the lateral portion is reattached to the cuboid.

Valgus deformity, if severe, requires stabilization in the form of a subtalar arthrodesis procedure. In younger children, there are many operations from which to choose. In the Grice procedure a tibial bone graft is used to fuse the talus to the calcaneus in order to eliminate motion of the subtalar joint. The modified Crawford technique achieves subtalar stabilization with arthrodesis by using a metal staple. With this technique, immediate weight bearing is allowed in a regular short leg cast (worn for 4–6 weeks). The most popular technique employs a screw through the neck of the talus into the calcaneus with iliac crest bone graft (Dennyson-Fulford method). However, a newer procedure, calcaneal lengthening, is gaining advocates because correction can be achieved without fusion (Sangeorzan, Mosca, & Hansen, 1993). The decision to perform a subtalar joint stabilization procedure is subjective, based on clinical rather than radiologic criteria. The presence of a flat, collapsed foot with a medial prominence, often with a callus, is the characteristic picture. Anywhere from 5 to 9 years is the usual age for

these procedures. Gait analysis with dynamic EMG may prove to be helpful in more objectively deciding when to do a procedure. In adults and adolescents, triple arthrodesis is the standard operation. Joints formed by the talus, calcaneus, navicular, and cuboid are all fused (Figure 8). Bleck (1987) preferred to add to this Grice's extra-articular fusion of the talus to the calcaneus to better keep the talus out of its plantar-flexed position. Long-term follow-up of patients undergoing triple arthrodesis reveals that many develop pain and osteoarthritis (Wetmore & Drennan, 1989).

In summary, the benefit of obtaining a plantar-grade foot is enhancement of sensory feedback and increased stability of the base of support, resulting in better equilibrium and decreased overall muscle tone.

Procedures About the Knee The indications for hamstring contracture surgery are a shortened step length, a popliteal angle measurement of greater than 45 degrees, and excessive knee flexion in mid- and terminal stance. Kyphosis in sitting, which also can be a consequence of hamstring spasticity, is another indication for hamstring lengthening. Thus nonambulators can also benefit from surgery. The

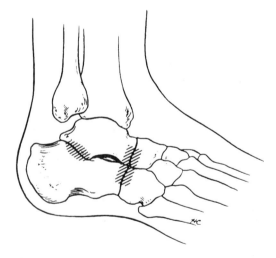

Figure 8. Ankle joint with triple arthrodesis. The hashed lines indicate fusion of the calcaneus and talus posteriorly and anteriorly plus fusion of the calcaneus and cuboid and the talus and navicular. (From Bleck, E.E. [1987]. *Orthopedic management in cerebral palsy* [Clinics in Developmental Medicine, No. 99/100, p. 376]. London: MacKeith Press; reprinted by permission.)

operation consists of fractional lengthening of the hamstring muscles (the biceps femoris, gracilis, semimembranosus, and semitendinosus). As noted previously, lengthening the hamstring muscles works by weakening each muscle and thereby reducing spasticity. Some surgeons prefer to lengthen only the medial hamstrings, leaving the biceps femoris intact. Excessive lordosis is a common—some say invariable—outcome when both the medial and lateral hamstrings are simultaneously lengthened. Postoperative management consists of long leg casting for 1 week or longer and intensive physical therapy. Following cast removal, part-time *knee immobilizers* (soft splints used day and night) have been employed for weeks to months, and some surgeons believe it may be worthwhile to persist with them over the long term to decrease recurrence. The recurrence rate of hamstring contractures is greater than that for hip adductor or heel cord contractures and is influenced greatly by type and severity of involvement. Recurrence may be largely secondary to positioning (chair, sleep), hence the utility of knee immobilizers and standing devices following cast removal. If the hamstrings are too loose, genu recurvatum and hyperlordosis may result. Because the hamstring muscles are powerful hip extensors in the first half of stance phase, one always pays a price for lengthening in terms of lost propulsive power during gait.

Internal tibial torsion (ITT) in the absence of cerebral palsy almost never requires surgical correction. In children with cerebral palsy, it is more likely to persist, although spontaneous correction can still occur. In some cases, derotational osteotomy of the tibia and fibula is required. Most surgeons favor a distal procedure because of the risk of neurovascular complications with proximal tibia surgery. Postoperative care includes long leg casting for 4 weeks followed by a short leg walking cast for another 4–8 weeks.

External tibial torsion (ETT) is actually more common than ITT in cerebral palsy, probably as a compensation for femoral anteversion or as a result of medial hamstring tendon lengthening. Surgical intervention is often required for ETT in ambulatory persons with cerebral palsy.

Procedures About the Hip Fixed and dynamic problems about the hip are the second most common orthopedic deformity in cerebral palsy. Indications for hip surgery include

1. Hip dysplasia and dislocation. Acquired hip dysplasia is never seen before 6 months. With dislocation, chronic hip pain ultimately follows. Pain is not a problem usually seen in younger children with relatively recent dislocations. It is a relatively late phenomenon and appears to be a consequence of arthritis in the dislocated hip joint.
2. Asymmetrical sitting base and pelvic obliquity caused by decreased mobility and hip stiffness from dislocation. Scoliosis is associated with the pelvic obliquity, and it is debated whether the curve is aggravated by this posture.
3. Difficult perineal care.
4. Decubitus ulcers and skin problems.

All of these problems are interrelated. With persistent muscle imbalance, both the acetabulum and the femoral head will become dysplastic—that is, deformed to such an extent that they do not structurally fit together. The femoral head migrates proximally and laterally, and the consequence of this is dislocation. Dislocation frequency increases with severity of spasticity. The incidence is 4% in ambulatory and 25% in nonambulatory individuals with spastic cerebral palsy. In ideal circumstances, frank hip dislocation should rarely happen because the indicators of progressive dysplasia are easy to recognize both clinically and radiographically, and preventive surgery is both safe and highly successful. In general, earlier surgery is associated with better long-term results.

Adductor tenotomy surgery involves cutting the tendons of the adductor longus, gracilis, and (in severe cases) adductor brevis muscles (Figure 9). Sectioning the anterior branch of the obturator nerve often is added, but only in more severely involved (i.e., nonambulatory) children. The adductor magnus is always left intact. The iliopsoas, although not an adductor, often is lengthened as well, at least in children with hip dysplasia, and produces a better result (Kalen & Bleck, 1985). The recurrence rate of contractures with adductor surgery is small, but children who have unilateral operations may ulti-

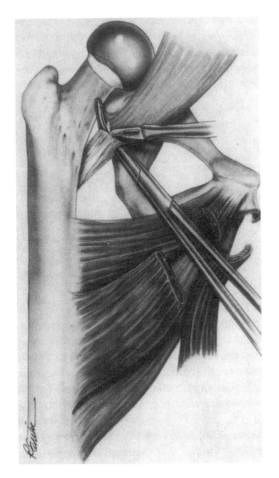

Figure 9. Releasing spastic muscles about the hip. Two adductor muscles (the adductor longus and the gracilis) have been sectioned and the iliopsoas tendon is being cut. (Courtesy of Michael D. Sussman, M.D.)

mately have problems with windswept hips. The windswept hip deformity, a combination of adduction contracture on one side (often with subluxation of the femoral head) and abduction posture (usually with contracture of the iliotibial band) on the other, often gives the mistaken impression of a leg length discrepancy. Windswept hips are not uncommon among more severely involved children with cerebral palsy. Adductor transfer rarely is done, although a few orthopedists do still favor it. Results of transfer are comparable to those of release, but transferring the adductors requires casting postoperatively, whereas release does not.

The functional benefits of hip surgery are improved gait as a result of diminished scissoring and crouching and improved sitting as a result of abolished pelvic tilt. Children do not need to have hip flexion or adduction contractures to benefit from this procedure. A relatively brief period of time is spent postoperatively in a body cast in most centers. However, the practice in a few facilities is to begin therapy 3–4 days postoperatively. The children do not require a body cast when such early positioning and handling techniques are used on an inpatient basis.

Complications of adductor surgery include the further progression of hip dysplasia, excessive abduction resulting from overweakening of the adductor muscle group, insufficient release so that the child still scissors, windswept hip deformity, and heterotopic ossification. Treatment of windswept hips involves surgical release of the adductors on one side and the iliotibial band contracture on the other. Heterotopic ossification refers to the unexplained deposition of bone in muscle tissue. A final issue is patient selection. Children with mixed quadriplegia with a predominant choreoathetoid component are at risk for a poor functional outcome if their lower extremity spasticity is relieved.

Torsional malalignment procedures include those for femoral anteversion and for tibial torsion (see above). Correction of increased femoral anteversion can be accomplished by proximal or distal osteotomy procedures. In proximal femoral varus derotational osteotomy, the femoral shaft is transected and rotated. This is a longer operation than the distal procedure, requires an internal fixation plate, and typically has a greater loss of blood. Nevertheless, proximal derotational osteotomy is the preferred procedure for hip dysplasia in association with anteversion. In distal femoral derotational osteotomy, the distal shaft of the femur is cut and rotated and held in place with removable pins. Postoperative spica casting for 4 weeks is necessary in both procedures. This is followed by long leg casts for about 4 more weeks and intensive physical therapy to promote mobilization and weight bearing. Casting is essential, and anything less, such as splinting, is ineffective. Some surgeons have sought to reduce non–weight-bearing time by using a pins-in-plaster casting technique.

Upper Extremity Procedures Upper extremity surgery in cerebral palsy is infrequent compared to the number of procedures done on the lower extremities. The main procedures considered are those on the spastic hand and wrist to relieve forearm pronation, wrist flexion, and thumb-in-palm deformities. The most frequent operations include small tendon releases, especially of the thumb; tendon lengthenings; and tendon transfers, most notably of the flexor carpi ulnaris. The goal is to improve positioning, especially wrist extension, in order to achieve better function and appearance.

In spastic hemiplegia, the upper extremity typically exhibits more functional impairment than the lower extremity. If sensation is relatively preserved, surgical treatment may well produce substantial functional gains. However, in the face of severe sensory loss, the lack of sensory feedback essentially nullifies any potential benefits from surgical procedures aimed at enhancing motor function (Goldner, 1974). Subjects must be old enough and cognitively intact enough (mental age of 5 years or better) to cooperate with sophisticated sensory testing (Bolanos, Bleck, Firestone, & Young, 1989). Evaluations of pain, touch, and temperature sensation are not relevant; rather, it is stereognosis, two-point discrimination, and other "parietal lobe" function that must be addressed. Some hand surgeons rely heavily on nerve blocks (lidocaine and related agents) and neuromuscular blocks (botulinum A toxin) to help determine potential for surgical benefit (Koman, Gelberman, Toby, & Poehling, 1990). Although it is difficult to predict which children are the best candidates for surgery, the best indicators are sensory testing, spontaneous hand use, absence of growth delay on the involved side, and possibly EMG studies (Hoffer, Lehman, & Mitami, 1989). The operations rarely prove to be as useful in children with spastic quadriplegia as they are in those with hemiplegia.

Postoperative Management

General principles of postoperative care—intensive monitoring, attention to fluids and electrolytes, and pain management—are the same for orthopedic surgery as they are for other types of surgery. However, a few special procedures that relate to the orthopedic patient are worth noting.

Caudal anesthesia using bupivacaine (Marcaine) to decrease postoperative pain has been advocated by some but abandoned by others because of complications. Caudal analgesia using narcotic agents such as fentanyl has been widely heralded as a major improvement in postoperative pain management. Risks include masking a compartment syndrome or skin pressure necrosis. Intravenous and oral narcotics have a definite place in pain control. Studies of self-administered narcotic analgesia have shown the advantages of this approach (Rodgers, Webb, Stergios, & Newman, 1988). The parents of children with disabilities actually control the administration based on their perception of the child's discomfort. Diazepam to decrease spasticity plays a major role in promoting comfort, and its muscle relaxant effect may prove to benefit the child even after the postoperative period. Traction, by maintaining muscle length with gentle (therefore painless) stretch, decreases spasticity as well. Physical therapy to achieve general mobilization is initiated as soon as possible after surgery. At first it must be limited and gentle, with a plan for gradually increased intensity in order to work up to the desired functional gains that engendered the surgery in the first place. One surgeon (Michael Sussman) conceives of the process in terms of "pre–physical therapy surgery" as opposed to "postoperative physical therapy."

Immobilization produces obvious muscle degeneration (atrophy) histologically after about 3 weeks. Because of this, some centers prefer early mobilization after many procedures, although longer duration cast immobilization is more traditional. Early mobilization has become possible mostly as a result of advances in solid internal fixation methods that make osteotomy sites stable and resistant to intrinsic and external forces. Appropriate positioning and handling techniques can be initiated on an inpatient basis 3–4 days after surgery, followed by weight bearing about 1 week postoperatively.

Temporary equipment—for example, an abductor pillow to maintain leg separation at night or an adaptive seating system for use until ambulation can be resumed—may need to be employed. Lower extremity casts, especially short leg casts, have been used for about 20 years specifically to immobilize the foot. They have been termed *inhibitive casts* because of observed decreases in spasticity after removal (Sussman & Cusick, 1979). Even upper extremities seem to benefit as a consequence of increased overall stability and resultant decreased overall tone. The casts can be split along the lateral and medial sides (bivalved) for use only during specified hours during the day. Bivalved short leg casts act like a rigid AFO and always require follow-up use of a plastic AFO. Gait improves in ambulatory children, and posture and general movements of nonambulatory children are said to improve as well. The disadvantage is that the casts and AFOs are cumbersome and unattractive.

Problems Associated with Surgery

Difficulties encountered with surgery fall into two major categories: complications common to surgical practice in general and errors in judgment related to specific orthopedic procedures. Pitfalls related to surgical technique revolve around the judgment as to how much to alter a tendon, muscle, or bone. For example, too much hip adductor release results in excessive abduction. Overlengthening the hamstrings results in genu recurvatum. Overlengthening the heel cord results in a floppy foot. In the other direction, insufficient release leaves the child with residual deformity and results in recurrence or persistence of the original problems: scissoring through the hips, knee flexion, or equinus deformity at the ankle. The functional consequence of these errors can be a worsened (or unimproved) gait or a loss of sitting support. Another consideration is timing. By waiting too long, the child loses developmental opportunity. Conversely, operating too soon may increase the likelihood of unnecessary procedures being done or the need for repeat surgeries as the child grows and changes.

Perhaps the single biggest reason for surgical failure relates to the mismatching of parental expectations with the surgeon's expectation of what can be accomplished. The most perfect, complication-free procedure is not satisfactory to the family or the child if it does not produce the functional outcome expected (Bleck, 1987).

Surgical complications are uncommon but potentially devastating. Potential complications, although rare, always should cause one to pause and reflect on the need for surgery. Among undesirable events to consider are the following:

1. Anesthesia always carries risks. There is an increased risk for malignant hyperthermia in neuromuscular diseases but not in cerebral palsy.

2. Wound infections, although rare in children under 10, may occur in older children, especially with adductor procedures. These infections probably are related to difficult perineal hygiene and perhaps to alterations in perineal flora that occur after puberty.

3. Other infections (pulmonary, urinary tract, decubiti, etc.) are more likely to develop in children with physical disabilities than in those without disabilities. The greater the motor impairment, the worse the oral–motor dysfunction, and so forth, the greater the risk is for these problems.

4. Immobilization, although essential, works against the child in several ways. Contracture formation and muscle atrophy will start to develop. In addition, hypercalciuria is uniformly present. Secondary stone formation (renal, gallbladder) occurs but the frequency is unknown. Symptomatic renal or gallbladder stones are quite rare. One study (Teele, Nussbaum, Wyly, Allred, & Emans, 1987) reported a 20% incidence of cholelithiasis, mostly asymptomatic, following immobilization after spine stabilization surgery. These subjects, however, were mostly older children and young adults.

5. Heterotopic ossification represents a rare and unexplained phenomenon in which osteogenesis takes place in nonskeletal tissue, most commonly muscle. It occurs in inherited and acquired forms, the latter being associated with a number of inciting events, including orthopedic surgery. Theories to explain each situation exist, but there is no one accepted explanation, let alone a unifying hypothesis (Smith & Triffitt, 1986). The incidence following surgery is very low, and the ossification is seen exclusively

around the hip. Heterotopic ossification appears to be related to extent of surgery and perhaps to overly aggressive or too early physical therapy following surgery.

6. Loss of gross motor skills is anticipated following surgery, but rapid recovery is to be expected. Developmental regression in non–gross motor areas also occurs. Oral–motor function, for example, may suffer substantially in a child kept unfed for days, and recovery may be a very slow process.

7. Disturbances in associated problem areas (e.g., seizure control) may occur. Careful attention must be paid to anticonvulsants and potential medication interactions. Preoperative drug levels become extremely valuable if seizure activity ensues in the postoperative period. Another example is the recognition of platelet dysfunction and unpredictable bleeding associated with valproic acid (Chambers, Mubarak, & Wenger, 1993; Tetzlaff, 1991).

SCOLIOSIS

Scoliosis is defined as a lateral curvature of the spine associated with rotation of the posterior vertebral elements into the concavity of the curve. This type of structural curvature is never "normal," although only a curve of greater than a 10-degree Cobb angle (see below) is designated as scoliosis. Nonstructural scoliosis refers to a visible curvature that does not have the true rotational component described above and is generally flexible back to normal when the offending cause resolves. Examples would be *splinting* (i.e., from thoracic or pleural pain); irritation of back soft tissues, especially the paraspinous muscles on one side; intervertebral disk disease; a hysterical situation; or simply poor posture. The term *fixed* scoliosis is sometimes used to indicate structural curvature, and *supple* or *postural* may be used to designate nonstructural curves. Any deformity may have a postural component added to a fixed degree of curvature.

Assessment

Screening for scoliosis on clinical examination is easy and reliable if the child can stand. Screening is unreliable in nonambulatory chil-

dren. Visual inspection of the back with the child standing erect ("at attention") allows several important observations:

1. The height of the shoulders (or extended hands)
2. The obvious position of the spine
3. Symmetry of the scapulae and the flanks
4. The level of the pelvis relative to the plane of the floor

Asking the child to bend forward, one can then note the height of the scapulae or the "rib hump" (see Figure 1). The *scoliometer* is a device constructed like a water bubble level that is useful for quantitating the rib hump in degrees, especially in the screening setting. One also can measure it in centimeters, as depicted in Figure 1. Of course, a good percentage of children with cerebral palsy will need to be viewed in sitting (often somewhat supported) to obtain a clinical impression of how straight the spine is. Objective measurement of the curve is only reliable when based on an upright standing (or minimally supported sitting) posteroanterior radiograph of the thoracolumbar spine. The angle of curvature is determined by the Cobb method (Figure 10). The uppermost and lower vertebrae delineating the curve (the ones that are most tilted) are identified and perpendiculars are constructed to them. The intersection of these lines reflects the curve's angle of concavity. (The concavity of the straight spine could be thought of as 180 degrees.) The Cobb angle then is the complement to the angle of concavity (e.g., 0 degrees in the straight spine).

Kyphosis refers to the posterior angulation of the spine normally seen in the thoracic region, whereas *lordosis* is the normal anterior curvature of the lumbar spine. As seen in Figure 11, a straightedge normally runs vertically between the sacrum and the normal thoracic kyphosis. An exaggerated hump (hyperkyphosis) can be visualized in terms of degrees of deviation from the vertical. Measurement is analogous to that of scoliosis utilizing the lateral spine radiograph. Normal thoracic kyphosis ranges from 15 to 50 degrees. The thoracic kyphosis may be exaggerated as a result of tight hamstrings in children with cerebral palsy. This rarely pro-

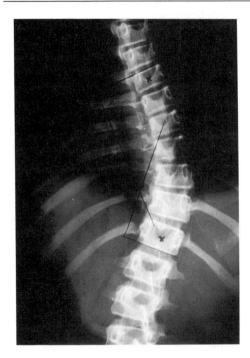

Figure 10. Posteroanterior spine film depicting construction of the Cobb angle. (Courtesy of John E. Lonstein, M.D.)

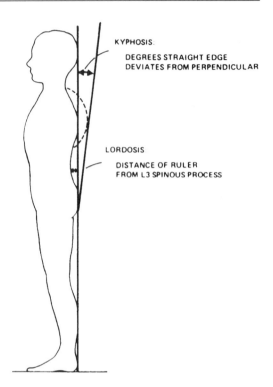

Figure 11. Assessment of standing posture. (From Bleck, E.E. [1987]. *Orthopedic management in cerebral palsy* [Clinics in Developmental Medicine, No. 99/100, p. 31]. London: MacKeith Press; reprinted by permission.)

gresses to a severe degree, and treatment consists of hamstring lengthening.

Lordosis is measured radiographically in the same manner as kyphosis. Clinically, it can be viewed in terms of distance from the L3 spinous process to the vertical, normally 3–4 cm at a maximum (Figure 11). Lordosis may be exaggerated in certain conditions, especially cerebral palsy and peripheral neuromuscular diseases that cause weakness about the pelvic girdle. In children with cerebral palsy, it usually develops in compensation for excessive hip flexion with contractures and forward pelvic tilt. In pelvic girdle weakness, one sees progressive lordotic (or hyperlordotic) posturing as a natural mechanism to maintain the center of gravity because, once again, the pelvis tilts forward, in this instance as a result of weakness (as opposed to spasticity). Initially flexible, it becomes increasingly fixed as the child grows. Quite disabling problems with low back pain may develop in young adults. Treatment in persons with cerebral palsy would be hip flexor contracture release. Unfortunately, there is no method to control hyperlordosis in persons with neuro-

muscular disease, although decreased ambulation and more time spent sitting will slow down or stop the rate of progression.

Classification

It is useful to classify structural scoliosis into four clinical subgroups:

1. *Idiopathic,* which is often familial and can have its onset in infancy, midchildhood, or adolescence
2. *Congenital,* in which anomalies of the vertebral bodies are invariably present and account for the development of the condition during intrauterine gestation
3. *Neuromuscular,* which is typically due to conditions such as cerebral palsy, myopathies, and peripheral nerve diseases with all their myriad variations
4. *Miscellaneous,* such as skeletal dysplasias, Marfan syndrome, hemihypertrophy syndromes, arthrogryposis, neurofibromatosis, and metabolic bone diseases

Curve types seen in cerebral palsy can be either double ("S"-type) or single ("C"-type) curves. Those that are primarily thoracic are seen in ambulatory children and during the adolescent growth spurt. Those that are primarily lumbar as a rule start earlier, tend to be more common in nonambulatory children, and are typically associated with pelvic obliquity. In ambulatory children with a double curve, there is generally a primary thoracic curve compensated by an opposite lumbar curve with little resultant pelvic obliquity. Interestingly, although scoliosis is common in hemiplegia, progression to the point of requiring intervention with bracing or surgery is uncommon.

Prevalence

The prevalence of scoliosis is best thought of in terms of the base population. In the general population, scoliotic curves (10 degrees or greater) have a prevalence of 3%–4%. Most of these are minor and are untreated. Idiopathic scoliotic curves greater than 20 degrees occur in about 0.25% of adolescents. Girls have a great predisposition for curves to progress: Whereas the female-to-male ratio for the mildest curves is about 1:1, for curves greater than 30 degrees it is 7:1. Among children with cerebral palsy, scoliosis is quite common. The prevalence ranges from 6% to 64%, depending on the type and severity of the disorder and the particular clinic population being surveyed. An overall incidence is hard to pinpoint, but in ambulatory children it is about 6%–7%; in nonambulatory children it is closer to 30%–40%. The more severely involved the child, the greater is the likelihood of progression. Hence, nonambulatory children are at high risk for progressive scoliosis, whereas ambulatory children infrequently require bracing or surgery.

Etiology and Progression

From a pathophysiologic standpoint the exact mechanism that triggers spinal curvature is not clear. Asymmetric spasticity, equilibrium reaction deficits, primitive reflexes (especially the Galant), sensory deficits, and positional factors have all been implicated in various theories. The time and cause–effect relationships between scoliosis, pelvic obliquity, and hip dislocation—which often coexist—are controversial. Scoliosis may develop regardless of the hip and pelvic positions. In simple terms, it is probably due to the inability of the back muscles to support the flexible spine against gravity. Muscle imbalance is probably a second important factor.

Regardless of etiology, scoliosis curves tend to progress most rapidly during the adolescent growth spurt. In most circumstances, curves less than 40 degrees at skeletal maturity will be stable in adulthood, whereas those greater than 50 degrees are likely to progress, albeit at a slower rate, after skeletal maturity (Thometz & Simon, 1988). Thus, degree of curvature, proximity to skeletal maturity, and linear growth rate are the key elements the surgeon considers in determining scoliosis management. The Risser sign (degree of capping of the iliac crest apophyses) is a convenient marker of skeletal maturity and can be readily evaluated on spine radiographs that include the pelvis. Signs of puberty (Tanner staging and other characteristics) are also very helpful indicators of expected growth rate and growth potential.

Treatment

Treatment of scoliosis in children with cerebral palsy is based on the following indications:

1. Maintenance of balance for sitting or walking
2. Pain, most often at the apex of the curve or at the pelvis, as a result of discomfort in sitting
3. Pressure sores, especially in the presence of pelvic obliquity
4. Cardiopulmonary function, which is compromised in all children with curves greater than 50 degrees. Pulmonary compromise does not become significant until the curve exceeds 100 degrees (which is seen rarely in cerebral palsy)

In general, curves less than 25 degrees in a child with remaining growth are followed regularly, usually at 4- to 6-month intervals, by means of the standard standing (or sitting) spine film. This would need to be continued until skeletal maturity is achieved in order to identify children with progressive curves. Curves between 25 and 45 degrees in children with significant skeletal growth remaining should be braced until skeletal growth is complete. Bracing in children with cerebral palsy is more efficacious in ambulatory than in nonambulatory children. It can slow the rate of progression and delay surgery until the adolescent growth spurt. This affords the child more time for linear growth and puts him or her in a better position to tolerate the operation if and when it becomes indicated, preferably after 10 years of age. Every effort is made to postpone spine fusion in younger children because of associated growth problems. Linear growth is compromised, but, with posterior fusion, the unfused anterior portion of the vertebrae will continue to grow, resulting in an increased rotational deformity. Fortunately, the need for spine fusion before age 10 rarely arises in children with cerebral palsy.

Modern spine orthoses are made of lightweight plastic materials carefully molded to the contours of the body. The utility of the TLSO (thoracolumbosacral orthosis) is in holding the curve for as long as possible, not in reducing it. The concept of "failing" brace treatment does not really hold; just gaining time by slowing the rate of progression is an advantage. The exception to this is the situation in progressive neuromuscular diseases in which pulmonary reserve deteriorates with time and therefore increases the surgical risk. Bracing should not be used because these children's curves are inexorably progressive, and delaying surgery only places the child at increased surgical risk (Sussman, 1984). There is no evidence that electrical stimulation is useful for the treatment of scoliosis.

Scoliosis surgery in children with cerebral palsy becomes indicated when correction of pelvic obliquity becomes increasingly urgent, when the curve progresses beyond 45–50 degrees, and when orthotics fail to hold a curve adequately. Surgical procedures are of two primary types. One type is posterior fusion and instrumentation involving a variety of stainless steel devices that are fixed directly to the spine. The purpose of these instruments is to straighten and hold the spine in place until bone graft material has time to heal and thereby form a rigid bridge between vertebrae. The most commonly used device today is the Luque seg-

mental device (Luque, 1982). Independent segmental attachment to each vertebra via a wire loop through the laminae is achieved with Luque rods. This provides excellent fixation and as a result permits early mobilization. Luque instrumentation also allows better control of the sagittal contour because it is easy to mold in desired lordosis and kyphosis. Harrington rods, two stiff rods that are fixed on each side of the spine, and Dwyer cables fixed to the anterior spine by means of screws, are now considered obsolete for fusion in children with cerebral palsy. Fixation of the instrument to the pelvis is controversial and a matter of the surgeon's preference. The advantage is said to be the prevention of additional pelvic obliquity. The disadvantages cited are added surgical morbidity, increased stress on the hardware, and greater limitation of spine flexion at the pelvis.

A second surgical procedure in scoliosis is anterior release of the intervertebral discs and the longitudinal ligaments and fusion by means of vertebral arthrodesis with autologous (generally rib) bone graft. For severe (greater than 90-degree) curves, anterior fusion is generally done in conjunction with the posterior procedure to increase correctability. Anterior fusion is never done in isolation in neuromuscular curves.

Nutritional assessment is a major preoperative consideration, especially the projected ability of the child to maintain good nutrition following surgery. Pulmonary care is the other critical factor. Postoperatively, orthoses sometimes are used on a temporary basis (for up to 6 months). Early ambulation, sitting in a swimming pool to minimize gravitational force, or both are adjuncts to early mobility and recovery.

Complications of spine surgery have improved dramatically in recent years, related mainly to the advent of segmental instrumentation and to continuing advances in pediatric anesthesiology. Mortality rates reported to be 3% in the past, seen mostly in the more severely involved cases, are now at or below 0.5%. Pseudarthroses represent failure of fusion and vary widely in different series, but now are reported to occur in less than 5% of the cases, and they rarely require reoperation. Neurologic complications caused by spinal cord stretching or vascular interruptions occur infrequently, with less than 0.5% having permanent sequelae. Postoperative hyperesthesia is a focal, transient neurologic phenomenon always resolving in about 2 weeks. Hardware failure refers to breakage of the instruments and is always associated with pseudarthoses. In some series, it is reported to be as high as 5%–10%, but current experience is closer to 1%. Infection is very rare.

With spine surgery, the back always loses flexibility in terms of anterior–posterior and lateral flexion, but gains stability. Because of the vertebral fusion, linear growth through the spine is severely limited and is a function of the number of segments fused. The loss in spinal growth can be roughly calculated before surgery (Bleck, 1987). Because major blood loss is expected, the surgeon can plan in advance to collect an autologous or a related donor supply for transfusion.

One final comment on the spine must be made. Bleck (1987) described several instances of persons with athetoid cerebral palsy who developed severe degenerative arthritis of the cervical spine. Symptoms of chronic neck pain and intermittent upper limb radicular pain completely resolved following anterior spinal fusion. Myelopathy with sudden quadriplegia has been reported to occur if there is a subluxation. Late radiculopathy is being recognized more frequently in adults as both survivorship increases and reporting improves. Others have not found the successful response to surgery reported by Bleck (Kidmon, Steiner, & Melamed, 1987).

NEUROSURGERY

Superficially, neurosurgery is appealing because it is hoped that the neurosurgeon can "fix" the brain by getting to the source of the problem, and a single surgery can affect all the joints and muscles. However, one must remember that these surgical procedures represent destructive lesions, not reparative ones. Neurosurgical techniques have had little application to children with cerebral palsy until the recent surge of interest in selective dorsal rhizotomy. Although the focus of this chapter is on orthopedic management, it is impossible to avoid the overlap

between these two surgical approaches to the same clinical condition, namely, spasticity, especially in the lower limbs.

Ventral posterolateral thalamotomy or dentate nucleus ablation represent old procedures pioneered in adults with movement disorders, particularly Parkinson's disease, that were applied to children with cerebral palsy. They achieved little long-term benefit for spasticity, which tended to recur. This type of stereotactic neurosurgery is more appropriate for cases of extrapyramidal cerebral palsy in which marked adventitious movement is the problem (Spelman & van Manen, 1989). This makes sense in view of the impressive past history of success in adults with Parkinson's disease.

Cerebellar stimulation, based on the century-old observation in animals that electrical stimulation of the anterior lobe of the cerebellum decreases spastic and rigid hypertonus, was advocated as a major therapeutic breakthrough in the early 1970s by Irving Cooper, the neurosurgeon who introduced thalamotomy for Parkinson's disease. Reduction in spasticity, increased ease of management, and improvements in speech (apparently as a result of better breath control) were claimed. Positive early results, however, are clouded by the very subjective nature of the assessments, and there is a high rate of malfunction of the apparatus. Spinal cord stimulation is a variation on the theme of cerebellar stimulation. Although now favored over cerebellar stimulation by its main, and possibly only, advocate (Joseph Waltz), there are virtually no data to support its use. Penn and his colleagues have appraised the limited benefits of this procedure carefully and fairly (Gottlieb et al., 1985; Ratusnick, Wolfe, Penn, & Schewitz, 1978).

Rhizotomy—cutting the dorsal roots of the spinal cord—is aimed specifically at eliminating spasticity and is one of a number of spinal cord and spinal root ablative procedures that have been used in limited settings for many years, mostly in adults with spinal cord injury or disease. By completely and permanently interrupting the spinal reflex arc, spasticity can be abolished. The technique involves gaining access to the lumbar spinal cord by performing a laminectomy. The dorsal roots are exposed and the point at which the dorsal root enters the cord is dissected. Each root consists of about 5–10 smaller rootlets rather than a single bundle. The rootlets, once they have been teased apart, are then individually electrically stimulated under constant EMG surveillance. Although all the rootlets will produce a muscle contraction when stimulated, a few tend to produce an exaggerated response (Phillips & Park, 1989). Presumably these rootlets are the ones mainly carrying reflex arc fibers that are implicated in spasticity, whereas the others are carrying different afferent fibers. Only those rootlets producing the abnormal response are sectioned; the others are left intact. Some neurosurgeons disagree even about this basic premise. The total number of rootlets that should be sectioned (regardless of electrical characteristics) is a matter of unresolved debate. Apparently, the stimulation procedure is extremely fickle and there is controversy about the validity of this selection process. Nonetheless, rhizotomy certainly works in the sense that spasticity is entirely or largely eliminated from the lower extremities and there has so far been very little recurrence.

Although popularized in Europe by Fasano in the 1970s (Fasano, Broggi, Barolat-Romana, & Sguazzi, 1978), the rejuvenation of selective dorsal rhizotomy can be attributed to Warwick Peacock's work in South Africa. In his hands, the procedure has been tremendously successful (Peacock & Arens, 1982; Peacock, Arens, & Berman, 1987). He has been careful to point out that the ideal candidate for this type of surgery appears to be the child with pure spastic diplegia. The more extrapyramidal involvement and the more asymmetry the child exhibits, the less acceptable the results. Prior orthopedic surgery is a relative contraindication, and the need for later orthopedic intervention to correct fixed alignment problems is quite high. Rhizotomy has not provided particular benefit for children with hemiplegia and has been abandoned for that population by some neurosurgeons. Children with spastic quadriplegia without ambulatory potential are offered the procedure by some groups for the purpose of improved sitting and easier care.

Postoperatively, the children are areflexic, hypotonic, and quite weak. There is occasionally some hyperesthesia of the legs, but this rapidly wears off. The duration of postoperative weakness and hypotonia is long, and children initially lose quite a bit of functional ground. Strength returns gradually but reflexes do not reappear, and there is typically need for ankle support (AFOs) when ambulation is resumed. Most centers demand long and intense rehabilitation programs, an issue that can become a limiting factor because of cognitive or other compliance problems, not to mention the arbitrary restrictions of insurance companies and other funding agencies.

Long-term concerns about this operation that will require years to answer include the following:

1.   Spinal column instability as a result of the laminectomy and the potentiation of scoliosis development. This is a great concern in children with quadriplegia and with asymmetrical spasticity. If they ever do come to need scoliosis surgery, they may no longer have posterior bony elements to use for a fusion. Pronounced lower lumbar hyperlordosis has been observed, but its long-term significance is unknown.

2.   Recurrence of spasticity. This is rarely a problem, although the data are incomplete.

3.   Rapid hip dislocation soon after rhizotomy. This has been reported mainly in children with spastic quadriplegia, but its true incidence and significance are unknown at present (Greene et al., 1991).

4.   Other changes resulting from weakness in the lower extremities, especially about the ankle. Children can exhibit impressive ankle valgus and a marked propensity for knee flexion when they begin to ambulate postoperatively. Long-term problems with ankle instability and crouch gait have yet to be defined.

5.   Potential for long-term degenerative joint arthropathy as a result of lost proprioceptive and other sensory feedback.

6.   Bladder dysfunction, which has not been a problem to date.

In conclusion, selective dorsal rhizotomy is a new procedure being widely offered for the management of spasticity in children with cerebral palsy. Its advantage over more traditional orthopedic approaches has not been demonstrated conclusively, and its long-term complications are unknown. Only a comparative study using sophisticated gait analysis and careful long term follow-up will clarify the relative advantages and disadvantages of these two approaches. Although few neurosurgeons and few orthopedists have been willing to collaborate on such a study, some efforts are beginning to appear. Given the paramount importance of patient selection, no child should undergo rhizotomy without evaluation by *at least* a three-member team of experienced clinicians.

REFERENCES

Albright, A.L., Cervi, A., & Singletary, J. (1991). Intrathecal baclofen for spasticity in cerebral palsy. *JAMA, 265,* 1418–1422.

Armstrong, R.W. (1992). Intrathecal baclofen and spasticity: What do we know and what do we need to know? *Developmental Medicine and Child Neurology, 34,* 739–745.

Bleck, E.E. (1987). *Orthopedic management in cerebral palsy* (Clinics in Developmental Medicine, No. 99/100). London: MacKeith Press.

Bolanos, A.A., Bleck, E.E., Firestone, P., & Young, L. (1989). Comparison of stereognosis and two-point discrimination testing of the hands of children with cerebral palsy. *Developmental Medicine and Child Neurology, 31,* 371–376.

Chambers, H.G., Mubarak, S.J., & Wenger, D.R. (1993). The effect of valproic acid on blood loss in patients with cerebral palsy. *Developmental Medicine and Child Neurology, 35*(Suppl. 69), 18.

Fasano, V.A., Broggi, G., Barolat-Romana, G., & Sguazzi, A. (1978). Surgical treatment of spasticity in cerebral palsy. *Child's Brain, 4,* 289–305.

Gage, J.R. (1991). *Gait analysis in cerebral palsy* (Clinics in Developmental Medicine, No. 121). New York: Cambridge University Press.

Goldner, J. (1974). Upper extremity tendon transfers in cerebral palsy. *Orthopedic Clinics of North America, 5,* 389–414.

Gottlieb, G.L., Myklebust, B.M., Stefoski, D., Groth, K., Kroin, J., & Penn, R.D. (1985). Evaluation of cervical stimulation for chronic treatment of spasticity. *Neurology, 35,* 699–704.

Greene, W.B., Dietz, F.R., Goldberg, M.J., Gross, R.N., Miller, F., & Sussman, M.D. (1991). Rapid progression of hip subluxation in cerebral palsy after selective posterior rhizotomy. *Journal of Pediatric Orthopaedics, 11,* 494–497.

Hoffer, M.M., Lehman, M., & Mitami, M. (1989). Surgical indications in children with cerebral palsy. *Hand Clinics, 5,* 69–74.

Inman, V.T., Ralston, H.J., & Todd, F. (1981). *Human walking.* Baltimore: Williams & Wilkins.

Kalen, V., & Bleck, E.E. (1985). Prevention of spastic paralytic dislocation of the hip. *Developmental Medicine and Child Neurology, 27,* 17–24.

Kidmon, D., Steiner, I., & Melamed, E. (1987). Late-onset progressive radiculomyelopathy in patients with cervical athetoid-dystonic cerebral palsy. *European Neurology, 27,* 164–166.

Koman, L.A., Gelberman, R.H., Toby, E.B., & Poehling, G.G. (1990). Cerebral palsy: Management of the upper extremity. *Clinical Orthopedics and Related Research, 253,* 62–74.

Luque, E.R. (1982). The anatomic basis and development of segmental spinal instrumentation. *Spine, 7,* 256–259.

Peacock, W., & Arens, L.J. (1982). Selective posterior rhizotomy for the relief of spasticity in cerebral palsy. *South African Medical Journal, 62,* 119–124.

Peacock, W.J., Arens, L.J., & Berman, B., (1987). Cerebral palsy spasticity: Selective posterior rhizotomy. *Pediatric Neuroscience, 13,* 61–66.

Phillips, L.H., & Park, T.S. (1989). Electrophysiologic studies of selective posterior rhizotomy patients. In T.S. Park, L.H. Phillips, & W.J. Peacock (Eds.), *Neurosurgery state of the art review: Management of spasticity in cerebral palsy and spinal cord injury.* (Vol. 4, pp. 459–469). Philadelphia: Hanley and Belfus.

Ratusnick, D.L., Wolfe, V.I., Penn, R.D., & Schewitz, S. (1978). Effects on speech of chronic cerebellar stimulation in cerebral palsy. *Journal of Neurosurgery, 48,* 876–882.

Reade, R., Hom, L., Hallum, A., & Lopopolo, R. (1984). Change in popliteal angle measurement in infants up to one year of age. *Developmental Medicine and Child Neurology, 26,* 774–780.

Rodgers, B.M., Webb, C.J., Stergios, D., & Newman, B.M. (1988). Patient-controlled analgesia in pediatric surgery. *Journal of Pediatric Surgery, 23,* 259–262.

Rose, S.A., DeLuca, P.A., Davis, R.B., Ounpuu, S., & Gage, J.R. (1993). Kinematic and kinetic evaluation of the ankle after lengthening of the gastrocnemius fascia in children with cerebral palsy. *Journal of Pediatric Orthopaedics, 13,* 727–732.

Rosenthal, R.K., Deutsch, S.D., Miller, W., Schumann, W., & Hall, J.E. (1975). A fixed-ankle, below-the-knee orthosis for the management of genu recurration in spastic cerebral palsy. *Journal of Bone and Joint Surgery, 57A,* 545–547.

Salenius, P., & Vankka, E. (1975). The development of the tibiofemoral angle in children. *Journal of Bone and Joint Surgery, 57A,* 256–261.

Sangeorzan, B.J., Mosca, V., & Hansen, S.T. (1993). Effect of calcaneal lengthening on relationships among the hindfoot, midfoot, and forefoot. *Foot and Ankle, 14,* 136–141.

Smith, R., & Triffitt, J.T. (1986). Bones in muscles: The problems of soft tissue ossification. *Quarterly Journal of Medicine, 61,* 985–990.

Spelman, J.D., & van Manen, J. (1989). Cerebral palsy and stereotactic neurosurgery: Long term results. *Journal of Neurology, Neurosurgery, and Psychiatry, 52,* 23–30.

Staheli, L.T. (1977). The prone hip extension test. *Clinical Orthopedics and Related Research, 123,* 12–15.

Staheli, L.T. (1985). Lower-extremity-specific rotational problems in children: Normal values to guide management. *Journal of Bone and Joint Surgery, 67A,* 39–47.

Sussman, M.D. (1984). Advantage of early spinal stabilization and fusion in patients with Duchenne muscular dystrophy. *Journal of Pediatric Orthopaedics, 4,* 532–537.

Sussman, M.D., & Cusick, B. (1979). Preliminary report: The role of short leg, tone reducing casts as an adjunct to physical therapy in patients with cerebral palsy. *Johns Hopkins Medical Journal, 145,* 112–114.

Sutherland, D.H. (1984). *Gait disorders in childhood and adolescence.* Baltimore: Williams & Wilkins.

Teele, R.L., Nussbaum, A.R., Wyly, J.B., Allred, E.N., & Emans, J. (1987). Cholelithiasis after spinal fusion for scoliosis in children. *Journal of Pediatrics, 111,* 857–860.

Tetzlaff, J.E. (1991). Intraoperative defect in hemostasis in a child receiving valproic acid. *Canadian Journal of Anesthesia, 38,* 222–224.

Thometz, J.G., & Simon, S.R. (1988). Progression of scoliosis after skeletal maturity in institutionalized adults who have cerebral palsy. *Journal of Bone and Joint Surgery, 70A,* 1290–1296.

Wetmore, R.S., & Drennan, J.C. (1989). Long-term results of triple arthrodesis in Charcot-Marie-Tooth disease. *Journal of Bone and Joint Surgery, 71A,* 417–422.

Glossary

Antalgic—to avoid pain (e.g., when there is a rock in one's shoe). The result is a shortened stance phase (quick and light step) on the affected side.

Anteversion (femoral)—internal rotation of the leg from the hip as a result of torsion of the femoral shaft such that the distal end (the intercondylar plane) is twisted medially relative to the proximal end (the plane of the femoral neck–shaft).

Cadence—in gait analysis, the number of steps per minute.

Calcaneus—largest of the seven tarsal bones; also used in reference to a deformity of the ankle whereby the foot is directed upward relative to its usual position (i.e., in dorsiflexion [*talipes calcaneus*]). Calcaneus gait is a short-step gait in which weight is borne primarily on the heel.

Cavus deformity—equinus posture of the foot only from the point of the midfoot, also referred to as a high-arched foot or *pes cavus*.

Cobb angle—the angle used to measure deformity in scoliosis. The measurement involves choosing the vertebrae at the top and at the bottom of the curve, drawing a line to mark their horizontal plane, and constructing the perpendiculars to those lines. The complement to the intersection of the perpendiculars represents the Cobb angle (see Figure 10).

Contracture—fixed limitation of passive muscle stretch as a result of soft tissue fibrosis (i.e., fibrosis of the muscle, tendon, or joint capsule).

Coxa—Latin for "hip," as in *coxa valga*, the straightening of the angle formed by the femoral neck and shaft.

Dysplasia—abnormal development with resultant distorted architecture.

Equinus—positioning of the foot whereby the plane of the toes is pointing downward.

Gait—walking.

Gait cycle—two steps (or one stride).

Genu—Latin for "knee," as in *genu varum* (bow legs) or *genu valgum* (knock knees).

Goniometer—a device resembling two rulers hinged together that is used to measure joint angles.

Hallux—Latin for the great toe, as in *hallux valgus* (a bunion deformity).

Hamstrings—the knee flexor muscles that originate from the ischium: the biceps femoris, semimembranosis, and semitendinosis; functionally, the gracilis could be included as well.

Heel cord—the Achilles tendon from the triceps surae inserting into the calcaneus.

Kinematics—the description of the geometry of movement without consideration for the underlying forces involved. Typically linear and angular displacements, velocity, and acceleration are the primary measures.

Kinetics—the description of movement in terms of the internal and external forces involved. These moment and power measurements of energy are not possible to appreciate by visual inspection alone.

Obliquity—being slanted, as in pelvic (also termed pelvic tilt).

Orthosis—a support (or brace) for correcting and stabilizing the position of a body structure. Nomenclature is derived from the portion of the body that is covered by the device: for example, AFO, ankle–foot–orthosis; KAFO, knee–ankle–foot orthosis; HKAFO, hip–knee–ankle–foot orthosis; TLSO, thoracolumbosacral orthosis.

Planus—flat, as in *pes planus*, a low-arched (or flat) foot.

Recurvatum—curved backward; mostly used exclusively with *genu*. Therefore, *genu recurvatum* is hyperextension of the knee joint, also known as back-kneeing.

Station—the position or posture assumed when standing (or sitting) erect.

Step length—the distance covered in one step; the distance between right foot initial contact and left foot initial contact in double-limb stance.

Stride length—the distance covered in two steps; the distance from heel strike (or initial contact) to the following heel strike with the same foot.

Subluxation—displacement of a joint from normal position, with some maintenance of continuity, that is to say, some direct contact. In contrast, dislocation indicates there is no contact.

Talipes—Latin for a deformed foot ("ankle–foot") (i.e., a clubfoot). Although sometimes used synonymously with *pes*, pes more correctly refers simply to the foot.

Talus—the tarsal bone that articulates with the tibia and fibula. Vertical talus refers to a congenital rigid flat (or "rocker-bottom") foot deformity.

Torsion—being twisted, as in tibial.

Trendelenburg—a German orthopedic surgeon whose name has been applied to several clinical entities:

    Trendelenburg gait—with each step the upper trunk sways toward the side on which the patient puts weight. This is due to insufficient hip abductor muscle function (i.e., weakness) or to hip pain.

    Trendelenburg test—the subject is asked to stand on one leg. Normally the powerful hip abductors of the stance leg will maintain the pelvis horizontal and parallel to the floor. If these abductors are weak, the pelvis will tilt, with the opposite side dropping below the stance leg side. This would be a positive Trendelenburg test indicating hip abductor weakness.

Valgus (feminine form *valga*, neuter *valgum*)—Latin for "turned or bent out"; that is, the angulation of the distal segment of the body part being described is away from the midline of the body.

Varus (feminine form *vara*, neuter *varum*)—Latin for "turned in"; that is, the angulation is pointed toward the midline of the body.

Windswept hips—a deformity consisting of adduction contracture on one side and abduction posture, usually with an iliotibial band contracture, on the other side.

Chapter 8

The Neurophysiology of Cerebral Palsy

Larry W. Desch, M.D.

The clinical features displayed by patients with prenatal or perinatal central nervous system (CNS) insults resulting in cerebral palsy are extremely diverse in both the character and degree of symptoms expressed. In infants and young children especially, the neurologic findings often change with time, which can delay the complete descriptive diagnosis of the type of cerebral palsy. Although cerebral palsy is due to a nonprogressive CNS lesion, neural development and reorganization do occur, especially in young children, and this can alter the neurologic findings. In adults with cerebral palsy, even though a complete clinical description of abnormal neurologic functioning can usually be made, this does not necessarily imply complete understanding of the underlying neuropathology.

At present, patients with cerebral palsy are classified according to their neurologic findings. Such a classification is briefly summarized in Table 1, although others have been suggested (e.g., Alberman, 1984; Holt, 1966). Such clinical classification systems are useful; however, it has been recognized for decades that such systems are less than completely satisfactory because they do little to lead to an understanding of the abnormal physiology that is occurring.

Likewise, the morphologic changes of the brain that can be seen by modern imaging techniques such as computerized tomography (CT) or magnetic resonance imaging (MRI) have been found to be inadequate in increasing our understanding of the neurophysiologic changes that occur as a result of cerebral palsy. In one study by Molteni, Oleari, Fedrizzi, and Bracchi (1987), patients were found by CT to have apparently identical brain pathology despite having different clinical presentations. Some of the

patients who had small lesions on CT, for example, had worse neurologic disabilities than some of the patients who had larger areas.

However, new techniques of noninvasive neurophysiologic measurement, especially those coupled to computerized data acquisition and analysis, have begun to lead to definite increases in our understanding of the pathophysiology of cerebral palsy. Some of these techniques have been applied directly to patient care. Techniques such as gait and movement analysis and electromyography (EMG) have been found useful in assessment and treatment. Invasive techniques, usually done as part of a treatment, have also led to important new knowledge. This chapter summarizes and interprets the results from a sampling of the major published reports that have used these invasive and noninvasive techniques in order to elucidate how this work has added to our knowledge about normal and abnormal neurophysiology. In addition, a variety of results and concepts based on animal research are discussed in the context of their possible application to the understanding of neurologic findings that may be seen in humans.

This chapter concludes by exploring the gaps in our understanding about the neurophysiology of cerebral palsy and suggesting ways in which our knowledge may be improved. In addition, some directions that the use of the newest, "high-technology" techniques and treatments may take in the future are discussed.

HUMAN EXPERIMENTAL RESEARCH

Anatomic and basic physiologic studies relating to the brain and spinal cord have led to knowledge about how the different central nervous

Table 1. Classification of cerebral palsy (topographic and neurologic)

Spastic cerebral palsy
  Quadriplegia
  Diplegia
  Hemiplegia
  Double hemiplegia
  Monoplegia
  Triplegia

Extrapyramidal cerebral palsy (dyskinetic, athetoid)
  Choreoathetosis
  Tension
  Rigidity
  Dystonia

Mixed cerebral palsy (features of both spasticity and
    dyskinesia)
  Ataxic cerebral palsy
  Hypotonic cerebral palsy (may be an early finding in
    some infants before progressing to another type)
  Tremor type (rare or nonexistent)

structures are interconnected; however, only recently have studies been able to assess the dynamics of the system in humans (Figure 1). What has become unequivocal is that there are ongoing changes in the brain throughout one's lifetime as old connections are lost and new ones develop. People who have cerebral palsy, especially children, will often have changing clinical pictures secondary to these normal processes.

The clinical description of people with motor dysfunction has been augmented by such techniques as EMG. Although much of the research has focused on responses seen with spinal or segmental reflexes, it should always be kept in mind that these neurologic abnormalities are secondary to dysfunction in descending pathways.

Spinal Segmental
Responses (Reflexes and Movement)

Spasticity (Noninvasive Studies) Noninvasive techniques have confirmed that spasticity in cerebral palsy is due to a lack of supraspinal control of spinal circuits. Earlier, from about 1970 to 1975, it was theorized that this lack of central inhibition may directly cause increased excitability of the fusimotor–spindle system (the gamma motoneuron system). Gamma motoneurons are small, slow neurons that control small muscles in the muscle spindle itself to provide compensation for changes in length of the muscle spindles so that the spindles maintain their sensitivity. However, enough proof has been developed since the early 1980s to implicate a faster neuronal system, which has essentially eliminated the gamma system as the cause for the type of spasticity seen with cerebral palsy (Figure 2).

Perhaps one of the best early examples of evidence to refute the *gamma-release theory* was that provided by Delwaide (1973), involving research on vibratory reflex inhibition (VRI) and the tonic vibration reflex (TVR). Essentially, it had been discovered decades previously that vibration could reduce monosynaptic reflexes (VRI) and also cause contraction of muscles (TVR). In his work with people who had hemiplegia, Delwaide noted that the VRI was absent on the affected side and normal on the unaffected side. If a gamma-release phenomenon was involved, vibration would have been expected to have caused some inhibition of reflexes (through causing decreased output from muscle spindles).

More important, Delwaide also developed a paradigm in which passive sinusoidal mechanical stretching of muscles around the ankle led to decreased H-reflex (electrical stimulus induced) responses without evidence of stimulation of the spindles in antagonist muscles (which occurs normally with the VRI). Even slight phasic stretching led to some inhibition of the H-reflex responses. Therefore, this mechanical analog to the VRI added considerable evidence that large sensory (Ia) afferents had to be involved in the creation of the type of spasticity seen in cerebral palsy.

Following these early studies, Delwaide and others have solidified the evidence that what is actually occurring is Ia inhibition of the involved reflex arc (see Figure 1) (Delwaide, 1973; Desmedt, 1983). This inhibition most likely is due to decreased inhibitory influences coming from Ia interneurons on the reflex arc. The interneurons are less inhibitory secondary to the lack of descending control from supraspinal centers. A comprehensive review of this subject by Burke (1983) provided added evidence for the Ia pathway and concluded that the gamma system seems most likely to be involved only with voluntary motor activity.

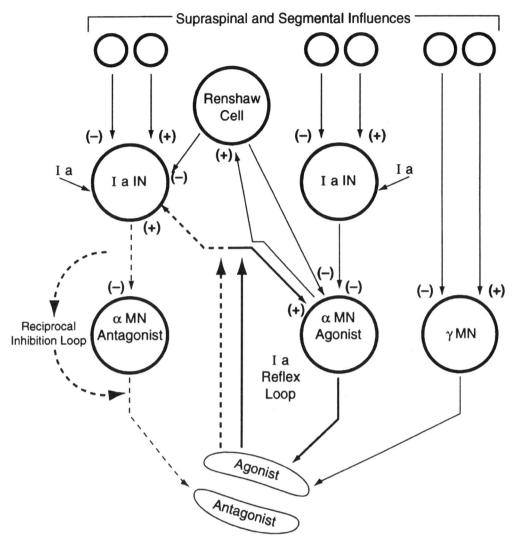

Figure 1. Diagram of the stretch reflex loop (myotatic reflex), reciprocal inhibition, gamma fusimotor system, and Renshaw circuit. (IN, inhibition; MN, motoneuron.)

Other research done since the 1970s provides corroborative data to support this *large afferent theory* as well. Neilson (1972) studied the tonic stretch reflex by evaluating biceps activity during voluntary as well as imposed sinusoidal flexion/extension movements at the elbow. Tonic stretch reflexes are essentially the reflexive response to movement of a muscle across a joint and are abnormal responses in subjects without neuromuscular disorders because muscles that are relaxed can be moved passively without resistance. A method was used that isolated the reflex EMG responses from those of the voluntary contraction. In sub-

jects without spasticity, the tonic stretch reflex became apparent with voluntary contraction, and modulation (decreases and increases) of the amplitude of the tonic stretch reflex occurred for some changes in frequency of the sinusoidal movements. In subjects with spasticity, no increase in the tonic stretch response with voluntary contraction was found, and the modulations in the reflex with changes in frequency of movement were not seen. These results indicate that the significant increases in spinal reflexes seen in persons with spasticity overwhelm any inhibition from descending supraspinal pathways, as would be seen in nor-

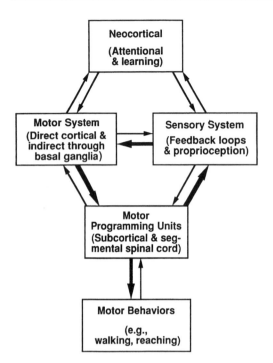

Figure 2. Simplified representation of the processes involved with motor skill learning. The influence of motor behaviors as well as sensory feedback should be noted. Thicker arrows indicate the major direction of the pathways.

mal subjects, a phenomenon that was called *short circuiting* by Neilson.

Since these earlier experiments by Neilson and similar ones by other researchers, other studies have demonstrated that subjects with spastic cerebral palsy are unable to inhibit antagonist muscles (i.e., triceps relaxation during biceps activity) during voluntary contractions. This abnormal co-activation of antagonistic muscles has been called by some researchers a *reciprocal excitation*, in contrast to the normal pattern of agonist excitation coupled with reciprocal inhibition of the antagonistic muscle (Gottlieb, Myklebust, Penn, & Agarwal, 1982). It is important to note from this research that the high degree of reciprocal excitation seen with people who have cerebral palsy is not seen in people who have adult-onset spasticity (e.g., secondary to stroke). Injury to an immature nervous system, subsequent changes in the CNS as a result of that injury, or both are somehow necessary for the extreme degree of reciprocal excitation to occur.

A study of normal infants by Myklebust, Gottlieb, and Agarwal (1986) demonstrated what appears to be reciprocal excitation as a result of tendon taps to elicit stretch reflexes. Although the researchers offer alternative possibilities for their findings, such as "hyperexcitable motor neuron pools" or "hypersensitive" motor units of the antagonistic muscles, these data add considerable evidence for the reciprocal excitation in spasticity being a "primitive" neuromotor program. These researchers provide evidence that this reciprocal excitation is due to decreased supraspinal inhibition of Ia interneurons that are usually responsible for normal reciprocal inhibition.

Myklebust (1990) has expanded on this work in studying infants and children both with and without spasticity. Much of this research has looked at the ratio of EMG responses from the tibialis anterior (TA) muscle to that of the soleus (SOL) muscle in response to stretch of the Achilles tendon (using tendon tap).

In infants without spasticity, the TA–SOL ratio is significantly larger than in adults. As a child matures, this TA–SOL ratio gradually decreases (especially during the first 3 years) until it is at adult values. Myklebust (1990) found that, in children and adults with cerebral palsy, this TA–SOL ratio remains large and is often larger than that seen in infants without cerebral palsy. Myklebust surmised, therefore, that in cerebral palsy either the normal reciprocal inhibition pathways are prevented from developing or, alternatively, there are facilitory pathways that persist. Although not mentioned by Myklebust, these findings could also be due to facilitory pathways that could be developing over time as a result of the abnormal supraspinal input.

This theory of reciprocal excitation has been challenged by results from a study done by Berbrayer and Ashby (1990). In their study of subjects with and without cerebral palsy, they did not find evidence of reciprocal excitation. In fact, the reciprocal inhibition found in subjects with cerebral palsy was as great as or greater than that seen in the subjects without cerebral palsy. This study used a paradigm of weak electrical stimulation to the tibial nerve, which was below the strength needed to cause contraction of the soleus muscle. Single motor unit recordings were done using a needle electrode into the TA muscle. This paradigm was chosen because of the concerns raised with the studies by Myklebust and Gottlieb that either vibratory effects (from the tendon tap) or volume conduction from one muscle group to another caused the EMG responses that were believed to be representing reciprocal excitation.

The results of both Berbrayer and Ashby's research and that by Myklebust and colleagues may not be contradictory. In addition to the different paradigms used, the subject population had more severe disabilities and was younger in the research by Myklebust. These are perhaps the most important distinctions. However, another distinction is that, in the study by Berbrayer and Ashby, the subjects voluntarily contracted the TA during the experiment to keep the single motor unit's firing rate as constant as possible. Although this report states that voluntary contraction should favor the presence of facilitation if it occurs with reciprocal excitation, facilitation on top of voluntary contraction may be seen only in "normal" motor systems. Thus, the voluntary contractions performed by those subjects with cerebral palsy may have "loaded" the supraspinal circuitry, causing the occurrence of TA inhibition subsequent to the stimulation of the alpha motoneuron to the soleus.

At this point in time, therefore, it is not certain that reciprocal excitation truly exists as a feature of spastic cerebral palsy or other conditions. Perhaps when and if reciprocal excitation occurs in a "damaged" motor control system, it is important primarily in situations in which supraspinal control over movements is not that helpful, such as walking. With typical gait, spinal segmentally generated motor programs may be partially to wholly at work (Joseph, 1985).

An alternative explanation that might explain how reciprocal excitation and reciprocal inhibition could both be taking place in spastic cerebral palsy is offered by looking at the possible function of another pathway called the Renshaw circuit (see Figure 1). Although our knowledge of the Renshaw circuit is incomplete, this circuit has been described as a "neural brake" for both agonist and antagonist alpha motoneurons (through inhibitory interneurons) (Brooks, 1986).

It is possible that, in cerebral palsy, it is the lack of descending control from supraspinal centers on this Renshaw circuit that is responsible for occasional reciprocal excitation as well as the high gain seen in the reflex loop (i.e., agonist spasticity). Limited studies done by a number of researchers, such as Katz and Pierrot-Deseilligny (1982), have led to some proof that decreased control over this Renshaw circuit seen in people with spasticity leads to problems with control over voluntary movement and in gauging the strength of contractions.

A theory incorporating the Renshaw circuit functions also might be useful to help explain why many people who have spastic cerebral palsy also have clonus. The theory of reciprocal excitation alone would seem to contradict the occurrence of clonus (thus, the presence of clonus in these individuals weakens the reciprocal excitation theory). Other researchers believe that other pathways, such as those involving Golgi tendon organs (located within muscle tendons), are more likely involved in clonus, especially because the time course of the Golgi tendon organ pathway is relatively long (Dimitrijevic, Nathan, & Sherwood, 1980). Such a "slow" pathway would be needed to set up the oscillations needed for clonus.

Spasticity (Invasive Studies) Surgical approaches to the treatment of cerebral palsy, although mainly orthopedic at present, may soon include more neurosurgical procedures. Spastic cerebral palsy is characterized by a lack of inhibition of monosynaptic reflexes, allowing all of the proprioceptive afferent impulses to influence the motoneuron pools directly, thus leading to spasticity. Similarly unmodulated polysynaptic pathways account for the more widespread abnormal motor responses. Because of these neural abnormalities, neurosurgical methods to change spinal cord sensory and motor nerve impulses have been seen as possible ways to improve overall motor functioning.

In persons with spasticity, Barolat-Romana and Davis (1980) found a direct relationship between the number of abnormal responses to rootlet stimulation and the degree of spasticity, and to more widespread motor problems such as startle reactions. Because of these monosynaptic and, more importantly, abnormal polysynaptic reflexes, a person with cerebral palsy apparently has limited alternatives for movement because of stereotyped response patterns.

Since this early research, several groups of researchers have improved on this technique of dorsal rootlet stimulation in order to use it for an increasingly popular neurosurgical procedure (e.g., Peacock & Staudt, 1991). Selective functional dorsal rhizotomy is done by selecting abnormal dorsal roots or rootlets that are then cut in an attempt to decrease spasticity in lower limb muscles. This root/rootlet sectioning is believed to cause an increase in the inhibition of motoneurons or a reduction in their facilitation.

These new surgical techniques, which use intraoperative electrical stimulation of the dorsal roots prior to any sectioning of nerves, have improved outcomes and reduced the incidence of complications, such as large areas lacking sensation or proprioception. In one of the first reported studies of this technique, 20 children were treated by selective rootlet section (Peacock & Arens, 1982). All children showed significant reduction in tone along with improvement in motor function. Unexplainedly, even though lumbar rootlets were sectioned, improved upper extremity function was reported in some cases. This study is mentioned primarily because it is one of only a few studies that have presented long-term follow-up results as well (Arens, Peacock, & Peter, 1989). This and other long-term results have indicated that lower extremity spasticity remains significantly reduced; however, some children have developed hip instability and other conditions requiring orthopedic procedures. Pre- and postsurgical gait analysis has been used to determine the efficacy of this surgical approach by Peacock's group as well as others (Boscarino, Ounpuu, Davis, Gage, & DeLuca, 1993) (see later section on EMG Techniques).

However, the scientific basis to justify this selective dorsal rhizotomy technique has come under intense, often heated, scrutiny and debate. Perhaps the most worrisome data available to date are those provided by Cohen and Webster

(1991). In their study of 22 persons undergoing the selective rhizotomy procedure, they were unable to find any EMG response to stimulation of rootlets that could be called "normal." This finding is not entirely unexpected, given that spasticity is due to decreased supraspinal inhibition. Why some rootlets at the same cord level might be spared the effects of decreased supraspinal inhibition and other rootlets are affected is difficult to explain. However, there may be differences in rootlet responses resulting from as yet undefined trans-segmental collateral- or interneuron-mediated interactions causing some "normalization" of the EMG responses to rootlet stimulation. Additional studies urgently need to be done with persons undergoing selective dorsal rhizotomy to resolve this and other questions.

Although this surgery is rapidly becoming commonplace, especially in the United States, this procedure still should be considered a research procedure to ensure that the subjects will be studied investigatively. Numerous authors have advocated for controlled trials, such as comparing the results of randomly selected partial rhizotomy with those of the selective approach, or comparing results of intense prolonged physical therapy with either neurosurgical procedure just mentioned. A few controlled research trials, such as one at the University of Washington, are nearing completion, and the results of these should be interesting and, perhaps, provocative.

Spasticity—A Summary   As the above descriptions attest, because spasticity can be easily studied using both invasive and noninvasive techniques, this has led to numerous studies being done (some with conflicting results). There are some congruities in these studies, however, that now are addressed further.

A review by Harrison (1988) presented an extensive evaluation of results from studies that support the role of abnormal spinal interneuronal relationships in spastic cerebral palsy. Harrison stated that movement depends on a balance of excitatory and inhibitory forces that act in coordinated fashion in spinal motoneurons and interneurons. In spastic cerebral palsy, however, the limited repertoire of voluntary movements suggests that there is a predominance of spinal interneuronal activity.

The proper sequencing of activation of muscles, which again is a reflection of the balancing of interneuron function, is likewise critical to movement, as shown by Nasher and McCollum (1985). Their studies of children with spasticity have demonstrated that proper sequencing of muscle activity is critical for both the stabilization and initiation of movements. The abnormalities that are seen with the sequencing of contractions may also help to explain the discrepancies between studies investigating reciprocal excitation. Related to this, another study demonstrated a variety of reciprocal interactions (e.g., both excitation and inhibition) using H-reflex testing during active movements (Leonard, Moritani, Hirschfeld, & Forssberg, 1990).

Despite this advancing knowledge, there remains a critical question: Does spasticity in cerebral palsy occur because there is lack of inhibition of motoneurons (e.g., because of inhibitory neuron death), or is it due to the formation of aberrant excitatory pathways (e.g., with spinal interneurons) secondary to the damage of the brain? Large longitudinal studies of subjects, preferably beginning during infancy, that evaluate both voluntary and reflex responses will undoubtedly be needed to answer such complex questions.

Extrapyramidal Influences

Athetosis (Extrapyramidal Cerebral Palsy, Dyskinesia, Dystonia)   Andrews, Neilson, and Knowles (1973) studied subjects with athetoid cerebral palsy using a research paradigm similar to that used by Neilson (1972) to study spasticity (see previous section). Measurement of the tonic stretch reflex activity in various muscles revealed an interesting differentiation between subjects with athetosis and those with spasticity. In contrast to subjects with spasticity, the subjects with athetosis showed inhibition of stretch reflexes as biceps length increased. Also, biceps EMG activity was increased at rest; this was considered to be due to alpha motoneuron hyperactivity. This work, and that of others (Narabayashi, Nagahata, Nagao, & Shimazu, 1965), has led to a clearer differentiation of patients with athetosis. Clinical subtypes of athetosis (rigid and rigidospastic) were suggested by Narabayashi and co-workers.

In their study of over 400 children who had different types of cerebral palsy, Narabayashi's group demonstrated that, when the affected muscles are stretched, a characteristic EMG pattern develops in response. With the rigid type of hypertonicity, EMG activity continues as long as the muscle remains stretched. With spastic hypertonicity, the EMG response occurs only or mainly during the initial stretching (the phasic response, described previously). This group found that subjects who had athetotic cerebral palsy had a combination of both rigidity and spasticity with considerable fluctuation in both degree and duration (especially of the rigidity). This fluctuation was the most characteristic EMG feature differentiating persons with a clinical diagnosis of athetoid versus spastic cerebral palsy.

Further research into the neurophysiologic basis of extrapyramidal cerebral palsy has addressed the abnormal involuntary movements that are often seen. Using a method that employed voluntary rapid flexion at the elbow of subjects, Hallett and Alvarez (1983) examined the EMG activity during these movements. They found the expected excessive muscular activity, but also found inappropriate activity, such as in the opposite limb. Different patterns of EMG activity were found, often in the same subject, that included patterns of co-contraction of both biceps and triceps muscles (often of long duration) or contraction of the triceps leading to extension rather than flexion.

Work by Neilson and O'Dwyer (1984) added further proof to this view that problems with the extrapyramidal system cause the abnormalities seen with voluntary movements. Their research, using extensive EMG recordings of muscles involved with speech production, has demonstrated that both the timing and amplitude of voluntary activity are abnormal in persons with cerebral palsy. These abnormalities therefore likely do not involve changes in segmental systems (as with spasticity) but are more likely due to problems with supraspinal control mechanisms. Incidental evidence for this can be found by contrasting the type of spasticity seen in cerebral palsy with adult-onset spasticity. In contrast to the vastly different symptomatology of these spastic states, extrapyramidal cerebral palsy resembles adult extrapyramidal disorders (e.g., Parkinson disease). An explanation for this difference may be the relatively late maturation of the basal ganglia (and "delayed" connections to it from other centers, such as the brain stem and cerebellum).

The abnormal movement patterns seen with athetoid cerebral palsy lend further credence to the hypothesis that damage to the basal ganglia is ultimately responsible. There are other areas of proof for this. For example, one study evaluated neuropathologic findings in children with athetoid cerebral palsy (Rutherford, Pennock, Murdoch-Eaton, Cowan, & Dubowitz, 1992). These children had hypoxic–ischemic encephalopathy during the neonatal period, and, on later brain imaging studies, most had cysts in the putamen and, occasionally, in other basal ganglia areas as well.

Central Motor Areas (Cortical Interactions)

Somatosensory Cortex   The motor disturbances seen in cerebral palsy have been shown to be the result of deficits in cortical processing of both motor output and sensory input. A child or adult with cerebral palsy can correct movement only if there is accurate awareness of the movement.

In addition to the numerous studies of the motor correlates of cerebral palsy, there have been a number of investigations of the sensory systems of patients with cerebral palsy. Early clinical studies by a number of investigators (e.g., Tachdjian & Minear, 1958) utilized subjective sensory measurements such as temperature, pain, and stereognosis to demonstrate that 40%–50% of children with cerebral palsy had sensory disturbances.

Later studies have improved on these early reports by use of more objective measurement techniques. For example, a study of children who have hemiplegic cerebral palsy demonstrated that a spectrum of sensory deficiencies can be found (Van Heest, House, & Putnam, 1993). In addition, this study demonstrated that the size of the limb (especially the arm and hand) is inversely related to the degree of the deficit (i.e., a smaller extremity is related to worse deficits).

In people with hemiplegic cerebral palsy, disturbances in peripheral sensory nerve conduc-

tion velocities have also been found by some researchers (Lang, Sillanpaa, & Hynninen, 1983), although not by others (Sutton, Cohen, & Krusen, 1967; Takebe & Basmajian, 1976). Nonetheless, if there truly is a difference in velocities, the responsible mechanism remains unclear. Peripheral nerve velocity changes, if they exist, may well be secondary to the damage in the sensory or motor cortex or both, or may be simply due to atrophy of muscles or temperature decrease of the affected limb. However, as Lang and co-workers pointed out, the decreased temperature or lesser muscle volume of a limb actually tends to increase the amplitude of the nerve conduction velocity rather than reduce it. This makes it more likely that changes in the cortex are primarily responsible for the decreased velocities observed (Lang et al., 1983).

Other work has found significant abnormalities in proprioception and other sensations related to movement. A study of kinesthetic recall in children with spastic or athetoid cerebral palsy compared to children without cerebral palsy was reported by Opila-Lehman, Short, and Trombly (1985). For this experiment, each of the children had their dominant arm moved in a specified amount of arc by internal or external rotation at the shoulder with the elbow held in 45 degrees of flexion. After each passive movement, the children were instructed to voluntarily return their arm to the same place. In this study, children with spastic cerebral palsy performed worse than children who had athetoid cerebral palsy, and both groups made significantly greater numbers of errors than controls.

Although there have been some studies of somatosensory evoked potentials in subjects without disabilities, including children, few data exist for subjects who have cerebral palsy. This may well be because these techniques are relatively new and somewhat difficult to perform reliably, although they are noninvasive. Wong, Lombroso, and Maysumiya (1982) reported on a small study that included a few children with hemiplegic cerebral palsy. They found that a larger amount of "noise," rather than clean signals, seems to be correlated with the degree of deficit.

Based on these interesting but limited results of studies that have examined the sensory changes that occur with cerebral palsy, it is hoped that further studies will be forthcoming. For example, longitudinal studies that would investigate sensory evoked potentials in children who have cerebral palsy should lead to very useful information about maturational effects and neural reorganization.

Motor Cortex Improvements in methods for noninvasive techniques have begun to provide information about motor functioning in children both with and without cerebral palsy. Revealing information can be obtained by methods for studying long latency transcortical responses and other changes that can be detected by precise EMG studies. Methods to study EMG responses have used such techniques as direct cutaneous electrical stimulation, uniform tendon taps, or imposed movement about a joint. Most of this work, however, has so far been done mainly with adult subjects without cerebral palsy.

A few studies of children have evaluated the normal development and maturation of long-latency (i.e., transcortical, M2 and M3) and short-latency (i.e., spinal reflex, M1) responses to imposed muscle stretch (Bawa, 1981) and to cutaneous stimulation (Issler & Stephens, 1983; Rowlandson & Stephens, 1985a, 1985b) (Figure 3). These studies have provided normative data that could be used with studies of individuals with cerebral palsy. Stephens' group showed a clear maturational sequence of short- and long-latency responses and suggested that the maturation of the long-latency pathway coincided with clinical observations of increased coordination in children's movements. As demonstrated in Figure 3, definite changes occur over time with the M1 and M2 (and M3) responses. These changes seem to reflect the expected developmental maturation in that the EMG activity seen with M1 (i.e., spinal reflexes) diminishes as cortically mediated motor control increases (as shown by the relative increase in M2 responses).

The recent work of Rowlandson and Stephens (1985a) demonstrates the potential of evaluating M1 and M2 responses as a way to help investigate the neurophysiologic problems of children with cerebral palsy. In their study, they examined children with various neuro-

logic abnormalities, including hemiplegia, spinal cord disorders, and learning disabilities. They found an increased short-latency response and an absent long-latency response on the affected side of the children with hemiplegia. The uninvolved side showed apparently normal reflexes.

There were other interesting results reported in this study. In subjects with learning disabilities, the long-latency response was usually abnormal, but changes in the short-latency response were also observed. Children who have learning disabilities often have subtle neurologic abnormalities ("soft signs") and have occasionally been diagnosed as having minimal cerebral palsy. The EMG findings in this study appear to lend some credence to this interpretation. Supportive evidence comes from preliminary data from a longitudinal study that demonstrated that EMG responses in some children who have learning disabilities and soft signs appear to continue (at least for 2 years) to be either delayed or abnormal compared to those of control children (Desch, 1989) (see also Figure 3).

Related research in individuals with neuromuscular disorders that might have bearing on future studies with individuals who have cerebral palsy (especially the athetoid type) has also been reported. Marsden, Merton, Morton, and Adam (1978) and Verrier, Tatton, and Blair (1984) reported the absence of long-latency responses in adult stroke patients. Patients with Parkinson's disease, however, had exaggerated and disordered long-loop responses. These and other researchers also found long-latency responses to be absent in Huntington's chorea, prolonged in dystonia musculorum deformans, and absent with dorsal column spinal lesions.

Cerebral Cortex—Summary The most important key to developing better understanding of the neurophysiology of cerebral palsy is the improvement of our knowledge of what occurs in typical developmental processes. As more is discovered concerning the usual neurodevelopmental changes, other studies will follow that will examine the specific effects of the damage to the brain that has led to cerebral palsy. It is most likely that, with further studies of cerebral palsy, a large variety of effects will be found that may be correlated to the multitude of differ-

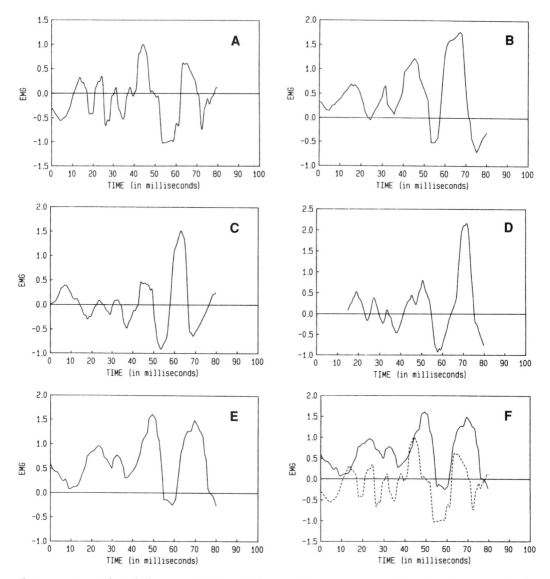

Figure 3.   Averaged rectified EMG activity (as multiples of background EMG) in subjects of different ages and with different disorders. Note that the M2 activity (around 60 msec) normally increases with age as M1 activity (spinal reflex loop) decreases. *A*, Normal exam in 3-year-old girl; *B*, normal exam in 5-year-old boy; *C*, normal exam in 7-year-old boy; *D*, normal exam in 12-year-old boy; *E*, minor soft signs in 9-year-old girl; *F*, comparison of subject in part A (dashed line) with subject in part E (solid line).

ent clinical findings that are seen with the various types of cerebral palsy.

Those days of enlightenment are still in the future. Nonetheless, in recent years, currently, and in the near future much will also be discovered about the neurophysiologic processes of cerebral palsy by research studies that are treatment and therapy oriented. In addition, these types of therapeutic studies often have served as

a guide for design of experimental controlled studies.

INSIGHTS FROM ANIMAL RESEARCH

Since the mid-1980s, a number of basic research endeavors using animal models have significantly improved our knowledge of the mechanisms underlying both normal and abnormal motor control. Extension of these findings to noninvasive measurement in human subjects provide a window into developmentally disordered brain function.

Spinal Segmental Responses

The search for animal models for the type of spasticity that is seen in cerebral palsy has not been very fruitful, mainly because of the difference between the brains of humans and of animals and because of the difficulty of producing injury to the brains of young animals. Often experimental injury to the brains of animals, such as rodents, leads to either the death of the animal or, in a short time, apparently full motor recovery. However, there is a type of hybrid mouse that has a genetic propensity for significant chronic spasticity. The use of these mice as an animal model for studying cerebral palsy was critiqued by Wright and Rang (1990). Their review concluded that this "spastic mouse model" is inadequate to study human disorders, mainly because the mice have a genetic alteration that causes an abnormally functioning neurotransmitter to be produced, whereas, in human disease, the pathophysiology is due to structural defects or damage. These researchers did point out that the spastic mouse model may be useful to help study the secondary effects of chronic spasticity on bones, joints, or muscles.

Researchers have also begun to develop investigations using intact animals. An example of this is work that evaluates whether spinal reflexes in animals can be modified by learning. Much of the recent research in this area has been done by Wolpaw and Dowman (1988) using neurologically intact animal models, including primates. The animals learned to control the level of EMG output in response to various degrees of stretch of a muscle. Spinal reflex amplitudes could be increased or decreased in this operant conditioning paradigm. At present, however, the utility of this approach with neurologically compromised persons, such as those with cerebral palsy, is difficult to assess.

Motor Cortex

Animal studies of the motor cortex have provided some information about possible mechanisms for dysfunction in humans, and in particular have provided us with considerable information about how injury or dysfunction of the corticospinal tract can relate to disturbances of motor performance.

Studies of the motor cortex of animal models have also elucidated feedback mechanisms that may be important in understanding cerebral palsy. The integrity and proper function of the motor cortex is important to govern the responses of movement and tone. This was demonstrated (primarily using the primate model) by Cheney, Fetz, and Mewes (1991). This and other research has demonstrated the importance of the long-latency (transcortical) responses that appear to be related primarily to control over muscle tone and fine movements (Porter, 1987).

Related to the neurophysiology of children (including those who have cerebral palsy) is recent work showing that the functioning of the motor cortex, specifically in relation to the long-latency transcortical loops, is a developmental process. These loops gradually develop over time and appear to be involved in the clinical development or appearance of improved balance and muscle control (Bruce & Tatton, 1980).

Research involving animal models of trans-synaptic degeneration may have particular significance to cerebral palsy in addressing what can happen as a result of early brain damage. Trans-synaptic degeneration refers to a phenomenon in which depriving target neurons of their inputs may result in the death of the post-synaptic cells. From this work, it has been concluded that trophic factors are necessary for the maintenance of target cells, most convincingly demonstrated in the neuromuscular junction, where muscle fibers degenerate in the absence of motoneurons or motoneuron activity (Lomo & Jansen, 1980).

In the adult CNS, however, most neurons receive afferents from more than one source, so that trophic factors from surviving structures combined with the sprouting of terminals from the intact source may help to preserve the post-synaptic cells. The *developing* CNS may respond differently to this process. If axons from the motor system, for example, fail to reach their primary targets as a result of trauma, do their targets in the other cortical areas degenerate, a process that is then repeated in both higher sensory and motor pathways? If this is so, then specific damage at a specific point in development could, by a cascade of transneuronal degeneration, produce symptoms of impairment in both somatic sensation and motor control. A striking example of such cascade effects was found in the kitten brain stem by Torvik (1956).

Another concern that has been raised based on results of animal research is concerned with possible effects of early brain damage to the occurrence and duration of critical developmental periods. In the cat visual system, for example, the normal development of cortical processing circuits depends on the kitten's exposure to a normal visual environment during a restricted time of a few weeks during postnatal life. If visual experience is restricted during this critical period, visual processing is permanently abnormal, whereas the same deprivation prior to or following this period has little or no permanent effect (Blakemore & Van Sluyters, 1975).

Extension of these findings about critical periods to the development of the motor system is as yet incomplete, but some hints that a motor critical period exists have been reported. Nissen, Chow, and Semmes (1951) encased the forelimbs of a newborn monkey in tubes, preventing tactile exploration of the world during early postnatal life. Subsequent testing of manual dexterity revealed impaired performance in the deprived animal. In addition to those results, there also appears to be a critical period in which forced movement can alter cortical neuronal development. Using a kitten model, a striking difference in cortical motor areas can be induced by forced exercise of a limb, but only if this exercise occurs sometime prior to 11 weeks (Spinelli & Jensen, 1979).

The existence of critical periods, directly shown only in animal models, has great implications for the treatment of cerebral palsy, because a knowledge of the critical periods for sensory and motor development would indicate those times during which therapeutic intervention would be most effective. Unfortunately, relatively little is known of human critical periods. Tychsen and Lisberger (1986) have provided data consistent with the presence of a crit-

ical period for normal binocular vision based on visual-pursuit testing of adults who had infantile strabismus.

There has also been concern about whether early brain damage can lead to motor and sensory impairments because of the creation of abnormal circuitry (Figure 4). This concern centers around the continuing controversy over what has been termed the *Kennard principle*. This theory states that a lesion early in development is less disruptive than the same lesion in an adult. This idea, based on lesion studies followed by behavioral observations such as those carried out by Kennard (1942) and refuted by others, such as Schneider (1979), cannot be reviewed fully here, but one of the theorized mechanisms, collateral sprouting, may be of direct relevance to how humans might recover from brain damage that occurs in early life.

It is well established that, in response to denervation, neighboring axon terminals may respond to a "signal" by growing branches to cover the denervated postsynaptic surfaces. This

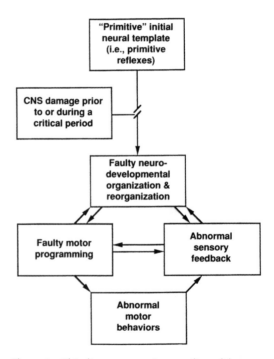

Figure 4. This diagram presents an outline of the possible manner in which early CNS damage can lead to abnormal motor behaviors. In this model, secondary neural abnormalities can occur as a result of erroneous motor behaviors and incorrect sensory feedback.

process occurs even in the adult nervous system but is more evident in the developing system, where a variety of analogous signals may be required for the normal innervation of target structures. These aberrant connections appear to make normal, functional synapses with inappropriate targets and so are likely to produce aberrant responses in those pathways. As noted previously, aberrant features of spinal pathways have been observed in children with cerebral palsy, and these may reflect such collateral sprouting following injury to, or the delayed growth of, descending tracts to the spinal segments.

Animal Studies—Summary

In this brief review, it is impossible to do justice to the extensive amount of work done with developing animal models, so attention has been focused on some of those features that appear to relate to the symptomatology of the different types of cerebral palsy. The three areas of research just presented, which have emerged from previous work with animal models, certainly need to be tested much further, but can be summarized as follows:

1. By the process of transneuronal degeneration, CNS damage may cause neuronal death in distant structures, resulting in motor and sensory deficits unrelated to the primary lesion.

2. Damage to a pathway may prevent a critical period or, more likely, have no functional sequelae until such a critical period occurs. Therefore, the neurologic symptoms may occur remotely in time from the occurrence of the insult (e.g., the appearance of athetosis after 12–13 months of age).

3. The response to injury by collateral sprouting may cause unpredictable behavioral effects, depending on the developmental state of axons near the denervated target. Axons in different pathways, therefore, may be differentially sensitive to the denervation signal as they approach or grow away from the target. Certain types of abnormal collateralization may be found that are induced by or occur as a *response* to feedback from the altered motor control, rather than secondary to the initial damage (see Figure 2).

It will remain uncertain for years to come which, if any, of the above theories are true. Ob-

viously much more research must be done to verify even one of these hypotheses. However, the implications are important. For example, a definitive answer regarding the third issue raises the possibility that suppression of sprouting, possibly by some type of medication, may be of therapeutic value in neurologic systems in which limited or no activity is "better" (in a functional sense) than is dysfunction.

NEUROPHYSIOLOGIC MEASUREMENTS IN TREATMENT REGIMENS

Much of the research that addresses the neurophysiology of cerebral palsy is carried out in the context of therapeutic interventions with humans. Some of the better research using the case study design has significantly added to our understanding of the developmental symptomatology of cerebral palsy. However, the use of this approach remains somewhat anecdotal and subjective, especially in those studies in which the assessment methods were not blinded or there are many confounding variables that are not controlled. Nonetheless, it is important to review some of these studies in order to examine certain current information and theories.

Electromyographic Techniques

Electromyographic techniques have been used to measure the effects of different therapies or interventions with people who have cerebral palsy. Almost every muscle that can be readily recorded has been studied in persons, usually adults, with cerebral palsy. This section takes an anatomic approach in reviewing the investigations by dividing studies into those centered on movements of the upper extremity, the lower extremity, and other areas.

Upper Extremity An important component of the overall functioning of a person who has cerebral palsy is the ability to control the hands and arms. Hand and arm function is not always simple to evaluate because of the variability of reflex pattern inhibition and ability to control involuntary movements, as in choreoathetosis. Electromyography has become one of the more reliable methods to assess improvements in hand function objectively.

A comprehensive study done by Mowery, Gelberman, and Rhoades (1985) used several methods to evaluate results of upper extremity tendon transfers in children with spastic hemiplegia. In that study, EMG and video recording of movement were used in addition to a clinical grading of muscles. In all 12 children studied, there was clinical improvement; however, a number of interesting changes took place in 4 of the 16 muscles studied with EMG following the tendon transfers. Three of these muscles that had been continuously firing preoperatively became phasic after the transfer. More important, one transferred muscle that was initially out of phase changed phase after operation to match that of the recipient muscle. In this study, as in similar research by Samilson and Morris (1964), there was no method found by which one could predict which muscles would change their electrical activity following tendon transfer.

At least one study failed to demonstrate any changes in phase of muscles after tendon transfer (Hoffer, Perry, & Melkonian, 1990). In that study, which was based on upper extremity transfers, the postoperative evaluations occurred somewhat earlier than in other reported studies. Although hypotheses have been raised to explain the probable alterations in the EMG of transferred muscles, such as being secondary to changes related to proprioception and sensory feedback from the muscles, a definite explanation is still forthcoming.

Although not employing EMG or other direct neurophysiological measurement techniques, Seeger, Caudrey, and O'Mara (1984) used an objective assessment of hand function to demonstrate that increasing the hip flexion angle of sitting does not appear to improve hand function in people with cerebral palsy. This is in contrast to widespread beliefs based on prior clinical impressions. Seeger et al.'s study used a microprocessor-controlled device that presents a series of target stimuli to which the subject being tested responds by moving a joystick. Accuracy and time of movements then were recorded and analyzed for different seating angles. It is likely that future studies will use EMG measurements in the upper extremity as well as similar computerized devices to objectify hand and arm movements.

Lower Extremity and Gait Analysis Locomotion in children and adults with cerebral palsy, and in controls without cerebral palsy, has been increasingly investigated using EMG (Gage, 1993). Spastic muscles are usually found to be dysphasic or to have prolonged phasic activity. The normal sequence of joint motion with muscle activity was also somewhat altered in children and adults with cerebral palsy, for example, with the presence of spastic cerebral palsy leading to a shorter stance phase (Berger, Quintern, & Dietz, 1985).

Chong, Vojnic, and Quanbury (1978) studied a specific type of gait pattern, internal rotation gait, which is often seen in children who have the spastic diplegic type of cerebral palsy. Three distinctive patterns of activity were found. The first was a diagnostic pattern in which the medial hamstring muscle group was primarily affected and caused the internal rotation. The second was a nondiagnostic pattern characterized by variability and inconsistencies in muscle groups involved. The third was a pattern called the *mass limb reflex* that involved many muscle groups. These workers concluded, as have numerous others studying EMG patterns since then, that EMG assessment is highly useful in distinguishing those persons most likely to benefit from orthopedic surgery from those unlikely to improve. The actual muscle activity is often not that distinctive on clinical examination, especially to physicians who lack extensive experience.

Improvements in EMG techniques have occurred recently that promise to enhance the analysis of gait using EMG. Winter and Yack (1987) were among the first groups to outline the "state of the art" of assessment using EMG to gather data on gait. Radiotelemetry was used to gather EMG and foot switch signals while subjects were walking. A video camera simultaneously recorded walking. A desktop personal computer was used to gather, average, and analyze EMG activity and collect other data. Using this system, the analyzed EMG data could be related directly to the video recording in order to gain further evidence about the types of abnormal gait that are seen. As a result of this and related studies, many researchers have concluded that such an approach should be used in both planning therapeutic procedures and assessing the results of treatments.

A promising new use of gait analysis, especially with studies incorporating EMG measurements, is in evaluating the treatment of individuals with cerebral palsy who are receiving antispastic medication, such as baclofen. Gait analysis employing integrated EMG and video recording has demonstrated that baclofen can reduce the co-contractions that are commonly seen with cerebral palsy (Knutsson, 1983).

This and other similar studies provide some indirect evidence of the neurophysiologic effects of baclofen. Baclofen is thought to have its major effects on spinal cord functions, especially in suppressing the motoneuron facilitation resulting from afferent input from muscles and possibly other sensory input. It is hoped that research in the basic pathophysiology of cerebral palsy as well as further therapeutic studies using baclofen or other medications will soon begin to answer the questions of how to predict and objectively evaluate the efficacy of those medications available now or ones that may be developed in the future.

Electromyographic activity during movements of the lower extremity in children and adults with cerebral palsy has also been used to determine the efficacy of physical therapy methods. Laskas, Mullen, Nelson, and Willson-Broyles (1985) used a single-subject experimental design to determine whether neurodevelopmental treatment would change the EMG activities of the lower leg muscles in a 2½-year-old boy with spastic quadriplegia. Recordings were made during movement to a standing position. Electromyographic activity in the dorsal flexors of the leg and heel contact increased after the therapy. Although this was a limited evaluation, it further supports the idea that EMG techniques can be useful in evaluating the outcomes of various types of treatment.

More needs to be done with gait analysis, especially in basic research. At the present time, gait analysis is used primarily to assess pre- versus postoperative improvement in individual subjects. Studies must be formulated in which the data from a large number of gait analyses are correlated to the clinical findings that are seen in the subjects. The data from gait analyses should also be compared to data from the same subject collected by experimental neurophysiologic measures such as averaged electroencephalography, magnetic stimulation, and EMG, as well as such evaluations as CT scans and MRI. Gait analysis will, for the foreseeable future, be plagued with the vast amounts of data being generated on each subject (e.g., movement, EMG, torque, pressure). Until artificial neural networks to analyze the data become available, much of the potential for gait analysis to answer many of the more complex questions about motor control will not be tapped.

Extraocular and Facial Muscles Cerebral palsy is also known to frequently affect the extraocular and facial muscles. Approximately 40% of children with cerebral palsy develop strabismus, and many require corrective surgery (Black, 1982). The neurophysiologic reasons for the development of strabismus in people with cerebral palsy are poorly understood; however, theories on the causes of strabismus have mainly considered strabismus to be due to either damage or maldevelopment in either the parietal–occipital or middle temporal cortical areas (Quick, Tigges, Gammon, & Boothe, 1989). Recently, a number of groups of researchers have demonstrated the permanent neurophysiologic changes that infantile strabismus can have on the visual system (e.g., Tychsen & Lisberger, 1986).

These studies often involve extensive analysis of such phenomena as visual pursuit and smooth eye muscle activity. For example, one neurophysiologic measurement technique involves attaching tiny magnetic coils to anesthetized eyes, with large pick-up coils around the subjects to receive impulses that then are converted into data concerning velocity and direction of eye movement (Tychsen & Lisberger, 1986). Studies such as these have reinforced the feelings of most clinicians that strabismus should be treated early and aggressively. At least one study has suggested that some of the later onset problems with visual tracking will be self-corrected if normal binocular vision can be restored before 6 months of age (Scheiman, Ciner, & Gallaway, 1989). This result reinforces the theories previously discussed regarding critical periods for development.

Even without the overt development of strabismus, other visual-motor problems may develop because of the presence of cerebral palsy, such as difficulties in accommodation or tracking. Abercrombie, Davis, and Schackel (1963) were among the first to report on abnormalities of pursuit eye movements in children with cerebral palsy by using electro-oculography. Pursuit eye movements are usually accompanied by such abnormalities as irregular head or eye movements, poor fixation, and poor visual-motor performance (Abercrombie et al., 1963; Mayberry & Gilligan, 1985).

Other facial muscles affected by cerebral palsy include those of speech production. Investigations of stretch reflexes and long-latency response mechanisms in the muscles of the face and neck have been carried out by Neilson and O'Dwyer (1984). They found that tonic stretch reflexes were probably not important causative agents in the dysarthric speech seen in spastic cerebral palsy. The study did find some increase in tonic stretch reflexes in jaw muscles.

Further work by O'Dwyer and Neilson (1988) revealed that dysarthria in patients with athetoid cerebral palsy may be due to abnormal *voluntary* activity rather than to involuntary activity. Each subject showed an idiosyncratic pattern of abnormal muscle activity on repetition of the same phrase. This adds further evidence to the growing impression that many of the normal movements seen in patients with cerebral palsy are motor programming defects that are often very consistent and replicable in each subject. Similar deficits have been found in nonspeech muscle coordination as well.

Electrical Stimulation

Although basic research has increasingly improved our understanding of CNS pathophysiology, few therapeutic studies have attempted to directly modulate the altered CNS. One such approach involves chronic stimulation of the cerebellum through implanted electrodes, a technique first introduced by Cooper beginning in 1972 (Cooper & Upton, 1978).

When the use of this technique was being implemented, it was thought that the relief of spasticity and improved motor control was due to increased output from stimulated Purkinjie cells, a theory mainly based on results from animal studies of epilepsy. Subsequent to that time, however, other more reasonable explanations have been brought forth. It has been theorized, for example, that cerebellar stimulation may actually cause effects on the ascending reticular formation and possibly some thalamic nuclei by activation of neurons in cerebellar nuclei and cerebellar inputs into the reticular formation. The effect may also be due to a more widespread excitation of the reticular formation, so that there is an overall increased cortical activation. However, one fact that would seem to dispute this theory of a widespread cortical activation increase is that there has been no report of any changes in sleep patterns or problems with sleep occurring with these subjects. In contrast, one group of researchers has found some evidence that there may be neurohumoral mechanisms at work to cause the clinical improvements seen after cerebellar stimulation (Wood et al., 1977). They base this theory on finding changes in norepinephrine and other metabolites measured while subjects were undergoing cerebellar stimulation.

In the early studies of cerebellar stimulation, improvement in symptoms was assessed by subjective means. More recent studies began to use methods such as EMG to improve the objectivity of postoperative assessment. In a study by Penn, Gottleib, and Agarwal (1978), an EMG system was developed to aid in objective evaluation of muscle tone. A reduction in tone is perhaps the most frequent subjective finding in individuals following cerebellar stimulation, although other effects, such as improved speech, have also been reported (Cooper, Upton, Rappoport, & Amin, 1980). In the study by Penn's group, an apparatus was made that used a computer-controlled motor to oscillate the foot of each subject while measurements of torque and angular velocity as well as EMG were recorded. Of the four persons studied (ranging in age from 5 to 28 years), three had decreased muscle stiffness as measured using the device and one did not improve. Interestingly, according to the authors, the one person who did not improve "closely resembled" clinically the subject who showed the most improvement. Possible faults of this study are that there were no controls without spasticity, nor were the researchers blinded to the fact that the subjects had received cerebellar stimulation.

At about the same time that this study was published, a number of clinicians and researchers began questioning the efficacy and safety of chronic cerebellar stimulation (Gillman, 1977). In 1981, a well-designed study using a double-blind crossover technique and follow-up for 12 months was done to evaluate the use of cerebellar stimulators in eight children and young adults ranging in age from 10 to 22 years (Gahm, Russman, Cerciello, Fiorentino, & McGrath, 1981). Standard clinical measures were used for this study, including occupational, physical, and speech therapy evaluations. None of the subjects in this study showed any significant improvement secondary to the cerebellar stimulation.

In this last study, as well as others such as that by Wong, Hoffman, and Froese (1979), the importance of monitoring the equipment for failure or nonoptimal function has been emphasized. This is usually done somewhat indirectly by such methods as reports of tingling from the subject when threshold current is delivered. However, it is important that more objective measures be used, if possible, to ensure that any difference in success rates can be shown to be due to factors other than problems with technique (e.g., electrode placement).

One group of investigators has developed a method by which to "biocalibrate" the cerebellar stimulators used by doing testing of somatosensory evoked potentials (SEPs) prior to and after implantation. Cooper and colleagues (1980) evaluated 87 subjects using such a technique and found that changes in SEPs were somewhat predictive of benefit from cerebellar stimulation, but that some subjects tested had clinical improvement (e.g., decreased muscle tone) but no changes in SEPs. Future research studies may be able to find other neurophysiologic techniques that will be of assistance in determining efficacy of cerebellar or other cortical stimulation.

The previous studies deal with results using the most common method of cerebellar stimulation, cerebellar cortical stimulation using large electrode arrays. It has been theorized by some

clinicians and researchers that the mixed results seen with use of such a "crude" system are due to the widespread excitation of several different types of neurons and that improved results would occur from more selective excitation. It is somewhat unfortunate that the ban on cerebellar stimulation occurred at about the same time that researchers were beginning to perfect both the technique and the methods of monitoring for effectiveness.

CONCLUSIONS

Until recently, although cerebral palsy was known to be due to brain pathology, most of the treatment modalities, including surgery, concentrated on secondary problems such as contracture development. The further refinement and use of the newer techniques described here will add to our understanding of the pathophysiology of cerebral palsy and may help to explain why certain pathologic findings in the brain may or may not be reflected in particular clinical manifestations. For example, people with cerebral palsy have been found by cranial CT to have identical pathology in the brain even though they have different clinical manifestations. People with similar clinical presentations of cerebral palsy also do not always share analogous CT findings. On occasion, those with smaller lesions may actually have worse neuropathologic findings than those with evidence of larger areas of damage. This "apparent paradox" has been explained in the past as a reflection of an alteration in the level of inhibition and excitation in the CNS (Molteni et al., 1987).

There continues to be a definite need for a better classification system for cerebral palsy. Clinical classifications have been used for many years, and several attempts have been made to try to improve them (Alberman, 1984; Holt, 1966; Narabayashi et al., 1965). Holt (1966) recommended the development of a physiologic classification. Even though a classification based on neurophysiologic patterns is becoming more developed, such a system is not commonly used. Although improvements in technology have now made such a system more attainable than in 1966, there appears to be little concentrated effort to perfect such a system.

The challenges of perfecting a neurophysiologic classification system may be especially severe in dealing with infants and very young children who have cerebral palsy. These children are undergoing continued neural development and probably regeneration occurring with time and maturation. The nervous systems of infants and young children with or without cerebral palsy are in a highly plastic state, and developmental changes of the CNS gradually occur over a period of years.

In the child who has cerebral palsy, this normal developmental maturation, which involves such anatomic changes as myelinization and axon branching, undoubtedly continues despite the damage done previously that caused the cerebral palsy. In some cases, normal developmental processes may make the clinical problems worse (see Figure 4).

Research on the process of developing motor control and the ways in which it is altered as a result of cerebral palsy is vastly important, both for our basic understanding and for therapeutic considerations. For a number of reasons, research with children who have cerebral palsy has been minimal and good longitudinal studies have not been done. However, this situation may be changing because a number of noninvasive measurement techniques are now available, such as those employing surface electrodes with computer averaging and analysis of less than optimal signals.

However, it will be impossible to perfect a neurophysiologic classification system for cerebral palsy until the typical physiologic processes are better understood. Basic human and animal research that uses these newer evaluative techniques will continue to improve our understanding of some of the motor output and motor–sensory linkages that must be present for typical function.

One hypothesis deriving from this research deals with the development of *motor programs* (Tatton & Bruce, 1981). In this model, adult motor function is viewed as an interaction of motor and sensory systems much in the way that a computer might work with various routines and subroutines. *Interaction* between sensory and motor systems is the key word here, because it is theorized that these systems are more integrated than may have been previously recognized. As Tatton and Bruce (1981) pointed out, "the only neuronal populations that can be unambiguously labeled as motor and sensory are the motor neurons and the primary sensory afferents" (p. 698).

One future hope for patients with profound cerebral palsy and average or near-average intelligence may lie in *neuroprostheses*, defined by Hambrecht (1979) as a "device or technique used to supplement, or replace, lost or missing function in neurologically impaired individuals" (p. 240). Hambrecht described the state of the art for biomaterials that currently are being used for different types of neuroprostheses. At present, crude forms of neuroprostheses such as cerebellar or spinal stimulation affect large populations of neurons. Work by such groups of researchers as Robertson, Lee, and Jacobs (1984) has shown that it is possible to use biofeedback techniques to control single motor units. This degree of fine control likely would be needed to provide for useful functioning of neuroprostheses.

The future of neuroprostheses therefore seems to depend on improved biofeedback techniques and sophisticated electronic technology. Multichannel, multifunction neuroprostheses will appear as advances and improvements are made with implantable electronics. Electronics may be developed to respond to single motor unit control, which individuals with cerebral palsy may be able to learn using biofeedback techniques. Thus, undamaged portions of the brain may be able, through indirect means by using electronic devices, to control muscles that would be otherwise unusable. In people with cerebral palsy, this would entail using undamaged parts of the brain to control muscles through totally artificial means by using electronic technology that is, perhaps, only decades in the future.

Another possible scenario that is currently being researched is the use of transplanted neuronal tissues in damaged brains. Although there have been no reports of use with patients who have cerebral palsy, success has been seen in patients with Parkinson's disease following fetal brain or adrenal tissue transplants. There is also some research demonstrating that connections between nerves can also be induced (Murakami, Song, & Katsumaru, 1992). Obviously, this type of research is very preliminary, and it remains to be seen whether or not it can be applied to the treatment of cerebral palsy or other chronic brain disorders.

Until neuroprosthetic bypass circuitry, neural transplants, or neural regeneration are available, if they ever are, much can and needs to be done utilizing *current* technology to evaluate both children and adults with cerebral palsy. This in-

cludes the use of the sophisticated EMG, electroencephalographic, and movement assessment techniques already available, as well as further refinements of these methods. It is important to note that, by aggressively using today's techniques to further understand both the abnormal and normal neurophysiology of movement, we will be that much better prepared for a future in which truly functional neuroprostheses can be developed for those who may benefit the most from them.

REFERENCES

Abercrombie, M.L., Davis, J.R., & Schackel, B. (1963). Pilot study of version movements of eyes in cerebral palsied and other children. *Vision Research*, *3*, 135–153.

Alberman, E. (1984). Describing the cerebral palsies: Methods of classifying and counting. In F. Stanley & E. Alberman (Eds.), *The epidemiology of the cerebral palsies* (pp. 27–31). Philadelphia: J.B. Lippincott.

Andrews, C.J., Neilson, P., & Knowles, L. (1973). Electromyographic study of the rigidospasticity of athetosis. *Journal of Neurology, Neurosurgery, and Psychiatry*, *36*, 94–103.

Arens, L.J., Peacock, W.J., & Peter, J. (1989). Selective posterior rhizotomy: A long-term follow-up study. *Child's Nervous System*, *5*, 148–152.

Barolat-Romana, G., & Davis, R. (1980). Neurophysiological mechanisms in abnormal reflex activities in cerebral palsy and spinal spasticity. *Journal of Neurology, Neurosurgery, and Psychiatry*, *43*, 333–342.

Bawa, P. (1981). Neural development in children: A neurophysiological study. *Electroencephalography and Clinical Neurophysiology*, *52*, 249–256.

Berbrayer, D., & Ashby, P. (1990). Reciprocal inhibition in cerebral palsy. *Neurology*, *40*, 653–656.

Berger, W., Quintern, J., & Dietz, V. (1985). Stance and gait perturbations in children: Developmental aspects of compensatory mechanisms. *Electroencephalography and Clinical Neurophysiology*, *61*, 385–395.

Black, P. (1982). Visual disorders associated with cerebral palsy. *British Journal of Ophthalmology*, *66*, 46–52.

Blakemore, C., & Van Sluyters, R.C. (1975). Innate and environmental factors in the development of the kitten's visual cortex. *Physiology (London)*, *248*, 553–716.

Boscarino, L.F., Ounpuu, S., Davis, R.B., Gage, J.R., & DeLuca, P.A. (1993). Effects of selective dorsal rhizotomy on gait in children with cerebral palsy. *Journal of Pediatric Orthopedics*, *13*, 174–179.

Brooks, V.B. (1986). *The neural basis of motor control*. New York: Oxford University Press.

Bruce, I.C., & Tatton, W.G. (1980). Synchronous development of motor cortical output to different muscles in the kitten. *Experimental Brain Research*, *40*, 349–353.

Burke, D. (1983). Critical examination of the case for or against fusimotor involvement in disorders of muscle tone. In J.E. Desmedt (Ed.), *Motor control mechanisms in health and disease* (pp. 133–169). New York: Raven Press.

Cheney, P.D., Fetz, E.E., & Mewes, K. (1991). Neural mechanisms underlying corticospinal and rubrospinal control of limb movements. *Progress in Brain Research*, *87*, 213–252.

Chong, K.C., Vojnic, C.D., & Quanbury, A.O. (1978). The assessment of the internal rotation gait in cerebral palsy: An electromyographic gait analysis. *Clinical Orthopedics*, *132*, 145–150.

Cohen, A.R., & Webster, H.C. (1991). How selective is selective dorsal rhizotomy? *Surgical Neurology*, *35*, 267–272.

Cooper, I.S., & Upton, A.R. (1978). Use of chronic cerebellar stimulation for disorders of disinhibition. *Lancet*, *1*(8064), 595–600.

Cooper, I.S., Upton, A.R., Rappoport, Z.H., & Amin, I. (1980). Correlation of clinical and physiological effects of cerebellar stimulation. *Acta Neurochirurgica, Supplementum 43*, 339–344.

Delwaide, P.J. (1973). Human monosynaptic reflexes and presynaptic inhibition. In J.E. Desmedt (Ed.), *New developments in electromyography and clinical neurophysiology* (pp. 508–522). Basel: Karger.

Desch, L.W. (1989). Assessing neurodevelopmental aspects of motor control by use of a non-invasive electromyographic technique. *Pediatric Research*, *25*, 355A.

Desmedt, J.E. (1983). Mechanisms of vibration-induced inhibition or potentiation: Tonic vibration reflex and vibration paradox in man. In J.E. Desmedt (Ed.), *Motor control mechanisms in health and disease* (p. 671). New York: Raven Press.

Dimitrijevic, M.R., Nathan, P.W., & Sherwood, A.M. (1980). Clonus: The role of central mechanisms. *Journal of Neurology, Neurosurgery, and Psychiatry*, *43*, 321–332.

Gage, J.R. (1993). Gait analysis: An essential tool in the treatment of cerebral palsy. *Clinical Orthopaedics and Related Research, 8,* 126–134.

Gahm, N.H., Russman, B.S., Cerciello, R.L., Fiorentino, M.R., & McGrath, D.M. (1981). Chronic cerebellar stimulation for cerebral palsy. *Neurology, 31,* 87–90.

Gillman, S. (1977). Ban proposed on cerebellar electrical stimulation. *Neurology (Minneapolis), 27,* 998.

Gottlieb, G.L., Myklebust, B.M., Penn, R.D., & Agarwal, G.C. (1982). Reciprocal excitation of muscle antagonists by the primary afferent pathway. *Experimental Brain Research, 46,* 454–456.

Hallett, M., & Alvarez, N. (1983). Attempted rapid elbow flexion movements in patients with athetosis. *Journal of Neurology, Neurosurgery, and Psychiatry, 46,* 745–750.

Hambrecht, F.T. (1979). Neural prostheses. *Annual Reviews of Biophysics and Bioengineering, 8,* 239–267.

Harrison, A. (1988). Spastic cerebral palsy: Possible spinal interneuronal contributions. *Developmental Medicine and Child Neurology, 30,* 769–780.

Hoffer, M.M., Perry, J., & Melkonian, G. (1990). Postoperative electromyographic function of tendon transfers in patients with cerebral palsy. *Developmental Medicine and Child Neurology, 32,* 789–791.

Holt, K.S. (1966). The physiological classification of cerebral palsy. *Developmental Medicine and Child Neurology, 8,* 337–339.

Issler, H., & Stephens, J.A. (1983). The maturation of cutaneous reflexes studied in the upper limb of man. *Journal of Physiology, 335,* 643–654.

Joseph, J. (1985). Neurological control of locomotion. *Developmental Medicine and Child Neurology, 27,* 822–826.

Katz, R., & Pierrot-Deseilligny, E. (1982). Recurrent inhibition of alpha-motoneurons in patients with upper motor neuron lesions. *Brain, 105,* 103-124.

Kennard, M.A. (1942). Cortical reorganization of motor function: Studies on a series of monkeys of various ages from infancy to maturity. *Archives of Neurology and Psychiatry, 48,* 227–240.

Knutsson, E. (1983). Analysis of gait and isokinetic movements for evaluation of antispastic drugs or physical therapies. *Advances in Neurology, 39,* 1013–1034.

Lang, A.H., Sillanpaa, M., & Hynninen, P. (1983). Asymmetric function of peripheral nerves in children with cerebral palsy. *Acta Neurologica Scandinavica, 67,* 108–113.

Laskas, C.A., Mullen, S.L., Nelson, D.L., & Willson-Broyles, M. (1985). Enhancement of two motor functions of the lower extremity in a child with spastic quadriplegia. *Physical Therapy, 65,* 11–16.

Leonard, C.T., Moritani, T., Hirschfeld, H., & Forssberg, H. (1990). Deficits in reciprocal inhibition of children with cerebral palsy as revealed by H reflex testing. *Developmental Medicine and Child Neurology, 32,* 974–984.

Lomo, T., & Jansen, J.K.S. (1980). Requirements for the formation and maintenance of neuromuscular connections. *Current Topics in Developmental Biology, 16,* 253–281.

Marsden, C.D., Merton, P.A., Morton, H.B., & Adam, J. (1978). Cerebral control in man: Long-loop mechanisms. In *Progress in clinical neurophysiology* (Vol. 4, pp. 334–341). Basel: Karger.

Mayberry, W., & Gilligan, M.B. (1985). Ocular pursuit in mentally retarded, cerebral-palsied, and learning disabled children. *American Journal of Occupational Therapy, 39,* 589–595.

Molteni, B., Oleari, G., Fedrizzi, E., & Bracchi, M. (1987). Relation between CT patterns, clinical findings and etiological factors in children born at term, affected by congenital hemiparesis. *Neuropediatrics, 18,* 75–80.

Mowery, C.A., Gelberman, R.H., & Rhoades, C.E. (1985). Upper extremity tendon transfers in cerebral palsy: Electromyographic and functional analysis. *Journal of Pediatric Orthopedics, 5,* 69–72.

Murakami, F., Song, W.J., & Katsumaru, H. (1992). Plasticity of neuronal connections in developing brains of mammals. *Neuroscience Research, 15,* 235–253.

Myklebust, B.M. (1990). A review of myotatic reflexes and the development of motor control and gait in infants and children: A special communication. *Physical Therapy, 70,* 188–203.

Myklebust, B.M., Gottlieb, G.L., & Agarwal, G.C. (1986). Stretch reflexes of the normal infant. *Developmental Medicine and Child Neurology, 28,* 440–449.

Narabayashi, H., Nagahata, M., Nagao, T., & Shimazu, H. (1965). A new classification of cerebral palsy based upon neurophysiologic considerations. *Confinia Neurologica, 25,* 378–392.

Nasher, L.M., & McCollum, G. (1985). The organization of human postural movements: A formal basis and experimental synthesis. *Behavioral and Brain Science, 8,* 135–172.

Neilson, P.D. (1972). Interaction between voluntary contraction and tonic stretch reflex in normal and spastic subjects. *Journal of Neurology, Neurosurgery, and Psychiatry, 35,* 853–860.

Neilson, P.D., & O'Dwyer, N.J. (1984). Reproducibility and variability of speech muscle activity in athetoid dysarthria of cerebral palsy. *Journal of Speech Hearing Research, 27,* 502–517.

Nissen, H.W., Chow, K.L., & Semmes, J. (1951). Effects of restricted opportunity for tactual, kinesthetic, and manipulative experience on the behavior of a chimpanzee. *American Journal of Psychology, 54,* 485–507.

O'Dwyer, N.J., & Neilson, P.D. (1988). Voluntary muscle control in normal and athetoid dysarthric speakers. *Brain, 111,* 877–899.

Opila-Lehman, J., Short, M.A., & Trombly, C.A. (1985). Kinesthetic recall of children with athetoid and spastic cerebral palsy and of non-handicapped children. *Developmental Medicine and Child Neurology, 27,* 223–230.

Peacock, W.J., & Arens, L.J. (1982). Selective posterior rhizotomy for the relief of spasticity in cerebral palsy. *South African Medical Journal, 62,* 119–124.

Peacock, W.J., & Staudt, L.A. (1991). Functional outcomes following selective posterior rhizotomy in children with cerebral palsy. *Journal of Neurosurgery, 74,* 380–385.

Penn, R.D., Gottlieb, G.L., & Agarwal, G.C. (1978). Cerebellar stimulation in man: Quantitative changes in spasticity. *Journal of Neurosurgery, 48,* 779–786.

Porter, R. (1987). The Florey le lecture, 1987: Corticomotoneuronal projections: Synaptic events related to skilled movement. *Proceedings of the Royal Society of London (Biology), 231,* 147–168.

Robertson, D.W., Lee, W.A., & Jacobs, M. (1984). Single motor-unit control by normal and cerebral-palsied males. *Developmental Medicine and Child Neurology, 26,* 323–327.

Rowlandson, P.H., & Stephens, J.A. (1985a). Cutaneous reflex responses recorded in children with various neurological disorders. *Developmental Medicine and Child Neurology, 27,* 434–447.

Rowlandson, P.H., & Stephens, J.A. (1985b). Maturation of cutaneous reflex responses recorded in the lower limb of man. *Developmental Medicine and Child Neurology, 27,* 425–433.

Rutherford, M.A., Pennock, J.M., Murdoch-Eaton, D.M., Cowan, F.M., & Dubowitz, L.M. (1992). Athetoid cerebral palsy with cysts in the putamen after hypoxic-ischaemic encephalopathy. *Archives of Diseases of Children, 67,* 846–850.

Samilson, R.L., & Morris, J.M. (1964). Surgical improvement of the cerebral-palsied upper limb: Electromyographic studies and results of 128 operations. *Journal of Bone and Joint Surgery, 46,* 1203–1216.

Scheiman, M., Ciner, E., & Gallaway, M. (1989). Surgical success rates in infantile esotropia. *Journal of the American Optometric Association, 60,* 22–31.

Schneider, G.E. (1979). Is it really better to have your brain lesion early? A revision of the "Kennard Principle." *Neuropsychology, 17,* 557–583.

Seeger, B.R., Caudrey, D.J., & O'Mara, N.A. (1984). Hand function in cerebral palsy: The effect of hip-flexion angle. *Developmental Medicine and Child Neurology, 26,* 601–606.

Spinelli, D.N., & Jensen, F.E. (1979). Plasticity: The mirror of experience. *Science, 203,* 75–78.

Sutton, L.R., Cohen, B.S., & Krusen, U.L. (1967). Nerve conduction velocities in hemiplegia. *Archives of Physical Medicine and Rehabilitation, 48,* 64–67.

Tachdjian, M.O., & Minear, W.L. (1958). Sensory disturbances in hands of children with cerebral palsy. *Journal of Bone and Joint Surgery, 40,* 85–90.

Takebe, K., & Basmajian, J.V. (1976). Motor and sensory nerve conduction velocities in cerebral palsy. *Archives of Physical Medicine and Rehabilitation, 57,* 158–160.

Tatton, W.G., & Bruce, I.C. (1981). Comment: A schema for the interactions between motor programs and sensory input. *Canadian Journal of Physiology and Pharmacology, 59,* 691–699.

Torvik, A.E. (1956). Transneuronal changes in the inferior olive and pontine nuclei in kittens. *Journal of Neuropathology and Experimental Neurology, 15,* 119–145.

Tychsen, L., & Lisberger, S.G. (1986). Maldevelopment of visual motion processing in humans who had strabismus with onset in infancy. *Journal of Neuroscience, 6,* 2495–2508.

Van Heest, A.E., House, J., & Putnam, M. (1993). Sensibility deficiencies in the hands of children with spastic hemiplegia. *Journal of Hand Surgery, 18,* 278–281.

Verrier, M.C., Tatton, W.G., & Blair, R.D. (1984). Characteristics of EMG responses to imposed limb displacement in patients with vascular hemiplegia. *Canadian Journal of Neurological Sciences, 11,* 288–296.

Winter, D.A., & Yack, H.J. (1987). EMG profiles during normal human walking: Stride-to-stride and inter-subject variability. *Electroencephalography and Clinical Neurophysiology, 67,* 402–411.

Wolpaw, J.R., & Dowman, R. (1988). Operant conditioning of primate spinal reflexes: Effect on cortical SEPs. *Electroencephalography and Clinical Neurophysiology, 69,* 398–401.

Wong, P.K.H., Hoffman, H.J., & Froese, A.B. (1979). Cerebellar stimulation with management of cerebral palsy. *Neurosurgery, 5,* 217–224.

Wong, P.K., Lombroso, C.T., & Maysumiya, Y. (1982). Somatosensory evoked potentials: Variability analysis in unilateral hemispheric disease. *Electroencephalography and Clinical Neurophysiology, 54,* 266–274.

Wood, J.H., Lake, C.R., Ziegler, M.G., Sode, J., Brooks, B.R., & Van Buren, J.M. (1977). Elevations in cerebrospinal fluid norepinephrine during unilateral and bilateral cerebellar stimulation in man. *Neurology, 27,* 260–265.

Wright, J., & Rang, M. (1990). The spastic mouse, and the search for an animal model of spasticity in human beings. *Clinical Orthopaedics and Related Research, 5,* 12–19.

PART III

THE SPECTRUM OF MOTOR DYSFUNCTION

Chapter 9

Neuromuscular Disorders

Thomas O. Crawford, M.D.

Children with neuromuscular disorders have a spectrum of motor difficulties that extend from mild weakness to total immobilization and are often burdened with associated complications that range from the near-trivial to the profound and life threatening. Physicians who care for these children thus need an equally wide range of skills. The neuromuscular specialist must be part neurologist, orthopedist, pulmonologist, cardiologist, geneticist, psychiatrist, counselor, and friend. At many large centers, children with neuromuscular disorders are cared for in neuromuscular clinics where many different specialists are available for consultation; however, each of these children also needs the interest and attention of a general practitioner, who ultimately delivers much of the care.

Children with neuromuscular disorders should be distinguished from the broader group of children with neuromotor dysfunction. A neuromotor dysfunction is defined as an abnormality of movement, tone, or coordination that originates from pathology of the brain or spinal cord. In contrast, a neuromuscular disorder involves dysfunction of the *motor unit,* a functionally defined entity that consists of all the cellular elements responsible for the mediation of movement and tone by the central nervous system (CNS). The motor unit is composed of the motor neuron, its associated nerve fiber, and all the individual muscle fibers innervated by that nerve fiber.

Because a neuromuscular disorder is defined as some dysfunction involving the motor unit, the various types of neuromuscular disorders are classified by which portion of the motor unit is primarily affected. Neuronopathies involve the motor neuron; neuropathies, the nerve (either the axon or the ensheathing Schwann cells); myasthenic disorders, the neuromuscular

junction; and the myopathies and the muscular dystrophies, the muscle. The neurologist's first task when diagnosing a child with a potential neuromuscular disorder is to identify whether or not there is dysfunction of the motor unit; if so, the second task is to localize which portion of the motor unit is primarily affected. This two-step process is done largely with the history and physical examination. Once a hypothesis about the nature of the dysfunction has been generated, ancillary tests such as electromyography or muscle biopsy can be chosen wisely to confirm or further narrow the diagnosis.

CLINICAL EVALUATION

Children with neuromotor problems are often described as being *hypotonic*, a word that unfortunately means different things to different people. Neurologists use the term specifically to describe a child with diminished tone, whereas others may use it more generally to describe a child with diminished motor ability. The term *floppy*, although colloquial, may be more useful given its unambiguously inclusive meaning. To determine whether the floppy child has a neuromotor or a neuromuscular problem, the child is evaluated according to the six different distinguishing characteristics outlined in Table 1. When this is possible, a good portion of the diagnostic localization follows easily.

Distinguishing Characteristics of Motor Function

A first distinguishing characteristic of motor function is *muscle tone*, a potentially complicated concept that even experts may not define with unanimity. For the purpose of diagnosis, however, muscle tone can be defined simply as the amount of force with which an awake and

Table 1. Important descriptive features of motor dysfunction

	Increased	Diminished
Tone	Hypertonia (spasticity, rigidity, dystonia)	**Hypotonia**
Power	Strength	**Weakness**
Range of motion	**Laxity, hypermobility**	**Contracture, arthrogryposis**
Fatiguability	Endurance	**Fatiguability**
Muscle bulk	**Muscular hypertrophy and pseudohypertrophy**	**Muscle atrophy**
Deep tendon reflexes	Hyperreflexic, clonus	**Hyporeflexic, areflexic**

Note: Items in **bold** typeface may be associated with neuromuscular disorders.

cooperative child resists passive movement (manipulation by the examiner). The level of consciousness is important, because resistance to passive movement is naturally diminished in sleep and in some forms of stupor or coma. Excessive alertness is equally problematic because the underlying muscle tone of a crying or fussy and fighting child is difficult to evaluate. It is similarly important, although sometimes difficult, to distinguish between voluntary resistance and the reflexive resistance that a child cannot suppress. As defined by the neurologist, only one form of reduced tone, or *hypotonia,* exists. In contrast, it is possible to distinguish several different forms of increased tone—spasticity, rigidity, and dystonia to name three—based on the nature of the resistance and the type of passive movement that most provokes it.

A second distinguishing characteristic of motor function is the available *muscle power*, a more easily understood concept defined as the maximum force that a child can produce. Usually this is not difficult to elicit, because many children are unwittingly provoked into active resistance and vigorous crying during the clinical evaluation (or during phlebotomy). Occasionally, a child, especially one with certain genetic disorders characterized by profound passivity, such as Down or Prader-Willi syndrome, cannot or will not resist passive movement or produce any effort despite the presumed ability to do so. It is then difficult to demonstrate full muscle power, even though its presence may be intuited by experienced clinicians.

Although muscle power is usually easy to demonstrate, in children it is often difficult to quantitate reliably. The Medical Research Council (MRC) has developed a 5-point scale for grading muscle power, but the most clinically important designations (Grade 4 and Grade 5) are difficult to determine reliably in children, even for experienced clinicians, because of the shifting baseline of development. Many investigators thus take a more functional approach to grading of muscle power (Brooke, 1994). I find it useful to seek out intrinsically rewarding tasks that are just within, and just beyond, the child's ability. Describing at least one such skill for the arms, legs, and trunk/head is worthwhile. In general, weak children are exquisitely aware of their limits and cannot be enticed to attempt a task beyond their ability. Refusal to try given apparent interest is thus almost equivalent to a demonstration of inability. Examples of quantifiable skills are included in Table 2.

A third distinguishing feature of motor function is the *range of available movement* at any joint. Normally, joint mobility is limited by both muscle tone and the physical features and surrounding ligamentous structures of the joint. Thus, hypotonia or weakness can manifest as an apparent increase in the range of joint movement. With profound hypotonia or weakness, apparent laxity of the joints is sometimes so remarkable that it is mistakenly thought to be the primary defect, leading to the incorrect diagnosis of Ehlers-Danlos syndrome, a disorder ordinarily not associated with diminished tone or muscle power.

The opposite problem, *restrictions of joint mobility*, may also result from abnormalities of tone or muscle power. Contractures are a well-known complication of spasticity; however, they can also arise in patients with decreased strength or tone, especially if the joints are not frequently ranged or are subject to unequal tone.

Thus, hypotonia and weakness can lead either to immobility or to hyperextensibility. On

Table 2. Muscle power evaluation tasks in children

	Infants	Children
Head control	Head lag Ability to roll head while supine or prone	Amount of lateral head tilt from which child can recover upright posture
Trunk	Paradoxic breathing Log rolling/resistance to torsion	Independent sit (slouched or upright) Sit-up (document manner, whether lateral, required use of arms, etc.)
Arm	Ability to get hand to mouth while on side/supine/seated Heaviest toy brought to mouth Heaviest toy of interest Resting posture	Highest point reaches for a toy Highest "high five" Adjustments in trunk posture to enable arm elevation Longest throw of ball from chair Heaviest toy of interest
Leg	Ability to elevate knees/feet/ entire leg from table	Longest standing broad jump Time to run / walk 30 feet Time to stand up from the floor

occasion, severe contractures make diagnostic evaluation difficult, especially in newborns, in whom prolonged in utero immobility, whether from weakness or from any other cause, can lead to *arthrogryposis*, a form of contracture that involves underdevelopment of the joint. With complete contracture of a joint, there is substantial secondary loss of muscle bulk. In such circumstances, determining whether a severe deformity is primarily neurologic or orthopedic in origin can be difficult.

A fourth characteristic to be evaluated is *resistance to muscle fatigue*. In adults, early muscle fatigue can be demonstrated by the patient's inability to sustain 5 minutes of forward arm abduction or of head flexion while supine. Because children and infants will refuse to perform such a test, unusual muscle fatigue often must be intuited from a history of difficulty sustaining everyday activities such as chewing; of weakness, hoarseness, or slurring of the voice after exercise or even vigorous laughing or crying; or of the inability to sustain bottle or breast feeding despite initial vigor and coordination. Fatigue can be intuited sometimes from signs of vacillating weakness, as when ptosis is interrupted by flickers of lid elevation (Cogan's sign).

Another characteristic to evaluate in a child with abnormal motor function is the *appearance and firmness of the muscle itself*. The muscular hypertrophy that results from sustained vigorous exercise in adults is not seen in children. In several forms of muscular dystrophy or denervating disease, abnormal firmness with pseudohypertrophy ("pseudo" because the increased bulk is due to fibrosis, not to muscle tissue) is seen in the calves. More generalized muscle hypertrophy may result from abnormalities of muscle relaxation, as seen in some of the myotonic disorders.

Diminished muscle bulk can be the consequence of either denervation or primary muscle disease. It is important to be familiar with normal variation, however, because a slender, tall, prepubescent child can easily be mistaken to have reduced muscle mass. When muscle atrophy is combined with strength that is more than expected for the available bulk, the child most often is constitutionally slender or has a chronic disorder or recent disuse atrophy. In babies, even profound muscle atrophy can be missed because the caliber of the limbs is relatively preserved with abundant baby fat. Thus, diminished muscle bulk is best appreciated in babies by deep palpation of the midshaft of the long bones: With atrophy, bony definition can be easily felt in a way not possible in infants without muscle atrophy.

Finally, it is important to characterize the child's *deep tendon reflexes*. Successful elicitation of reflexes requires that the child be quiet and relaxed and that the tendon percussion be delivered unexpectedly. Even with children without neuromuscular disorders, this scenario may be difficult to achieve, and so even skilled examiners may disagree about the vigor of the reflexes. The most that can be expected to be reliable is a determination of their presence or absence, and some measure of intensity relative to the available muscle power. It is probably more reliable to evaluate the ease of reflex elicitation than the vigor of the response. Usually the knee and ankle jerks are the easiest, and most reliable, reflexes to elicit.

Localization of Motor Unit Pathology

Once the clinician has evaluated these six characteristics, a preliminary diagnosis is usually possible. The most consistent finding in disorders of the motor unit is weakness. Because a weak child cannot resist passive manipulation, weakness is always accompanied by hypotonia. Hypotonia without weakness, or hypotonia with relative preservation of muscle power, however, strongly implies that the disorder stems from dysfunction of the CNS. Such a clinical picture should suggest a general disorder of brain, metabolism, or genetics rather than a more restricted problem of the motor unit. Thus, tests such as nerve conduction studies and muscle biopsy, which are typically used to understand dysfunction in the motor unit, are likely to be useful only as they elucidate a generalized disorder of neural function involving both the CNS and the motor unit.

As indicated, weakness strongly implies involvement of the motor unit, either in the neuron, nerve, or muscle. Significant clues about the location of the pathology within the motor unit come from where the weakness is within the body (Table 3). Thus, patients with myopathic disorders often present with a waddling gait or difficulties in rising from the floor or climbing stairs because these tasks rely heavily on the largest muscles of the leg. For reasons not fully known, disorders of the neuromuscular junction are often associated with weakness predominantly in the bulbar and extraocular muscles. Because of their length-dependent pathology, neuropathies produce weakness that is largely distal in the extremities. Finally, children with disorders of the motor neuron (e.g., spinal muscular atrophy) will have diffuse weakness, although often eye movements, facial expression, and movement of the diaphragm and anal and urethràl sphincters will be relatively preserved.

Any form of increased tone, in any degree or in any portion of the body, even in combination with hypotonia elsewhere, implies some pathology of the CNS. Children with disorders of the CNS predominantly involving the cerebral hemispheres are hypotonic in infancy, but even at these early times they develop regional signs of spasticity in motor functions controlled principally by the hemispheric corticospinal tracts. Thus, primate adaptations such as thumb abduction, hand supination, and foot dorsiflexion give way to the quadrupedal (ontologically more primitive) pattern of tone (i.e., adduction of the thumb into a pronated hand resembling a quadruped's forepaw, and equinus deformity of the foot resembling the quadrupedal stance on the metatarsus).

Increased deep tendon reflexes in the floppy child (or disproportionately typical reflexes in the setting of weakness or hypotonia) have nearly the same implications as regional hypertonia: probable involvement of the CNS. Almost all neuromuscular disorders of children, with the exception of disorders of the neuromuscular junction in which fatigue is the only presenting sign, have diminished reflexes. In the myopathies, axonal neuropathies, and neuronopathies, diminution of the reflexes is commensurate with weakness. In demyelinating neuropathies, however, reflexes are diminished more than the degree of weakness would suggest, because the afferent signal of sudden tendon shortening from the hammer tap loses coherence in the demyelinated nerve as it ascends to the spinal cord. The signal is dispersed by the time it arrives at the spinal cord because each axon has a slightly different slow conduction velocity. Because of this dispersion, the stimulus does not provoke a compensatory muscle reflex.

Special Tests of the Motor Unit

Once there is reasonable suspicion of a disorder within the motor unit, ancillary tests can be focused on the problem to obtain a specific diag-

Table 3. Clinical clues to the location of motor unit pathology

Region of motor unit pathology	General regions of greatest dysfunction	Chief complaint	Frequent or diagnostically important signs
Muscle	Proximal muscles of leg and arm	Slowness of gait; difficulty with stairs; difficulty with arising from chair or floor	Proximal muscle weakness; waddling gait, Gower's sign
Neuromuscular junction	Extraocular and bulbar muscles	Double vision; sleepy eyelids; hoarse voice; difficulty with chewing, swallowing, or choking	Variable ptosis or extraocular muscle weakness; excessive fatigue for available muscle power
Nerve	Distal muscles, distal sensory loss	Easily twisted ankles; difficulty walking at night or on uneven ground	Disproportionate weakness of feet and hands; atrophy of intrinsic hand muscles; distal hyporeflexia; distally diminished large-fiber sensation (vibration and proprioception)
Neuron	Diffuse symmetrical weakness	Generalized weakness	Generalized weakness

nosis. These tests, especially electrophysiologic tests and biopsies, require the assistance of a neuromuscular specialist.

Nerve conduction tests on children (Miller & Kuntz, 1986) in particular require special expertise because the results from each nerve will determine the nature of, and indications for, further testing. In nerve conduction studies, a nerve (either motor or sensory) is electrically stimulated and the resulting signal is recorded as it is conducted to a distant site. Motor nerves are studied by comparing the effect of stimulation of the same nerve in two places, typically at a distal site at the wrist or ankle and a more proximal site at the elbow or knee, with recordings made over the innervated muscle. The velocity of nerve conduction between these sites is obtained by dividing the difference in times necessary to evoke a muscle potential from the two sites by the distance between the stimulus sites. The amplitude of the evoked muscle potential is also important, as a decrease in amplitude results from a diminished number of axons (axonal neuropathy or motor neuron disease); from a diminished number of conducting axons (conduction block from a demyelinating neuropathy); or, to a lesser degree, from a severe myopathy. Special tests with rapid repetitive stimulation of the nerve are necessary to diagnose defects of transmission across the neuromuscular junction (Cornblath, 1986).

To test a sensory nerve, either the stimulus or the recording electrode is placed over a pure sensory nerve, usually in the fingers or the dorsum of the foot, beyond where the motor branches have departed the nerve for muscles in the calf or forearm. Recordings are taken directly from the nerve, so that the amplitude of the signal is much lower than that of the signals recorded from muscle with motor nerve stimulation. As with motor nerve studies, the recording of diminished sensory nerve amplitude suggests an axonal disease or conduction block, whereas slowed conduction velocity suggests a demyelinating disorder.

Electromyography (EMG) frequently is done in tandem with nerve conduction tests as part of the electrophysiologic evaluation of the motor unit. This test evaluates the electrical activity received by a recording needle electrode that is inserted into muscle. As with the nerve conduction tests, the performance of the EMG on children requires special expertise by a physician who is aware of the indications for the test and the specific questions being asked (Jones, 1990; Russell, Afifi, & Ross, 1992). Doing a thorough EMG evaluation takes time and, on the part of the child, cooperation, something that is often not forthcoming because the test involves repeated needle sticks. Sedation of the child helps with some portions of the test but hinders other portions. Thus, EMG evaluation of the child is oftentimes incomplete, but, if the diagnostic question is properly framed, it is still possible to obtain much useful information. It is best to be sensitive to the child's (and the parents') tolerance for the test as well as to the quality and usefulness of the information obtained. Given these difficulties, it is sometimes better to limit the study and repeat, or extend, the test at later times if important answerable questions remain.

Important features of the EMG valuation include assessment of resting activity and partial voluntary activity. At rest, the muscle should be silent. The firing of single muscle fibers is seen as a fibrillation potential or positive sharp wave. The presence of either indicates the muscle fiber is denervated and firing spontaneously because it is orphaned from its parent motor neuron or that it is in some way damaged. The presence of fibrillation potentials thus implies there is nerve damage or an irritable myopathy. A small amount of voluntary activity makes it possible to identify the firing of single motor units. A small and short-duration motor unit suggests a disorder of muscle. Motor unit potentials that are large and of prolonged duration suggest that motor units have been lost, and the resulting orphaned muscle fibers were rescued by sprouting from the surviving motor neurons to produce enlargement of the remaining motor units. As the child increases the force of muscle contraction, the pattern of recruitment of the first and subsequent motor units will reveal much about whether the weakness stems from the nerve or the muscle.

Muscle biopsy can reveal much about the nature of motor unit dysfunction, but like the electrophysiologic tests is subject to important limitations and cautions, the most important of which is the need for experience (Dubowitz, 1989). Muscle biopsy, particularly biopsy of children, should be done by physicians practiced in the preparation and evaluation of frozen tissue by special histochemical stains specific to this tissue. Too often important information is lost when specimens are handled improperly or are prepared only with standard formaldehyde-fixed, paraffin-embedded, pathologic methods. The age of the child at the time of biopsy is an important limiting factor because pathologic

features may not have developed yet in an infant's immature muscle. As with the use of electrophysiologic tests, the questions to be answered by the biopsy must be correctly framed, because errors of interpretation are most likely when the diagnostic question is too broad.

We are entering an era when specific *DNA tests* are becoming increasingly important, offering diagnostic information of much higher quality than those available from electrophysiology or biopsy. DNA testing, however, first requires a strong hypothesis about the nature of the disease, a hypothesis that must often be developed through these more preliminary tests. Table 4 lists important genetic neuromuscular diseases of children and the current potential for DNA diagnosis.

TREATMENT

Certain themes recur across the treatment spectrum of neuromuscular disease. These disorders are usually lifelong in nature, implying that the long view of intervention is warranted. A substantial fraction of the children with motor unit disorders have a static or very slowly progressive disorder; however, despite the stability of the underlying disease, these children often continue to worsen with time. This worsening is often a treatable consequence of complications rather than a change in the underlying disease. For children with both static and progressive disorders, anticipation and treatment of the complications caused by weakness is the most important theme in their care.

One of the potentially most difficult aspects of therapy is knowing *when* to intervene. In many areas of care, whether orthopedics, physical or occupational therapy, education, or parenting, there is a natural conflict between doing more for a child and doing less. On the one hand, a child may accomplish more with the assistance of a brace, device, or helping hand; on the other hand, this assistance may beget dependence, to the detriment of future function. In many cases, the physician's experience and knowledge of the condition will be crucial in striking the proper balance. In other cases, everyone concerned—physicians, therapists, teachers, and parents alike—must be aware of

Table 4. DNA diagnostics for important neuromuscular diseases of children

Disease	Inheritance	Chromosome location (gene product)	Nature of mutation	Useful genetic tests[a]
Duchenne muscular dystrophy	X linked	XP21.2 (dystrophin)	Deletion (60%)	PCR deletion screen
			Duplication (6%)	
			Point mutation	Southern blot
				RFLP analysis of family
Becker muscular dystrophy	X linked	XP21.2 (dystrophin)	Deletion (85%)	PCR deletion screen
			Duplication	
			Point mutation	Southern blot
				RFLP analysis of family
Malignant hyperthermia	Dominant	19q13.1 (ryanodine receptor)	Point mutation	DNA sequencing (research only)
Central core disease	Dominant	19q13.1 (ryanodine receptor)	Point mutation	DNA sequencing (research only)
Myotonic dystrophy	Dominant	19q13	Triplicate repeat (100%)	PCR
Myotonia congenita (Thompson disease)	Dominant	7q35 (muscle chloride channel)	Point mutation	DNA sequencing (research only)
Becker myotonic disease	Recessive	7q35 (muscle chloride channel)	Point mutation	DNA sequencing (research only)
Charcot-Marie-Tooth disease, type 1a (demyelinating form)	Dominant	17p11.2-12 (peripheral myelin protein, pmp-22)	Duplication	Southern blot
			Point mutation	DNA sequencing (research only)
Charcot-Marie-Tooth disease, type 1b (demyelinating form)	Dominant	1q21-23 (myelin protein P_0)	Point mutation	DNA sequencing (research only)
Dejerine-Sottas disease, type A	Dominant or recessive	17p11.2-12 (peripheral myelin protein, pmp-22)	Point mutation, homozygous duplication	DNA sequencing (research only) or Southern blot
Dejerine-Sottas disease, type B	Dominant	1q21-23 (myelin protein P_0)	Point mutation	DNA sequencing (research only)
Charcot-Marie-Tooth disease, type X (demyelinating form)	X linked	Xq13 (connexin 32)	Point mutation	DNA sequencing (research only)
Spinal muscular atrophy types 1, 2, and 3	Recessive	5q13.2 (SMN or NAIP)	Deletion	RFLP analysis of family and/or deletion of SMN

Data from Chance and Reilly (1994) and "Neuromuscular Disorders" (1994).

[a]PCR, polymerase chain reaction; RFLP, restriction fragment length polymorphism.

the difficulties inherent in both over- and under-support, must acknowledge the need for trial and error, and must be willing to make adjustments based on experience.

As another important caveat, physicians and others must concentrate on things that matter. It is not unusual for caregivers to spend inordinate energy and time on unreachable goals, inadvertently losing sight of other valuable and attainable achievements. The worthiness of a goal (e.g., independent ambulation) should not substitute for a careful assessment of whether it can be achieved. Again, to know what is obtainable with effort requires experience. Also important is to be sure that the goals are meaningful to the child and his or her functioning; for example, attention to cosmetic details, such as the repair of contractures in the feet of a non–weightbearing child, may not be as important as some other forms of assistance that may be overlooked.

Orthopedics

Although children with weakness have a variety of bone and joint problems, one area in particular deserves special attention. Many children with weakness of the long back and other trunk muscles are at substantial risk for catastrophic scoliosis. The scoliosis of weakness differs from idiopathic scoliosis in the rate of progression, the wide arc of bending over the entire spine, and the potential life-threatening consequence of untreated progression. Neuromuscular scoliosis can occur with great speed once a small degree of curvature develops because the unopposed action of gravity on a tilted spinal column increases as the curve worsens. Children with weakness of the trunk sufficient to cause difficulty in sitting upright are at greatest risk and should be followed with frequent careful examinations and upright spine films. A curvature of greater than 30 degrees constitutes a high risk for further rapid collapse. In many children, a carefully fitted stiff body jacket (sometimes known as a TLSO, or thoracolumbosacral orthosis) can slow early progression but not reverse it. Unfortunately, these jackets are uncomfortable or may restrict some functions. The goal of trunk bracing is only to delay (not prevent) the need for operative spinal fusion until after growth is complete. When scoliosis becomes severe, operative spinal fusion is indicated to prevent compromise of vital functions; to maintain an upright posture; and to provide comfort, as the child with extreme scoliosis is often bedridden or suffers from painful pressure sores over the trunk (Phillips, Roye, Farcy, Leet, & Shelton, 1990; Shapiro & Specht, 1993a, 1993b).

Many children with neuromuscular disorders will develop deformities of foot posture that may destabilize standing and walking. Foot deformities generally evolve in one of three patterns. The first is the development of an *equinus deformity*, with shortening of the Achilles tendon leading to obligate toe walking. This is particularly common in disorders such as Duchenne muscular dystrophy, which are associated with calf pseudohypertrophy. Treatment involves regular passive stretching of the foot into dorsiflexion and nighttime bracing (with an ankle–foot orthosis, or AFO) to retard the development of contracture. If equinus becomes functionally significant, treatment with progressive casting or, if severe, tendon lengthening becomes necessary.

The second common foot deformity is the *valgus, pes planus foot*, often seen in myopathies or spinal muscular atrophy. Here, the weight of the body is borne on the inside flattened arch of the foot, which may cause pain under the medial malleolus. Therapy with carefully fitted in-shoe orthoses (University of California, Biomechanics Laboratory, or UCBL, orthoses) improves stability.

Finally, children with neuropathies may develop a *pes cavus foot*. The characteristic features of an exaggerated arch, hammer toe deformity, varus deformity of the calcaneus, and equinus all result from the length-dependent nature of the weakness. Weak distal muscles in the foot and calf are overcome at these joints by the action of more powerful proximal muscles of the calf. Therapy must be individualized for the deformity, but may include passive stretching exercises and special shoe inserts. When symptoms coincide with progressive deformity in a growing foot, selective tendon transfers to stabilize the unbalanced forces of the foot can be worthwhile. When symptoms coexist with fixed deformity, however, operative reconstruction of the foot with a triple arthrodesis may become necessary, although it is of limited benefit.

Nutrition and Metabolism

Children with neuromuscular disorders are at risk for nutritional difficulties for several reasons. First, intake may be difficult, especially if bulbar muscles are involved. Careful attention to swallowing, chewing, and the potential problems of aspiration and reflux in these children is warranted. Manipulation of diet can resolve many problems. Difficulty with swallowing can be minimized by using pureed food. Children often avoid meats or hard-to-chew foods when chewing is difficult. Making liquids thicker will minimize aspiration as well as suppress reflux. When indicated, the use of alternate routes of feeding, either with a nasogastric tube or a gastrostomy, can be very successful in assuring adequate caloric intake and frequently leads to increases in strength. In some rare situations, the primary muscle disorder may involve smooth muscles of the alimentary tract as well as skeletal muscle. The resulting pseudo-obstruction of impaired or diminished intestinal motility can become a major impediment to overall nutrition.

A second metabolic problem arises from the little-appreciated but paramount role of muscle as a repository of short-term energy stores. After a short fast and the depletion of liver glycogen stores, muscle protein becomes a major supplier of the carbon skeleton as well as the energy source for gluconeogenesis by the liver. The contractile elements of muscle as well as soluble proteins within the sarcoplasm contribute to this metabolic pathway. In healthy individuals, this shift from anabolic to catabolic states is a part of normal metabolism throughout the day and night. In the evening, the loss of a small percentage loss of total body weight in the form of muscle is unnoticed. However, with severely diminished muscle mass, as is seen in many patients with a neuromuscular disorder, mobilization of the same amount of muscle protein for energy dissipates a commensurately larger proportion of the remaining muscle. Although individuals with neuromuscular disorders rarely recognize weakness after a single overnight fast, establishing a routine, stable, and nutritious diet has in our experience often achieved real gains in available muscle power. Fasting combined with disuse is particularly detrimental; after a debilitating illness with fasting, many patients experience substantial losses of strength that may take weeks to recover.

Obesity is the third major nutrition problem faced by children with neuromuscular disease. In the setting of weakness, caloric expenditure is substantially diminished so that intake becomes the only regulator of weight. In particular, with progressive disease such as Duchenne muscular dystrophy, appetite remains stable. The consequence is a further deterioration of mobility. Obesity may also be worsened by corticosteroids used to slow the loss of muscle power. Because obesity precludes the effective use of an external body brace to retard the progression of scoliosis, it can also become a medical problem in itself. Unfortunately, there is no substitute for fastidious and progressive restriction of the diet to match diminishing caloric expenditure.

Respiratory Issues

The compromised power and endurance of the respiratory muscles is the major life-threatening feature of neuromuscular disease. The different neuromuscular disorders often lead to different forms of restrictive lung disease, each of which may require significantly different interventions and precautions, but the general respiratory problems include diminished vital capacity, total lung volume, and expiratory force with cough; inspiratory obstruction with collapse of the extrathoracic airway; atelectasis; and ventilation–perfusion mismatches, especially with severe scoliosis. Given these conditions, minor upper respiratory infections can progress rapidly to more serious respiratory compromise. They thus warrant early and close evaluation by primary care physicians, with early institution of therapies such as postural drainage and percussion, assisted cough, bronchodilators, and antibiotics. Unfortunately, the warning signs of respiratory insufficiency may be subtle, because diminished vital capacity and cough can suppress rales and overall breath sounds. In general, an increased resting respiratory rate is the most sensitive measure of diminished reserve in children with weakness.

Whether a child will be benefitted by the use of a ventilator in the setting of respiratory failure is a complex and painful decision for all involved, and one that must be individualized for each child (Bach, 1993; Keens, Jansen, DeWitt, & Ward, 1990). The tendency to choose one way, a priori, for any one community, institution, or disease should be resisted. Medical issues including the natural course of the disease, the degree of weakness, the availability of useful assistive devices, and the absence of other medical complications must be weighed. Nonmedical issues that are at least as important include the quality of life, the availability and willingness of family support, the logistics of support, and community standards. Unfortunately, financial concerns also play a role. Too often, a single supporting parent must choose the poverty of joblessness and limited public assistance in order to maintain the 24-hour care that a ventilator requires.

In general, if long-term ventilator support is initiated by emergency department or intensive care unit staff in a crisis without prior planning, such support is more difficult and often unsatisfactory. Ideally, the use of a ventilator is part of a long-term plan that evolves over time while the respiratory safety margin is monitored by experienced pulmonologists. Creation of an environment of informed involvement by all concerned, including the child as he or she is capable, is critical to the satisfactory use of the ventilator as a means to improve quality of life.

Many children with respiratory muscle weakness suffer from nighttime hypoventilation. This is due to the natural collapse of the throat during deep sleep being added to the underlying weakness of these muscles. Often a sign of this problem is the appearance of snoring with respiratory pauses. The associated hypercarbia and hypoxia of apnea produce an alerting response that disturbs natural sleep. The resulting daytime fatigue is often interpreted as weakness and attributed to the underlying disease.

Sleep apnea and hypoventilation are best evaluated with sleep studies, which include end-tidal CO_2 measurements, oxygenation, chest movement, electrocardiography (ECG), and electroencephalography. These problems can be effectively treated with nighttime ventilatory assistance, either with continuous positive airway pressure or positive airway pressure with an occlusive facial mask (bilevel positive airway pressure). Rather often, the daytime strength of children with nighttime hypoventilation is improved significantly by respiratory support. There is little concern about worsening respiratory muscle power, because daytime respiration provides more than enough training to maintain normal function. The use and monitoring of nighttime ventilation provides an important resource for evaluating the child's and family's response to respiratory support. A natural outgrowth of nighttime ventilatory support is that families become more aware of the benefits and burdens of assisted ventilation, which in turn becomes important to informed choice about additional steps in support (Heckmatt, Loh, & Dubowitz, 1990).

Cardiac Dysfunction

Cardiac muscle resembles skeletal muscle in physiology and structure and hence is often affected by diseases of skeletal muscle. Either the cardiac conduction system can be damaged, as in Friedreich's ataxia and Emery-Dreifuss muscular dystrophy, or the primary contractile function can be diminished, as in the dystrophin-deficient muscular dystrophies and mitochondrial myopathies. It is well to note that, in the absence of movement, it is not possible to manifest the exercise intolerance of cardiomyopathy until very late in the course. Children can remain asymptomatic in the setting of severe cardiomyopathy, only to become symptomatic when it is immediately life limiting. Children at risk should have routine ECG and echocardiographic studies, and early symptoms of cardiac insufficiency should be sought carefully because these symptoms, which may not be obviously cardiac in origin, are often treatable with afterload-reducing agents. Telltale complaints may include inability to tolerate a full meal, inability to tolerate the upright position in a wheelchair, and unusual fatiguability.

Role of Exercise and Therapy

Virtually all children with neuromuscular disease can be helped by physical and occupational and other therapists, who can play an important and constructive role. In most cases, children with limited active range of movement benefit from a regular program of passive stretching to retard or prevent the development of acquired joint contractures. In some diseases (e.g., Duchenne muscular dystrophy), contractures will restrict function unless addressed early and with vigor. The involvement of therapists is crucial in this effort, although their primary goal should be supervisory, to ensure that appropriately vigorous passive range-of-motion exercises be carried out regularly and well by the parents.

It is important to be clear, however, that in many of these disorders little is to be gained by exercise training directed toward the development of additional muscle power. This is true in the neuronopathies and neuropathies, partly because denervated muscle does not participate in exercise and partly because hypertrophy of the remaining innervated muscle occurs naturally in the setting of neighboring denervation. This is true of some myopathies as well, for unknown reasons. Strength training, although possibly successful in the short run, may be contraindicated in the dystrophin-deficient and dystrophin-associated muscular dystrophies. A corollary of a widely held (but unproved) theory—that, with malfunction of dystrophin, strain of the muscle plays a role in the pathogenesis of muscle fiber degeneration—is that exercise hastens the downward course of the disease. Thus, for many diseases, training specifically to increase strength is either not successful or not indicated.

More restricted exercise training can be useful, however. Muscle atrophy will occur when muscles are not used. For purely mechanical reasons, children may not work at certain tasks because these tasks are beyond their ability. Thus, substituting simpler tasks or providing partial assistance may lead to substantial gains in strength. For example, children who lack the strength to stand will not use antigravity muscles of the trunk and hips to full effect, but these children often enjoy using a prone standing board to maintain an upright posture at a table and may develop upper trunk muscle power or head control that was previously thought to be unavailable. Using a mobile arm support or exercising in the partial antigravity conditions of a pool may be effective for the same reasons. Sometimes, as with resistive-airway exercises, it is worthwhile to concentrate specifically on developing muscle power despite the large investment of time and energy this takes.

Enhancement of function should be the primary goal of therapy. To this end, the creative and correct use of braces, wheelchairs, and other aids is a primary task of the therapist. One of the therapist's most difficult jobs, however, is distinguishing between the use of such devices as aids and their contribution to dependency. For instance, overreliance on a wheelchair by a child capable of household or community ambulation may lead to disuse atrophy or contractures. Underreliance is seen just as often in children who refuse to give in to their disease by using a wheelchair or a crutch when it would clearly aid function. These children, and their parents, may not see or want to admit that the disease is already restricting function, and so they may need to be shown how the use of an aid extends range rather than defines limits. Thus, these devices should be prescribed and fitted by physicians who understand and can advise patients about these distinctions.

When a disease is known to be progressive, the physician should generally prescribe a wheelchair earlier than absolutely required, so as to introduce early the idea of it being a powerful means of extending the range of mobility rather than merely a poor substitute for independent ambulation. For very young nonambulatory children with generally nonprogressive disorders such as spinal muscular atrophy, it is worthwhile to prescribe a motorized wheelchair early (in the second or third year) and allow the child to use it progressively as interest in a wider geographic range develops.

Role of the Family

One of the most important emotional issues that the family must deal with, often unaddressed, is the distorting influence that a neuromuscular or any other severe chronic illness has on normal childhood development. These children are frail and so require much assistance and attention by their caregivers. Because everyone can easily see the dependency, the child too often adopts a chronic "sick role." Unfortunately, the sick role, although appropriate in acute illness, is disabling when embraced as a way of life. With time, such children may become so demanding or shrill in their interaction with others that they ultimately drive people away. Experienced physicians caring for patients with neuromuscular disease encounter many patients who are, over time, as disabled by elements of personality as by physical weakness. The ultimate result too often is a combination of isolation, dependency, and depression.

Because frequent interaction with health professionals forces parents to adopt a more clinical view of their child, these parents often inadvertently detach from their role as parents. Physicians and others must recognize this dilemma and help restore parents to their proper role. Although the child may have a severe chronic illness, he or she is fundamentally still a child and needs more than anything else the care, support, and especially structure of family. One of the more important roles of teachers and therapists is to emphasize the child's talents for all to see, so that the child's abilities are as evident as the disabilities.

Expectations and Performance

Every child deserves to be challenged by high expectations for independence and responsibility. This is especially true for children with physical and mental disabilities, for whom expectations are too often kept low because of pity, guilt, grief, inexperience, or fear of contributing to the child's sense of failure. A frequent conse-

quence of lowered expectations is that the child lives down to them or fails even to meet them. A clue that this is occurring comes when remarkably different levels of performance are elicited by different situations—whether at school, therapy, or home, and whether the issues are physical, intellectual, social, self-help, or independence. A crucial but often overlooked role of the caring physician is precisely in this area. Because the physician is not directly involved in caregiving, he or she is often in a better position to recognize these variations of performance, partly because many primary caregivers may at first feel defensive about responsibility for the environment in which diminished performance occurs. Moreover, if handled gently and persuasively, the physician's advice has a stature and credibility that few other individuals will possess.. Ironically, in a setting of long-term "incurable" illness, long-term issues are too often lost among the more immediate medical concerns. Physicians should not miss the opportunity to place the long- and short-term issues in perspective and to promote communication between, and humility among, all concerned in the care of these children.

REFERENCES

Bach, J.R. (1993). Pulmonary rehabilitation in neuromuscular disorders. *Seminars in Respiratory Medicine, 14,* 515–529.

Brooke, M. (1994). *A clinician's view of neuromuscular disease* (3rd ed.). Baltimore: Williams & Wilkins.

Chance, P.F., & Reilly, M. (1994). Inherited neuropathies. *Current Opinion in Neurology, 7,* 372–380.

Cornblath, D.R. (1986). Disorders of neuromuscular transmission in infants and children. *Muscle Nerve, 9,* 606–611.

Dubowitz, V. (1989). *Color atlas of muscle disorders of childhood.* Chicago: Year Book Medical Publishers.

Heckmatt, J.Z., Loh, L., & Dubowitz, V. (1990). Night-time ventilation in neuromuscular disease. *Lancet, 335,* 579–582.

Jones, H.R. (1990). EMG evaluation of the floppy infant: Differential diagnosis and technical aspects. *Muscle Nerve, 13,* 338–347.

Keens, T.G., Jansen, M.T., DeWitt, P.K., & Ward, S.L.D. (1990). Home care for children with chronic respiratory failure. *Seminars in Respiratory Medicine, 11,* 269–282.

Miller, R.G., & Kuntz, N.L. (1986). Nerve conduction studies in infants and children. *Journal of Child Neurology, 1,* 19–26.

Neuromuscular disorders: Gene location. (1994). *Neuromuscular Disorders, 4,* 277–283.

Phillips, D.P., Roye, D.P., Farcy, J.P., Leet, A., & Shelton, Y.A. (1990). Surgical treatment of scoliosis in a spinal muscular atrophy population. *Spine, 15,* 942–945.

Russell, J.W., Afifi, A.K., & Ross, M.A. (1992). Predictive value of electromyography in diagnosis and prognosis of the hypotonic infant. *Journal of Child Neurology, 7,* 387–391.

Shapiro, F., & Specht, L. (1993a). The diagnosis and orthopaedic treatment of inherited muscular diseases of childhood. *Journal of Bone and Joint Surgery, 75A,* 439–454.

Shapiro, F., & Specht, L. (1993b). The diagnosis and orthopaedic treatment of childhood spinal muscular atrophy, peripheral neuropathy, Friedreich ataxia, and arthrogryposis. *Journal of Bone and Joint Surgery, 75A,* 1699–1714.

Chapter 10

Pediatric Dysphagia

Brian T. Rogers, M.D., and Thomas M. Lock, M.D.

Successful feeding and swallowing are essential for normal growth and development. It is also important to recognize that effective feeding is dependent on a number of important biologic and environmental processes. Knowledge of these processes is essential for the accurate diagnosis and effective management of feeding and swallowing disorders in children. This chapter provides a diagnostic and management approach to these disorders.

FUNCTIONAL ANATOMY OF THE AERODIGESTIVE TRACT

The upper aerodigestive tract consists of the oral and nasal cavities, pharynx, larynx, trachea, and esophagus. The oral cavity and pharynx provide a common passage for both deglutition (swallowing) and respiration. This relationship emphasizes the importance of coordination between respiration and deglutition.

The anatomic landmarks and developmental changes of the aerodigestive tract that are important in the evaluation of deglutition are illustrated in Figures 1 and 2. In addition to the structures illustrated, the anterior and lateral sulci are important landmarks. The anterior and lateral sulci are spaces between the mandible and maxilla and the lip muscles and cheeks, respectively. In infants, the volume of the sulci is minimized by the presence of extensive buccal fat pads, the relatively greater space the tongue occupies at this age, and the absence of teeth (Bosma, 1986). The sulci are important in that they are potential spaces for food to accumulate in children with dysphagia and poor tongue control. The close proximity of the tongue, soft palate, pharynx,

and larynx during the first 4–6 months of life promotes the passage of food boluses through the oral and pharyngeal cavities (Figure 1). The base of the tongue and the larynx descend during the first 4 years of life (Caruso & Sauerland, 1990). Generally, by age 4, the base of the tongue forms part of the anterior wall of the oropharynx (Figure 2). These changes result in a greater distance that food boluses must traverse during the pharyngeal phase of deglutition. In patients with dysphagia, changes in both the size and the orientation of the pharyngeal cavity may result in decompensation of feeding.

Figure 3 is a posterior sketch of the upper aerodigestive tract. Food boluses normally pass on either side of the larynx via the pyriform sinuses. These sinuses are additional potential dead spaces for the accumulation of food boluses in the presence of dysphagia.

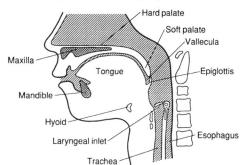

Figure 1. Schematic lateral view of the infant upper aerodigestive tract. Structures of the oral cavity and pharynx can be seen, as well as the laryngeal inlet, trachea, and esophagus. (From Arvedson, J.C., Rogers, B., & Brodsky, L. [1993]. Anatomy, embryology, and physiology. In J.C. Arvedson & L. Brodsky [Eds.], *Pediatric swallowing and feeding: Assessment and management*, p. 6. San Diego, CA: Singular Publishing Group. Copyright ©1993. Reprinted by permission.)

We thank Joan Arvedson, Ph.D., for her insightful comments and review of the manuscript. Secretarial assistance in the preparation of this manuscript was provided by Mary Jane Hall.

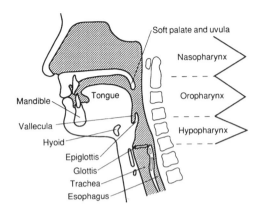

Figure 2. Schematic lateral view of the adult upper aerodigestive tract, demonstrating anatomic limitations of nasopharynx, oropharynx, and hypopharynx. (From Arvedson, J.C., Rogers, B., & Brodsky, L. [1993]. Anatomy, embryology, and physiology. In J.C. Arvedson & L. Brodsky [Eds.], *Pediatric swallowing and feeding: Assessment and management*, p. 6. San Diego, CA: Singular Publishing Group. Copyright ©1993. Reprinted by permission.)

PHYSIOLOGY OF SWALLOWING

Deglutition can be divided conveniently into the oral preparatory, oral, pharyngeal, and esophageal phases (Miller, 1982). The manipulation of food to form a bolus in the oral cavity represents the *oral preparatory phase*. Examples of food manipulation include expression of formula or breast milk from a nipple, lip closure around a spoon, the chewing of solid foods, and the collection of the food in the center of the tongue. This phase is entirely voluntary and varies considerably in duration. The *oral phase* begins with the posterior propulsion of the food bolus by the tongue and ends with the production of a swallow. A posteriorly directed sequential contact between the tongue and palate results in movement of the bolus toward the oropharynx. The soft palate subsequently moves in a superior and posterior direction while the pharyngeal wall moves medially and anteriorly, resulting in closure of the nasopharynx. Immediately prior to the pharyngeal phase, the hyoid bone is brought to a preparatory position by moderate elevation. The duration of the oral phase is normally less than 1 second and is not dependent on texture or density of the food bolus.

The sensory fields for the initiation of the *pharyngeal phase* are located at the level of the

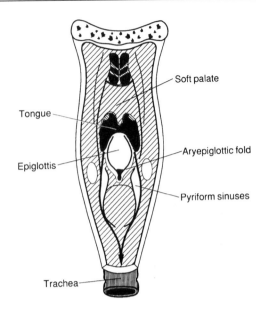

Figure 3. Posterior sketch of the upper aerodigestive tract (larynx and pharynx). Pathway for food is around the larynx through the pyriform sinuses to the esophageal inlet. (From Arvedson, J.C., Rogers, B., & Brodsky, L. [1993]. Anatomy, embryology, and physiology. In J.C. Arvedson & L. Brodsky [Eds.], *Pediatric swallowing and feeding: Assessment and management*, p. 10. San Diego, CA: Singular Publishing Group. Copyright ©1993. Reprinted by permission.)

pillars of the fauces, the posterior pharyngeal wall, and possibly the base of the tongue and preepiglottic sinus. Major components of the pharyngeal phase include elevation of the whole pharyngeal tube followed by a descending peristaltic wave. This engulfing action and subsequent peristalsis are quite forceful, generating food bolus speeds of 100 cm/sec (Miller, 1982). Simultaneously, the larynx elevates and is pulled anteriorly under the root of the tongue, and the epiglottis folds down over the laryngeal aperture. The epiglottis has a flattened lingual surface and acts to direct food laterally into the recesses formed by the pyriform sinuses. This movement of food is away from the midline and laryngeal inlet. The larynx is further protected by the medial movements of the arytenoid cartilages and aryepiglottic folds and by the anterior movement of the larynx under the mandible by the hyoid bone and musculature. Finally, the valvelike function of the bilateral superior (false) and inferior (true) vocal folds results in further protection against aspiration. During oral feedings, adult subjects without dysphagia occasionally show transient food spillage into the laryngeal vestibule (the space between the superior and inferior folds) but not through the true vocal folds (Ekberg, 1982).

The maintenance of respiration during swallowing appears to undergo some degree of developmental maturation. Normal preterm and term infants in the first week of life frequently experience decreases in minute ventilation, respiratory rate, and tidal volume during continuous nutritive sucking. This has been shown to persist in infants with various central nervous system abnormalities (Rosen, Glaze, & Frost, 1984). There is limited information regarding the coordination of respiration and deglutition in children. In adults, the onset of swallowing appears to interrupt expiration (Smith, Wolkove, Colacone, & Kreisman, 1989).

The *esophageal phase* begins with dilatation of the upper esophageal sphincter (UES) and movement of the food bolus into the upper esophagus. The dynamics of UES function during swallowing are dependent on the volume of the food bolus. Larger bolus volumes result in increased UES diameters and duration of relaxation (Kahrilas, Dodds, Dent, Logemann, & Shaker, 1988). At the end of the esophageal peristaltic wave, a momentary relaxation of the lower esophageal sphincter (LES) allows swallowed food to enter the stomach. Between swallows, the pressure generated by the LES is important in preventing gastroesophageal reflux. Anatomic factors important in promoting LES pressure include the phrenoesophageal ligaments, the angled entrance of the esophagus into the stomach (flap valve), and the partial location of the LES in the abdomen (Rossi, 1993). Gastric emptying and esophageal acid clearance also appear to be important. Delayed gastric emptying may be one factor that increases the likelihood of gastroesophageal reflux (Rossi, 1993). Some investigators have postulated that LES pressure changes may be the result of reflux and not the cause. Acid exposure of the esophageal mucosa may produce changes in both LES function and esophageal peristalsis. Reduced swallowing rate and esophageal peristalsis in patients with dysphagia may be important factors in the persistence of low pH in the lower esophagus, promoting

gastroesophageal reflux and esophagitis (Rossi, 1993).

DEVELOPMENT OF FEEDING BEHAVIOR

The acquisition of food and the oral preparatory phase are greatly influenced by central nervous system maturation. Suckling is first noted at 18–24 weeks' gestation. This type of nipple feeding consists of anterior–posterior rhythmic stripping movement of the tongue, and the lips may loosely approximate (Bosma, 1986). The tongue moves forward for half of the suckle pattern, but the backward phase is the more pronounced. This pattern persists for the first 4–6 months of life. These events make way for spoon feeding and sucking, which consists of more vertical movement of the tongue rather than the jaw (transition period). The transition period is also characterized by enlargement of the oral cavity and the development of lateral tongue movements. Munching or vertical jaw movements start at 6 months, followed by rotary chewing at 7 months (Arvedson, Rogers, & Brodsky, 1993).

Changes in gross motor function are also important in the development of feeding skills. At term gestation, the presence of equal amounts of passive flexor muscle tone in the arms and legs, and the balance of flexor and extensor tone of the axillary girdle, promote a semiflexed position for nipple feedings. Primitive reflexes, including the Moro, tonic labyrinthine, and asymmetric tonic neck, gradually dissipate during the first 4–6 months of life. These changes are associated with increased midline skills that are important for such activities as spoon and finger feeding. Midline hand play, bottle or cup holding, and extended reach and grasp can only occur after the palmar grasp and tonic labyrinthine reflexes are diminished. Improved equilibrium skills permit the development of sitting posture and the free use of the hands for self-feeding.

Functional feeding skills and parent–child interaction during meals are also greatly influenced by cognitive development. Table 1 summarizes the complex relations between streams of development and feeding abilities in the first 2 years of life.

Table 1. Neurodevelopmental milestones relevant to normal feeding

Age (months)	Cognitive	Sensory motor	Feeding skills
Birth to 2	Visual fixation and tracking	Balanced flexor and extensor tone of neck and trunk	Promotion of parent–infant interaction during feeding Maintenance of semiflexed posture during feeding
3 to 4	Visual recognition of parents	Head maintained primarily in midline and aligned with trunk in supported sitting	Parents preferred for oral feedings Upright supported position for spoon feeding
5 to 9	Visual interest in small objects Extended reach and grasp Object permanence Stranger anxiety	Independent sitting Extended reach with pincer grasp	Feedings more frequently in upright position Initiation of finger feeding Parents preferred for feedings
18 to 24	Use of tools Increasing attention and persistence in play activities Independence from parents Parallel or imitative play	Refinement of upper extremity coordination	Use of feeding utensils Prefer to feed self over longer periods of time Imitate others during meals

From Rogers, B., & Campbell, J. (1993). Pediatric and neurodevelopmental evaluation. In J.C. Arvedson & L. Brodsky (Eds.), *Pediatric swallowing and feeding: Assessment and management,* p. 55. San Diego, CA: Singular Publishing Group. Copyright ©1993. Reprinted by permission.

NEURAL CONTROL OF DEGLUTITION

Multiple levels of the nervous system are responsible for successful deglutition. Key peripheral and central nervous system areas include the cranial nerves, brain stem, midbrain, cerebellum, and cerebrum. More extensive reviews of this subject are available (Miller, 1982, 1986).

The peripheral afferents for deglutition include cranial nerves V, VII, IX, and X (Table 2). Successful bolus formation and transport are dependent on light touch and deep pressure innervation by the Vth (trigeminal) nerve. Cranial nerves IX (glossopharyngeal) and X (vagus) provide afferents to proposed areas of swallow initiation, including the anterior faucial pillars, pharynx, and posterior larynx (Miller, 1982). These cranial nerves also provide several sensory feedback loops that are involved in the modification of the pharyngeal peristaltic wave. Food boluses with higher viscosity result in increased duration of the pharyngeal peristaltic wave and UES relaxation (Dantas et al., 1990). The vagus nerve (cranial nerve X) also provides afferents to the larynx that contribute to effective airway protection during and between swallows.

There are also central afferents for deglutition. Sources of these afferents include the cerebrum, midbrain, cerebellum, and upper brain stem (Figure 4). These descending pathways are believed to provide much of the voluntary control of deglutition (Miller, 1982). Areas of the medulla comprising the nucleus tractus solitarius and ventral medial reticular formation form what is referred to as the "swallowing center" (Miller, 1982, 1986). This center, which is a complex network of interneurons, functions as a "central pattern generator" for deglutition, and

Table 2. Afferents for swallowing

Cranial nerve	Function
Trigeminal (V)	General sensation, anterior 2/3 of tongue
	Soft palate, nasopharynx, mouth
Facial (VII)	Taste, anterior 2/3 of tongue
	Touch sensation to lips and face
Glossopharyngeal (IX)	Taste and general sensation posterior 1/3 tongue
	Sensation to tonsils, pharynx, soft palate
Vagus (X)	Pharynx, larynx, viscera
	Base of tongue

From Arvedson, J.C., Rogers, B., & Brodsky, L. (1993). Anatomy, embryology, and physiology. In J.C. Arvedson & L. Brodsky (Eds.), *Pediatric swallowing and feeding: Assessment and management*, p. 37. San Diego, CA: Singular Publishing Group. Copyright ©1993. Reprinted by permission.

is responsible for the programmed series of neuronal discharges that are responsible for the reflexive motor components of deglutition (Miller, 1986).

Table 3 outlines the primary efferents for deglutition. In addition to cranial nerves V, VII, IX, X, and XII, cervical nerves 1 and 2 provide innervation for tongue, hyoid, and laryngeal movements.

ETIOLOGIES OF SWALLOWING AND FEEDING DISORDERS

There are numerous etiologies of feeding and swallowing disorders in childhood. Table 4 contains a convenient diagnostic outline based on clinical history and physical findings. Great care should be taken in determining the onset and natural history of any feeding problem. The majority of chronic conditions are static in nature. The feeding skills of children with static conditions generally remain the same or gradually improve with maturation. Although feeding efficiency may change during acute illnesses or transition feeding periods, persistent loss of previously acquired oromotor and swallowing skills does not occur. Regression or loss of previously mastered feeding skills is seen in progressive disorders and should prompt appropriate medical evaluation.

ASSESSMENT

Feeding History

The feeding history is the first step in evaluating feeding problems. Initially, the chief concerns of parents and other caregivers should be obtained. Feeding is an activity that requires a large amount of parental involvement and, consequently, reflects both the child's and the parents' feeding skills. Frequently the parents feel responsible for the feeding problems, and the history should be obtained in a manner that helps the parents feel involved in finding a solution rather than feeling that they are a part of the problem.

The feeding history should include the following questions. Do feedings produce symptoms? Frequent coughing and progressive "noisy" breathing during feeding may suggest residual food in the pharynx after swallows and laryngeal penetration or aspiration. Does the child become distressed or refuse feedings? This may suggest a painful swallow or the child's perception that the swallow is dangerous. Inquiries should be made regarding the onset, duration, and course of the feeding problem. Progressive or new feeding problems should be identified. An early onset of symptoms may suggest the presence of an anatomic abnormality. In contrast, gradually worsening of symptoms late in the first year or in the second suggest decompensation as oropharyngeal structures grow in a child with suprabulbar dysfunction. The duration of typical feedings should be determined. Abnormalities of any one of the three phrases of deglutition (oral, pharyngeal, and esophageal) may result in slowing or frequent interruptions of oral feedings. Oral feedings lasting longer than 30 minutes are often a sign of a clinically significant feeding disorder. The time of day in which feeding prob-

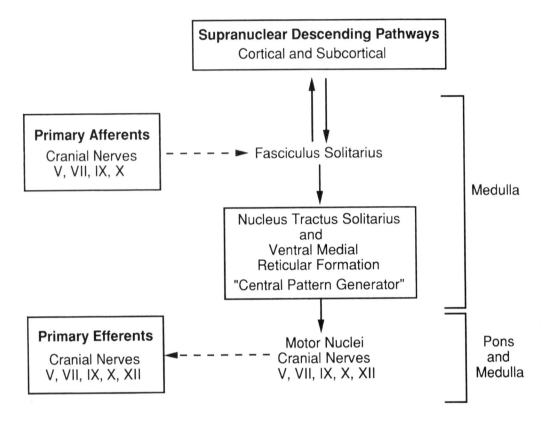

Figure 4. Diagrammatic representation of major peripheral and central nervous system pathways for deglutition. Afferents, including cranial nerves and cortical and subcortical pathways, send input through the fasciculus solitarius to the nucleus tractus solitarius and the ventral medial reticular formation (central pattern generator). Efferent nerves synapse with motor nuclei primarily of cranial nerves V, VII, IX, X, and XII. (From Arvedson, J.C., Rogers, B., & Brodsky, L. [1993]. Anatomy, embryology, and physiology. In J.C. Arvedson & L. Brodsky [Eds.], *Pediatric swallowing and feeding: Assessment and management*, p. 36. San Diego, CA: Singular Publishing Group. Copyright ©1993. Reprinted by permission.)

lems occur may clarify the roles of specific feeders as well as the child's mental status or appetite.

Specific food textures or the methods by which foods are given to the child may result in symptoms during feedings. Where and in what position do feedings occur? A comfortable, erect position is necessary for an efficient oral phase. Posterior tilt of the head increases the risk of premature leak of food into the pharynx and larynx. What is the food texture? Is the texture developmentally appropriate? Thickened textures may be easier for a child who has difficulty forming a bolus. Thin liquids are more frequently aspirated in children with dysphagia (Arvedson, Rogers, Buck, Smart, & Msall, 1994). Are liquids taken from a bottle or a cup? Are solids taken from a spoon or fork? Are the

utensils modified? How does the child participate in the feedings? The answers to these questions may suggest what feeding strategies have worked in the past, which have failed, and which have yet to be attempted.

Medical History

Both the sequelae and the management of epilepsy, behavioral disorders, and neurodevelopmental disabilities can result in disorders of feeding. Uncontrolled seizures can result in altered levels of consciousness and interfere with feeding. Commonly used anticonvulsants can also produce lethargy (barbiturates and benzodiazepines) or anorexia (valproic acid). Certain neuroleptics (e.g., thioridazine, chlorpromazine) used in the management of severe behavioral problems have been associated with

Table 3. Efferents for swallowing

Phase of swallow	Innervation
Oral	
Muscles of mastication	Trigeminal (V_3)—mandibular branch
Lip sphincter and face muscles	Facial (VII)
Tongue	Hypoglossal (XII)
Intrinsic muscles	Ansa cervicalis (C_1–C_2)
Palatoglossus	Vagus (X)
Pharyngeal	
Stylopharyngeus	Glossopharyngeal (IX)
Palate, pharynx, and larynx	Vagus (X)
Tensor veli palatini	Trigeminal (V_3)
Hyoid and laryngeal movement	V_3, VII, C_1–C_2
Esophageal	
Esophagus	Vagus (X)

From Arvedson, J.C., Rogers, B., & Brodsky, L. (1993). Anatomy, embryology, and physiology. In J.C. Arvedson & L. Brodsky (Eds.), *Pediatric swallowing and feeding: Assessment and management*, p. 39. San Diego, CA: Singular Publishing Group. Copyright ©1993. Reprinted by permission.

lethargy and the development of laryngeal–pharyngeal dystonia and esophageal dysmotility (Moss & Green, 1982). Dysphagia is common in children with severe cerebral palsy. Benzodiazepines, which have been used for increased passive muscle tone, have also been associated with the development of drooling, reduced pharyngeal peristalsis, and cricopharyngeal incoordination (Wyllie, Wyllie, Cruse, Rothner, & Erenberg, 1986).

Chronic or recurrent gastrointestinal or respiratory symptoms may suggest the presence of feeding dysfunction. One of the more common complications of significant dysphagia is reduced fluid intake. Acutely reduced fluid intake may result in dehydration during acute illnesses. Chronically low fluid intake, particularly when combined with immobility, often results in chronic constipation. Gastroesophageal reflux frequently presents as vomiting, but reflux to lower levels may produce symptoms such as frequent belching followed by a train of swallows or apparent discomfort. The relationship of these apparent reflux episodes to respiratory symptoms such as cough, cyanosis, retractions, or noisy breathing should be noted. Recurrent pneumonia or intractable asthma may be caused by chronic or intermittent aspiration. Stridor may be caused by laryngeal dysfunction resulting from a primary laryngeal disorder or inflammation secondary to gastroesophageal reflux (Nielson, Heldt, & Tooley, 1990).

Physical Examination

The physical examination, guided by the history, will usually provide the bulk of information needed to formulate a diagnosis and treatment plan. Evaluation of somatic growth; orofacial, cardiorespiratory, abdominal, cranial nerve, and neurodevelopmental examinations; and the observation of feeding all require special attention.

Somatic Growth Measurements of weight, height, head circumference, and weight for height, along with triceps skinfold thickness and midarm circumference, are quite helpful for assessing nutritional trends. Accurate measurements of height may be difficult in children with scoliosis and joint contractures. Standards for upper arm and lower leg lengths appear to be useful in assessing linear growth in children with severe cerebral palsy (Spender, Cronk, Charney, & Stallings, 1989). These measurements are most helpful in determining response to nutritional rehabilitation.

Stunted growth is a common complication in children with neurogenic dysphagia. Serial anthropometric measurements are preferable for the diagnosis of stunted growth. If previous growth data are limited, the interrelationship between height, weight, and head circumference measurements can still provide valuable information about nutritional history. Signs of acute protein–calorie malnutrition include re-

Table 4. Etiologies of dysphagia in childhood

Site of pathology	Acute	Chronic	
		Static	Progressive

Central nervous system	Hypoxic–ischemic encephalopathy
	Cerebral infarctions
	Intracranial hemorrhage
	Infections
	  Meningitis
	  Encephalitis
	  Poliomyelitis
	  Botulism
	  Syphilis
	Acute bilirubin encephalopathy
	Metabolic encephalopathies
	  Aminoacidopathies
	  Disorders of carbohydrate metabolism
	Neonatal withdrawal syndrome (heroin, barbiturates)
	Traumatic encephalopathies and brain stem injuries
		Arnold-Chiari malformation
		Genetic disorders
		Familial dysautonomia (Riley-Day syndrome)
		Möbius sequence
		Developmental disorders of the brain
		Cerebral palsy
		Chronic postkernicteric bilirubin encephalopathy
			Arnold-Chiari malformation
			Intracranial malignancies
			  Tumors
			  Leukemia
			  Lymphoma
			Degenerative white and gray matter diseases
			Lysosomal storage diseases
			Metachromatic leukodystrophy
			Adrenoleukodystrophy
			Leigh's encephalomyelopathy
			Neuroaxonal degeneration
			Zellweger's disease
			Wilson's disease
			HIV encephalopathy
			Rett syndrome
			Spinocerebellar disorders
			Dystonia musculorum deformans
			Multiple sclerosis
			Amyotrophic lateral sclerosis
			Syringobulbia

Anterior horn cell			Infantile spinal muscular atrophy
Peripheral nervous system	Acute inflammatory polyradiculoneuropathy	Polyneuropathies	Polyneuropathies
Neuromuscular junction	Hypermagnesemia		Myasthenia gravis

Muscles	Polymyositis
	Dermatomyositis
		Congenital myopathies
		  Nemaline rod
		  Myotubular
		  Fiber type disproportion
		Myotonic dystrophy
		Congenital muscular dystrophy
		Infantile fascioscapulohumeral dystrophy
			Metabolic myopathies
			  Glycogen storage disease
			  Mitochondrial
			Duchenne muscular dystrophy

Respiratory tract	Otitis media Sinusitis Adenotonsillitis/pharyngitis	Severe chronic lung disease Bronchopulmonary dysplasia Structural anomalies of upper respiratory tract	

Cardiovascular disorders		Congenital heart disease
		  Cyanotic
		  Congestive heart failure
			Congenital heart disease (may be progressive at times)

(continued)

Table 4. (continued)

Site of pathology	Acute	Chronic	
		Static	Progressive
Gastrointestinal tract		Gastroesophageal reflux Peptic ulcer	Gastroesophageal reflux and esophagitis Peptic ulcer
Psychological		Disorders of parent–child interaction	

Adapted from Rogers and Campbell (1993).

duction of weight to below the 5th percentile for age and weight for height less than the 10th percentile (Rossi, 1993). Chronic protein–calorie malnutrition in children with cerebral palsy and dysphagia can result in reductions of fat stores, fat-free mass (muscle area), and linear growth (Stallings, Charney, Davies, & Cronk, 1993).

Orofacial Examination Orofacial examination may reveal congenital and secondary anomalies of the structures involved in feeding. Obstructive lesions of the nose, such as choanal atresia, nasal polyps, and foreign bodies, interfere with the coordination of oral activities and respiration. Midline defects ranging from complete cleft lip and palate to subtle submucous clefts produce leakage of food into the nasopharynx and result in progressive nasal congestion during feedings. These defects may also disturb the continuity of the alveolar ridge and shape of the palatal vault, resulting in disruption of their relationship to one another or of the tongue to the palate. Partial respiratory obstruction and mouth breathing may result from tonsillar and adenoidal hypertrophy. Retraction of the lips can contribute to drooling and, in combination with mouth breathing, can result in the drying of teeth and gums, plaque formation, gingival hyperplasia, and gingivitis. Mandibular hypoplasia may be associated with disruption of the relationship of the tongue and palate, interfering with suckling in infants or producing malocclusion of the teeth in older children. Acute lesions of the oral mucosa may be responsible for acute deterioration in oral feeding.

The oral examination may be greatly aided by the use of a lollipop. Sorbitol-based sugarless lollipops are preferable to sugar-based ones because the sorbitol is much less brittle and does not shatter under the pressure of a tonic bite reflex. Careful stroking of the lips will often initiate mouth opening and tongue protrusion. Stroking the tongue will stimulate salivation, and the handling of oral secretions can be observed. Gentle pressure on the tongue will often facilitate mouth opening and the examination of intraoral structures. Just before removal of the lollipop, it can be moved posteriorly into the oropharynx in an attempt to initiate a gag reflex.

Auscultation of the swallow can be a helpful adjunct to the oral examination. Swallows can be either spontaneous or stimulated by the examiner. The normal swallow involves the total closure of the glottis and vestibule followed by a brisk opening. On auscultation this is heard as a period of total silence (glottis closed) followed by a brisk "snap" (glottis opens) followed by the flow of air. With dysfunction of the vocal folds, the movement of air may be audible throughout the swallow, or, if the vestibule closes partially, it may form an echo chamber amplifying the sounds of the partial closing and opening of the larynx, resulting in a loud swallow. If swallows fail to clear the entire bolus from the larynx and vestibule, breathing will become progressively more noisy through a feeding unless the throat is cleared by repeated swallows between bites or by a cough.

Cardiorespiratory Examination Examination of the heart and lungs may reveal important signs of chronic effects of dysphagia and aspiration. Cyanosis is a sign of severe hypoxemia. Clubbing may result from longstanding hypoxemia. Central nervous system disorders and neuromuscular disease can result in reduced chest wall compliance and diminished chest excursion during inspiration. Respiratory rate may be elevated in the presence of chronic aspiration. Careful auscultation of the lungs, with special attention to asymmetrical findings, is necessary to differentiate intrapulmonary sounds such as rales and wheezes from ubiquitous upper respiratory tract sounds heard in children with dysphagia. In the absence of wheezes or tachypnea, a prolonged expiratory phase of the respiratory cycle may be due to chronic aspiration. On cardiac examination, a pulsus paradoxus, or an accentuated pulmonary component or fixed splitting of the second heart sound, may be clues to chronic pulmonary disease. Finally, primary cardiopulmonary disease may interfere with feeding. Infants and children who are short of breath will feed poorly. Heart failure can result in progressive fatigue during oral feedings.

Abdominal Examination Constipation is a common complication of a diet low in fiber and water combined with immobility. Stool is often palpable or detected by dullness on percussion in the left upper and lower quadrants and suprapubic region. The rectal examination will provide evidence of retained hard stool in the rectum and will also provide evidence of neurogenic dysfunction in spinal cord lesions and Hirschsprung disease. A positive stool guaiac test provides evidence of occult bleeding, frequently as a consequence of esophagitis.

Examination of Cranial Nerves The examination of the cranial nerves involved in deglutition includes assessment of the trigeminal (Vth), facial (VIIth), glossopharyngeal (IXth), vagus (Xth), and hypoglossal (XIIth) nerves. A summary of physical examination findings useful in localizing the site of cranial nerve deficits that may be seen in patients with dysphagia is found in Table 5. Nuclear or peripheral cranial nerve deficits usually result from traumatic or ischemic injuries (Möbius sequence, traumatic head injury), destructive lesions (syringobulbia, neoplasms), or infectious processes (polio, acute inflammatory polyradiculoneuropathy).

The mandibular division of the trigeminal nerve innervates the muscles of mastication. Nuclear or peripheral lesions of the nerve will produce drooping or opening of the jaw and weakness of jaw movements in the absence of the jaw jerk reflex. Supranuclear lesions may result in poorly coordinated jaw movements and exaggerated jaw jerk. The trigeminal nerve also carries sensory fibers to the face and pain and light touch sensation to the mucous membranes of the nose and mouth.

The facial nerve innervates the muscles of facial expression. Nuclear or peripheral lesions are associated with weakness resulting in flattening of the nasolabial folds and paralysis of forehead and lower face muscles. In contrast, unilateral supranuclear lesions produce only paresis of the lower face, because the rostral portion of the facial nucleus that innervates the forehead receives bilateral descending input. Paralysis of the lower facial muscles can result in drooling and accumulation of food in the sulci between the alveolar ridges and the cheeks. The facial nerve also sends fibers to the stylohyoid muscle and posterior belly of the digastric muscle. Paralysis of these muscles can result in malfunction of the pharyngeal swallow, with delayed passage of the bolus and aspiration. The facial nerve also provides sensory fibers for taste to the anterior two thirds of the tongue and parasympathetic innervation to the salivary glands and oral mucosa.

The glossopharyngeal nerve innervates the stylopharyngeus muscle and provides general sensation to the mucous membranes of the soft palate, tongue, and posterior pharyngeal wall. The sensory component of the gag reflex is carried by the glossopharyngeal nerve, and its motor component by the trigeminal, vagus, and hypoglossal nerves.

The vagus nerve provides efferent fibers to the soft palate, larynx, and pharynx. The dorsal motor nucleus of the vagus contributes to sensorimotor coordination of swallowing, breathing, phonation, cardiovascular responses, and vomiting. Lesions of the vagus or its nucleus produce severe dysphagia with palatal weakness and vocal fold paralysis.

The hypoglossal nerve innervates the muscles involved with the movement of the tongue, hyoid bone, and larynx. The most obvious signs of peripheral or nuclear damage to the hypoglossal nerve are wasting, immobility, or fasciculations of the tongue. In unilateral lesions, the tongue will deviate toward the side of the lesion. Supranuclear lesions may result in dysfunctional tongue movements such as prolonged and exaggerated tongue thrusting.

Neurodevelopmental Examination The neurodevelopmental examination is important in the evaluation of the feeding process.

Table 5. Clinical localization of cranial nerve deficits associated with dysphagia

Cranial nerve	Supranuclear	Nuclear or peripheral
Trigeminal (CN V)	Mandible movements are well preserved but often immature or poorly coordinated	Mandible movements are usually minimal or absent
	Jaw jerk reflex present or exaggerated	Jaw jerk reflex is usually absent
	Tonic bite reflex may be present	Tonic bite reflex is absent
Facial (CN VII)	Paralysis of lower half of face	Paralysis of upper (forehead) and lower half of face
	Paralysis is almost always unilateral	Paralysis can be unilateral or bilateral
Glossopharyngeal (CN IX) and vagus (CN X)	Muscular palate has normal strength	Weakness of muscular palate
		Asymmetry of muscular palate movement is common
	Normal appearance of palatopharyngeal folds	Flattening of palatopharyngeal folds
	Vocal fold movement preserved	Vocal fold paralysis
Hypoglossal (CN XII)	Tongue movements are dysfunctional but present	Unilateral or bilateral absence of tongue movement
	Tongue protrusion reflex can be exaggerated and prolonged in duration	Tongue fasciculations Tongue atrophy

From Rogers, B., & Campbell, J. (1993). Pediatric and neurodevelopmental evaluation. In J.C. Arvedson & L. Brodsky (Eds.), *Pediatric swallowing and feeding: Assessment and management*, p. 74. San Diego, CA: Singular Publishing Group. Copyright ©1993. Reprinted by permission.

Suprabulbar dysphagia is more common in choreoathetoid or mixed cerebral palsy than in spastic cerebral palsy. Mental retardation and communication disorders are important risk factors in the development of behavioral food refusal and in the maintenance of maladaptive feeding behaviors after an intercurrent illness.

Observation of Feeding The etiology of a feeding problem can usually be deduced from a detailed history and a careful physical examination. An observation of an oral feeding will help confirm the diagnosis and form the basis for an effective management plan.

Disorders affecting the oral preparatory phase will generally result in displacement or loss of food from the oral cavity. Bottle feeding may be complicated by slow extraction of milk or formula from the nipple. During a sucking sequence, lack of a steady series of bubbles in the bottle may be observed. The strength of the suck can be estimated by pulling the nipple from the oral cavity during a sucking sequence. Paresis of the facial and masseter muscles will often result in poor lip closure and loss of liquids from the oral cavity. In older infants (greater than 12 months) and children, pocketing of food in the lateral sulci may indicate poor tongue lateralization, lack of chewing, or both. Abnormally prominent oral reflexes can also be detrimental in bolus formation. The tonic bite reflex is often quite strong with central nervous system disorders. Contact of feeding instruments (nipples, spoons) with the alveolar ridges and tongue will result in a forceful, uncontrolled bite that may last for a number of seconds.

Oral-phase abnormalities are manifested by slow and inefficient movement or misdirection of the food bolus into the oropharynx. Normally, the movement of the food bolus through the oral cavity to the pharynx takes approximately 1 second. Children with oral-phase disorders will often have portions of food boluses on the dorsum of their tongue for long periods of time. Fragmentation of food boluses by inefficient tongue movements can result in multiple swallows per bolus. Children with serious oral-phase abnormalities often utilize extensor posturing of the neck and trunk to facilitate movement of food boluses from the oral cavity to the pharynx. Persistence of the bolus on the dorsum of the tongue can also result in the dissolution of part of the bolus and "drooling" posteriorly into the vallecula and laryngeal vestibule.

Disorders of the pharyngeal phase are characterized by delays and misdirected movements of food boluses through the pharynx. Delays in swallow initiation can result in frequent coughing and gagging during oral feedings. Aspiration before swallow initiation can occur. Delay in swallow initiation is a very common finding in children with dysphagia and cerebral palsy. This abnormality may be observed only while swallowing specific food textures (Rogers, Arvedson, Buck, Smart, & Msall, 1994). The action of pharyngeal constrictors may be poorly coordinated or weak. This frequently results in food residue in the vallecula, pyriform sinuses, and laryngeal vestibule after swallows. The presence of food residue can result in multiple swallows, noisy breathing, and aspiration during feeding. Videofluoroscopic modified barium swallow studies have demonstrated that aspiration during oral feedings of children is usually of trace amounts and does not result in a cough (Arvedson et al., 1994). Thus, coughing cannot be relied on to identify aspiration. Dysfunction of the cricopharyngeus muscle can result in blockage of the food bolus in the hypopharynx and rapid expulsion through either the nasal or oral cavities. Serious pharyngeal-phase abnormalities may lead to compensatory responses, including extension of the neck to promote food passage and opening of the airway. Irregular respiration and gasping may be observed during oral feedings.

Common abnormalities of the esophageal phase include esophageal dysmotility and gastroesophageal reflux. Food refusal and signs of irritability or discomfort toward the end of meals can be manifestations of gastro-esophageal reflux and esophagitis. Finally, abnormal posturing and movement, including extensor arching of the neck and trunk during or after feeding suggesting a movement disorder or seizures, can result from gastroesophageal reflux (Kinsbourne, 1964; Werlin, D'Souza, Hogan, Dodds, & Arndorfer, 1980).

Consultations

Once a differential diagnosis is formulated, a number of special studies and consultations may be helpful in establishing definitive diagnoses and formulating a treatment plan. In addition to performing specific therapies, consultants are often essential for the performance of diagnostic tests. Strong interdisciplinary relationships are necessary to avoid useless repetition and improper performance of these tests. Consultants from several other disciplines may be involved in the care of children with dysphagia.

Speech-Language Pathologists Speech-language pathologists are integral members of interdisciplinary teams for pediatric dysphagia because of their expertise in the broad aspects of communication and in oral-motor function. Communication is basic to all human interaction and must be taken into account in both assessment and intervention decision making. Oral-motor function for swallowing and for speech motor production requires coordination of the same structures (lips, tongue, palate, mandible, pharynx, and larynx).

In many medical centers, speech-language pathologists conduct the radiographic evaluation of swallowing with radiologists. Speech-language pathologists are valuable resources in the interpretation of radiographic studies and in the clinic observations of feeding and swallowing, as well as for oral-motor treatment recommendations and follow-up.

Occupational Therapists Occupational therapists have a long history of evaluating and treating feeding disorders in individuals with developmental disabilities. They have particular expertise in positioning and adapting equipment for feeding and in the treatment of oral-phase disorders. In some centers, they also are active in radiographic evaluation of swallowing. The skills of speech-language pathologists and occupational therapists are closely related and have evolved into complimentary functions at many centers.

Nutritionists Nutritionists are important in the evaluation of the diets of children with feeding problems. They are able to assess the nutritional adequacy of diets, both before and after the institution of therapy. Nutritionists are often essential in addressing constraints of volume, food texture, route of delivery, taste, and caloric intake.

Nurses Nurses are helpful in the care of children with special medical needs for feeding. They can provide essential support for the child who cannot take oral feedings and requires nasogastric or gastrostomy feedings.

Behavior Therapists Disordered communication at meals can result in significant behavioral feeding problems. Preexisting dysphagia can also result in secondary behavioral problems including food refusal. These behavioral problems, may persist even after causes of dysphagia, including esophagitis and gastroesophageal reflux, have been successfully treated. Behavior therapists, in conjunction with the feeding team, can assist in addressing these important issues.

Gastroenterologists Disorders of gastroesophageal function are important causes of dysphagia. Gastroenterologists can provide invaluable consultation in cases of severe and persistent gastroesophageal reflux, esophagitis, and peptic ulcer disease. Gastroenterologists can also perform useful diagnostic and management procedures, including endoscopy and percutaneous endoscopic gastrostomy placement.

Otorhinolaryngologists Otorhinolaryngologists are essential in the diagnosis and management of upper and lower airway tract disorders that can compromise oral feedings. They can be invaluable in the diagnosis of conditions resulting in airway obstruction. Anomalies of the upper respiratory tract that may result in misdirected food boluses, including clefts of the palate and larynx, can be effectively diagnosed and treated by otolaryngologists and other professionals.

Pediatric Surgeons Pediatric surgeons are involved in the treatment of congenital anomalies of the digestive tract. They are involved in tracheotomy care in some centers, and they

place gastrostomies and perform surgical procedures for the treatment of gastroesophageal reflux. Good communication with these specialists is important to assure timely and appropriate performance of these procedures.

Dentists Dentists are important for the treatment of congenital dental anomalies and for the maintenance of oral health in children with dysphagia, who often present great difficulties in oral hygiene and may have diets that affect the oral bacterial flora differently than the usual diet of children.

Special Studies

Special procedures are especially relevant to the pharyngeal and esophageal phases of the swallow, because these phases are not accessible to direct inspection. The most frequently useful studies are reviewed below.

Videofluoroscopic Swallow Studies The fluoroscopic observation of the swallowing of boluses impregnated with radiopaque material provides a dynamic view of the passage of a bolus from mouth to esophagus. These studies require careful coordination between the radiologist and the oral-motor specialist or clinician. The more faithfully the examiners can duplicate the child's usual feeding experience, the more valid will be the information obtained. Under optimal conditions, a clear view of the path taken by foods of a number of textures can be obtained. If the child is not comfortable and resists the feeding, or is fed in a manner that bears little resemblance to his or her usual feedings, the presence or absence of aspiration in the study may reveal little about the risk of aspiration outside of the radiology suite. These studies are especially helpful in evaluation of "silent" aspiration, those aspiration events not accompanied by coughing or obvious respiratory distress.

Upper Gastrointestinal Tract Series The radiologic evaluation of the esophagus, stomach, and small intestine using radiopaque contrast must be differentiated from the video oropharyngeal swallow study. This study is designed to fully evaluate anatomic structures, has different technical requirements, and usually cannot be done in the same room or at the same time as the video swallow study. This study provides evidence of severe gastroesophageal reflux, obstruction of the upper digestive tract, and the gross anatomy of the esophagus and stomach. Absence of gastroesophageal reflux in this study does not rule out reflux because it samples only a brief period of time, and reflux is an intermittent event. Most surgeons consider this study essential for planning for surgical approaches to the stomach and esophagus.

Scintiscan for Gastroesophageal Reflux
Infusion of radiolabeled tracer into the stomach allows for the assessment of the fate of stomach contents, including gastric emptying and gastroesophageal reflux. This is the only study that can give direct evidence of passage of stomach contents into the lung fields. If an insufficient volume is placed in an empty stomach and the patient experiences reflux only at greater volumes, no reflux may be observed. In addition to the evaluation of reflux, this study also can provide evidence of delayed gastric emptying.

pH Probe   The pH probe provides evidence of excessive and prolonged acidification of the esophagus in gastroesophageal reflux. This study can provide an assessment of periods of reflux over many hours. Prolonged clearance of acid from the esophagus, even in the presence of normal clearance of radiotracers, is associated with the development of esophagitis. It is important that the study not be done while the child is receiving antacid therapy, such as histamine-2 blockers, which can result in false-negative tests. The pH probe is most easily done in older or immobile children because small, active children have a tendency to remove the probe. When properly performed, this is probably the most sensitive test for gastroesophageal reflux. A certain amount of reflux occurs in normal individuals. The number and duration of reflux events observed during a study are compared with normal controls. Whether a normal amount of reflux in an individual who has an inability to protect the airway can result in pulmonary problems and whether available antireflux therapy could be effective in this situation are unanswered questions.

Esophagoscopy   The direct examination and biopsy of the esophagus by esophagoscopy is the most sensitive test for esophagitis. If symptoms are more suggestive of esophagitis than reflux, as

in cases of painful swallowing or hematemesis, this test may be preferable to radiologic, radionuclide, or pH probe evaluation of the esophagus. However, in the presence of massive reflux, the high frequency of concomitant esophagitis and the similarity of treatment of the two conditions often render esophagoscopy unnecessary.

Oximetry   Many children with dysphagia have marginal pulmonary reserve. The availability of pulse oximetry provides the opportunity to monitor arterial oxygen saturation during feeding. These studies may be useful when evaluating the feeding of premature infants with bronchopulmonary dysplasia. Their use in older children with previously occult hypoxemia is investigational.

COMPLICATIONS AND MANAGEMENT STRATEGIES

The diagnosis and proper management of feeding and swallowing disorders are important in the provision of hospital and outpatient pediatric health care to a wide variety of children and their families. At all times, feeding must be viewed in the context of each child's general health, developmental status, and environment. A brief review of important complications and primary and secondary prevention strategies is presented here.

Dysphagia frequently results in a general decreased intake of all macronutrients rather than specific nutritional restrictions (primary protein–energy malnutrition [PEM]). Serum protein and vitamin concentrations are usually well preserved (Rossi, 1993). Chronic PEM is a relatively common complication in children with quadriplegic cerebral palsy (Stallings et al., 1993). In children with severe dysphagia and cerebral palsy, gastrostomy tube feedings have been effective in increasing weight-for-height ratios (Shapiro, Green, Krick, Allen, & Capute, 1986). Placement of a gastrostomy tube also permits the separation of nutritional and oral-motor therapies when the demands of these interventions come into conflict. Further investigations are needed to examine the efficacy of other nutritional interventions, including oral-motor therapy and high-caloric oral feedings.

Children with severe dysphagia are at risk for a variety of respiratory complications (Loughlin, 1989). Symptoms range from mild cough during feeding to bronchospasm, recurrent pneumonia, bronchiectasis, and respiratory failure. Children with significant pharyngeal-phase abnormalities, including delayed initiation of swallow, food residue, and decreased pharyngeal motility, are at high risk for aspiration before, during, or after swallows. In some children with dysphagia, the occurrence of aspiration is often dependent on the texture of food swallowed (Arvedson et al., 1993). There is evidence that aspiration during oral feedings in adults with multiple severe developmental disabilities is associated with chronic lung disease (Rogers, Stratton, et al., 1994). Additionally, gastroesophageal reflux in patients with severe dysphagia may be an important factor in the development of respiratory complications (Loughlin, 1989). Finally, it is important to note that not all patients who aspirate during videofluoroscopic swallow studies have recurrent pulmonary disease. Further clinical investigations of the pathophysiology of pulmonary complications in children with dysphagia are needed.

The safety of oral feedings is the prime consideration in the evaluation of children with dysphagia. Nonoral or tube feedings are an appropriate consideration for a child with severe dysphagia. Isolated abnormalities of deglutition are rarely an indication for nonoral feeding. Infants and children with severe dysphagia who are at risk for or have a history of health complications, including acute and chronic lung disease, airway obstruction, and malnutrition, are potential candidates for nonoral feedings. Finally, particular attention should be paid to the influence of various feeding programs on the quality of life of children and their families.

The undertaking of nonoral feeding should not result in the abandonment of oral-motor interventions. In some children with developmental disorders, oral-motor function will improve with time and oral feeding may be resumed. In others with a poor prognosis for oral feedings, the absence of oral stimulation seems at times to be associated with further decrease in spontaneous swallowing and increased pooling of oral secretions. Finally, the experience of numerous tastes is pleasurable to most children with dysphagia. Nonnutritive quantities of flavorful foods can add to their daily experience without endangering their health.

Any feeding problem should be interpreted in its social or family context. A great deal of verbal and nonverbal communication occurs between parents and children during meals. This interaction can influence the willingness or desire for oral feedings (Huber, 1991). Disordered communication during meals may result in primary feeding problems or complicate the meals of children with dysphagia. The communicative and nurturing aspects of meals must be recognized and promoted in all feeding programs for children and their families.

REFERENCES

Arvedson, J.C., Rogers, B., & Brodsky, L. (1993). Anatomy, embryology, and physiology. In J.C. Arvedson & L. Brodsky (Eds.), *Pediatric swallowing and feeding: Assessment and management* (pp. 5–51). San Diego: Singular Publishing Group.

Arvedson, J.C., Rogers, B., Buck, G., Smart, P., & Msall, M. (1994). Silent aspiration prominent in children with dysphagia. *International Journal of Pediatric Otorhinolaryngology, 28,* 173–181.

Bosma, J.F. (1986). Development of feeding. *Clinical Nutrition, 5,* 210–218.

Caruso, V.G., & Sauerland, E.K. (1990). Embryology and anatomy. In C.D. Bluestone, S.E. Stool, & M.D. Scheelz (Eds.), *Pediatric otolaryngology* (Vol. 2, 2nd ed., pp. 807–815). Philadelphia: W.B. Saunders.

Dantas, R.O., Kern, M.K., Massey, B.T., Dodds, W.J., Kahrilas, P.J., Brasseur, J.G., Cook, I.J., & Lang, I.M. (1990). Effect of swallowed bolus variables on oral and pharyngeal phases of swallowing. *American Journal of Physiology, 258 (Gastrointestinal Liver Physiology, 21),* G675–G681.

Ekberg, O. (1982). Closure of the laryngeal vestibule during deglutition. *Acta Otolaryngologica, 93,* 123–129.

Huber, C.J. (1991). Documenting quality of parent–child interaction: Use of the NCAST Scales. *Infants and Young Children, 4*(2), 63–75.

Kahrilas, P.J., Dodds, W.J., Dent, J., Logemann, J.A., & Shaker, R. (1988). Upper esophageal sphincter function during deglutition. *Gastroenterology, 95,* 52–62.

Kinsbourne, M. (1964). Hiatus hernia with contortions of neck. *Lancet, 1,* 1058.

Loughlin, G.J. (1989). Respiratory consequences of dysfunctional swallowing and aspiration. *Dysphagia, 3,* 126–130.

Miller, A.J. (1982). Deglutition. *Physiological Reviews, 62,* 129–184.

Miller, A.J. (1986). Neurophysiological basis of swallowing. *Dysphagia, 1,* 91–100.

Moss, H.B., & Green, A. (1982). Neuroleptic associated dysphagia confirmed by esophageal manometry. *American Journal of Psychiatry, 139,* 515–516.

Nielson, D.W., Heldt, G.P., & Tooley, W.H. (1990). Stridor and gastroesophageal reflux in infants. *Pediatrics, 85,* 1034–1039.

Rogers, B., Arvedson, J., Buck, G., Smart, P., & Msall, M. (1994). Characteristics of dysphagia in children with cerebral palsy. *Dysphagia, 9,* 69–73.

Rogers, B., & Campbell, J. (1993). Pediatric and neurodevelopmental evaluation. In J.C. Arvedson & L. Brodsky (Eds.), *Pediatric swallowing and feeding: Assessment and management* (pp. 53–91). San Diego: Singular Publishing Group.

Rogers, B., Stratton, P., Msall, M., Andres, M., Champlain, M.K., Koerner, P., & Prazza, J. (1994). Long-term morbidity and management strategies of tracheal aspiration in adults with severe developmental disabilities. *American Journal on Mental Retardation, 98,* 490–498.

Rosen, C.L., Glaze, D.C., & Frost, J.D. (1984). Hypoxemia associated with feeding in the preterm infant and full-term neonate. *American Journal of Diseases of Children, 138,* 623–628.

Rossi, T. (1993). Pediatric gastroenterology. In J.C. Arvedson & L. Brodsky (Eds.), *Pediatric swallowing and feeding: Assessment and management* (pp. 123–156). San Diego: Singular Publishing Group.

Shapiro, B.K., Green, P., Krick, J., Allen, D., & Capute, A.J. (1986). Growth of severely impaired children: Neurological versus nutritional factors. *Developmental Medicine and Child Neurology, 28,* 729–733.

Smith, J., Wolkove, N., Colacone, A., & Kreisman, H. (1989). Coordination of eating, drinking and breathing in adults. *Chest, 96*(3), 578–582.

Spender, Q.W., Cronk, C.E., Charney, E.B., & Stallings, V.A. (1989). Assessment of linear growth of children with cerebral palsy: Use of alternative measures to height or length. *Developmental Medicine and Child Neurology, 31,* 206–214.

Stallings, V.A., Charney, E.B., Davies, J.C., & Cronk, C.C. (1993). Nutritional related growth failure of children with quadriplegic cerebral palsy. *Developmental Medicine and Child Neurology, 35,* 126–138.

Werlin, S.L., D'Souza, B.J., Hogan, W.J., Dodds, W.J., & Arndorfer, R.C. (1980). Sandifer syndrome: An unappreciated clinical entity. *Developmental Medicine and Child Neurology, 22,* 374–378.

Wyllie, E., Wyllie, R., Cruse, R.P., Rothner, A.D., & Erenberg, G. (1986). The mechanism of nitrazepam induced drooling and aspiration. *New England Journal of Medicine, 314,* 35–38.

Chapter 11

Spina Bifida and Hydrocephalus

Peter J. Chauvel, M.B., M.P.H., and
Stephen L. Kinsman, M.D.

Spina bifida and hydrocephalus represent a major challenge to the developmental pediatrician. The physical impairments associated with paraplegia are often combined with the social impairment of urinary and fecal incontinence. The presence of hydrocephalus adds a developmental dimension. With so many different facets in management involving different medical and surgical specialities, as well as allied health disciplines, the pediatrician must continually draw all the parts into a whole so that the child and family are dealt with in a holistic and appropriate manner.

TERMINOLOGY

Spina bifida is a term that was first used by the anatomist Nicholas Tulp in 1652 to describe a group of developmental defects characterized by the separation of the posterior elements of the vertebral arch. This descriptive term remains in popular use. Geneticists postulate a neural tube defect spectrum that includes anencephaly, encephalocele, and spina bifida, with these conditions being etiologically related by a presumed failure in closure of the neural tube during early embryonic development.

Anencephaly results from failure of closure of the cephalic end of the neural tube, with complete or partial absence of the cranial vault and overlying tissues and consequent destruction of the exposed neural rudiments. Infants with this condition are stillborn or die very soon after birth. *Cranium bifidum* includes encephalocele and cranial meningocele. This is a defect in the skull, often in the occipital area, with herniation of neural tissue into a meningeal sac.

Spina bifida refers to those conditions that result from failure of neural tube closure in that part of the neural tube that will become the spinal cord. Spina bifida is further classified as *cystica* (or aperta) or *occulta*. Spina bifida cystica describes 1) the herniation of a meningeal sac containing neural elements (meningomyelocele); 2) flat, exposed neural tissue without a protective sac (myeloschisis); or 3) the protrusion of a meningeal sac through the vertebral defect without overt spinal cord involvement (meningocele). Spina bifida occulta is a skin-covered bone defect in the vertebral arch without overt spinal cord involvement. A relatively common defect, it is usually without accompanying neurologic impairment. The only clue to its presence may be an overlying skin dimple or hairy tuft.

Other rarer forms of spina bifida include the lipomeningoceles and lipomyelomeningoceles, in which fatty tissue is also contained in the sac. Dermoid tracts may also be included in this group. These lesions have been classified as spina bifida occulta (Aicardi, 1992; Anderson, 1975) because they are usually skin covered and less obvious. However, they are often symptomatic and require management similar to that for the more classic spina bifida cystica group.

Hydrocephalus is a dilatation of the cerebral ventricles caused by an obstruction in the flow of cerebrosinal fluid (CSF). Noncommunicating hydrocephalus results from obstruction to the flow of CSF between the choroid plexuses and the foramina of Luschka and Magendie at the outlet of the fourth ventricle. There is dilatation of the ventricular system proximal to the obstruction with normal ventricular size distally. In communicating hydrocephalus, there is obstruction to CSF flow within the sub-arachnoid space between the outlet of the fourth ventricle and the arachnoid granulations, leading to failure of resorption of CSF. The most common causes are hemorrhage and infection, with adhesions and scarring of the meninges and subarachnoid spaces. There is usually a moderate degree of dilatation of the lateral ventricles and mild enlargement of the third and fourth ventricles.

ETIOLOGY

The etiology of neural tube defects appears to be multifactorial, with genetic and environmental factors being most prominent (Carter, 1969). A familial tendency has been identified, with the risk of recurrence of neural tube defects among siblings estimated at 5% higher after the first affected child and rising to 10% higher after two affected children (Milhan, 1962). Several environmental factors have been implicated in the etiology of these defects. Recently an association between folic acid and neural tube defects has been demonstrated. The multicenter Medical Research Council (MRC) Vitamin Study (1991) confirms a protective effect of periconceptual folic acid intake in preventing neural tube defects in over 70% of at-risk pregnancies. Other observed associations are with valproic acid intake during early pregnancy, maternal hyperthermia, and diabetes mellitus. Neural tube defects are also associated with a variety of rare syndromes, including Meckel syndrome, Dandy-Walker syndrome, and trisomy 13.

The actual teratogenic process that leads to a neural tube defect continues to be controversial. Defects may occur in the processes of neurulation or canalization. Neurulation occurs at about the 4th week of gestation when the embryo converts the flat plate of the *neural plate* into the cylinder that we know as the *neural tube*. This cylinder is essentially closed off from the amniotic cavity. However, neurulation does not account for the whole length of the neural tube; the caudal portion of the tube forms its lumen through a process of cavitation of small clusters of cells. This is known as canalization. Thus neural tube defects can be classified into 1) neu-rulation defects (upper neural tube defects) and 2) canalization defects (lower neural tube defects). The demarcation line between these two types has been set at the T11–T12 level. The two types may represent differing causes (Seller, 1990).

EPIDEMIOLOGY

The actual incidence of neural tube defects is not known because many affected pregnancies terminate as spontaneous abortions that are neither detected nor recorded. Asymptomatic neural tube defects such as occult spina bifida may miss detection. However, the birth prevalence (i.e., infants with a neural tube defect as a proportion of all live and stillbirths) has been extensively studied. There are geographic and temporal variations. The highest prevalences of neural tube defects have been recorded in Ireland (4 per 1,000 live births) (EUROCAT Working Group, 1987) and in China (up to 10 per 1,000 live births) (Xiao et al., 1990). The lowest prevalences occur in the United States (0.6 per 1,000 live births) (Yen et al., 1992), continental Europe (EUROCAT Working Group, 1987, 1991), and Japan (1 per 1,000 live births) (Hobbins, 1991). In the United Kingdom (Smithells, 1991) and Australia (Bower, Hobbs, Carney, & Simpson, 1984), the prevalence is approximately 2 per 1,000 live births.

A decrease in the birth prevalence of neural tube defects has been recorded in many countries over the past 20 years that is not totally explained by the increase in prenatal diagnosis with termination of neural tube defect–affected pregnancies (Smithells, Sheppard, & Wild, 1989). This decrease has not been consistent or universal throughout the world (Bower, Raymond, Lumley, & Bury, 1993).

Eighty-five percent to 90% of neural tube defects consist of equal proportions of anencephaly and spina bifida. Seventy percent to 85% of spina bifida cases are meningomyeloceles, and 10%–15% of neural tube defects are encephaloceles. Neural tube defects are more prevalent in women, with a consistently higher prevalence being observed in women of lower socioeconomic status (Bower et al., 1984).

PRENATAL SCREENING

Prenatal screening programs have commenced in many parts of the world based on a raised serum α-fetoprotein level as a marker for an open neural tube defect (Robertson, 1991). Ultrasonic demonstration of a spinal defect or hydrocephalus also is used in prenatal detection programs, but this is unreliable when used in isolation or nonspecifically. Regions that have introduced screening programs report a significant decrease of births of infants with spina bifida (Robertson, 1991). Most screening programs carry out serum α-fetoprotein level determinations at 16 weeks' gestation. Those women with significantly elevated levels then have ultrasonography. If this is not definitive in detecting a lesion despite raised serum α-fetoprotein levels, amniocentesis is performed, with estimations of amniotic α-fetoprotein and acetylcholinesterase levels. This approach can detect open meningomyelocele with a 95%–98% probability (Haddow & Macri, 1979), but, by the time these procedures are completed and the results are returned, the mother is well into the pregnancy, sometimes even 20 weeks. At this stage, termination is not a simple process and carries a health and emotional toll.

THE NEONATE WITH SPINA BIFIDA

The pediatrician is often involved with the affected baby and its family soon after its birth. So that the prognosis and appropriate management can be determined, a complete physical and neurologic examination of the baby is required, with special attention to the degree of spinal cord dysfunction and hydrocephalus.

The skull is examined as the fontanel and sutures are palpated for evidence of distention of the cerebral ventricles. Careful measurement and charting of the head circumference allows the clinician to detect and estimate the rate of development of any hydrocephalus.

The length and width of the lesion visible over the spinal column is measured because this will aid the surgeon in planning the repair and the area of skin cover that will be needed. The integrity of the sac of the meningomyelocele or meningocele is assessed. Any infection at this site must be treated because this will affect the timing of any repair. Other deformities may be present along the spine, such as scoliosis and kyphosis. Active leg movements are observed. Muscle power assessment is subjective at this age and is largely an observation of power against gravity. Usually there are signs of a lower motor lesion below the spinal level of the cord disruption. However, upper motor neuron signs may be present, with increased tone and brisk reflexes. These may be superimposed onto the flaccid paralysis and may reflect further cord abnormality, such as hydrosyringomyelia or diastatomyelia.

A reasonable assessment of the sensory level can be made by pinprick and observation. Anal sphincter tone and anal reflex are examined. The bladder is palpated and any urinary dribbling is observed.

A radiologic examination of the head and spine is usually done prior to the repair. Cranial ultrasonography reveals the presence of hydrocephalus, and serial ultrasound examinations will allow the progression of any hydrocephalus to be documented. Ultrasonic examination of the lesion itself is not recommended because it is possible that "unsplinted" neural tissue and its blood supply may be further traumatized by additional pressure over the area (Hobbins, 1991).

Although early closure of the meningomyelocele has been advocated to prevent further spinal cord damage and infection, there appears to be no disadvantage to waiting 1 or 2 days so that the parents can bond with their child and become aware of the possible problems and outcomes. Usually the back lesion is closed by covering the defect with skin, either directly or by a flap. The parents must be aware that this initial surgery will not cure their child.

SPECTRUM OF MORBIDITY WITH SPINA BIFIDA AND ITS MANAGEMENT

Following the initial surgery, continuing management addresses the various manifestations and complications of spina bifida. Different problems predominate at different ages, and the pediatrician must ensure that the child's overall needs are met. The ultimate goal in the management of an individual with spina bifida is for that person to achieve independence and self-respect. Because there are a number of different organ systems involved with this disorder, management is better handled in a multidisciplinary setting. The pediatrician must work with the neurosurgeon, the orthopedic surgeon, and the urologic surgeon. The array is widened by the allied health team, usually consisting of a physical therapist, occupational therapist, incontinence nurse, orthotist, psychologist, dietician, speech pathologist, and social worker. The costs of caring for people with spina bifida can be considerable. With 1,500 infants with spina bifida being born in the United States annually, about 1,000 would be expected to survive into childhood. The annual cost of surgical and medical care for all these people is estimated to be in excess of $200 million ("Economic Burden," 1989). In Western Australia, the hospital costs of the first 10 years of life were estimated to be $51,000 per child (Bower, 1988).

The pediatrician has a central role in the team by acting as an advocate for the patient and the parents. The family needs a consistent person to take their problems to, and the pediatrician is the logical person to meet this role. The pediatrician must have an understanding of the underlying disorder, of child development, and of the contributions that the other medical, surgical, and allied health personnel make to the child's care. Despite the expertise that is involved in this team, the upbringing of the child must remain the responsibility of the parents. They must make the ultimate decisions on behalf of their child, and it is the duty of each team member to develop a reasonable working relationship with the family. It is unproductive for a professional to usurp the decision-making role from the parents because this will diminish parental responsibility and interest in the child. The consequences are social isolation of the child and a family that may either overprotect or reject the affected child. The child needs to be raised as an integral family member to grow into a fulfilled adult.

The value of a team approach is that it allows the various aspects of spina bifida to be addressed in a coordinated manner (see Chapter 24, Volume I). The major areas of morbidity encountered in the spina bifida clinic include mobility, hydrocephalus, intellectual and learning problems, nutritional and incontinence difficulties, orthopedic deformities, and possible progression of disability. The treatment plan must always take into account the quality of life of the child.

A 1988 review article summarizing the management of spina bifida in an American center is an excellent outline from which to begin an analysis of the best practice in the care of individuals with spinal dysraphism and related disorders (Liptak et al., 1988). First, it is imperative to state the principles on which the care is based:

1. Minimize the degree of disabilities caused by the child's impairments.
2. Prevent the disabilities from becoming handicaps by removing those environmental barriers that can further impair function.
3. Prevent the occurrence of secondary conditions (i.e., those preventable conditions that are related to the underlying disorder).

Liptak et al. stated that, to achieve these goals, a system of comprehensive and coordinated care is required. A multidisciplinary spina bifida clinic can be the hub of such a system. Such a clinic should provide a number of important services, including

1. Routine comprehensive medical evaluations that include ongoing communication with the family and the patient
2. Preventive health care and anticipatory guidance
3. Nursing services, especially to evaluate, plan, and coordinate the child's needs within the school
4. Psychosocial support, which includes evaluation and therapeutic and informational services

Neurologic/Neurosurgical Management

Serious pathology often accompanies the complaints of individuals with spinal dysraphism. Several neurologic aspects of spina bifida require an index of suspicion on the part of the physician and a high degree of vigilance in management. Imaging studies and prompt referral for neurosurgical consultation frequently are indicated.

Serial assessment of the neurologic level (motor and sensory) of impairment is necessary to detect deterioration from such potentially reversible problems as tethered cord, hydromyelia, spinal cord compression from lumbar stenosis, or arachnoid cysts. Associated intraspinal pathology can also present as a progression of disability, such as a decrease in functional mobility. The degree of complete or incomplete paraplegia of the muscle groups below the level of the spinal lesion will determine the subsequent motor impairment.

There are four functional categories of ambulation (Hoffer, Feiwell, Perry, Perry, & Bonnett, 1973):

1. *Community ambulators* are able to walk indoors and outdoors for most activities, although a wheelchair may be used for longer trips outside the immediate vicinity of the home.
2. *Household ambulators* are able to walk indoors and transfer to a wheelchair for community use and most outdoor activity.
3. *Nonfunctional ambulators* may walk as part of a therapy session or in a gymnasium with orthotic devices, but use a wheelchair for most mobility needs.
4. *Nonambulators* use a wheelchair for all indoor and outdoor activities.

Other neurologic changes of potential importance include decrease of muscular strength within a muscle group of one grade or more, or a change in tone.

In assessment of upper extremity function, decreased hand grip strength, change in reflexes, evidence of hand atrophy, pain or parathesia in the hands and/or arms, or the onset of upper extremity weakness should raise the suspicion of a Chiari malformation, syringomyelia, or both. Problems with coordination may signify changes in the status of the hydrocephalus or the Chiari malformation.

The child with spina bifida must be monitored for symptoms and signs of increased intracranial pressure, including headache, nausea, vomiting, lethargy, irritability, and personality change. Changes in school and other functional performance also must be monitored. These may be nonspecific indicators of a new problem arising, such as uncompensated hydrocephalus (shunted or unshunted) or depression (see Chapter 12, this volume). Medical disturbances such as electrolyte imbalances or renal failure may also present this way. Complex psychological adjustment reactions may come to the forefront as educational disturbances. However, medical causes must be investigated and ruled out at the same time as the psychosocial issues are pursued.

Finally, care of the child with spina bifida includes management of neurologic problems that may manifest themselves at different ages. Seizures may occur in up to 15% of individuals with myelomeningocele by adolescence (Bartoshesky, Haller, Scott, & Wojick, 1985). Certain neurologic aspects of spina bifida are important in the first year of life, especially the development of hydrocephalus. Because of increased skull (and possibly brain) compliance at this age, prior to the fusion of the cranial sutures, shunt failure may not be detected for a significant period unless head growth is monitored carefully, at least monthly. Some infants with spina bifida will develop early difficulties from Chiari malformation. Most of these problems have been described as the *infant brain stem syndrome*. Prominent symptoms include apnea, stridor, and dysphagia. Most authorities recommend that such infants undergo surgical decompression of the Chiari malformation, but this approach is not universally supported. Some neurosurgeons may recommend shunt replacement in this situation, thus ensuring that the hydrocephalus is adequately treated.

Urologic Management

Treatment of urologic abnormalities is high on the list of management priorities. At the top of this list is the maintenance of renal health. Those individuals who are at high risk for renal deterioration must be identified. This includes those individuals with high-pressure bladder systems, vesicoureteric abnormalities leading to reflux and hydronephrosis, and recurrent urinary tract infections (Ehrlich & Brem, 1982). It is important to emphasize that urologic status is rarely static in people with spinal dysraphism.

Frequent monitoring and aggressive management centered around clean intermittent catheterization (CIC) are needed to prevent such complications as hypertension and renal failure. Prior to the introduction of CIC in the early 1970s, the most common neural tube defect–related cause of death over the age of 1 year was renal failure (Rickwood & Thomas, 1984).

Another major aspect of urologic care is the management of urinary incontinence. The care of incontinence has advanced considerably over the last two decades, particularly with the acceptance of CIC. A rational management plan must be based on adequate information on voiding function. This usually requires a cystometrogram to determine bladder tone and pressure, outlet function, and the coordination or degree of synergy between the two. Management of urinary continence often includes the use of medications such as oxybutinin for bladder relaxation, sympathomimetics (e.g., ephidrine) to promote bladder outlet contraction, and imipramine to do both. Doses must be titrated and side effects monitored. Some authors recommend intravesicular infusion of oxybutinin when side effects such as flushing become prohibitive with administration via the usual route. (Greenfield & Fera, 1991; Mizunaga, Miyata, Kaneko, Yachiku, & Chiba, 1994; Weese, Roskamp, Leach, & Zimmern, 1993).

Finally, issues of sexual function must be considered as children with spina bifida approach adolescence. The proper management of sexuality in this group goes beyond medical management and will involve disability-specific education, a supportive home and clinic environment, and parents and professionals working together to help the affected individuals meet their developmental milestones. More attention to these matters in spina bifida clinics might well go a long way toward helping people with childhood-acquired disabilities overcome some of the substantial barriers that exist for people with disabilities in achieving lives that include intimacy and sexuality.

Orthopedic Management

The management of orthopedic deformities in individuals with dysraphic states has been subject to much discussion, if not investigation, and management philosophies can differ drastically. The crux of the debate is how aggressively interventions to maintain ambulation should be pursued. Orthopedic interventions often required to maintain an upright posture and adequate hip-knee-ankle alignment include release of hip or knee contractures or both and procedures designed to manage dislocated hips. Proponents of aggressive maintenance of ambulation state that posture and alignment are critical components of child development (Gram, Kinnen, & Brown, 1981; Jackman, Nitschke, Haake, & Brown, 1980). Other factors supporting this approach include less skin breakdown, better renal health, and improved bowel function and continence. Others argue that the repeated surgical procedures required to maintain ambulation are too high a price to pay (Shurtleff, 1986). Risks and complications of these procedures can have lasting consequences (Drummond, Moreau, & Cruess, 1981). Many of these individuals do not remain ambulatory, even in the second decade of life. There are also data suggesting that the ambulatory group also has problems with skin breakdown, but in a different distribution (Liptak, Shurtleff, Bloss, Baltus, & Manitta, 1992).

The first orthopedic problem to be confronted in a newborn with myelomeningocele is the management of clubfoot, usually talipes equinovarus. Serial casting is the first line of treatment, with surgery being reserved until later, if it is necessary.

The proper alignment of the spine is indisputably an important area for the orthopedist. Scoliosis of greater than 40 degrees and kyphosis of greater than 60 degrees are considered indications for orthopedic correction by some method of vertebral fusion with instrumentation (Osebold, Mayfield, Winter, & Moe, 1982). Lesser degrees of scoliosis that may be progressing can be managed by a spinal jacket.

Lesions of the fifth lumbar nerve root and below (i.e., sacral lesions) are often associated with inversion/eversion and calcaneal deformities of the foot and may require tendon releases, transfers, and joint fusions.

Orthopedic management also includes the appropriate introduction of orthoses such as hip-knee-ankle-foot orthoses (HKAFOs), knee-ankle-foot orthoses (KAFOs), and ankle-foot orthoses (AFOs). Parapodium and reciprocating gait orthoses may be considered for youngsters with thoracic level lesions. Canes or crutches should also be offered. The evaluations and prescriptions for these devices are best done through a cooperative team that includes the orthopedist, orthotist, and physical therapist.

MEDICAL MANAGEMENT

Bowel Continence

The management plan of fecal incontinence is based on the individual assessment of the child. The history determines stool frequency and consistency, frequency and timing of toileting, level of functional independence, sensation for stool in the rectum, and diet. Physical examination should note external and internal sphincter tone, the ability for any voluntary sphincter contractions, presence or absence of an anal wink, and amount and consistency of stool in the rectal vault. The management plan is stepwise, including education and feedback. The major steps include the following:

1. Regular toileting, 15–20 minutes after meals, to take advantage of the gastrocolic reflex (sometimes behavioral therapy or biofeedback are of use)
2. Increase in the stool bulk with either a high-fiber diet or a stool softener such as Lactulose, Ducolux, or Metamucil.
3. Use of suppositories (Ducolux or glycerin) or cathartics (Senokot)
4. Enemas such as standard enemas or retention enemas (there is a danger in using repeated hypertonic phosphate enemas)

Most important is the need to approach each child and family as individuals, recognizing their resources and abilities to carry out the recommendations of a particular program used to achieve fecal continence.

Skin Integrity

Skin integrity is the most important cause of morbidity in these children. Prevention and early detection are the best approach to this problem. Methods of prevention include teaching self–skin checks and recognizing the signs of an early pressure ulcer. Early detection must be followed by relief of the inciting factors, such as pressure and wetness, as well as appropriate wound care.

Obesity

Like obesity in the general population, this is an extremely difficult problem to treat once it occurs. Excessive weight gain is best identified in the 4- to 6-year age group as a child is beginning to cross larger percentile curves for age. At this point nutritional and fitness counseling should be initiated. Weight should also be monitored after surgery.

Endocrinopathies

The most common endocrine problem identified in patients with myelomeningocele is precocious puberty (Meyer & Landau, 1984). There is some concern that the short stature seen in these children has lasting psychological consequences over and above those resulting from their other impairments. Treatment with growth hormone has been advocated by some. It should be noted that growth hormone treatment is not without potential side effects.

Latex Allergy

Latex allergy is now recognized as an important health issue for individuals with myelomeningocele. An incidence rate of up to 40% has been reported (Swartz & Leger, 1992), but other authors cite lower rates (Pearson, Cole, & Jarvis, 1994). Individuals allergic to latex can have life-threatening reactions to that substance. Exposure to latex during surgery represents a particular risk, with anaphylactic shock and death sometimes occurring. Screening for latex allergy prior to surgery is being carried out by most clinics by direct inquiry about previous latex reactions and by determining latex titers by radioallergosorbent test (RAST). Individuals with a high RAST antibody titer to latex are counseled about risk, exposure, and avoidance of latex products during and after surgery.

Genetic Counseling

It is important to have professional genetic counseling services available to families of newborn children with spina bifida. Particular attention should also be paid to folic acid education. It is now believed that over one half of cases of neural tube defects may be preventable by the use of folate supplementation before conception. This includes those cases occurring in families with a history of previous neural tube defects. The recommendation for women in this group currently is to take the 10-times higher daily dose of 4 mg folic acid under the guidance of a physician. Finally, it has become increasingly clear that adolescents and young adults with spina bifida are often not given sufficient personal information regarding the genetic aspects of their condition. These individuals also deserve and would benefit from genetic counseling.

ROLE OF THE MULTISPECIALTY CLINIC/SERVICE IN THE CARE OF INDIVIDUALS WITH SPINA BIFIDA

It would not be appropriate to complete a chapter on the care of individuals with spina bifida without further commenting on the methods used to deliver services to this population. Almost from the beginning of providing serious

services to this group, the advantages of using a multispecialty or multidisciplinary group to deliver care have been emphasized. A key feature of this approach is the greater potential for communication among providers, thus increasing coordination, comprehensiveness, and access. All of these elements are deemed important aspects of high-quality care. In 1990, the Spina Bifida Association of America developed the Guidelines for Spina Bifida Health Care Services Throughout Life, in which they emphasize the importance of the multispecialty spina bifida team. (The SBAA may be reached at 1-800-621-3141.) The guidelines also focus on expectant outcomes, with the goals of 1) maintaining health status and preventing secondary disabilities, 2) maximizing potential to participate in society, and 3) fostering independence according to individual abilities. The guidelines further stress a developmental approach that adds an anticipatory element to care. In this age of health care reform, these guidelines form the basis for a rational, coordinated, and comprehensive care plan for individuals with spina bifida.

REFERENCES

Aicardi, J. (1992). *Diseases of the nervous system in childhood*. London: MacKeith Press.

Anderson, F.M. (1975). Occult spinal dysraphism: A series of 73 cases. *Pediatrics, 55*, 826–835.

Bartoshesky, L.E., Haller, J., Scott, R.M., & Wojick, C. (1985). Seizures in children with meningomyelocele. *American Journal of Diseases of Children, 139*, 400–402.

Bower, C. (1988). *Screening for neural tube defects in Western Australia: A cost-benefit analysis*. Perth: Health Department of Western Australia.

Bower, C., Hobbs, M., Carney, A., & Simpson, D. (1984). Neural tube defects in Western Australia 1966–81 and a review of Australian data 1942–81. *Journal of Epidemiology and Community Health, 38*, 208–213.

Bower, C., Raymond, M., Lumley, J., & Bury, G. (1993). Trends in neural tube defects 1980–1989. *Medical Journal of Australia, 158*, 152–154.

Carter, C.O. (1969). Spina bifida and anencephaly: A problem in genetic-environmental interaction. *Journal of Biosocial Science, 1*, 71–83.

Drummond, D.S., Moreau, M., & Cruess, R.L. (1981). Postoperative neuropathic fractures in patients with myelomeningocele. *Developmental Medicine and Child Neurology, 23*, 147–150.

Economic burden of spina bifida—United States, 1980–1990. (1989). *MMWR. Morbidity and Mortality Weekly Report, 38*, 264–267.

Ehrlich, O., & Brem, A.S. (1982). A prospective comparison of urinary tract infections in patients treated with either clean intermittent catheterization or urinary diversion. *Pediatrics, 70*, 665–669.

EUROCAT Working Group. (1987). Prevalence of neural tube defects in 16 regions of Europe, 1980–1983. *International Journal of Epidemiology, 16*, 246–251.

EUROCAT Working Group. (1991). Prevalence of neural tube defects in 20 regions of Europe and the impact of prenatal diagnosis, 1980–1986. *Journal of Epidemiology and Community Health, 45*, 52–58.

Gram, M., Kinnen, E., & Brown, J.A. (1981). Parapodium redesigned for sitting. *Physical Therapy, 61*, 657–660.

Greenfield, S.P., & Fera, M. (1991). The use of intravesical oxybutynin chloride in children with neurogenic bladder. *Journal of Urology, 146*, 532–534.

Haddow, J.E., & Macri, J.N. (1979). Prenatal screening for neural tube defects. *JAMA, 242*, 515–516.

Hobbins, J.C. (1991). Diagnosis and management of neural-tube defects today [editorial; comment]. *New England Journal of Medicine, 324*, 690–691.

Hoffer, M.M., Feiwell, E., Perry, R., Perry, J., & Bonnett, C. (1973). Functional ambulation in patients with myelomeningocele. *Journal of Bone and Joint Surgery, 55A*, 137–148.

Jackman, K.V., Nitschke, R.O., Haake, P.W., & Brown, J.A. (1980). Variable abduction HKAFO in spina bifida patients. *Orthotics and Prosthetics, 34*, 3–9.

Liptak, G.S., Bloss, J.W., Briskin, H., Campbell, J.E., Hebert, E.B., & Revell, G.M. (1988). The management of children with spinal dysraphism [review]. *Journal of Child Neurology, 3*, 3–20.

Liptak, G.S., Shurtleff, D.B., Bloss, J.W., Baltus, H.E., & Manitta, P. (1992). Mobility aids for children with high-level myelomeningocele: Parapodium versus wheelchair. *Developmental Medicine and Child Neurology, 34*, 787–796.

Meyer, S., & Landau, H. (1984). Precocious puberty in myelomeningocele patients. *Journal of Pediatric Orthopedics, 4*, 28–31.

Milhan, S. (1962). Increased incidence of anencephalus and spina bifida in siblings of affected cases. *Science, 138*, 593.

Mizunaga, M., Miyafa, M., Kaneko, S., Yachiku, S., & Chiba, K. (1994). Intravesicular instillation of oxybutynin hydrochloride therapy for patients with neuropathic bladder. *Paraplegia, 32*, 25–29.

MRC Vitamin Study Research Group. (1991). Prevention of neural tube defects: Results of the Medical Research Council Vitamin Study [see comments]. *Lancet, 338*, 131–137.

Osebold, W.R., Mayfield, J.K., Winter, R.B., & Moe, J.H. (1982). Surgical treatment of paralytic scoliosis associated with myelomeningocele. *Journal of Bone and Joint Surgery, 64A*, 841–856.

Pearson, M.L., Cole, J.S., & Jarvis, W.R. (1994). How common is latex allergy? A survey of children with myelodysplasia. *Developmental Medicine and Child Neurology, 36*, 64–69.

Rickwood, A.M., & Thomas, D.G. (1984). The upper renal tracts in adolescents and young adults with myelomeningocele. *Zeitschrift für Kinderchirurgie, 2*, 104–106.

Robertson, E.F. (1991). Maternal serum screening for neural tube defects and Down's syndrome [see comments]. *Medical Journal of Australia, 155*, 67–68.

Seller, M.J. (1990). Neural tube defects: Are neurulation and canalization forms causally distinct? *American Journal of Medical Genetics, 35*, 394–396.

Shurtleff, D.B. (1986). Mobility. In D.B. Shurtleff (Ed.), *Myelodysplasias and extrophies: Significance, prevention, and treatment* (pp. 313–356). Orlando, FL: Grune & Stratton.

Smithells, R.W. (1991). Prevention of spina bifida and hydrocephalus. In C.M. Bannister & B. Tew (Eds.), *Current concepts in spina bifida and hydrocephalus* (pp. 1–15). New York: Cambridge University Press.

Smithells, R.W., Sheppard, S., & Wild, J. (1989). Prevalence of neural tube defects in the Yorkshire Region. *Community Medicine, 11*, 163–167.

Swartz, M.K., & Leger, R. (1992). Latex hypersensitivity. *Journal of Pediatric Health Care, 6*, 381–382.

Weese, D.L., Roskamp, D.A., Leach, G.E., & Zimmern, P.E. (1993). Intravesical oxybutynin chloride: Experience with 42 patients. *Urology, 41*, 527–530.

Yen, I.H., Khoury, M.J., Erickson, J.D., James, L.M., Waters, G.D., & Berry, R.J. (1992). The changing epidemiology of neural tube defects: United States, 1968–1989. *American Journal of Diseases of Children, 146*, 857–861.

Xiao, K.Z., Zhang, Z.Y., Su, Y.M., Liu, F.Q., Yan, Z.Z., Jiang, Z.Q., Zhou, S.F., He, W.G., Wang, B.Y., Jiang, H.P., Yang, H.G., Li, M.M., Ju, Z.H., Hong, S.Q., Yao, J.S., Xing, G.K., Li, H., Den, H.Y., Yu, D.V.Z., Chen, H.X., Liu, L.W., Bao, G.Z., Shang, H.Q., Zhou, M.M., Ciren, Z.M., Zhang, Y.J., Tan, X.L., Li, Y.Z., Zhou, G.Z., & Jia, W.G. (1990). Central nervous system congenital malformations, especially neural tube defects in 29 provinces, metropolitan cities and autonomous regions of China: Chinese Birth Defects Monitoring Program. *International Journal of Epidemiology, 19*, 978–982.

Chapter 12

Childhood-Acquired Hydrocephalus

Stephen L. Kinsman, M.D.

The progress seen in neurosurgical practice over the last few decades has greatly increased the survival and neurologic function of individuals with hydrocephalus. However, it is safe to say that many individuals with shunted hydrocephalus continue to have neurologic difficulties that bring them to the attention of the neurologist, the developmental pediatrician, or both. On the one hand, most often a neurosurgeon has ruled out the possibility that shunt malfunction is the cause of the child's presenting problems, such as headaches, seizures, school problems, lethargy, and behavior changes. The problems still exist, however, and must be diagnosed and managed. On the other hand, problems related to shunt malfunction or new-onset hydrocephalus have not been considered or were missed and require identification and referral for proper neurosurgical management. For these reasons, it is important to review the proper management of hydrocephalus. There is also a growing literature on the neuropsychological abnormalities found in children with hydrocephalus. The second part of this chapter reviews this literature and makes some recommendations about how to evaluate and manage the developmental/neurologic problems found in these individuals.

MANAGEMENT OF HYDROCEPHALUS

Proper management of individuals with hydrocephalus requires the physician to be familiar with the following:

1. Basic anatomy and physiology of cerebrospinal fluid (CSF) circulation
2. Pathophysiology of abnormal CSF circulation
3. Etiologic issues

4. Neurologic and clinical problems associated with hydrocephalus
5. Management issues
6. Prognosis
7. Shunt failure and its management

Using the information provided in the following sections, one can properly assess the individual with hydrocephalus who presents with a neurologic symptom, sign, or both. The reader should also develop an understanding of when referral to a neurosurgeon is indicated. The ideal management of the patient with hydrocephalus requires a team approach so that parents can rely on all health professionals they encounter to be knowledgeable about the issues related to the management of hydrocephalus.

Cerebrospinal Fluid Circulation

Basic Physiology and Anatomy The circulation of CSF requires both a balance between CSF formation and absorption and unimpeded flow of CSF through its normal travel routes. Most (at least 80%) of the formation of CSF takes place in the choroid plexus (McComb, 1989). This complex tissue is found in the lateral ventricles, the third ventricle, and the fourth ventricle, with some extending via the foramina of Luschka into the cerebellopontine angles. The bulk of this tissue resides within the lateral ventricles. The cellular composition of the tissue includes endothelial cells forming capillaries and specialized cuboidal epithelium. Specialized tight junctions present at the apical sides of the epithelial cells provide the blood–CSF barrier. This barrier provides for the chemical integrity of the CSF. It appears that brain extracellular fluid is the source of nonchoroidal CSF. Brain extracellular space accounts for about 15% of brain volume under normal conditions (McComb, 1989). Cerebrospinal fluid is formed by the 1) ultrafiltration of plasma through choroidal capillary epithelium and 2) uptake of the ultrafiltrate and secretion of CSF (by an active metabolic process). Detailed review of this process is beyond the scope of this chapter. The reader is referred to McColb (1989) for a detailed review. It should be noted that several enzymes are believed to be important in the process of CSF formation, with sodium/potassium–adenosine triphosphatase (Na^+/K^+-ATPase) pumps and carbonic anhydrase being particularly prominent.

Pathophysiology of Abnormal Circulation
It is important to note that the pathophysiology of hydrocephalus is extremely varied. Etiology plays a critical role in determining such factors as the age of onset, presence and degree of blockade to CSF circulation, degree and course of ventricular dilatation, brain/cranial compliance, and type of associated intracranial pathology. It should be emphasized at this juncture that the term *congenital hydrocephalus* can be deceiving; presentation of this entity has been reported at almost any age. Therefore, age of onset does not always lead immediately to easy determination of the etiology.

It is important to note a caveat of terminology pointed out by McCollough (1989). He considered the terms *internal/external* hydrocephalus and *obstructive* and *nonobstructive* hydrocephalus to be outdated and related to such obsolete diagnostic tools as pneumoencephalography. He advocated the use of a more elaborate classification system to describe the type of hydrocephalus present in an individual. The hydrocephalus should be classified with respect to 1) site of the blockage of CSF circulation; 2) probable or precise etiology, as well as the state of progression; and 3) dynamic status of the disorder (i.e., progressive or arrested). McCollough alluded to the clinical problem that not all ventriculomegaly, even if progressive, is hydrocephalus. It is sometimes difficult to determine whether a case of progressive ventriculomegaly is due to hydrocephalus or atrophy.

Etiologic Issues

Many classification systems for the etiology of hydrocephalus have as their main branch point a separation between congenital cases and hydrocephalus of other causes, such as inflammatory or neoplastic. However, it would be better to abandon the term *congenital hydrocephalus* when discussing etiology. The issue is really whether the cause of the hydrocephalus is

1. A malformation, such as Chiari malformation
2. A genetic process, such as X-linked or autosomal recessive types
3. Inflammation, of either the leptomeninges or ventricular lining
4. Chemical irritants, such as subarachnoid or ventricular blood
5. Neoplasms

As noted above, it is important to identify first the site of the blockade to CSF circulation, reabsorption, or both. Terms originating from the era of pneumencephalography, such as internal versus external or obstructive versus nonobstructive, are confusing and outdated (McCullough, 1989). External hydrocephalus is sometimes confused with subdural hygromas, and all hydrocephalus is to some degree caused by obstruction to normal CSF circulation. The terminology that best describes CSF blockade is *communicating* versus *noncommunicating*. Noncommunicating hydrocephalus denotes a blockade of CSF pathways at or proximal to the outlet foramina of the fourth ventricle (foramina of Lushka and Magendie). Communicating hydrocephalus denotes a blockade distal to this point, either in the basal subarachnoid cisterns, in the subarachnoid spaces over the brain surface, or within the arachnoid granulations (specialized units where CSF is absorbed back into the circulation) (McCullough, 1989).

The next step in proper diagnosis is to determine the etiology of the blockade. The site of the blockade is often helpful in narrowing the search for causes of the hydrocephalus. However, a given pathologic process will often demonstrate elements of both communicating and noncommunicating hydrocephalus, although one type usually predominates. Tables 1 and 2 summarize potential etiologies for hydrocephalus.

Table 1. Causes of noncommunicating hydrocephalus

Aqueductal stenosis
Chiari malformation with or without myelodysplasia
Dandy-Walker malformation
Atresia of the foramen of Monroe
Skull base anomalies
Mass effect from
    Neoplasia
    Benign intracranial cysts
Inflammatory ventriculitis from
    Infection
    Hemorrhage
    Chemical irritation
    Ruptured cysts (e.g., arachnoid cyst)

Table 2. Causes of communicating hydrocephalus

Congenital anomalies that sometimes cause
    hydrocephalus without obvious blockade of
    proximal CSF pathways:
    Chiari malformation with or without myelodysplasia
    Dandy-Walker malformation
    Encephalocele
    Benign cysts
Incompetent arachnoid villi
Leptomeningeal inflammation from
    Viral infection
    Bacterial infection
    Subarachnoid hemorrhage from
        Vascular malformation
        Trauma
        Surgery
    Chemical arachnoiditis
Neoplasia causing carcinomatous meningitis

Neurologic and Clinical Problems Associated with Hydrocephalus

The clinical presentation of hydrocephalus is different in newborns and infants than in older children and adults. Also of importance in determining the symptoms and signs of hydrocephalus are the accompanying conditions. Such things as the rate of onset and the degree of increased pressure, etiology, associated malformations, and additional insults contribute to determine the clinical presentation.

The diagnosis of hydrocephalus is based on one of the following situations:

1. Ventriculomegaly with signs/symptoms of increased intracranial pressure, such as vomiting, headaches, irritability, lethargy, poor feeding, and changes in muscle tone. In a newborn, this is usually accompanied by a bulging fontanel, a large and/or enlarging head, and splitting of the sutures. Some newborns present with forced downward deviation of the eyes, the so-called sunset sign. Other deficiencies of eye movements with uncompensated hydrocephalus, such as internal strabismus, can occur.
2. Progressive increase in head or ventricle size or both without signs and symptoms of increased intracranial pressure.
3. Static ventriculomegaly in an individual with a large head. Some authors refer to this situation as arrested or compensated hydrocephalus (McLone & Aronyk, 1993). However, these concepts do not appear to add to the clinical care or understanding of indi-

viduals cases. A situation more difficult to determine is the condition of an individual with normocephaly but enlarged ventricles. The concomitant presence of increased extraaxial CSF space points to atrophy as the cause of the ventriculomegaly. Sometimes it can be difficult to completely rule out hydrocephalus in these cases, and serial examinations and images are required. Hammock, Milhorat, and Baron (1976) reported improvement in seven patients with spina bifida with "normal pressure hydrocephalus" who were previously unshunted and improved after shunting.

The presentation of hydrocephalus in older children differs from that of newborns and infants in that, after 3 years of age, abnormal changes in head measurements are less likely. Hydrocephalus of acute onset in older children usually presents with headaches, often worse in the morning; vomiting (often protracted); deficiencies of eye movements (particularly VIth nerve and gaze palsies); and altered levels of consciousness. If onset is particularly rapid or the condition is unrecognized, coma and herniation syndromes can ensue. Papilledema is seen frequently.

Along with helping to identify new-onset hydrocephalus or episodes of shunt failure in a timely manner, the pediatric neurologist and developmentalist can benefit the child with hydrocephalus and his or her family best by helping them to understand the proper evaluation, interpretation, and treatment/management of the cognitive/academic problems associated with hydrocephalus. Often these issues are unresolved by school personnel and others not familiar with the neuropsychological deficits common in this condition. Individuals with hydrocephalus often do not meet the strict diagnostic criteria school systems set for learning disability and therefore qualify for little or no supportive educational services. However, these children often show patterns of learning deficiencies, inefficiencies, or both that severely affect their ability to reach their educational and ultimately vocational potential. In addition, these individuals can have evidence of deficits in the so-called executive functions. Difficulties in such areas of function as attention, organizational skill, and problem solving can have a profound effect on a child's day-to-day school functioning and stamina for academic work. It is imperative that the clinician help families and schools to recognize these impairments as being neurologically based and steer them from labeling a child with hydrocephalus as lazy, unmotivated, or attention seeking. These labels imply a conscious decision on the part of the child to fail, and this is usually not the case. Conversely, it is important to recognize that children with hydrocephalus are at risk for concomitant social and emotional problems. These must also be diligently screened for, identified, and addressed if we are to help these individuals achieve their maximal potential.

Management Issues

The following issues must be addressed in the management of childhood-acquired hydrocephalus:

1. Diagnosis and evaluation of suspected cases of hydrocephalus (both neonatal and childhood). The gold standard test to evaluate a patient for the presence of hydrocephalus is either a computerized tomography (CT) scan or magnetic resonance imaging (MRI). MRI is particularly useful for diagnosing the presence of congenital

malformations such as Chiari, Dandy-Walker, or heterotopias (see Chapter 22, Volume I).

2. Recognition of acute shunt failure and prompt referral to a neurosurgeon for definitive treatment of the increased intracranial pressure. It is also important to recognize situations in which individuals are at increased risk for repeated shunt failures, such as the slit ventricle syndrome (McLaurin, 1989).

3. Recognition of chronically "uncompensated" hydrocephalus requiring evaluation of the integrity of any in-place shunt system. These situations can be difficult to manage. Some neurosurgeons occasionally monitor intraventricular or intrathecal pressure (for cases of communicating hydrocephalus) in an intensive care unit in an attempt to predict whether shunting or shunt replacement is likely to alleviate any of the presenting problems.

Sometimes ventricular size remains stable in these cases. Ventricles can be statically enlarged or slit. Although there is currently no clear set of neuropsychological tests that can predict, with sensitivity and specificity, which children indeed are suffering from increased intracranial pressure, at least some authors suggest that serial ordering behavior may be affected by hydrocephalus status. Such tests as timed motor tasks, verbal fluency, and word retrieval and such complex timed motor tasks as the Wechsler Intelligence Scale for Children–Revised (WISC–R) (Wechsler, 1974) Picture Arrangement may be particularly useful (Wills, 1993, p. 253). The importance of solid baseline measures is stressed by Wills (1993) in her review of the neuropsychological consequences of hydrocephalus.

4. Awareness of the seriousness of shunt infections and how to evaluate and treat them. For a review of identification and treatment of shunt infections, the reader is directed to McLaurin (1989).

5. Reinforcing to individuals with shunts and their families the life-threatening nature of shunt problems and the need to take all symptoms and signs of potential shunt failure or infection seriously.

Prognosis

The advent of the valve-regulated shunt system has radically changed the prognosis for individuals with most forms of hydrocephalus. In the United States, virtually all children with hydrocephalus, with the possible exception of some with massive in utero–acquired hydrocephalus, receive intervention. Laurence and Coates' (1967) series of 182 untreated individuals gives us some idea of the prognosis for untreated cases. There was only a 20% chance of an infant reaching adulthood in this series. Many of the deaths occurred in the first 1½ years of life. In those children with untreated hydrocephalus who lived, 1) 60% had intellectual impairment; 2) some had IQ scores in the normal range, but often with significant disparities between verbal and performance scores; 3) 25% were labeled "completely ineducable"; and 4) 25% had *cocktail party syndrome* (see below). Also of concern was the finding that some cases with compensated hydrocephalus experienced sudden death or a downhill spiral of deterioration.

There is little question that, for most individuals, untreated hydrocephalus is bad for the health and intellect. How well do patients do with treatment? Studies show that a postshunting mantle of about 3 cm or greater is important for normal intellectual development (Nulsen & Rekate, 1982). Preshunt scans do not appear predictive of ultimate function. The most important prognostic factors are 1) the cause of the hydrocephalus, 2) the duration of the condition prior to shunting, and 3) associated brain abnormalities.

A key question remains: Is there a critical point during the development of hydrocephalus when irreversible damage occurs? The evidence is clear that shunt infections are a risk factor for below-average IQ scores (McLone, Czyzewski, Raimondi, & Sommers, 1982). When children with infection and related complications are excluded from the sample, studies yield average IQ scores within groups of children with uncomplicated, shunted hydrocephalus. Wills (1993), in her review of the neuropsychological function of children with hydrocephalus, pointed out that the effects of infection, as well as serious birth trauma, are so robust that they are likely to "wash out" more subtle or complex influences of other medical factors on neuropsychological function. She also pointed out that there appears to be an association between slit ventricle syndrome and lowered IQ scores (Lonton, 1979).

It has been difficult to longitudinally study the effects of hydrocephalus on cognitive development. As Wills (1993) pointed out, it is inappropriate to compare or merge similar results from various tests given to children of various ages. When studies examine a more select and appropriate group, some findings do seem to emerge. As Wills summarized,

> Overall, the consensus of these findings appears to be that it is the presence of brain anomalies, cytoarchitectonic defects, or a history of trauma or infection rather than the presence and extent of HC [hydrocephalus] per se that accounts for most cognitive deficits. The "pure" effect of HC, if such exists, seems to impair visuospatial and visuomotor performance specifically and may depend on selective compression of posterior brain regions. (1993, p. 252)

These issues are further reviewed below.

Shunt Failure and Its Management

The most important aspect of assuring prompt detection and management of shunt failure is thorough education. First, it is critical that families take seriously any symptoms or signs of shunt malfunction and seek evaluation. Evaluation should be undertaken in a center that is aware of the proper workup. Most patients will have a CT scan and shunt radiographic series done. Many neurosurgeons recommend a shunt tap to evaluate the CSF for signs of infection. It is critical to identify and treat infection when it is present. It is not recommended that new hardware be placed when infection is present. Shunt failure occurs most frequently in the first several months after a shunt has been placed. However, this does not negate the fact that a shunt can fail after many years, possibly even decades.

NEUROPSYCHOLOGIC FUNCTIONING IN CHILDREN WITH HYDROCEPHALUS

First, when considering the neuropsychologic functioning of children with hydrocephalus, it is important to remember that this is a diverse group of children. Many variables can influence the development of these children, including physiological and medical factors; innate and acquired traits; and family, school, and social experiences (Wills, 1993). One important variable that has only begun to be investigated is the anatomic brain differences seen in children with hydrocephalus. Investigators have noted a complex set of developmental neuropathologic abnormalities within the brains of individuals with spina bifida and hydrocephalus (Gilbert, Jones, Rorke, Chernoff, & James, 1986). Certain of these findings have now been extended to a wider population of these children using MRI scanning to detect these abnormalities (Gammal, Mark, & Brooks, 1987; Just, Swartz, Ludwig, Ermert, & Thelen, 1990; see also Chapter 22, Volume I).

A 1992 study found that dysgenesis (partial agenesis or hypoplasia) of the corpus callosum may be of particular importance (Fletcher, et al., 1992). Fletcher and co-workers found that the cross-sectional area of the corpus callosum correlated with concurrent measures of verbal and nonverbal cognitive skill, with the correlation being higher for nonverbal measures. The size of the corpus callosum was not only smaller for children with myelomeningocele, but for those with aqueductal stenosis as well. In addition, Fletcher et al. found that cognitive skill was also influenced by hydrocephalus-related changes in the lateral ventricles and other cerebral white matter tracts. They found larger ventricles and smaller internal capsules in both of the hydrocephalus groups (myelomeningocele and aqueductal stenosis) when compared to age-matched healthy controls. Another large cerebral white matter tract, the centrum semiovale, was the same size in all groups. Nonverbal measures correlated with the right, but not the left, lateral ventricle size and with the area of the right *and also* left internal capsules. Verbal measures correlated with the left, but not the right, lateral ventricle size and with the left, but not the right, internal capsule. These authors hypothesized that the decreased size of both the internal capsules may reflect the degree to which the brain was distended by hydrocephalus during critical periods of myelination.

Fletcher et al. (1992) presented their findings as being consistent with current theories that suggest that the development of nonverbal skills is dependent on the integrity of central nervous system white matter in both hemispheres (Rourke, 1989). They believe that the correlations found in their study between the corpus callosal abnormalities and the cognitive deficiencies are consistent with a failure of posterior parietal areas to develop as a result of reduced interhemispheric communication. This reduced communication would then prevent the normal specialization of these areas, particularly the right hemisphere. Finally, they pointed out that children with hydrocephalus may have other central nervous system abnormalities that influence development. It is not yet clear what those abnormalities might be. It should also be noted that children with hydrocephalus are not exempted from inheriting learning disabilities from their parents. This combination of hydrocephalus-related learning problems and inherited learning disabilities can have particularly devastating consequences.

Specific Domains of Neuropsychologic Functioning

IQ   Verbal and nonverbal skill discrepancies, such as verbal-performance IQ score mismatches, frequently are seen in children with hydrocephalus (Badella-Ribera, Shulman, & Paddock, 1966; Lonton, 1979; Wills, Holmbeck, Dillon, & McLone, 1990). Often it is appropriate to judge intellectual potential on the usually higher verbal IQ scores of these individuals.

Verbal Skills   Early in the 1960s, some children with hydrocephalus and spina bifida were noted to exhibit hyperverbal behavior. This led Hadenius and co-workers to coin the term *cocktail party syndrome* to describe such individuals (Hadenius, Hagberg, Hyttnas-Bensch, & Sjogren, 1962). Several groups subsequently have studied this entity (Dennis, Hendrick, Hoffman, & Humphreys, 1987; Hurley, Dorman, Laatsch, Bell, & D'Avignon, 1990; Tew, 1979). This syndrome consists of 1) verbosity; 2) a high frequency of irrelevant, inappropriate, nonconstructive, even bizarre utterances; 3) poor exploratory or descriptive speech, analogical reasoning, and language comprehension; and 4) social disinhibition (Wills, 1993, p. 255). Despite common knowledge of this syndrome among clinicians, it is actually less common than more generalized learning deficiencies in these children and is probably declining in incidence (Wills, 1993). It should also be noted that children with hydrocephalus who are persistently hyperverbal after age 10 are more likely to have mental retardation (Tew & Laurence, 1979).

Memory Several studies of memory function in children with hydrocephalus have been done, and they do not show any specific deficits in this domain. Wills (1993) suggested that teacher and parental complaints of learning and memory problems are more likely attributable to difficulties with attention, executive functioning, or both, than to dysfunctional memory.

Executive Functioning There are some studies that suggest that hydrocephalic children have attentional problems on tasks requiring visual scanning and analysis (Horn, Lorch, Lorch, & Culatta, 1985; Landry, Copeland, Lee, & Robinson, 1990; Tew, Laurence, & Richards, 1980).

Visual-Motor Ability Children with spina bifida and hydrocephalus appear to have the most trouble in this domain. It is likely that this relates to the common finding of brain stem and cerebellar abnormalities (such as the Chiari malformation) in these individuals. These troubles are particularly manifested in low WISC-R Performance IQ scores, with the weakest subsets being Object Assembly (puzzles) and Coding (a timed digit–symbol association task) (Wills, 1993). As discussed above, Fletcher and colleagues (1992) suggested that posterior parietal lobe deficiencies may also play a role.

Tactile-Perceptual Ability Both children with spina bifida and hydrocephalus and those with hydrocephalus from other causes can have difficulties with such tactile tasks as tactile matching and graphesthesia (Grimm, 1976; Miller & Sethi, 1971). It is not clear what role these kinds of problems play in any observed academic difficulties.

Visuoperceptual Abilities Wills (1993) reviewed the reported work in this area and concluded that the results are conflicting. It appears that some studies found deficits because of confounding visuomotor problems. She also pointed out that distractibility and impulsivity, regardless of visuoperceptual ability, may have affected results.

Academic Skills Several studies have shown impairment in reading comprehension for children with hydrocephalus, when a child's IQ or single-word reading recognition is compared to his or her comprehension level (Carr, Halliwell, & Pearson, 1981; Lonton, 1981; Tew & Laurence, 1975). A study by Barnes and Dennis (1992) suggested that children with hydrocephalus use a different strategy for deriving meaning from printed paragraphs. The strategy appears to rely on word knowledge rather than contextual information to derive meaning (Wills, 1993).

It is well established that children with spina bifida/hydrocephalus have difficulty with arithmetic. Their achievement scores can in fact decrease with age (Wills et al., 1990). At least some of these difficulties relate to problems with paper-and-pencil skills caused by the visuomotor impairments noted above. Handwriting can also be a distinct problem, with difficulties in speed, alignment, and spacing as well as endurance. Finally, Wills (1993) noted that, in clinical practice, there are children who have done well in the elementary grades who begin to have difficulties as schoolwork becomes more complex and demanding.

Neuropsychologic Management

The management of school and life functioning of the individual with childhood-acquired hydrocephalus, regardless of the etiology, should take into account the high likelihood of underlying cognitive impairments contributing to any observed problems. Proper management should start with a complete assessment of the individual's neuropsychologic function. A degree of flexibility is necessary in interpreting the results. Some of these children will have combinations of deficits that are below the threshold for special educational services within the school system. However, clinicians with experience with this group have noted that these same children are at high risk for school failure. It is this author's opinion that they would be better served if these impairments were anticipated and recognized and interventions carried out and studied.

CONCLUSIONS

The care of children with hydrocephalus, of any etiology, has advanced dramatically as a result of improved neurosurgical interventions. However, children with hydrocephalus continue to exhibit nervous system–based problems that often bring them to the attention of neurologists and developmental pediatricians. In order to contribute to the management of these children, physicians should be familiar with the basic principles outlined in this chapter. Finally, the areas of impairment in higher cortical function in children with hydrocephalus should receive increased attention from clinicians if we are to help these individuals to improve their functional outcomes.

REFERENCES

Badella-Ribera, A., Shulman, K., & Paddock, N. (1966). The relationship of non-progressive hydrocephalus to intellectual functioning in children with spina bifida cystica. *Pediatrics, 37,* 787–793.

Barnes, M., & Dennis, M. (1992). Reading in children and adolescents after early onset hydrocephalus and in normally developing age peers: Phonological analysis, word recognition, word comprehension, and passage comprehension skills. *Journal of Pediatric Psychology, 17,* 445–466.

Carr, J., Halliwell, M.D., & Pearson, A.M. (1981). Educational attainments of spina bifida children attending ordinary and special schools. *Zeitschrift für Kinderchirurgie, 34,* 364–370.

Dennis, M., Hendrick, E., Hoffman, H., & Humphreys, R. (1987). Language of hydrocephalic children and adolescents. *Journal of Clinical and Experimental Neuropsychology, 2,* 593–621.

Fletcher, J.M., Bohan, T.P., Brandt, M.E., Brookshire, B.L., Beaver, S.R., Francis, D.J., Davidson, K.C., Thompson, N.M., & Miner, M.E. (1992). Cerebral white matter and cognition in hydrocephalic children. *Archives of Neurology, 49,* 818–824.

Gammal, T.E., Mark, E.K., & Brooks, B.S. (1987). MR imaging of Chiari II malformation. *American Journal of Neuroradiology, 8,* 1037–1044.

Gilbert, J.N., Jones, K.L., Rorke, L.B., Chernoff, G.F., & James, H.E. (1986). Central nervous system anomalies associated with meningomyelocele, hydrocephalus, and the Arnold-Chiari malformation: Reappraisal of theories regarding the pathogenesis of posterior neural tube closure defects. *Neurosurgery, 18,* 559–564.

Grimm, R. (1976). Hand function and tactile perception in a sample of children with myelomeningocele. *American Journal of Occupational Therapy, 30,* 234–240.

Hadenius, A.M., Hagberg, B., Hyttnas-Bensch, K., & Sjogren, I. (1962). The natural prognosis of infantile hydrocephalus. *Acta Paediatrica Scandinavica, 51,* 117–123.

Hammock, M.K., Milhorat, T.H., & Baron, I.S. (1976). Normal pressure hydrocephalus in patients with myelomeningocele. *Developmental Medicine and Child Neurology, 37,* 55–68.

Horn, D.G., Lorch, E.P., Lorch, R.F., Jr., & Culatta, B. (1985). Distractibility and vocabulary deficits in children with spina bifida and hydrocephalus. *Developmental Medicine and Child Neurology, 27,* 713–720.

Hurley, A., Dorman, C., Laatsch, L., Bell, S., & D'Avignon, J. (1990). Cognitive functioning in patients with spina bifida, hydrocephalus, and the "cocktail party syndrome." *Developmental Neuropsychology, 6,* 151–172.

Just, M., Swartz, M., Ludwig, B., Ermert, J., & Thelen, M. (1990). Cerebral and spinal MR findings in patients with postrepair myelomeningocele. *Pediatric Radiology, 20,* 262–266.

Landry, S.H., Copeland, D., Lee, A., & Robinson, S. (1990). Goal-directed behavior in children with spina bifida. *Developmental and Behavioral Pediatrics, 11,* 306–311.

Laurence, K.M., & Coates, S. (1967). Spontaneously arrested hydrocephalus: Results of re-examination of 82 survivors from a series of 182 unoperated cases. *Developmental Medicine and Child Neurology, 13*(Suppl.), 4–13.

Lonton, A.P. (1979). The relationship between intellectual skills and the computerized axial tomograms of children with spina bifida and hydrocephalus. *Zeitschrift für Kinderchirurgie, 28,* 368–374.

Lonton, A.P. (1981). The integration (mainstreaming) of spina bifida children into ordinary schools. *Zeitschrift für Kinderchirurgie, 34,* 356–364.

McComb, J.G. (1989). Cerebrospinal fluid formation and absorption. In Section of Pediatric Neurosurgery of the American Association of Neurological Surgeons and R.L. McLaurin (Ed.), *Pediatric neurosurgery: Surgery of the developing nervous system* (2nd ed., pp. 159–169). Philadelphia: W.B. Saunders.

McCullough, D.C. (1989). Hydrocephalus: Etiology, pathologic effects, diagnosis, and natural history. In Section of Pediatric Neurosurgery of the American Association of Neurological Surgeons & R.L. McLaurin (Ed.), *Pediatric Neurosurgery: Surgery of the developing nervous system* (2nd ed., pp. 180–199). Philadelphia: W.B. Saunders.

McLaurin, R.L. (1989). Ventricular shunts: Complications and results. In Section of Pediatric Neurosurgery of the American Association of Neurological Surgeons & R.L. McLaurin (Ed.), *Pediatric neurosurgery: Surgery of the developing nervous system* (2nd ed., pp. 219–229). Philadelphia: W.B. Saunders.

McLone, D.G., & Aronyk, K.E. (1993). An approach to the management of arrested and compensated hydrocephalus. *Pediatric Neurosurgery, 19*(2), 101–103.

McLone, D.G., Czyzewski, D., Raimondi, A.J., & Sommers, R.C. (1982). Central nervous system infections as a limiting factor in the intelligence of children with myelomeningocele. *Pediatrics, 70,* 338–342.

Miller, E., & Sethi, L. (1971). Tactile matching in children with hydrocephalus. *Neuropaediatrie, 3,* 191–194.

Nulsen, F.E., & Rekate, H.L. (1982). Results of treatment for hydrocephus as a guide to future management. In Section of Pediatric Neurosurgery of the American Association of Neurological Surgeons & R.L. McLaurin (Ed.), *Pediatric neurosurgery: Surgery of the developing nervous system* (2nd ed., pp. 229–241). Philadelphia: W.B. Saunders.

Rourke, B.P . (1989). *Nonverbal learning disability: The syndrome and the model.* New York: Guilford Press.

Tew, B. (1979). The "cocktail party syndrome" in children with hydrocephalus and spina bifida. *British Journal of Disorders of Communication, 14,* 89–101.

Tew, B., & Laurence, K.M . (1975). The effects of hydrocephalus on intelligence, visual perception, and school attainments. *Developmental Medicine and Child Neurology, 17*(Suppl. 35), 129–135.

Tew, B., & Laurence, K. (1979). The clinical and psychological characteristics of children with "cocktail party" syndrome. *Zeitschrift für Kinderchirurgie, 28,* 360–367.

Tew, B., Laurence, K., & Richards, A. (1980). Inattention among children with hydrocephalus and spina bifida. *Zeitschrift für Kinderchirurgie, 31,* 381–385.

Wechsler, D. (1974). *Wechsler Intelligence Scale for Children–Revised.* New York: The Psychological Corporation.

Wills, K.E. (1993). Neuropsychological functioning in children with spina bifida and/or hydrocephalus. *Journal of Clinical Child Psychology, 22,* 247–265.

Wills, K.E., Holmbeck, G.N., Dillon, K., & McLone, D.G. (1990). Intelligence and attainments among children with myelomeningocele. *Journal of Pediatric Psychology, 15,* 161–176.

Chapter 13

The Spectrum of Mild Neuromotor Disabilities

Thomas A. Blondis, M.D.

Two longitudinal clinical studies have demonstrated that children who experience mild neuromotor dysfunction—the so-called clumsy child syndrome (Taft & Barowsky, 1989)—more often than not have comorbid neurodevelopmental deficits (Hellgren, Gillberg, Gillberg, & Enerskog, 1993; Losse et al., 1991). One of these studies (Losse et al., 1991) clearly demonstrated significant other associated disabilities in learning and social and emotional development among adolescents who in the early elementary period were diagnosed as having motor control and output deficits. These newer studies demonstrate the continuing neural dysfunction and poor adaptation that clumsy children experience as adults and make it clear that mild neuromotor developmental delay and dysfunction is not mainly a phenomenon affecting only the child's motor domain. Because this area is often ignored by the educational system, it becomes exceedingly important for the developmental pediatrician to consider minor motor deficits that are pinpointed by the neurodevelopmental assessment.

The longtime notion that elementary children outgrow early motor and achievement delays has been challenged (Blondis, Snow, Roizen, Opacich, & Accardo, 1993; Snow, Blondis, Accardo, & Cunningham, 1993; Snow, Blondis, & Brady, 1988). An apparent problem with previous studies, leading to results that favored the maturational theory, may have been that the baseline measures employed were the same as those used for much older children. Since these earlier studies, it has been demonstrated that what were viewed as soft neurologic signs in the past must be viewed from a developmental framework (Wolff, 1985). A separate issue that is under investigation is whether or not mild motor dysfunction underlies a specific learning disability (Berninger & Rutberg, 1992; Hooper & Willis, 1989).

HISTORY OF CHILDHOOD INCOORDINATION

Nicholas Oseretsky investigated motor incoordination in Russia during the 1920s and published tests in 1923 that have been translated and revised in the United States (Doll, 1946). His studies focused on static and dynamic coordination of the hands, motor speed, dynamic coordination related to gross motor activity, and the neuroinhibition of associated movements. Orton (1937) is perhaps the first investigator to describe motor clumsiness in terms of dyspraxia or poor motor planning. Walton, Ellis, and Court (1965) expanded on Orton's conceptualization. In *The Clumsy Child*, Gubbay (1975) published longitudinal data on incoordination that linked dyspraxia to clumsiness. Deuel and Robinson (1987) defined two possible causes of childhood clumsiness: 1) poor motor expression resulting from the inability to alter joint angles accurately and quickly and 2) poor motor expression because of dysfunctional spatial processing.

NOSOLOGY

The term *mild neuromotor dysfunction* is used to refer to a serious impairment in the development of motor coordination that cannot be explained by mental retardation or any other specific congenital or acquired neurologic disorder (World Health Organization, 1992). This disorder has received various labels that currently include *specific developmental disorder of motor function* (SDDMF), *developmental coordination disorder* (DCD) (American Psychiatric Association, 1994), *clumsy child syndrome* (Gubbay, 1975), and *minimal cerebral palsy* (Capute & Accardo, 1991). Children with such dysfunction who do not qualify for another neurologic diagnosis could be labeled with any one of these terms to describe their condition. This nosology is based on a dimensional diagnostic approach.

Currently, the *International Classification of Diseases* (10th ed.) (World Health Organization, 1992) lists certain symptoms and signs that the child must demonstrate to be diagnosed as having SDDMF. He or she must show documented fine or gross motor abilities significantly below the expected level on the basis of his or her cognitive function. In addition, the problem must have been present early in development. Finally, and most importantly, the child must not have a diagnosable neurologic disorder that underlies the motor deficits. The diagnostic criteria for DCD are consistent with these but also require that the motor deficit interferes with either academic achievement or adaptive development. A consensus conference on the subject *Children and Clumsiness* was held in London, Ontario, Canada. Forty-one scientists from Europe, Australia, the British Isles, Netherlands, the United States, and Canada came to the conclusion that the term *developmental coordination disorder* should be used in the clinical settings in order to get recognition and payment (Fox & Polatajko, 1995). However, I will substitute the generic clumsy children nomenclature with the World Health Organization SDDMF classification because it is a more accurate and descriptive classification.

INCIDENCE AND ETIOLOGY

Johnston, Crawford, Short, Smyth, and Moller (1987) carried out an epidemiologic study in Australia to determine the incidence of poor coordination among primary school children between the ages of 5 and 7 years. They began by screening approximately 1,500 children and then determining whether or not the children had coordination deficits on the basis of the Mc-

Carthy Motor Scale (McCarthy, 1972). A total of 6.4% of the children had scores below 45 on the McCarthy scale and were classified as poorly coordinated. Cases with McCarthy scores between 40 and 45 were included, although the investigators acknowledged that these were borderline cases. This is probably the most accurate of four studies that attempted to determine the prevalence of SDDMF. If one looks at all incidence studies, the percentage ranges from 5 to 15.

In Johnston et al.'s study, a history of clumsiness in close relatives was given for 20% of the 5-year-olds identified as being clumsy and for 13% of the 7-year-olds. Johnston et al. obtained birth histories from parents of all but two poorly coordinated children who were screened and determined that perinatal complications occurred more frequently in this group of poorly coordinated children when compared to birth statistics available in South Australia. This difference reached statistical significance when the 5-year-old group was compared but not when the 7-year-old children were compared. All epidemiologic studies of this clinical population that have looked at a broad range of possible etiologies have speculated that a high percentage of clumsy children have birth histories associated with high-risk factors, including prematurity. Although familial incidence of clumsiness has been described in this Australian study and elsewhere, no prospective and/or controlled genetic studies currently exist.

PATHOPHYSIOLOGY

Regional cerebral blood flow studies and magnetic resonance imaging studies have been carried out on subjects with normal motor function (Kim et al., 1993; Roland, Larsen, Lassen, & Sknhoj, 1980), but to date this has not been done with a group of children diagnosed as having SDDMF. Supplementary motor and primary motor and sensory areas are activated during learned sequential movements. The supplementary motor area participates in assembling a central motor program. If a planned sequence of movements is not being carried out, blood flow to the supplementary motor cortex does not increase. These supplementary motor areas, which appear to be programmed areas for motor subroutines, have also been shown to be more active during speech. Studies of children with SDDMF could possibly elucidate the underlying cause of the children's dysfunction.

In a controlled study involving 51 clumsy children and 33 children with typical motor function, Knuckey, Apsimon, and Gubbay (1983) studied the neuroanatomy of both groups to determine if differences existed. The ventricular area index was significantly smaller in the clumsy group ($p < .001$). Altogether, 39% of the clumsy group had abnormal scans, versus 9% of the controls. These results were highly nonspecific, and no specific area of the brain could be correlated with clumsiness.

CLINICAL FINDINGS

Dyspraxia

Numerous forms of dyspraxia have been described that include ideomotor, ideamotor, speech, oralmotor, constructional, and dressing. Controversy surrounds the professed difference between ideomotor and ideamotor dyspraxia. *Ideomotor dyspraxia* refers to the inability to perform simple single-action gestures, whereas *ideamotor dyspraxia* refers to the inability to execute a sequence of multistep motor acts.

DeRenzi, Pieczoro, and Vignolo (1968) studied aphasic adults as well as control subjects and concluded that ideamotor apraxia is associated with lesions of the dominant hemisphere and especially the retrorolandic areas subserving language. Walton et al. (1965) described five cases of clumsy children who had no evidence of pyramidal tract, cerebellar, or extrapyramidal dysfunction. All of these children had at least average intelligence on the verbal scale of the Wechsler Intelligence Scale for Children (Wechsler, 1974), and in each case there was a significant discrepancy between the measurement of verbal and performance intelligence. The investigators concluded that in three of the cases praxis was the underlying dysfunction, and in the other two cases gnosia was dysfunctional. Deuel, Feely, and Bonskowski (1984) studied 20 controls and 20 children with learning disabilities described to have motor

dysfunction and found that these children with disabilities differed ($p = .0001$) from the controls on three different apraxia scales. They could not discriminate ideomotor from ideamotor dyspraxia in this study.

Sensory Relationships to Motor Control

Some neurophysiologists have proposed a closed-loop system to explain a sensory relationship to motor control. According to this theory, sensory feedback (afferent systems) provides second-to-second information with regard to the position of body parts in space during a movement.

Kinesthetic sense has previously been defined to be the discrimination of positions and movements of body parts via data coming from a system other than verbal, visual, or auditory (Howard & Templeton, 1966). Peripheral proprioception is sensitivity to the contraction of single muscles or tension on tendons. Using this framework, some scientists propose a hierarchical framework in which arranged sequences of incrementally complicated cells become involved in control over motor movement. The central question, proposed by Kalaska (1988), becomes, "Do the postcentral and parietal cortex contain an encyclopedic single cell compilation of all the typical combinations of posture?" Gardner's (1987) studies with monkeys support this theory.

Several studies have been reported that evaluated the importance of kinesthetic inputs with both clumsy children and typically coordinated control children. Bairstow and Laszlo (1981) reported a deficiency in kinesthetic sensation among clumsy children. They developed a closed-loop model (one that proposes that sensory feedback is directly related to motor responses) and concluded that the performance of skilled motor acts is dependent on intact kinesthesis. Studies by Henderson (1993) have also demonstrated striking differences between the kinesthetic ability of the clumsy child group when compared to controls. A study by Lord and Hulme (1987) concluded that the visual system is more responsible for clumsiness than is kinesthesis. They also demonstrated that the Kinaesthetic Sensitivity Test (Laszlo & Bairstow, 1985) did not distinguish between a group of clumsy children and an age-matched control group. Another recent study of clumsy children was unable to duplicate the striking differences found by Laszlo and Bairstow (Hoare & Larkin, 1991).

In recent studies by van der Meulen, Denier van der Gon, Gielen, Gooskens, and Willemse (1991a, 1991b), results indicated that the whole notion of a closed-loop system and lack of sensory feedback underlying the clumsy motor output performance of children with SDDMF may be completely inaccurate. Clumsy children had poorer visual tracking quality and longer delays than did control children, and the disparity between groups did not change significantly if visual feedback was removed. The study speculates that findings by Wann (1987) indicating that poor writers are more dependent on visual feedback than good writers related more to a strategy developed by poor writers than to an adaptation that made any difference to the poor writers' performance.

The relationship of kinesthetic input in children with SDDMF remains uncertain. If such input should be determined to play a role in SDDMF, given the clinical research that is now available, it seems highly unlikely that a deficit of kinesthetic feedback represents a problem among a large segment of the population of children with SDDMF.

Motor Learning Disabilities

It is apparent that children with learning disabilities frequently have associated motor dysfunction, most easily demonstrated among children with learning difficulties in kindergarten and first grade (Snow et al., 1989; Wolff, 1985). Whether motor dysfunction is the underlying dysfunction for a particular learning disability subtype is a question that cannot yet be answered. Empirical studies that have sought to subtype learning disabilities have generally utilized variables that are neurocognitive, academic, or neurolinguistic. If the investigator utilizes neurolinguistic variables in a hierarchical agglomerative cluster analysis, it is unlikely that motor dysfunction will show up as a primary neuroprocessing problem underlying the child's disability. In fact, none of the empirical

cluster analysis studies include motor processing as an underlying factor (Hooper & Willis, 1989). Both Denckla (1972) and Mattis (1981) have described motor disability subtypes using a clinical inferential model. Table 1 summarizes studies that have asserted that a motor or sensory mechanism was entirely or in part responsible for a specific learning disability.

In a cluster-analytic study of 99 children with writing disorder and 63 children without writing disorder, six subtypes emerged, two non–writing disorder control clusters and four writing disorder clusters. The writing disorder subtypes were 1) fine motor and linguistic deficits, 2) visuospatial deficits, 3) attention and memory deficits, and 4) sequencing deficits (Sandler et al., 1992).

Developmental Gerstmann syndrome has been reported by several clinical investigators (e.g., PeBenito, Fisch, & Fisch, 1988). It does not vary with respect to the cardinal signs of finger agnosia, right–left disorientation, dysgraphia, and dyscalculia. In the largest recent case study, all the children had learning disabilities but only one had a language deficit. Investigators debate whether constructional dyspraxia or dysgraphia underlies the poor handwriting. Although adult Gerstmann syndrome is attributable to a specific lesion in the dominant parietal lobe, there is no proof that this is true of the developmental syndrome.

Although controversy still surrounds the linkage of motor and sensory dysfunctions to a learning disability, there appears to be little doubt that these neurodevelopmental dysfunctions are frequently associated with developmental output failure (Berninger & Rutberg, 1992; Levine, Oberklaid, & Meltzer, 1981). The developmental output disorder study found that half of the sample had finger agnosia and that all of the subjects with agnosia had fine motor problems.

In order to determine whether or not motor or sensory deficit(s) account for a viable learning disability subtype, it will be necessary to utilize variables from a valid test of motor function as part of an empirical study. Such a study should also include achievement variables as well as cognitive variables. At this time there is reason

Table 1. Learning disability subtype studies

Investigator	Method	Disability subtypes	Problems
Kinsbourne and Warrington (1963)	Clinical inferential	Gerstmann, language retarded	Small sample size
Denckla (1972)	Clinical inferential	Specific language, visuospatial, motor dyscontrol	70% mixed type or don't fit any type
Mattis (1981)	Clinical inferential	Phonemic sequencing, specific language, articulatory and graphomotor, visuospatial, mixed	Articulatory and graphomotor subtype represents only 10%
Myklebust (1978)	Clinical inferential	Auditory processing, visual processing, language integration, intermodal processing	
Satz and Morris (1981)	Cluster analysis	Specific language, global language, visual-perceptual, mixed	A nonspecific disability subtype generalizes deficiencies through various academic areas
Snow, Cohen, and Holliman (1985)	Cluster analysis	Global, attention, language, mild language; 2 normal subtypes	No visuospatial subtype
Sandler et al. (1992)	Cluster analysis	Fine motor and linguistic, visuospatial, attention and memory, sequencing	Subtypes limited to written language failure

to believe that motor dysfunction may underlie some learning disabilities of written expression.

OUTCOME

The only longitudinal study to document all phases of outcome is the study by Losse et al. (1991). The results of this study indicate why the SDDMF condition should be taken seriously. The children with SDDMF showed significant statistical differences in physical education performance, neuromotor performance, self-concept, and academic achievement. Of children with SDDMF, 82% had documented emotional or behavioral problems by adolescence. More specific outcome information is provided in Table 2.

DIAGNOSIS

The developmental pediatrician should always begin with a careful medical history that includes developmental milestones. The developmental history should take into account both motor deviancy and delay. The child with SDDMF in some cases has deviant development during infancy, sometimes missing the rolling or crawling stages of locomotion. In some cases, the child cannot walk by 14 months. To document early motor milestones,

Table 2. Neurobehavioral outcome of teenagers diagnosed at age 6 to be clumsy children

	Poor performance in physical education	Poor performance on neuromotor exam	Poor physical self-concept	Poor academic attainment	All emotional/ behavior problems[a]
% of clumsy group as teens	65	73	73	71	82
Clumsy versus control groups	$p = .001$	$p = .001$	$p = .01$	$p = .05$	b

Adapted from Losse et al. (1991).

[a]A total of 53% of the clumsy group were reported to have problems with attention, concentration, or both as adolescents.

[b]No statistical comparison was made between the control and the clumsy groups; 36% of the control group had problems.

it is generally a good idea to have the family complete a questionnaire that asks them to refer to the child's baby book. Typically, the child may be failing to progress in gross motor, fine motor, and adaptive skills during the early elementary years. Such delays are often reflected by the failure to ride a bicycle without training wheels by the age of 6 years if the child lives in an area where most children begin riding a bike by 5 years. Other delayed gross motor milestones may include catching a bounced ball (typically acquired by 5 years), catching a ball with the hands when it is thrown to the child (6 years), skipping (5 years), and hopping forward on one foot 10 consecutive times (5 years). Typical delays in fine motor skills include failure to develop the use of a tripod pencil grasp by 5 years, inability to print the child's complete name by 6 years, lack of skill to color within lines by 5 years, and inability to cut a paper along a line by 5 years. Adaptive milestone delays may include failure to button and unbutton shirts by 4 years, inability to put shoes on the correct foot by 4 years, and failure to tie shoes by 6 years.

The general physical examination should include anthropometric measurements, dysmorphology evaluation, physical observation (ptosis, diplegic facies, etc.), and a complete extremity examination. Numerous soft sign batteries may be used. The list is exhaustive, but some of the more noteworthy include the Physical and Neurological Examination of Soft Signs, the Neurological Evaluation Schedule, the Examination of the Child with Minor Neurological Dysfunction, the Test of Motor Impairment, and the Neurodevelopmental Test Battery (Stokman et al., 1986; Stott, Moyes, & Henderson, 1984; Touwen, 1979; Tupper, 1987). The developmental pediatrician should choose a soft sign battery that tests a variety of motor and sensory functions, including motor coordination, gestures that require motor planning ideation, motor speed, pencil control, right–left orientation, finger gnosia, kinesthetic/proprioceptive function, and inhibition of associated movements. Table 3 matches some well-known motor and sensory skills with the average age of appearance and the *chief* mechanism(s) underlying

each skill. If one of these skills does not appear at the expected age, it would be considered a developmental soft sign (significant delay would generally be considered to be >1.5 standard deviations beyond the mean age of appearance of the skill).

Developmental soft signs vary with regard to reliability. Most standardized soft sign assessments take a minimum of 25 minutes to complete (this includes scoring), and variability in administration time may be related to the child's ability to follow the verbal directions given by the examiner or may reflect a child's slow processing tempo. Any motor assessment should begin with the determination of handedness, because it is the primary clinical marker for determining laterality. Mild hemiparesis has been described as an underlying cause of clumsiness. Clinical investigators have demonstrated that several of these tests have reasonable reliability but that the validity data are usually less than adequate. Nevertheless, developmental soft sign tests offer neurodevelopmental medicine the most useful clinical method for establishing motor and sensory developmental delays.

Although children with SDDMF do not have focal neurologic findings, one should always rule out mild cerebral palsy as well as muscular dystrophy. Whether or not clumsy children have typical tone has been a matter of controversy (Abbie, Douglas, & Ross, 1978; Johnston et al., 1987). Blondis, Roizen, Stein, Zier, and Opacich (1994) conducted a prospective controlled study using a battery that included a tone scale and a reflex scale to determine if elementary school children with SDDMF had abnormal neurologic findings. This investigation identified an association between axial hypotonia and SDDMF. No clear differences between children from a middle-class school district and a clinic population of children with SDDMF were noted with respect to neurologic reflexes. The use of developmental soft sign tests and other developmental tests does not substitute for a complete neurologic examination, but these tests may augment and refine both neuromotor and sensory findings.

The developmental pediatrician can gain further insight into the motor, sensory, and

Table 3. Motor and sensory skills as related to average age of attainment and mechanism underlying ability

Name of skill	Age of appearance (years)[a]	Mechanism underlying skill			
		Kinesthesia/ sensory	Motor A, B, C[b]	Praxis	Neural inhibitory
Localize touch	4	x			
Stand on one foot for 15 seconds	5	x	x (A)		
Hop on one foot 20 times	5	x	x (A)		
Catch ball thrown to hands with hands	5		x (B)	x	
Identify right and left side	5			x	
Successive finger-to-finger, smooth movements (5 cycles)	6		x (B, C)		x
Recognition of touch of finger	6	x			
Rhythmic skipping	6		x (B)	x	
Rapid alternating movements	7		x (B, C)		
Rhythmic alternate hopping in place (sequential)	7		x (B)		x
Imitation of a "V": hands raised, index and middle finger form "V," and other fingers are flexed	8			x	
Move toward and catch ball	8		x (B, C)	x	
Suppression of intense and frequent mirror movements	8				x
Finger gnosia	8	x			
Persistent tandem stance with eyes closed (15 seconds)	9	x			
Stereognosis	10				x
Absence of choreiform movements during motor stance (eyes closed)	10				x
Absence of arm overflow during stressed gait on outside and inside of feet	11				x
Imitation of "junior birdman" gesture	12			x	

[a]Age of appearance is the age at which approximately 85% of children attain the skill.

[b]A, balance; B, coordination; C, speed.

visual–motor processes of the child by using several developmental tests of fine motor, gross motor, and visual-motor processing. During a task that asks the child to copy a figure or print/write his or her name, the clinician can gain insight into the awkwardness of the child's pencil grasp, the smoothness of his or her pencil stroke, and the frequency and intensity of associated movements, as well as observing other behaviors such as the child's impulsivity. The clinician also must consider other neurodevelopmental areas that may reveal a deficit and utilize tasks and tests to evaluate cognitive and academic abilities. The developmental pediatrician should also evaluate the adaptive development of the child with SDDMF.

If SDDMF is suspected, then a referral to a pediatric occupational therapist or adaptive physical educator should be considered. The Bruininks-Oseretsky Test of Motor Performance evaluates fine and gross motor development in children 4–14 years of age. This test is well standardized and has been shown to have fair to good reliability. Construct validity studies that included children with learning disabilities and mild mental retardation clearly show that this test differentiates between children with or without disabilities. The long form is required, however, for use as a clinical diagnostic tool. The test yields both a fine motor and a gross motor composite score. A short-form version of the test has been used as a screening measure (R.H.

Bruininks, 1978; V.L. Bruininks & Bruininks, 1977; Sabatino, 1985).

MANAGEMENT

In North America, two different interventions are primarily being utilized for children with SDDMF: individualized physical therapy and sensory integration therapy. If the school addresses this problem, it is usually through a physical educator who has expertise in individualizing a physical education program for children with motor delay. Some schools employ pediatric occupational or physical therapists for intervention, but very few have the resources to hire a certified "sensory integration" therapist or to pay for the equipment and space needed to conduct a sensory integration treatment program.

Two randomized intervention studies that investigated the efficacy of sensory integration therapy have been published. Humphries, Wright, Snider, and McDougall (1992) administered two different forms of occupational therapy (perceptual motor and sensory integration) to children with learning disabilities. At the end of the study, the subjects who received either form of occupational therapy had improved motor skills compared to subjects in the no-treatment group. None of the groups made academic gains. Another study that examined the effects of two different forms of occupational therapy on children with learning disabilities failed to replicate the improvement in motor performance, but the results were in agreement with regard to the failure of the treatment group to make academic gains (Polatajko, Law, Miller, Schaffer, & Macnab, 1991). Because the latter investigation had significant losses from the no-treatment/control group, the results did not represent a sufficient group of untreated children with learning disabilities. Neither of these studies focused on children with SDDMF.

It seems reasonable, without sufficient clinical studies to support or negate the efficacy of adaptive physical education or pediatric occupational therapy, for the developmental pediatrician to continue to refer children with SDDMF for individualized services. Some clinicians and therapists suggest that these children do not get sufficient practice in motor games because they are not included by their school-age peers. This theory advances the argument that, through practice, children are able to recall motor movement and thus may be better able to perform in games played at school during play time. Given the results of the outcome study by Losse et al. (1991), developmental pediatricians should refer children with SDDMF for services until studies clearly show that individualized interventions cannot benefit these children. However, in doing so, the developmental pediatrician should caution the family about some of the claims made by sensory integration therapists. The developmental pediatrician can help the family to identify particular skills they would like their child to develop, and can also specify by prescription that these targeted skills should be the primary focus of the intervention. Future clinical research should help discriminate which skills should be targeted for greatest efficacy.

REFERENCES

Abbie, M.H., Douglas, H.M., & Ross, K.E. (1978). The clumsy child: Observations in cases referred to the gymnasium of the Adelaide Children's Hospital over a three-year period. *Medical Journal of Australia, 1,* 65–69.

American Psychiatric Association. (1994). *Diagnostic and statistical manual of mental disorders* (4th ed., pp. 53–55). Washington, DC: American Psychiatric Press.

Bairstow, P.J., & Laszlo, J.I. (1981). Kinesthetic sensitivity to passive movements and its relationship to motor development and motor control. *Developmental Medicine and Child Neurology, 23,* 606–617.

Berninger, V., & Rutberg, J. (1992). Relationship of finger function to beginning writing: Application to diagnosis of writing disabilities. *Developmental Medicine and Child Neurology, 34,* 155–172.

Blondis, T.A., Roizen, N.J., Stein, M., Zier, A., & Opacich, K. (1994). Axial tone in children with developmental coordination disorder (DCD). *Pediatric Research, 35,* 19.

Blondis, T.A., Snow, J.H., Roizen, N.J., Opacich, K.J., & Accardo, P.J. (1993). Early maturation of motor-delayed children at school age. *Journal of Child Neurology, 8,* 323–329.

Bruininks, R.H. (1978). *The Bruininks-Oseretsky Test of Motor Proficiency.* Circle Pines, MN: American Guidance Service.

Bruininks, V.L., & Bruininks, R.H. (1977). Motor proficiency of learning disabled and nondisabled students. *Perceptual and Motor Skills, 44,* 1131–1137.

Capute, A.J., & Accardo, P.J. (1991). Cerebral palsy: The spectrum of motor dysfunction. In A.J. Capute & P.J. Accardo (Eds.), *Developmental disabilities in infancy and childhood* (pp. 344–345). Baltimore: Paul H. Brookes Publishing Co.

Denckla, M.B. (1972). Clinical syndromes in learning disabilities: The case for "splitting" vs. "lumping." *Journal of Learning Disabilities, 5,* 401–406.

DeRenzi, E., Pieczoro, A., & Vignolo, L. (1968). Ideational apraxia: A quantitative study. *Neuropsychologia, 6,* 41–52.

Deuel, R., Feely, C., & Bonskowski, C. (1984). Manual apraxia in learning disabled children. *Annals of Neurology, 16,* 388.

Deuel, R.K., & Robinson, D.J. (1987). Developmental motor signs. In D.E. Tupper (Ed.), *Soft neurological signs* (pp. 95–130). New York: Grune & Stratton.

Doll, E.A. (1946). *The Oseretsky Tests of Motor Proficiency* [Translated from the Portuguese adaptation]. Circle Pines, MN: American Guidance Service.

Fox, A.M., & Polatajko, H.J. (1995). *Children and clumsiness: An international consensus meeting. The London Consensus.* Canada: University Press.

Gardner, E.P. (1987). Somatosensory cortical mechanisms of feature detection in tactile and kinesthetic discrimination. *Canadian Journal of Physiology and Pharmacology, 66,* 439–454.

Gubbay, S.S. (1975). *The clumsy child: A study of developmental apraxia and agnosic ataxia.* Philadelphia: W.B. Saunders.

Hellgren, L., Gillberg, C., Gillberg, I.C., & Enerskog, I. (1993). Children with deficits in attention, motor control and perception almost grown up: General health at 16 years. *Developmental Medicine and Child Neurology, 35,* 881–892.

Henderson, S.E. (1993). Motor development and minor handicap. In A.F. Kalverboer, B. Hopkins, & R. Geuze (Eds.), *Motor development in early and later childhood: Longitudinal approaches* (pp. 286–306). Cambridge, England: Cambridge University Press.

Hoare, D., & Larkin, D. (1991). Kinaesthetic abilities in clumsy children. *Developmental Medicine and Child Neurology, 33,* 671–678.

Hooper, S.R., & Willis, W.G. (1989). Empirical classification models. In S.R. Hooper & W.G. Willis (Eds.), *Learning disability subtyping* (pp. 62–91). New York: Springer-Verlag.

Howard, I.P., & Templeton, W.B. (1966). *Human spatial orientation.* New York: John Wiley & Sons.

Humphries, T., Wright, M., Snider, L., & McDougall, B. (1992). A comparison of the effectiveness of sensory integrative therapy and perceptual-motor training in treating children with learning disabilities. *Journal of Developmental and Behavioral Pediatrics, 13,* 31–40.

Johnston, D., Crawford, J., Short, H., Smyth, T.R., & Moller, J. (1987). Poor co-ordination in 5 year olds: A screening test for use in schools. *Australian Pediatric Journal, 23,* 157–161.

Kalaska, J.F. (1988). The representation of arm movements in postcentral and parietal cortex. *Canadian Journal of Physiology and Pharmacology, 66,* 455–463.

Kim, S.G., Ashe, J., Hendrich, K., Ellermann, J.M., Merkle, H., Ugurbil, K., & Georgopoulos, A.P. (1993). Functional magnetic resonance imaging of motor cortex: Hemispheric asymmetry and handedness. *Science, 261,* 615–617.

Kinsbourne, M., & Warrington, E.K. (1963). Developmental factors in reading and writing backwardness. *British Journal of Psychology, 54,* 145–146.

Knuckey, N.W., Apsimon, T.T., & Gubbay, S.S. (1983). Computerized axial tomography in clumsy children with developmental apraxia. *Brain and Development, 5,* 14–19.

Laszlo, J.L., & Bairstow, P.J. (1985). *Kinaesthetic Sensitivity Test.* London: Holt, Rinehart & Winston.

Levine, M.D., Oberklaid, F., & Meltzer, L. (1981). Developmental output disorder: A study of low productivity in school-aged children. *Pediatrics, 67,* 18–25.

Lord, R., & Hulme, R. (1987). Kinesthetic sensitivity of normal and clumsy children. *Developmental Medicine and Child Neurology, 29,* 720–725.

Losse, A., Henderson, S.E., Elliman, D., Hall, D., Knight, E., & Jongsmans, M. (1991). Clumsiness in children—Do they grow out of it? A 10-year follow-up study. *Developmental Medicine and Child Neurology, 33,* 32–39.

Mattis, S. (1981). Dyslexia syndromes in children: Toward the development of syndrome-specific treatment programs. In F.G. Pirozzolo & M.C. Wittrock (Eds.), *Neuropsychological and cognitive processes in reading* (pp. 93–107). New York: Academic Press.

McCarthy, D.A. (1972). *Manual for the McCarthy Scales of Children's Abilities.* New York: Psychological Corporation.

Myklebust, H.R. (1978). Toward a science of dyslexiology. In H.R. Myklebust (Ed.), *Progress in learning disabilities* (Vol. 4, pp. 1–39). New York: Grune & Stratton.

Orton, S.T. (1937). *Reading, writing, and speech problems in children.* New York: W.W. Norton.

PeBenito, R., Fisch, C.B., & Fisch, M.L. (1988). Developmental Gerstmann's syndrome. *Archives of Neurology, 45,* 977–982.

Polatajko, H., Law, M., Miller, J., Schaffer, R., & Macnab, J. (1991). The effect of a sensory integration program on academic achievement, motor performance, and self-esteem in children identified as learning disabled: Results of a clinical trial. *Occupational Journal of Research, 11,* 155–176.

Roland, P.E., Larsen, B., Lassen, N.A., & Sknhoj, E. (1980). Supplementary motor area and other cortical areas in organization of voluntary movements in man. *Journal of Neurophysiology, 43,* 118–136.

Sabatino, D.A. (1985). Review of Bruininks-Oseretsky Test of Motor Proficiency. In J.V. Mitchell (Ed.), *The ninth mental measurement yearbook* (pp. 235–236). Lincoln, NE: University Press.

Sandler, A.D., Watson, T.E., Foote, M., Levine, M.D., Coleman, W.L., & Hooper, S.R. (1992). Neurodevelopmental study of writing disorders in middle childhood. *Journal of Developmental and Behavioral Pediatrics, 13,* 16–23.

Satz, P., & Morris, R. (1981). Learning disabilities subtypes: A review. In F.J. Pirozzolo & M.C. Wittrock (Eds.), *Neuropsychological and cognitive processes in reading* (pp. 109–141). New York: Academic Press.

Snow, J.H., Blondis, T.A., Accardo, P.J., & Cunningham, K.J. (1993). Longitudinal assessment of motor and sensory skills in academically disabled and control children. *Archives of Clinical Neuropsychology, 8,* 55–68.

Snow, J.H., Blondis, T.A., & Brady, L. (1989). Motor and sensory abilities with normal and academically at-risk children. *Archives of Neuropsychology, 3,* 227–238.

Snow, J.H., Cohen, M., & Holliman, W.B. (1985). Learning disability subgroups using cluster analysis of the WISC–R. *Journal of Psychoeducational Assessment, 4,* 391–397.

Stokman, C.J., Shafer, S.Q., Shaffer, D., Ng, S.K.C., O'Conner, P.A., & Wolff, R.R. (1986). Assessment of neurological soft signs in adolescence. *Developmental Medicine and Child Neurology, 28,* 428–439.

Stott, D.H., Moyes, F.S., & Henderson, S.E. (1984). *The Henderson Revision of the Test of Motor Impairment.* San Antonio, TX: Psychological Corporation.

Taft, L.T., & Barowsky, E.I. (1989). Clumsy child. *Pediatrics in Review, 10,* 247–253.

Touwen, B.C.L. (1979). *Examination of the child with minor neurological dysfunction* (2nd ed.). Philadelphia: J.B. Lippincott.

Tupper, D.E. (1987). Appendix D. In D.E. Tupper (Ed.), *Soft neurological signs* (pp. 381–388). New York: Grune & Stratton.

Van der Meulen, J.H.P., Denier van der Gon, J.J., Gielen, C.C.A.M., Gooskens, R.H.J.M., & Willemse, J. (1991a). Visuomotor performance of normal and clumsy children. I: Fast goal-directed arm-movements with and without visual feedback. *Developmental Medicine and Child Neurology, 33,* 40–54.

Van der Meulen, J.H.P., Denier van der Gon, J.J., Gielen, C.C.A.M., Gooskens, R.H.J.M., & Willemse, J. (1991b). Visuomotor performance of normal and clumsy children. II: Arm-tracking with and without visual feedback. *Developmental Medicine and Child Neurology, 33,* 118–129.

Walton, J., Ellis, E., & Court, S. (1965). Clumsy children: Developmental apraxia and agnosia. *Brain, 85,* 603–612.

Wann, J.P. (1987). Trends in the refinement and optimization of fine-motor trajectories: Observations from an analysis of the handwriting of primary school children. *Journal of Motor Behavior, 19,* 13–37.

Wechsler, D. (1974). *Wechsler Intelligence Scale for Children–Revised.* New York: Psychological Corporation.

Wolff, P.H. (1985). Neuromotor maturation and psychological performance: A developmental study. *Developmental Medicine and Child Neurology, 27,* 344–354.

World Health Organization. (1992). Specific developmental disorder of motor function, F82 (pp. 250–252). In *International Classification of Diseases* (10th ed.). Geneva: Author.

PART IV

MENTAL RETARDATION

Chapter 14

Mental Retardation

Pasquale J. Accardo, M.D., and Arnold J. Capute, M.D., M.P.H.

Mental retardation refers medically to organic brain dysfunction syndromes that are accompanied by significant cognitive limitation. The significance of the cognitive limitation is reflected by an IQ that is more than 2 standard deviations below the mean for age on the test instrument used. Because most such tests have a mean of 100 and a standard deviation of 15 points, an IQ of 70 is the typical cutoff for establishing the cognitive component for a diagnosis of mental retardation. However, a standard error of the mean of about 5 points for most instruments allows this cutoff point to be expanded into a range of 65–75. This means that clinical judgment can determine that one child with an IQ of 66 does not have mental retardation while another with an IQ of 74 does. Some of the factors that will influence such clinical judgments include the child's medical, social, and educational history; specific neurodevelopmental diagnoses; and the pattern of past developmental progress and adaptive skill acquisition. It must be noted that biologic risk factors are similar to sociobehavioral risk factors in that both are merely risk factors: Neither Down syndrome nor low family socioeconomic status can predict the IQ of a given child accurately.

Lack of skill of the examiner, inappropriateness of the test, and missed medical diagnoses may invalidate the test score. For example, in the absence of cognitive impairment secondary to brain damage, IQs in the range of mental retardation range may indicate pseudoretardation secondary to undetected deafness or psychosis. When the underlying brain dysfunction is reflected by an accurate measure of cognitive limitation, a similar degree of social–adaptive impairment almost automatically follows. Significant discrepancies between intellectual and social–adaptive age levels suggest the need for more careful differential diagnostic assessment.

The different levels of mental retardation also are defined largely by IQ ranges (Figure 1). The lower the IQ, the greater the long-term predictive validity of the developmental level. Among children between ages 1 and 5 with developmental disabilities, the ratio developmental quotient (DQ) derived from the pediatric neurodevelopmental assessment appears to be more stable (and to have better predictive validity) than the standard scores derived from formal infant psychometrics.

The latest American Association on Mental Retardation (AAMR) definition of mental retardation has retained an age of onset by 18 years but has raised the IQ cut off from 70 to 75

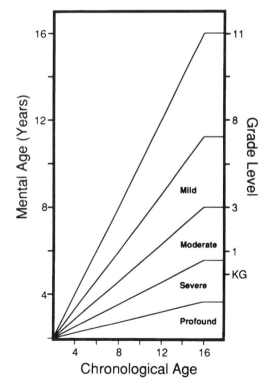

Figure 1. Levels of mental retardation.

(Luckasson et al., 1992). This 5-point elevation of the IQ score will more than double the population eligible for a diagnosis of mental retardation, and this increase (in the millions of persons) will include a markedly disproportionate representation of minority group children (MacMillan, Gresham, & Siperstein, 1993). Levels of severity have been replaced in the AAMR reformulation by levels of needed supports. In rough equivalency, people with mild mental retardation (IQs of 50–75) will require intermittent supports; people with moderate mental retardation (IQs of 35–50) will require limited supports; people with severe mental retardation (IQs of 20–35) will require extensive supports; and people with profound mental retardation (IQs below 20) will require pervasive supports. In fact, the support levels are defined not by IQ ranges but rather by a detailed assessment of 10 social skill areas. The absence of acceptable instruments to assess these social skill areas, however, makes this definition operationally difficult at the present time. This attempt to introduce greater individualization into programming and service provision for people with mental retardation has opened the door to a serious lack of objectivity. Such a move away from a neuropsychological and biomedical perspective is more striking when viewed from the perspective of dramatic advances in behavioral genetics (O'Brien, 1992; Rosen, 1993).

Mental retardation is frequently an associated deficit in the presence of other developmental diagnoses, such as specific genetic syndromes, cerebral palsy, autism, and communication disorders. The decision as to which condition should be given prominence in the diagnostic formulation may change as clinical goals change. Genetic counseling, school placement, and problem solving for behavioral deterioration will necessitate a comprehensive review of all the specific neurodevelopmental diagnoses that are contributing to the child's disability. An extreme bias toward the behavioral aspects of mental retardation, with a focus on learned helplessness, the Pygmalion effect, institutional experiences, verbal mediation, and social reinforcement theories, has led to a relative neglect of the contribution of organic factors not merely to cognitive delay but also to the complex rela-

tionships that produce developmental dissociation and deviance (Figure 2).

ASSESSMENT

There is no routine medical evaluation for mental retardation. The tests and procedures listed in Table 1 must be considered in each case in the light of history, physical, and neurodevelopmental findings. For example, of all the associated deficits, those of vision and hearing potentially have the greatest impact on development and behavior in people with mental retardation. These deficits occur in persons with retardation approximately 10 times as often as they do in the general population, with some degree of visual and auditory impairment occurring in 10%–20% of people with mental retardation (Ellis, 1986). Self-injury, stereotypies, and aggression appear to be more common when the impairment presents with unique difficulties, and it is here that a familiarity with the various medical risk factors can be of assistance (see Chapter 21, this volume). Many genetic syndromes associated with mental retardation identify an increased risk for disorders of vision and hearing. Hearing aids or eyeglasses are much less invasive treatments for behavior disorders than pharmacologic or physical restraints.

The first step in the evaluation of a child with mental retardation is an accurate assessment of developmental level (see Chapter 18, Volume I). A detailed developmental history can be supported by birth records, baby books, family photographs, and videotapes. This developmental history of past and current milestones, along with a neurodevelopmental examination of language, motor, and problem-solving abilities, can generate a comprehensive profile of the child's various functional levels in these areas (see Chapters 14 and 21, Volume I). Motor age tends to be the least helpful; language assessment generally represents the most sensitive early screening device for mental retardation. The clinician must be careful not to equate severe language delay with mental retardation even in the presence of significant dysmorphology. The significance of language delay within mental retardation and its implications for service delivery remain controversial (Cole, Dale,

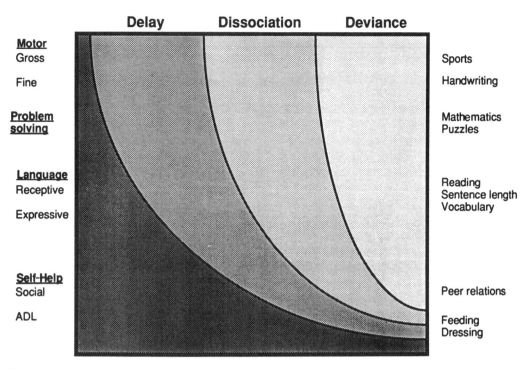

Figure 2. Delay, deviance, and dissociation and the spectrum of development disabilities.

& Mills, 1992). In the 2- to 5-year-old child, the pediatric neurodevelopmental assessment may be supplemented by formal psychometric testing; for school-age children, it *should* be supplemented by formal psychometric testing (see Chapters 17, 19, and 20, Volume I).

In exploring genetic contributions to mental retardation, the family history should focus on the entire spectrum of developmental disor-

Table 1. Sample tests and procedures to be considered in the biomedical assessment of the child with mental retardation

Amino acids: serum and urine

Audiologic assessment

Chromosome studies: sex chromatin, karyotype, banding, fragile X, DNA probes

Consultations: ophthalmologic, dermatologic, genetic

Electroencephalogram

Evoked potentials: auditory, visual

Fibroblast cultures

Metabolic screening

Skull radiographs, computerized tomography scan, (quantitative) magnetic resonance imaging

Thyroid function tests

Titers for infectious agents

ders, rather than on mental retardation alone. The pregnancy, labor, and delivery should be investigated for markers of both intrinsic and extrinsic influences on the fetus and infant. Fetal alcohol syndrome is a syndrome of low birth weight, short stature, microcephaly, short palpebral fissure lengths, and cardiac and bone abnormalities (see Chapter 19, this volume). However, it is often very difficult to confirm the critical history of maternal alcohol consumption during pregnancy. Exposure to other chemicals also can affect prenatal development (see, e.g., Chapter 10, Volume I), and the potential number of chemical exposures that can affect fetal brain development is limitless. A more surprising association between maternal urinary tract infection during pregnancy and otherwise unexpected mental retardation has been reported (Leviton & Giles, 1984).

Relative fetal hypoactivity provides some support for a prenatal origin of mental retardation (see Chapter 2, this volume). Perinatal difficulties, in contrast, may be the result of congenital or intrauterine fetal problems rather then the cause of the retardation. Although Costeff,

Cohen, and Weller (1983) and Hagberg, Hagberg, Lowerth, and Lindberg (1981) have argued that perinatal events rather than a polygenetic etiology are more important in explaining mild mental retardation, this interpretation was not supported by the results of the Perinatal Collaborative Study (Broman, Nichols, Shaughnessy, & Kennedy, 1987).

Low birth weight can accompany prematurity and intrauterine growth retardation (see Chapter 7, Volume I). Low birth weight for gestational age suggests a genetic syndrome, a congenital infection, or some other chronic toxic influence on the developing fetus. Persistent poor growth is a frequent finding in severe mental retardation with or without oral–motor dysfunction. Serious developmental disabilities always should be considered in the differential diagnosis of failure to thrive. High birth weight and mild mental retardation are observed in Wiedemann-Beckwith syndrome and cerebral gigantism (Sotos-Dodge syndrome). Children with Prader-Willi and Laurence-Moon-Bardet-Biedl syndromes have normal birth weights and moderate mental retardation but later show excessive weight gain. Minor malformations (dysmorphic features) may point to a specific syndrome (Buyse, 1990; Jones, 1988; Wiedemann, Kunze, Gross, & Dibbern, 1992), or at least a prenatal onset (see Chapter 15, Volume I). Physical stigmata, such as the facies of Down syndrome, microcephaly, and other dysmorphic features are associated with a halo effect in which a child's developmental level will tend to be underestimated. Vomiting, fluid and electrolyte imbalance, and dramatic variations in behavior and alertness may suggest a metabolic etiology (see Chapter 5, Volume I).

Microcephaly accompanies many genetic syndromes (see Chapter 15, Volume I). Proportional microcephaly, in which the head circumference and the height are both proportionally small, represents a lower risk for mental retardation. Even the more severe degrees of microcephaly do not automatically imply mental retardation but do support the presence of some type of developmental disorder. Macrocephaly requires that hydrocephalus be ruled out; skin lesions may help identify phakomatoses (see Chapter 15, Volume I; Chapters 11 and 12, this

volume). Postnatal etiologies such as meningitis, encephalitis, and severe head injuries are relatively easy to identify (see Chapters 8 and 12, Volume I). However, the usual mild head traumas suffered by toddlers during early walking have only a coincidental association with the first perception of developmental delay.

The age at which parents suspect a developmental problem usually correlates with the degree of mental retardation. Children who are identified before 1 year of age usually have DQs below 50; those diagnosed after age 2 usually have DQs above 50. Regardless of the presence or absence of hard or soft neurologic signs on physical examination (Birch, Richardson, Baird, Horobin, & Illsley, 1970), children with mental retardation are not neurologically "normal." Mental retardation is presumptive evidence of organic brain dysfunction (see Chapter 13, this volume).

A medical diagnostic workup should be performed on children with mental retardation for three main reasons. First, identification of a genetic contribution to the etiology allows a better prediction of the risk of recurrence for mental retardation and other developmental disorders for the parents, for the child, and for other blood relations. Second, the clarification of organic contributions to etiology can permit more accurate prediction of long-term developmental outcomes as well as the potential for later medical complications as a result of the involvement of other organ systems that is found in different syndromes. The presence of associated deficits in addition to the mental retardation will affect this aspect of the pediatric neurodevelopmental assessment. Finally, some medically diagnosable conditions are amenable to treatment intervention that might, in rare cases, reverse a downward developmental trend, but more commonly might foster maximum progress. This relates especially to the associated deficits present.

These specific goals must be identified and kept in mind when counseling parents as to how far to pursue a specific etiology. A test that does not contribute to the above goals and that might, for example, produce information that does not suggest the risk of recurrence or indicate prognosis or treatment should not be presented to parents as part of the indicated workup. The purpose of each test and the probability that it will contribute to a specific goal identified by the family must be discussed before a test is ordered. The fact that the electroencephalogram (EEG) frequently exhibits nonspecific abnormalities in people with mental retardation rarely recommends it to the parents of children with mental retardation. Such parents are often angry when they are informed that the EEG could not have been expected to answer their concerns about etiology and treatment. The EEG has its place in the evaluation of children with mental retardation who are suspected of having seizure disorders, or as a baseline study for children with syndromes or risk factors for the later development of seizures or mental retardation. These cautions must be heeded at a time when research on brain function and localization is making use of results of tests covered by third-party insurers. Parents of children with mental retardation may act in loco parentis for their children. Professionals may *not* act in loco parentis for the parents of children with mental retardation, but rather should interact with the parents as adults who have a right to collaborate in the evaluation and decision-making process. Unfortunately, the style for later professional communication is, for many families, often determined by this initial interaction.

STATIC VERSUS PROGRESSIVE RETARDATION

One of the major reasons for close developmental follow-up in early infancy and the taking of a detailed developmental history when a child presents with developmental delay is to distinguish between mental retardation in which development proceeds at a relatively fixed slow rate and mental retardation in which development proceeds at a decreasing rate, with actual regression and skill loss secondary to a progressive central nervous system lesion, such as a metabolic defect, storage disease, brain tumor, or other degenerative process. In the latter case, treatment might halt the progress of the disease and allow development to continue at a more normal rate. (Shunting an active hydrocephalus would be an example of effective treatment.)

Table 2 lists some of these progressive conditions and highlights the fact that these disorders can appear at various ages. Indeed, several of these diseases have genetically heterogeneous infantile- and juvenile-onset forms.

Although it is important to discriminate static from progressive encephalopathies, the distinction between the two categories is of diminishing significance. For example, in its onset, Rett syndrome is a degenerative disorder that, from the point of view of biomedical research, should be investigated with all the specialized techniques appropriate to that diagnostic category; however, from the point of view of the life cycle of girls with severe to profound mental retardation and autistic features, the principles of habilitation are not different from those of any other static encephalopathy of similar severity. Close observation of intelligence and social quotients in Down syndrome reveals a steady if slow deterioration over decades, a decline that appears to be independent of living arrangements (Brown, Greer, Aylward, & Hunt, 1990). If this decline were restricted to childhood and early adolescence, it might be attributed to an early plateauing of learning capabilities; its persistence into the later decades, however, supports an actual loss of adaptive skills. The degree to which this degeneration

Table 2. Age of onset of various degenerative conditions

Condition	Age of onset (years)
Phenylketonuria	0–1
Galactosemia	
Maple syrup urine disease	
Homocystinuria	
Hypothyroidism	
Hyperammonemia	
Lesch-Nyhan syndrome	
Menkes' kinky hair syndrome	
Tay-Sachs disease	
Metachromatic leukodystrophy	1–6
Mucopolysaccharidoses	
Tuberous sclerosis	
Ataxia–telangiectasia	
Sturge-Weber syndrome	
Subacute sclerosing panencephalitis	
Rett syndrome	
Neurofibromatosis	6–adolescence
Wilson's disease	
Sea blue histiocyte syndrome	
Hallervorden-Spatz disease	

relates to the learning style of people with Down syndrome, to a preprogrammed genetic decline, to early Alzheimer's syndrome changes, or to some combination of these factors requires further research. This subtle pattern, however, suggests that Down syndrome should be placed in the category of degenerative disease and raises the question of how many less common, less well-studied "static" encephalopathies also eventually will reveal a more progressive pattern. Blatt (1987) has reminded professionals in the mental retardation field that the educability hypothesis remains unproven. The emphasis placed here on the potentially degenerative aspect of the organic substrate to mental retardation should not be labeled as pessimistic; rather, it should be seen as a neutral reality against which the educability hypothesis must prove itself (see Chapter 1, this volume).

THE CONTINUUM
VERSUS THE TWO-GROUP THEORY

In the past, the biomedical assessment placed special emphasis on the developmental cutoff between mild and moderate mental retardation (Accardo & Caputo, 1994; Schaefer & Bodensteimer, 1992). This accurately reflected the clinical observation that, in the absence of obvious organic pathology—in the form of gross dysmorphology or severe neurologic damage—there would be a much higher yield of positive laboratory findings in those children whose IQs or DQs were below 50. In contrast, when the history and physical examination did not suggest specific diagnostic leads, an extensive laboratory investigation for the etiology of mental retardation in those children with DQs above 50

(i.e., in the range of mild mental retardation)—was frequently unrewarding. This clinical rule of thumb contributed to a misunderstanding of the "two-group theory" of mental retardation (Table 3). There seemed to be implicit acceptance of the fact that only people with the most severe retardation had an organic etiology and that the vast majority of people with mild retardation merely had sociocultural or cultural–familial retardation or deprivation. The possibility was allowed that this latter group might have a polygenetic etiology, but this was medically irrelevant because the heritability of intelligence in the normal population was not accepted (Zigler & Balla, 1982).

However, using an IQ of 50 as a cutoff for the selection of an assessment battery was never intended to support the interpretation of mild mental retardation as a nonorganic behavioral syndrome. Medically, the group with moderate to profound retardation traditionally yielded a high proportion (75%) of specific diagnostic etiologies (either brain localization or genetic metabolic syndromes) (Asthana, Sinha, Haslam, & Kingston, 1990), whereas the group with mild retardation yielded a low proportion of specific etiologies whenever a broad array of nonspecific tests was applied indiscriminately (the "shotgun" approach). Clinical, laboratory, and epidemiologic advances now suggest that more vigorous biomedical investigations are warranted even in the area of mild mental retardation (Al-Ansari, 1993; Lamont & Dennis, 1988). Fetal alcohol and fragile X syndromes are only two examples of relatively new and apparently common syndromes whose full impact on the incidence of mental retardation has yet to be defined. The complete mapping of the human

Table 3.   The two-group theory of mental retardation

	Mild retardation	Severe retardation
Incidence	2.5%	0.5%
Age at diagnosis	1–10 years	Birth–1 year
Stability of IQ	Fair	Very high
Familial occurrence	Common	Rare
Socioeconomic status/maternal education, IQ	Low	High
Genetic/metabolic syndrome/organ malformations	Very rare	Common
Seizures, neurologic complications, expanded Strauss syndrome	Infrequent	Common
Identifiable etiology	<50%	>75%

genome over the next several decades undoubtedly will expand the genetic contribution to the prevalence of mild mental retardation and even borderline intelligence.

The effect on the central nervous system of a variety of factors also supports a continuum of cognitive effects rather than the existence of two discrete groups. The two-group theory remains a positive contribution as a first approximation, but the more closely the population with mental retardation is investigated, the less tenable the approach appears. Pre- and postnatal toxins such as alcohol, lead, and radiation can cause severe mental retardation, mild mental retardation, and subtle disorders of learning and behavior in children with average intelligence. Although some risk factors, etiologies, and associated deficits vary with the level of mental retardation, there are benefits to be gained from viewing these conditions on a continuum. Not only people with mild retardation but also people with more severe retardation are continuous with the population without retardation. Learning disabilities occur in the population without retardation with a relatively high frequency. Almost everything that is known about brain factors influencing learning suggests that the same learning disability patterns—uneven cognitive development—should be at least as (if not more) common in the population with mental retardation and actually should increase in prevalence as IQ decreases. Nevertheless, almost all the research on the psychological differences between people with mild and people with severe retardation focuses on factors with homogeneous relationship to mental or chronologic age. The measures that show the least variance are assumed to be the most accurate descriptors of the group.

Children with average intelligence or retardation but similar mental ages often reach a given functional level by different pathways. Children with mental retardation and with similar mental ages reflect a variety of medical etiologies. Some are at the higher functional level for a given diagnosis while others will be at the lower level, usually because of the presence of associated deficits. Children with degenerative disease will be at a particular cognitive level only transiently. The association of given genetic syndromes with specific IQ ranges tends to minimize the (sometimes) extreme variability that occurs in practice. The behaviorist orientation that etiology and prognosis are irrelevant to diagnosis of mental retardation, which is simply a descriptor of current functional levels, assumes that the population without retardation is homogeneous and cedes many of the lessons students of each of these groups of children can learn from each other.

OUTCOME

With some exceptions (that relate to misdiagnosis and professional incompetence rather than a change in the condition itself), children with mental retardation grow up to be adults with mental retardation. On the one hand, the stability of IQ and the level of mental retardation is striking. On the other hand, as the child with mental retardation matures, social and personal interaction skills assume a greater importance in determining the degree of independence that can be assumed. Discrepancies between IQ and functional independence most often relate to the presence of associated deficits, and these in turn are influenced strongly by the specific medical syndrome.

For example, Prader-Willi syndrome is characterized by mental retardation, hypotonia, hyperphagia, obesity, and a deletion on the long arm of chromosome 15 (Cassidy, 1984; Greenswag & Alexander, 1988) (see also Chapter 16, this volume). Mild to moderate mental retardation is present in only two thirds of these cases, but severe learning disabilities are frequent in children with Prader-Willi syndrome without mental retardation. Adult outcome of this syndrome is not predictable by IQ alone. With regard to associated deficits, the syndrome can be divided into three stages. Stage one (infancy) presents with hypotonia, failure to thrive, and dysmorphic features. Stage two (from preschool to adolescence) exhibits uncontrollable hyperphagia, obesity, mental retardation, and learning disabilities. Stage three (adolescence) is characterized by increasingly severe behavior problems, excessive daytime somnolence, increased skin picking, perseverative and compulsive thought processes, and sexual identity issues (Whitman & Greenswag, 1995).

Two important lessons can be learned from Prader-Willi syndrome. First, a distinct behavioral pattern has been identified that has its onset at the upper limit of the pediatric age group. This leads one to question how many other late-developing stages exist in other less common syndromes. Second, this syndrome highlights the importance of associated deficits on into adulthood. Many adults with Prader-Willi syndrome and normal intelligence but continuing severe eating problems cannot live independently and function best in group homes.

The history of mental retardation in the 20th century has been a discontinuous movement toward normalization (Kanner, 1964). The most successful medical focus has been prevention (Crocker, 1992), with little in the way of genuine cure (Spitz, 1986). Increasing longevity (Eyman, Grossman, Chaney, & Call, 1993) is coupled with a reluctance on the part of society to fund medical care at the extremes of the life span. Increasing community placement without adequate support services has accelerated the development of a new series of problems. Women with mental retardation living in the community are having children and contributing significantly to the incidence of homeless families. Although few children of mothers who have mental retardation have retardation themselves, they are at high risk for deprivation, abuse, neglect, sexual abuse, developmental delay, language disorder, and failure to thrive

(Whitman & Accardo, 1993). Novel problems continue to challenge successful past solutions.

CONCLUSIONS

There is no single IQ or mental retardation label to which a child can or should be reduced; there are only quantitative and qualitative descriptors of strengths and weaknesses for children and adults with average intelligence or mental retardation. When we allow for the medical complications and associated deficits of various mental retardation syndromes, the predominant disability in mental retardation remains societal acceptance. The primary vehicle for achieving greater societal acceptance of people with mental retardation remains education—appropriate education for people with mental retardation and community education for people without mental retardation.

As a behavioral psychological and psychiatric diagnosis, mental retardation describes current functional deficits irrespective of past development and behavior and with no pretensions of predictive power. The medical model that interprets mental retardation as a brain damage syndrome can understand the functional deficit only in terms of past neurodevelopmental insult and progress, and in view of an urgent necessity for a prognosis of sufficient accuracy to allow for intelligent diagnostic and therapeutic choices. From this perspective, the developmental pediatrics approach would appear to be the only true genetic psychology.

REFERENCES

Accardo, P.J., & Capute, A.J. (1994). Mental retardation. In F.A. Oski, C.D. DeAngelis, R.D. Feigin, & F.B. Warshaw (Eds.), *Principles and practice of pediatrics* (pp. 673–679). Philadelphia: J.B. Lippincott.

Al-Ansari, A. (1993). Etiology of mild mental retardation among Bahraini children: A community-based case control study. *Mental Retardation, 31,* 140–143.

Asthana, J.C., Sinha, S., Haslam, J.S., & Kingston, H.M. (1990). Survey of adolescents with severe intellectual handicaps. *Archives of Disease in Childhood, 65,* 1133–1136.

Birch, H.G., Richardson, S.A., Baird, D., Horobin, G., & Illsley, R. (1970). *Mental subnormality in the community: A clinical and epidemiologic study.* Baltimore: Williams & Wilkins.

Blatt, B. (1987). *The conquest of mental retardation.* Austin, TX: PRO-ED.

Broman, S., Nicols, P.L., Shaughnessy, P., & Kennedy, W. (1987). *Retardation in young children: A developmental study of cognitive deficit.* Hillsdale, NJ: Lawrence Erlbaum Associates.

Brown, F.R., III, Greer, M.K., Aylward, E.H., & Hunt, H.H. (1990). Intellectual and adaptive functioning in Down syndrome in relation to age and environmental placement. *Pediatrics, 85,* 450–452.

Buyse, M.L. (1990). *Birth defects encyclopedia.* Dover, MA: Center for Birth Defects Information Services.

Cassidy, S.B. (1984). Prader-Willi syndrome. *Current Problems in Pediatrics, 14*, 1–55.

Cole, K.N., Dale, P.S., & Mills, P.E. (1992). Stability of the intelligence quotient–language quotient relations: Is discrepancy modeling based on a myth? *American Journal on Mental Retardation, 97*, 131–143.

Costeff, H., Cohen, B.E., & Weller, L.E. (1983). Biological factors in mild mental retardation. *Developmental Medicine and Child Neurology, 25*, 580–587.

Crocker, A.C. (Ed.). (1992). Symposium on prevention of mental retardation and related disabilities. *Mental Retardation, 30*, 303–369.

Ellis, D. (1986). *Sensory impairments in mentally handicapped people.* San Diego: College-Hill Press.

Eyman, R.K., Grossman, H.J., Chaney, R.H., & Call, T.L. (1993). Survival of profoundly disabled people with severe mental retardation. *American Journal of Diseases of Children, 147*, 329–336.

Greenswag, L.R., & Alexander, R.C. (Eds.). (1988). *Management of Prader-Willi syndrome.* New York: Springer-Verlag.

Hagberg, B., Hagberg, G., Lowerth, A., & Lindberg, U. (1981). Mild mental retardation in Swedish school children. II. Etiologic and pathogenetic aspects. *Acta Pediatrica Scandinavica, 70*, 445–452.

Jones, K.L. (1988). *Smith's recognizable patterns of human malformation.* Philadelphia: W.B. Saunders.

Kanner, L. (1964). *A history of the care and study of the mentally retarded.* Springfield, IL: Charles C Thomas.

Leviton, A., & Giles, F.H. (1984). Acquired perinatal leukoencephalopathy. *Annals of Neurology, 16*, 1–8.

Luckasson, R., Coulter, D.L., Polloway, E.A., Reiss, S., Schalock, R.L., Snell, M.G., Spitalnik, D.M., &

Stark, J.A. (1992). *Mental retardation: Definition, classification, and systems of supports* (9th ed.). Washington, DC: American Association on Mental Retardation.

MacMillan, D.L., Gresham, F.M., & Siperstein, G.N. (1993). Conceptual and psychometric consensus about the 1992 AAMR definition of mental retardation. *American Journal on Mental Retardation, 98*, 325–335.

O'Brien, G. (1992). Behavioral phenotypy in developmental psychiatry. *European Child and Adolescent Psychiatry, Supplement 1*, 1–61.

Rosen, M. (1993). In search of the behavioral phenotype: A methodological note. *Mental Retardation, 31*, 177–178.

Schaefer, G.B., & Bodensteimer, J.B. (1992). Evaluation of the child with idiopathic mental retardation. *Pediatric Clinics of North America, 39*, 929–943.

Spitz, H.H. (1986). *The raising of intelligence: A selected history of attempts to raise retarded intelligence.* Hillsdale, NJ: Lawrence Erlbaum Associates.

Whitman, B.Y., & Accardo, P.J. (1993). The parent with mental retardation: Rights, responsibilities and issues. *Journal of Social Work and Human Sexuality, 8*, 123–136.

Whitman, B.Y., & Greenswag, L. (1995). The psychological management of Prader-Willi syndrome. In L. Greenswag & L. Alexander (Eds.), *Management of Prader-Willi syndrome* (pp. 125–141). New York: Springer-Verlag.

Wiedemann, H.R., Kunze, J., Gross, F.R., & Dibbern, H. (1992). *An atlas of clinical syndromes.* St. Louis: Mosby–Year Book Medical Publishers.

Zigler, E., & Balla, D. (Eds.). (1982). *Mental retardation: The developmental-difference controversy.* Hillsdale, NJ: Lawrence Erlbaum Associates.

Chapter 15

Down Syndrome

Paul T. Rogers, M.D., Nancy J. Roizen, M.D., and
George T. Capone, M.D.

Down syndrome is the most common genetic cause of mental retardation and congenital malformation, and accounts for 25%–30% of persons with severe mental retardation (IQ < 50) worldwide (McLaren & Bryson, 1987). The birth of a child with Down syndrome is usually an unexpected event. Parents often turn to their child's pediatrician for both information and support. The child with Down syndrome presents a challenge because of numerous, complex medical problems intertwined with changing developmental needs. This chapter reviews selected information that is useful for understanding the genetic and neurobiologic basis for the mental retardation and associated neurodevelopment dysfunction in Down syndrome. We also present the major medical concerns and management strategies for a person with Down syndrome from birth to young adulthood. This chapter also presents methods to educate and assist parents through their child's life cycle.

HISTORICAL BACKGROUND

John Langdon Down, an Englishman, published the first clinical description of Down syndrome. While working in 1866 as superintendent of the Earlswood Asylum for Idiots, he described patients with similar Asiatic or "Mongolian" features in his classic article "Observations on an Ethnic Classification of Idiots." The term *mongolism* prevailed until the late 1960s. Objection to the term and its ethnic allusion led to the preferred use of the eponym Down syndrome. Early investigations attributed Down syndrome to maternal tuberculosis or hypothyroidism. In 1932, Waardenburg suggested that the syndrome was a consequence of a chromosomal abnormality. In 1959, Lejeune, Gautier, and

Turpin confirmed the presence of trisomy 21 chromosome abnormality in Down syndrome.

CYTOGENETICS

Down syndrome is a genetic disorder that occurs in approximately 1 in 800 live births. It is caused most often by an abnormality during cell division called nondysjunction (Hook, 1981). This abnormality occurs during the production of the sperm or egg cells. Because of nondysjunction, the egg (or, in some cases, the sperm cell) divides improperly and passes two chromosomes instead of one to each of the daughter cells. At fertilization, the zygote receives a third copy of chromosome 21, resulting in a total of 47 chromosomes rather than the normal complement of 46. The term *trisomy 21* refers to this extra chromosome 21 in addition to the two normally occurring chromosomes. Of all the causes of Down syndrome, trisomy occurs the most frequently, accounting for 93%–95% of all cases. Translocation, which occurs when an extra piece of chromosome 21 attaches to another chromosome (usually number 13, 14, 15, or 22), accounts for less than 5% of the children with Down syndrome. Trisomy 21 mosaicism is a mixture of trisomic and normal cells and accounts for about 2% of children with Down syndrome. Children who have mosaic Down syndrome may exhibit fewer of the physical characteristics of the syndrome and may function higher developmentally.

The rate of Down syndrome increases with maternal age by about 30% after the age of 30. Maternal age also relates to the type of chromosome abnormality. For example, translocation occurs 10% of the time in children born to mothers between 15 and 19 years of age. Whenever chromosome analysis reveals a transloca- tion, both parents should have chromosome analysis to check for a balanced translocation. If present, the risk is greatly increased for Down syndrome in later conceptions. The magnitude of the risk increase will depend on whether the mother or the father has the translocation, as well as the type of translocation. The increased risk of recurrence for parents who are not translocation carriers is about 1%–2%. All chil- dren suspected of having Down syndrome should have chromosome analysis because of the recurrence risk of translocation.

MOLECULAR GENETICS

Advances in molecular biology are furthering our understanding of the pathogenesis of Down syndrome. In Down syndrome, as in other tri- somic conditions, the developmental expression of normal genes present in triplicate results in altered patterns of development and ultimately abnormal morphology, physiologic function, or both (Epstein, 1990). Chromosome 21, one of the smallest human autosomes, contains ap- proximately 54 million base pairs of DNA and constitutes approximately 1.7% of the haploid human genome. Chromosome 21 is acrocentric, with two arms joined at its centromere close to one end. The short arm (21p) consists of the nu- cleolar organizer region, which contains multi- ple copies of genes coding for ribosomal RNA, and a more proximal region composed of highly repetitive DNA sequences. The genes on 21p do not appear to be essential for normal develop- ment because duplications or deletions in this region usually have few observable phenotypic manifestations. All of the other genes on chro- mosome 21 map to the long arm (21q). It is esti- mated that the long arm contains between 500 and 1,000 genes, many or all of which may con- tribute to the pathogenesis and phenotype of Down syndrome (Gardiner, 1990). Approxi- mately 30 genes of known function and over 100 unique DNA sequences of unknown signifi- cance have been mapped to the long arm (McKusick, 1994).

Advances in understanding the genes impli- cated in Down syndrome are due, in part, to technological advances during the past decade

that have allowed researchers to isolate and clone genes and construct detailed maps of chromosome 21. Several types of maps have been developed. *Physical maps* convey infor- mation about gene location relative to subre- gions of the chromosome as defined by tradi- tional cytogenetic banding (Watkins, Tanzi, Cheng, & Gosella, 1987). Using techniques such as fluorescent in situ hybridization using labeled DNA probes or by direct measurement of gene dosage, it has become possible to map genes and anonymous DNA sequences to spe- cific subregions of the chromosome (Koren- berg, 1993) (Figure 1). *Genetic maps* convey in- formation about the order and distance between genes and their linkage relationships (Haines et al., 1993; Warren, Slaugenhaupt, Lewis, Chakravarti, & Antonarakis, 1989). Linkage in-

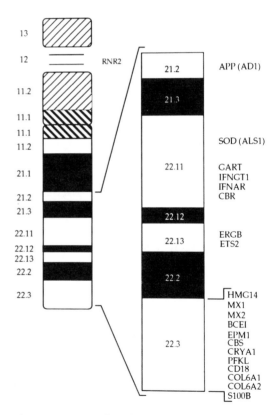

Figure 1. Regional assignment of genes to chromo- some 21. (From Korenberg, J.R. [1993]. Toward a mo- lecular understanding of Down syndrome. In C. Epstein [Ed.], *The phenotypic mapping of Down syndrome and other aneuploid conditions*, p. 94. New York: Wiley- Liss. Copyright ©1993 by Wiley-Liss. Reprinted by per- mission of John Wiley & Sons.)

formation is derived from the analysis of recombination frequency between sister chromatids during meiosis and is influenced by such factors as age and sex (Tanzi, Haines, & Gosella, 1990). A map composed of continuous units of overlapping sequences of cloned DNA covering the entire long arm has been reported (Chumakov et al., 1992). These *contig maps* are constructed from relatively large pieces of DNA (100–2,000 kb) and provide information not readily obtained from either physical or genetic maps. One major advantage of contig maps is that they provide an ordered set of markers that can be stored as sequence information on a computer data base. Newly isolated genes from 21q then can be assigned to a specific genomic segment once that gene has been localized by linkage or cytogenetic methods. This strategy will greatly enhance efforts to identify new genes and derive sequence data for the entire long arm.

In an attempt to assign the individual phenotypic features of Down syndrome to specific subregions of the chromosome, investigators have started to construct a fourth type of map. *Phenotypic maps* are constructed using DNA from individuals with rare partial duplications of 21q (partial trisomy) and correlating this cytogenetic information with clinical phenotype. The conceptual basis for phenotypic mapping of conditions resulting from aneuploidy has been advanced by Epstein (1990). The most important a priori assumption is that the phenotype of any aneuploid condition results from the abnormal number of gene copies present on the unbalanced chromosome, and that specific components of the phenotype are attributable to imbalance of specific genes. Thus, in trisomy 21 the phenotype is a direct consequence of gene dosage imbalance of specific genes on chromosome 21, which are present in three copies. The existence of a minimal or "critical region" on 21q that is responsible for most of the physical features of the Down syndrome phenotype also has been advanced (Epstein, 1990; Korenberg et al., 1990). As studies of genotype–phenotype correlation have progressed, the available evidence supports the concept that each of the specific phenotypic features commonly seen in Down syndrome may be associated with a critical region or gene cluster along 21q. Many of the nonspecific features of Down syndrome, however, may be less amenable to phenotypic mapping. The most currently published phenotypic map shows 26 commonly observed features of Down syndrome and their approximate location on chromosome 21 (Figure 2). Notice that the segments of chromosome 21 that contribute to the nonspecific features of the phenotype (mental retardation, microcephaly, and hypotonia) are widely distributed along 21q. In comparison, the chromosomal segment responsible for congenital heart disease (CHD) is more localized, mapping distal to band q22.12. A gene cluster within the distal portion of band q22 is proposed to constitute the critical region for the expression of CHD in Down syndrome (Korenberg, 1993). It may be concluded, then, that a relatively large number of genes (or gene combinations) on chromosome 21, when present in triplicate, can result in mental retardation and microcephaly, whereas CHD may result from triplication of one or only a small number of genes.

NEUROBIOLOGY

Trisomy 21 as the cause of Down syndrome has been recognized since 1959 (Lejeune et al., 1959). However, our understanding of how an extra copy of chromosome 21 leads to the development of microcephaly, mental retardation, hypotonia, and other neurodevelopmental sequelae remains poorly understood. The effects of gene dosage imbalance on the normal cellular, molecular, and biochemical processes that regulate neuronal proliferation, migration, differentiation, and organization will continue to be an active area of research for the future.

Developmental Neuropathology

The neurobiologic sequelae of trisomy 21 include a variety of morphologic and histopathologic alterations. No single finding, however, is pathognomic for Down syndrome, because many of these alterations are seen in the brains of individuals with other mental retardation/major congenital anomaly syndromes. Additionally, no single individual with Down syndrome will necessarily demonstrate all of these changes to the same degree.

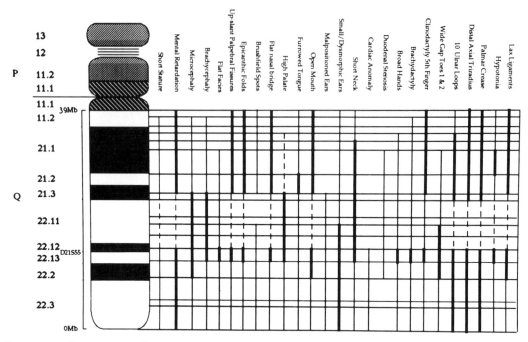

Figure 2. A phenotypic map of trisomy 21, based on the clinical and molecular analysis of 16 individuals with partial trisomy 21 and no other significant aneuploidy. Note the various sizes for 26 common phenotypic features of varying specificity. Thick lines indicate minimal regions, thin lines indicate maximal regions, dashed lines indicate a subset of maximal regions that are not within the region of minimal overlap, and open spaces indicate regions whose duplication has not been associated with a given phenotype. (From Korenberg, J.R. [1993]. Toward a molecular understanding of Down syndrome. In C. Epstein [Ed.], *The phenotypic mapping of Down syndrome and other aneuploid conditions*, p. 104. New York: Wiley-Liss. Copyright ©1993 by Wiley-Liss. Reprinted by permission of John Wiley & Sons.)

The Down syndrome brain is said to have a characteristic morphologic appearance, which permits it to be easily identified at autopsy. Decreased size and weight with foreshortening of the anterior–posterior diameter, flattening of the occiput, and a narrow superior temporal gyrus are most characteristic. Primary cortical gyri may appear wide while secondary gyri are often poorly developed or absent, with shallow sulci (Davidoff, 1928). The cerebellum and brain stem frequently are noted to be markedly reduced in size compared to forebrain structures (Crome, Cowie, & Slater, 1966).

Brain growth during the first half of gestation does not appear to be markedly different in fetuses with Down syndrome (Schmidt-Sidor, Wisniewski, Shepard, & Sersen, 1990). Commonly, the rate of brain growth is normal up to 5 or 6 months postnatally before decelerating later in the first year of life (Palmer et al., 1992). Hypoplasia of the brian is probably best reflected by changes in head growth during the first year

of life. Detailed neuropathologic studies reveal generalized hypocellularity of the brain. Reductions in neuronal number and neuronal density have also been demonstrated for most regions examined (Wisniewski, Laure-Kamionowska, Connell, & Wen, 1986). In the cerebral cortex, there are reductions in neuronal number in all cortical layers, with a striking paucity of small interneurons from cortical layers II and IV (Ross, Galaburda, & Kemper, 1984). These interneurons use the neurotransmitter γ-aminobutyric acid and provide the primary inhibitory influence to the pyramidal cells of the cerebral cortex. Reductions in this interneuron cell population may have particular significance for understanding the co-occurrence of seizures in individuals with Down syndrome (Stafstrom, 1993). Additionally, these interneurons are thought to play a critical role in the higher order information-processing capabilities of the cerebral cortex. The actual percentage reduction of interneurons, which probably differs among individuals, may explain in part the variability of cognitive impairment seen in persons with Down syndrome. Ultrastructural studies of pyramidal neurons from the cerebral cortex reveal abnormalities of dendritic arborization and reduced numbers of postsynaptic spines (Becker, Armstrong, & Chan, 1986; Marin-Padilla, 1976; Suetsugu & Mehraein, 1980). Surviving spines are often abnormally long, thin, or irregular in contour and appearance (Marin-Padilla, 1972). As would be predicted, reductions in synaptic density and synaptic surface area are also present (Wisniewski et al., 1986). Such reductions with accompanying alterations of spine morphology almost certainly result in dysfunctional electrochemical signaling in the cerebral cortex and further contribute to the cognitive and neuromotor impairments observed in children with Down syndrome.

Delays in myelination are also commonly observed in Down syndrome (Wisniewski & Schmidt-Sidor, 1989). During the first year of life, decreased myelination is observed throughout the cerebral hemispheres, basal ganglia, cerebellum, and brain stem. After the first year, myelination delays affect primarily those fiber tracts with a late beginning and slow myelination cycle. The intercortical fibers and U fibers of the frontal and temporal cortices are especially vulnerable.

Neuropathology and Aging

Several important age-related changes in the brain have been described in association with Down syndrome. Basal ganglia calcification (BGC) has been described in several reports (Takashima & Becker, 1985; Wisniewski et al., 1982). Typically, the globus pallidus and putamen are affected. Massive calcium deposition in the brain parenchyma is most frequently observed in those children with Down syndrome who die during the first decade of life. Those surviving beyond this period and into the fourth decade usually show perivascular calcium deposition in and around the vessel walls themselves. Using computerized tomography (CT), Wisniewski demonstrated that 27% of individuals with Down syndrome of various ages showed BGC. None of these individuals had any clinical evidence of movement disorder or

dysfunction of serum calcium homeostasis, parathyroid hormone secretion, or vitamin D regulation. In contrast, 100% of postmortem Down syndrome brains showed histopathologic evidence of BCG. Interestingly, only 11% of these postmortem brains showed evidence of BCG when evaluated by CT scan prior to autopsy. Thus, BCG seems to be a universal finding in all individuals with Down syndrome, the pathogenesis and clinical significance of which remain obscure.

The neuropathologic stigmata of Alzheimer's disease is another universal finding in Down syndrome. All persons with Down syndrome develop senile plaques, neurofibrillary tangles, and granovacuolar bodies, which is virtually identical to the Alzheimer's pathology seen in the general population (Burger & Vogel, 1973; Ellis, McCulloch, & Corely, 1974). Senile plaques are composed of extracellular deposits of amyloid protein fragments (β-amyloid), as well as remnants of degenerating neuronal perikarya. Neurofibrillary tangles are composed of the hyperphosphorylated cytoskeletal protein *Tau*, which forms precipitates intracellularly with a characteristic paired-helical configuration. Granovacuolar bodies consist of clear areas of vacuolization containing clusters of dense, granular material within the neuronal perikaryon. Alzheimer-type neuropathologic changes are most pronounced throughout the cerebral cortex and limbic structures. Autopsy studies have convincingly demonstrated that senile plaques and neurofibrillary tangles are present in all individuals with Down syndrome by the fourth decade of life (Wisniewski, Wisniewski, & Wen, 1985), with some individuals showing a much earlier onset (Rumble et al., 1989; Wisniewski et al., 1985).

In addition to histopathologic similarities between Alzheimer's disease and aged persons with Down syndrome, a similar pattern of neurochemical deficits is seen. Presynaptic markers for cholinergic, noradrenergic, and serotonergic markers are all reduced in the brains of aged individuals with Down syndrome (Godridge, Renyolds, Czudek, Calcutt, & Benton, 1987; Yates et al., 1983). These neurochemical changes appear to be caused by degeneration and cell loss of the cortical projection neurons arising from the nucleus basalis of Meynert (cholinergic), locus ceruleus (noradrenergic), and dorsal raphe nuclei (serotonergic). Progressive degeneration and loss of neurons from these nuclei is associated with the appearance of senile plaques and neurofibrillary tangles within the cerebral cortex and hippocampus (Mann, Yates, & Marcyniuk, 1984).

Central Nervous System Gene Expression

It is believed that one third to one half of the estimated 100,000 genes in the human genome contribute to the development or function, or both, of the central nervous system (CNS). Accordingly, between 330 and 500 of the estimated 1,000 genes that map to the long arm of chromosome 21 would be expressed in the CNS. In trisomy 21, these genes are all present in an extra copy resulting in dosage imbalance. Theoretically, one extra copy of each of these genes should lead to a 50% increase in messenger RNA (mRNA) and gene product (protein). It is not understood currently whether increased intracellular concentrations of mRNA or protein can exert a primary effect on development events directly or whether these excess products initiate a cascade of secondary and tertiary responses that are then manifested as abnormal development. The developmental consequences of increased gene dosage probably depend, in part, on the biologic function of the gene product itself (e.g., enzyme, structural protein, transcription factor, receptor subunit), as overexpression of certain proteins is more likely to result in disturbance(s) of the major developmental events that occur during brain development (see Chapter 2, Volume I).

Of the approximately 30 known genes that map to chromosome 21, at least 12 appear to have some role in the nervous system (Table 1). A number of these genes have been particularly well characterized and have been implicated in the neuropathogenesis of Down syndrome.

Amyloid Precursor Protein   The gene for amyloid precursor protein (APP) maps to band 21.2. Mutations in the APP gene are associated with some cases of familial Alzheimer's disease, as well as one form (Dutch type) of cerebral amyloid angiopathy (Clark & Goate, 1993). The APP gene codes for a large transmembrane protein expressed in both neurons and astrocytes. Although the function of APP is not precisely known, various fragments are associated with cellular adhesion, neuronal outgrowth, neurotoxicity, and serine protease inhibition (Hardy & Allsop, 1991). APP expression is regulated during CNS development and has been found to be overexpressed in the brain in at least one fetus with Down syndrome (Neve, Finch, & Dawes, 1988). It is not currently known if overexpression of APP by itself can result in significant impairment in CNS development. The small 42-amino-acid fragment of APP, referred to as the β-amyloid protein (βAP) is found in the senile plaques associated with Alzheimer's disease and the Alzheimer-type pathology observed in Down syndrome. It is hypothesized that overexpression of APP leading to increased βAP formation is a central event in the development of Alzheimer-type pathology in Down syndrome (Hardy & Allsop, 1991; Rumble et al., 1989). Improved understanding of APP synthesis, as well as the formation of βAP and its subsequent metabolism, should provide new insights into the mechanism of precocious βAP deposition in persons with Down syndrome.

Superoxide Dismutase   The gene for superoxide dismutase–1 (SOD-1) maps to band 22.1. Mutation of SOD-1 is associated with a familial form of amyotrophic lateral sclerosis (Deng et al., 1993). SOD-1 is a cytoplasmic enzyme that catalyzes the dismutation of superoxide radicals $(O_2 \cdot^-)$, a product of normal oxidative metabolism, to produce hydrogen peroxide (H_2O_2) (Sinet, 1982). Generally, SOD-1 is regarded as a protective enzyme, but under certain conditions it may prove detrimental. The H_2O_2 generated by SOD-1 action is itself toxic and may, in combination with $O_2 \cdot^-$, form the highly toxic hydroxyl radical $(OH \cdot)$, with resultant cellular damage. $OH \cdot$ can cause peroxidation of lipid membranes as well as direct damage to proteins and DNA molecules. SOD-1 activity has been demonstrated in a variety of tissues, including the brain, where it is expressed in both neurons and glia (Takashima et al., 1990). A gene dosage effect for SOD-1 has been documented in Down syndrome. Elevations in SOD-1 activity and increased lipoperoxidation are observed in the Down syndrome brain as early as 15–25 weeks'

Table 1. Genes mapped to chromosome 21

Symbol	Location on chromosome	Name
AABT	Unknown	β-Amino acid renal transport
AML1	q22	Acute myeloid leukemia oncogene
APP	q21.3-22.05	Amyloid β precursor protein
ASNSL2	Unknown	Asparagine synthetase–like 2
BAS	Unknown	β-Adrenergic response
BCEI	q22.3	Breast cancer, estrogen inducible sequence
CBR	Unknown	Carbonyl reductase
CBS	q22.3	Cystathionine-β-synthetase
CD18	q22.3	Integrin (antigen CD18)
COLA6A1	q22.3	Collagen, type VI α 1
COLA6A2	q22.3	Collagen, type VI α 2
COLA18A1	q22.3	Collagen, type XVIII, α 1
CRFB4	q22.1	Cytokine receptor, family II
CRYA1	q22.3	Crystallin, α-polypeptide 1
EPM1	q22.3	Epilepsy, progressive myoclonic 1
ERG	q22.3	Avian erythroblastosis virus E26 oncogene
ETS2	q22.3	Avian erythroblastosis virus E26 oncogene homolog 2
GART	q22.1	Phosphoribosylglycinamide formyltransferase
		Phosphoribosylglycinamide synthetase
		Phosphoribosylaminoimidazole synthetase
GLUR5	q21.1-22.1	Glutamate receptor, subunit 5
GPXP2	Unknown	Glutathione peroxidase pseudogene 2
HMG14	q22.3	Nonhistone chromosomal protein HMG-14
HSPA3	Unknown	Heat shock 70-kD protein 3
HTOR	Unknown	5-Hydroxytryptamine oxygenase regulator
IFNAR	q22.1	Interferon, α receptor
IFNGT1	q22.1-22.2	Interferon, γ transducer 1
KCNE1	Unknown	Potassium voltage-gated channel
MACSL1	Unknown	Myristoyrated alanine-rich protein kinase 1 substrate
MST	q11.2	Myeloproliferative syndrome, transient
MX1,2	q22.3	Myxovirus (influenza) resistance 1 and 2
PKFL	q22.3	Phosphofructokinase, liver type
RNR4	p12	Ribosomal RNA-4
S14	Unknown	Surface antigen (chromosome 21)
S100B	q22.2-22.3	S100 protein, β subunit
SOD1	q22.1	Cu/Zn superoxide dismutase, soluble form
SML1	q22.3	Spasmolytic protein–1
VDAC2	Unknown	Voltage-dependent anion channel

Adapted from McKusick (1994).

gestation (Brooksbank & Balazs, 1984). Alterations in the antioxidant system have also been hypothesized to play a role in the Alzheimer-type pathology observed in Down syndrome. Interestingly, adults with Down syndrome and Alzheimer-type pathology have significantly lower SOD-1 activity in erythrocytes compared to age-matched controls with Down syndrome without Alzheimer-type pathology (Percy et al., 1990). The neurobiologic manifestations of ele-

vated SOD-1 activity, and therapeutic strategies to counter the effects of disturbances in antioxidant diffuse mechanisms in Down syndrome, will continue to be an important and active area of research (Dickinson & Singh, 1993).

S100 Protein   The gene for the S100 protein (β-subunit) maps to band 22.3. S100 is a low-molecular-weight, dimeric, calcium-binding protein implicated in the signal transduction pathways that regulate the cell cycle and neuronal differentiation (Kligman & Hilt, 1988). Levels of S100 are especially high in nervous tissue. In the brain, the β subunit is found primarily in glial cytoplasm, although large amounts also are secreted extracellularly. In cultured cells, β S100 possesses neurotrophic properties (Kligman & Hsieh, 1987). S100 protein is detectable in the human brain by about 10 weeks' gestation, and levels increase in specific regions concomitant with advancing maturation (Zuckerman, Herschman, & Levine, 1970). Elevated levels of S100 protein and increased numbers of S100 immunopositive astrocytes have been detected in the Down syndrome brain. Although the significance of these findings is unclear, a role for β S100 has been proposed in the pathogenesis of mental retardation and the Alzheimer-type pathology seen in Down syndrome (Griffin et al., 1989; Jorgensen, Brooksbank, & Balazs, 1990; Mito & Becker, 1993).

Future Directions in Research   The task of isolating and mapping the genes on the 21st chromosome is still in its earliest stages. As improved methods of DNA analysis become available, this process will accelerate significantly (Casey, 1993). These efforts, however painstaking, represent the most rational starting point for understanding the pathogenesis of Down syndrome. Since the mid-1980s, it has become apparent that a small portion of mouse chromosome 16 shares genetic homology with human chromosome 21. Thus there now exist several animal models that can be used to understand the genetic basis for the Down syndrome phenotype (Davisson et al., 1993; Reeves, Gearhart, & Littlefield, 1986). Mice that are either wholly or partially trisomic for chromosome 16 have proven especially promising in studies describing the developmental consequences of gene dosage imbalance as it relates to the brain (Bendotti et al., 1988; Capone, Bendotti, Oster-Granite, & Coyle, 1991; Coyle et al., 1991).

CLINICAL MANAGEMENT: A LIFE CYCLE APPROACH

Birth

Diagnosis   Specific dysmorphic features usually bring the possibility of the diagnosis of Down syndrome to the attention of the clini-

cian. A clinical diagnosis of Down syndrome, can be complicated by the fact that a newborn may have fewer of the distinguishing stigmata than generally found in older children. The principle physical findings in the newborn with Down syndrome, as described by Hall (1966), are listed in Table 2. At least four of these abnormalities were present in all of the 48 newborns studied. A pelvic radiograph demonstrates a reduced iliac index (the angle between the acetabular and the iliac angles) in 80% of newborns with Down syndrome.

Informing the Parents   Although the diagnosis will need to be confirmed by chromosome analysis, after a complete examination, the clinician can be reasonably confident of the diagnosis and should present the information to the parents.

The manner in which the clinician presents the diagnosis of Down syndrome to the parents is critical and will be remembered by the parents for a long time. The clinician should display tact, truthfulness, sympathy, and hope. Some guidelines for informing the parents are provided in Table 3. The clinician should provide the parents with the names of other families with children with Down syndrome or refer them to parent support organizations. Other families often provide support as well as information about community resources. The clinician should refer the family to an early intervention program and encourage them to enroll but stress the importance of the family taking time to adjust to the new baby with Down syndrome. Information about national organizations that can provide support as well as educational in-

Table 2.   Clinical signs associated with Down syndrome

Hypotonia
Poor Moro reflex
Hyperflexibility of joints
Flat facial profile
Slanted palpebral fissures
Anomalous auricles
Dysplasia of pelvis
Dysplasia of midphalanx of fifth finger
Simian crease
Excess skin on back of neck

Adapted from Hall (1966).

Table 3. Suggestions for informing parents of a diagnosis of Down syndrome

Have both parents present or mother with a supportive person.

Have the baby present and point out the positive physical findings.

Discuss diagnosis with the parents within the first 24 hours in a private setting.

Adopt a direct, honest, hopeful, and unrushed manner.

Discuss specific implications of diagnosis for the child.

Discuss specific ways the parents can facilitate their child's developmental outcome.

Provide information about community resources and programs.

Provide relevant reading material.

Provide names of other parents with a child with Down syndrome.

Suggest ways in which to share the diagnosis with friends and relatives.

Provide the opportunity for return visits for further discussions and questions.

Table 4. Pediatric management of the newborn with Down syndrome

Perform chromosome analysis.

Provide genetic counseling.

Screen for cataracts.

Screen for thyroid dysfunction.

Assess cardiac function.

Perform complete physical examination to detect congenital anomalies.

Provide parent education and support.

formation to families also should be provided (see Appendix).

Medical Problems   The pediatric management of the newborn with Down syndrome is summarized in Table 4.

Congenital Heart Disease and Pulmonary Hypertension   Congenital heart disease (CHD) occurs in 40%–60% of children with Down syndrome. CHD in Down syndrome consists mainly of the following five defects: atrial–ventricular canal defect (51%), ventricular septal defect (28%), atrial septal defect (11%), tetralogy of Fallot (7%), and patent ductus arteriosus (2%). Pulmonary artery hypertension with rapid progression to irreversible vascular disease frequently complicates CHD in Down syndrome. The increased incidence of pulmonary artery hypertension is related, in part, to the high incidence of left-to-right shunts and also may be related to chronic upper airway disease.

Children with Down syndrome and severe CHD exhibit reduced growth velocity and weight, increased hypotonia, and greater gross motor delay, as well as reduced life expectancy, compared to the child with Down syndrome without CHD. CHD accounts for 30%–35% of the deaths in Down syndrome. The 1-year expected survival rate for those children with CHD is 76.3%, compared to 90% for those without heart disease.

To identify CHD and to avoid complications of irreversible pulmonary vascular obstructive disease, newborns with Down syndrome should have a complete cardiac assessment, including an echocardiogram and pediatric cardiology consultation. A serious cardiac defect may be present in the absence of a murmur, and the majority of CHD in children with Down syndrome is acyanotic.

Gastrointestinal Malformations   In Down syndrome, congenital malformations of the gastrointestinal tract usually present in the newborn period with symptoms of bowel obstruction, such as vomiting and abdominal distention. Gastrointestinal malformations are identified in 5% of children with Down syndrome and include most frequently duodenal atresia or stenosis (2.4%), imperforate anus (1%), aganglionic megacolon or Hirschsprung disease (0.5%), tracheoesophageal fistula (0.4%), and pyloric stenosis (0.3%). Although many of these malformations present in the neonatal period with symptoms of bowel obstruction, a partial obstruction can occur later in life. Aganglionic megacolon is associated with congenital anomalies in 77% of cases and should be considered in any child with Down syndrome whose constipation is unresponsive to conventional therapy. Children with pull-through operations for aganglionic megacolon generally develop satisfactory continence.

Newborns with Down syndrome are more likely to have neonatal jaundice. One study reported that 71% of newborns with Down syndrome had elevated serum bilirubin levels, compared to only 4% of infants without Down syndrome.

Growth   Children with Down syndrome tend to have slow initial weight gain and must have their growth plotted on a growth chart specific for children with Down syndrome. Several factors can contribute to this poor weight gain, including low caloric intake as a result of weak suck and slow feeding, difficulty with breast feeding, and extra caloric requirements resulting from CHD. Infants with poor weight gain as a result of ineffective feeding may be helped by a consultation with an infant feeding specialist, such as an occupational therapist or speech pathologist.

Ophthalmologic Problems   Ophthalmologic minor malformations and functional disorders occur frequently in children with Down syndrome. The most frequent ophthalmologic malformations include almond-shaped palpebral fissures (58%); an oblique slant to the palpebral fissures (62%); and Brushfield spots (50%), which are of nonfunctional significance. In the neonatal period, the most important ophthalmologic disorder to identify is congenital cataracts, which are found in 3% of children with Down syndrome and may present with absence or distortion of a red reflex. Any suspicion of a congenital cataract is sufficient cause for immediate referral to a pediatric ophthalmologist.

Laboratory Studies   All children suspected of having Down syndrome should have chromosomal analysis to confirm the diagnosis, rule out other syndromes, and help assess recurrence risk by determining if a translocation is present. A medical genetics consultation can be helpful in discussing the recurrence risk and genetic basis of Down syndrome. Because the incidence in newborns with Down syndrome of persistent primary congenital hypothyroidism is 0.7% and that of transient congenital hypothyroidism is 0.3%, neonatal hypothyroid screening is indicated.

1–12 Months

The pediatric management of the 1- to 12-month-old infant with Down syndrome is summarized in Table 5.

Medical Problems

Audiology   Between 60% and 80% of children with Down syndrome have hearing loss. The loss may be conductive, sensorineural, or mixed. Conductive hearing loss can be due to middle ear fluid or abnormalities of the ossicular chain. Because of the high incidence of hear-

Table 5.   Pediatric management of the 1- to 12-month-old infant with Down syndrome

Reassess for cardiac problems.

Assess hearing by ABR test.

Assess vision (by a pediatric ophthalmologist if possible).

Monitor growth.

Continue to provide parent support and education.

Refer to an early intervention program.

ing loss and difficulty in obtaining reliable responses to behavioral testing, all children with Down syndrome should have an auditory brain stem response (ABR) test conducted in the first 6 months. Based on the results of the ABR, management of a hearing loss may include antibiotic therapy, placement of ventilation tubes in the middle ear, and/or amplification. Because of the high incidence of hearing loss, all children with Down syndrome should have an annual evaluation of their hearing until 3 years of age and then every other year thereafter.

Growth   A growth chart developed for children with Down syndrome can be used to monitor growth (Cronk, Crocker, & Pueschel, 1988). Growth failure requires an evaluation for congenital malformations of the heart, gastrointestinal malabsorption (specifically, celiac disease), an endocrinopathy such as hypothyroidism, and gastroesophageal reflux. A pediatric nutritional assessment may be helpful to diagnose low calorie intake and to plan dietary management. All children with Down syndrome require growth monitoring because they may be underweight for their height in infancy.

Infections   Children with Down syndrome are susceptible to upper and lower respiratory infections that cause significant morbidity and mortality. Children with Down syndrome have anatomic, cardiac, and immunologic factors that make them prone to infections. Otitis media, pneumonias, and sinus infections are common in children with Down syndrome and must be diagnosed and treated promptly. In addition to the usual treatment regimen for an infection, the child with Down syndrome and a chronic infection may need management that includes 1) switching the infant to a home-based education program during peak incidence of upper respiratory infections to decrease contact with infected infants, 2) using prophylactic antibiotics when upper respiratory infections are epidemic in the community, and 3) immunizing older children with Pneumovax and an influenza vaccine.

Ophthalmic Problems Thirty-five percent of infants with Down syndrome have an ophthalmic disorder that requires treatment or monitoring. All infants with Down syndrome should have an evaluation by a pediatric ophthalmologist within the first 6 months of life, with the evaluation occurring earlier if they have signs or symptoms of an ophthalmic disorder. Strabismus occurs in 23%–44% of children with Down syndrome and is most frequently an accommodative esotropia. Although strabismus occurs commonly in children with Down syndrome, amblyopia is reported in less than 10% of the children with strabismus. Nystagmus occurs in about 15% of children with Down syndrome and can be secondary to central nervous lesions, lens opacities, or refractive errors, although typically the nystagmus is unrelated to pathology. Nystagmus may be part of the symptom complex of spasmus nutans, a benign disorder with onset in infancy that also includes head tilt and head nodding. Blepharitis, a chronic condition that is typically first symptomatic in infancy, is diagnosed in 36% of people with Down syndrome. Rubbing the eyes with blepharitis may contribute to the development of keratoconus in the teenage and adult years. Vigorous treatment of the blepharitis is important to prevent the rubbing of the eyes. Blocked tear ducts are found in about 20% of infants with Down syndrome. Primary infantile glaucoma is rare but considerably more frequent in infants with Down syndrome than in the general population. Signs and symptoms of infantile glaucoma (tearing, blepharospasm, and photophobia) should prompt a referral to a pediatric ophthalmologist for treatment before serious visual impairment occurs.

Orthopedic Problems Although congenital dislocation of the hips does not appear to be more prevalent in newborns with Down syndrome, the hips are hypermobile and may be dislocated at 2 months to 10 years of age.

Seizure Disorders As many as 5% of children with Down syndrome less than 1 year of age may develop infantile spasms. Fortunately,

children with Down syndrome and infantile spasms may respond favorably to treatment with adrenocorticotropic hormone and maintain developmental progress similar to that prior to onset of seizures.

Development Virtually all children with Down syndrome manifest neuromotor dysfunction (hypotonia, hyporeflexia, and reduced primitive reflexes) and gross motor delays during the first year of life. However, there is considerable variation in the attainment of early motor milestones in children with this condition (Zausmer & Shea, 1984). Several factors have been implicated as sources of variability in the attainment of early motor milestones, including home versus institutional rearing (Centerwall & Centerwall, 1960); associated medical conditions, especially severe CHD (Yessayan & Pueschel, 1984); seizures (Stafstrom & Konkol, 1994); severity of hypotonia (Yessayan & Pueschel, 1984); and delayed sensorimotor reaction times (Anwar, 1981). Of all these factors, degree of hypotonia appears to be the most studied, and the best predictor of later motor skill attainment (Reed, Pueschel, Schnell, & Cronk, 1984). The presence of serious CHD is thought to exert its negative impact on motor skill acquisition by further decreasing muscular tone. Muscle tone, which is often defined as the slight tension that offers a steady resistance to passive stretching, is largely influenced by the functional integrity of the brain, spinal cord, and peripheral nerves. Dygenesis of the cerebral cortex and cerebellum, as well as delays in myelination during the first few years of life, probably constitute the primary neurobiologic substrate of hypotonia and neuromotor dysfunction in children with Down syndrome. The organization and functional integrity of these structures are themselves determined by both genetic and epigenetic developmental factors, which may also represent a significant source of individual variability.

Delays in early prelinguistic language and visual-perceptual milestones are usually apparent by the end of the first year. Unlike gross motor milestones, delays in these areas often go unnoticed by parents and professionals, who may tend to focus more on motor skill achievement during the first year of life.

Supporting the Family   As the family begins to adjust and is able to formulate more specific questions, the clinician should review with the parents all the medical information. The clinician should offer to meet with concerned extended family members, such as grandparents and siblings, to discuss medical information and answer questions. Parents with particularly strong or longstanding feelings of anger, guilt, or depression should be referred for supportive counseling (see Chapter 26, Volume I). Occasionally, adoption is necessary for the child when the family is unable to cope.

Early Intervention   Early intervention services attempt to maximize the developmental potential of children with Down syndrome. By the second month of life, the early intervention program should evaluate the family and child. Depending on the model of the individual program, early intervention therapies may include infant education, speech and language therapy, occupational therapy, and physical therapy. In the first year of life, the individual therapists monitor the infant's development, set therapeutic goals, and plan an intervention program that will facilitate the accomplishment of these goals. Intervention goals for the young infant include educating and supporting the family as well as working directly with the child. The therapist who manages feeding programs should work with those infants who exhibit poor suck and swallow, tongue protrusion, and chewing difficulties. A feeding therapist can assist in the management of an infant who refuses an advance in the texture of the diet or certain foods.

Controversial Therapies   Parents of children with Down syndrome may become frustrated with the lack of a cure, the incomplete success of educational interventions, and the chronic nature of the disorder. Parents frequently will hear about nontraditional interventions and want information about the efficacy of these interventions. The parents will appreciate it if the clinician presents a balanced view of nontraditional therapies for children with Down syndrome.

Controversial therapies often have several shared characteristics, which include a theoretical basis not completely consistent with modern scientific knowledge; a claim of effectiveness for a broad range of problems; the use of "natural" substances, dietary therapy, exercise, and simple manipulations; a treatment with no adverse side effects; data not presented in peer-reviewed journals; and lay organizations that develop and support the use of the treatment (see Chapter 33, Volume I). Controversial therapies used in children with Down syndrome include megavitamins, cell therapy, and patterning.

Megavitamin, or orthomolecular, therapy attributes mental retardation to a congenital lack of trace minerals and vitamins, and advocates replacement with large doses of vitamins to correct the mental retardation. The initial study of megavitamin therapy was flawed by small sample size and unfounded by the use of thyroid hormone. Several follow-up studies that were better designed did not replicate the results. The American Academy of Pediatrics Committee on Nutrition (1993) has concluded, based on the lack of scientific evidence, that the unselected administration of megavitamins to all children with mental retardation is not warranted.

Cell therapy consists of implantation or injection of fetal sheep brain cells (produced by Cybila under the brand name "Sicca Cell") and reportedly activates brain growth, improves intelligence, and reduces the frequency of infections. Cell therapy is not licensed by the Food and Drug Administration, but some parents travel to Canada or Germany for this hazardous therapy. Potential problems include foreign body reaction as well as acquisition of a slow virus. Beneficial effects have not been proved.

Patterning, or the Doman-Delacato treatment, consists of a dominating and inflexible regimen of flash cards and patterned movements developed by the Institute for Achievement of Human Potential. Advocates of patterning assert that less than 100% effort is cause for failure of the treatment. Critics of patterning express concern about the restrictions placed on age-appropriate activities and the responsibility for lack of success being placed on the parents' lack of rigor in pursuing the regimen. Successful outcomes of patterning are frequent in children who have sustained an acute insult to the CNS. Patterning has not proven to be efficacious in children with Down syndrome.

First Year to Puberty

The pediatric management of children between the ages of 1 and puberty is summarized in Table 6.

Medical Problems

Dental Problems   Common dental aberrations include delayed eruption of the first tooth until 13.67 months as well as abnormal sequence of eruption. The incidence of missing teeth, malformed teeth, fused teeth, and microdontia is greatly increased in children with Down syndrome and, although there are no biologic factors that contraindicate orthodontic intervention, a lack of cooperation may complicate treatment. Periodontal disease is the most serious dental concern and is due to malocclusion, tooth dysmorphology, bruxism, and a lack of normal masticatory function. Routine dental evaluation and treatment as well as twice-daily dental care is indicated for prevention of periodontal disease and dental caries.

Endocrine Problems   The incidence of hypothyroidism is increased in children with Down syndrome because of an autoimmune process. The clinical signs and symptoms may be subtle and attributed to the Down syndrome itself. Therefore, annual screening for hypothyroidism with thyroxine (T_4) and thyroid-stimulated hormone (TSH) should begin at 12 months of age. Compensated hypothyroidism with mild transient elevations of TSH and normal T_4 levels is an indication for a repeat screening to make sure that the child's laboratory values do not progress to hypothyroidism. The incidence of diabetes mellitus is increased in children with Down syndrome, occurring in 1 in 250 children. The clinician should lower the threshold of suspicion in relation to the presence of diabetes

Table 6.   Pediatric care of the child with Down syndrome from age 1 to puberty

Arrange for dental care.
Obtain cervical spine film.
Monitor weight and height.
Reassess vision annually.
Screen for thyroid dysfunction annually.
Monitor school progress.
Perform annual physical and neurologic examination.
Continue to provide family education and support.

mellitus in children with Down syndrome. Growth hormone therapy for children with Down syndrome is still considered experimental, and further assessment of the safety, efficacy, and ethical ramifications is needed.

Nutrition   Children with Down syndrome tend to be underweight for their height in infancy but in early childhood may become overweight and develop obesity. By the age of 3 years, 30% of boys and girls with Down syndrome develop obesity. Factors that contribute to obesity include excessive caloric intake, decreased physical activity, and a low resting metabolic rate. Anticipatory guidance should include the early establishment of patterns of daily exercise, low caloric intake, a balanced diet, and high-bulk/low-calorie snacks. Clinicians should encourage parents to modify eating behavior by prohibiting snacks while watching television, permitting eating only at the table, and setting limits on time spent watching television.

Ophthalmic Problems   In children with Down syndrome, a yearly eye examination by a pediatric ophthalmologist is indicated because the incidence of ophthalmic disorders increases with age, and such disorders can occur in 70% of children with Down syndrome (Gaynon & Schimek, 1977). Refractive errors, which tend to increase with age, occur in 30%–70% of people with Down syndrome (Jaeger, 1980; Lowe, 1949), with a substantial number of children exhibiting high myopia (8.00 diopters); two studies found high myopia in 35%–40% of people with Down syndrome (Roizen, Mets, & Blondis, 1994). Astigmatism and hyperopia are also common.

Orthopedic Problems   Atlantoaxial instability occurs in 10%–30% of children with Down syndrome, and they are at increased risk for atlantoaxial subluxation. Atlantoaxial instability is defined as more than 5 mm of space between the atlas and odontoid process of the axis when measured on lateral cervical spine radiographs in flexion, neutral, and extension. In one large study, atlantoaxial instability was observed in 15% of individuals with Down syndrome.

The radiograph of the cervical spine, however, is only a screening tool and should be interpreted as part of an overall assessment that includes a careful neurologic and physical examination. In some cases, there have been reports (Selby et al., 1991) of a cervical spine film being abnormal while a repeat study is normal. In addition, information is incomplete about the natural history of atlantoaxial instability. Studies are currently underway to determine how reliable and predictive radiographic results turn out to be. Until we have complete information, the current practice is to monitor children with atlantoaxial instability with careful annual examinations and limit physical activities that involve somersaults, trampoline exercises, and diving.

A small number of children with atlantoaxial instability identified radiographically develop atlantoaxial subluxation, with symptoms and signs of spinal cord compression. The symptoms include torticollis, long track neurologic signs, gait disturbances, and neck pain. Symptomatic patients require immediate surgical stabilization.

The incidence of hip dislocation in children and young adults is reported to be 2%–5%. The hips of children with Down syndrome are hypermobile, with the laxity of the ligaments and muscle hypotonia predisposing to hip dislocation. The child's habit of sitting with the hips abducted, flexed, and externally rotated ("reverse tailor") may also contribute to the dislocation. Orthopedic surgeons recommended surgery rather than less aggressive modes of therapy. Hip dislocation can present with gait disturbances, delayed ambulation, or hip dislocation on physical examination.

Facial Plastic Surgery   The facial plastic surgery advocated for children with Down syndrome includes tongue resection to improve speech and appearance, silicone implants for the saddle nose and micrognathia, and removal of the epicanthal folds. Published series report few complications (Lemperlie, 1985). Studies on cosmetic surgery have revealed no evidence that the surgery actually improves a child's social acceptance, clarity of speech, or intelligence. Nevertheless, many parents believe that the surgery is beneficial and is one way they can improve the quality of life of their child. If parents are strongly in favor of cosmetic surgery, they can be referred to an experienced plastic

surgeon for more information when the child is between 2 and 4 years of age.

Development   Developmental abilities vary greatly in children with Down syndrome. Average milestones include walking unsupported by 24 months, first word at 24 months, and toilet training by 34 months. Intelligence quotients typically range from 40 to 55, although occasionally children score at lower or higher levels.

As expectations for language and cognitive growth increase during the second year of life, delays in these areas are usually apparent to both parents and professionals. It is difficult to address what constitutes "typical" cognitive development for children with Down syndrome. Simply stated, no two children with this condition are quite alike. Possible sources of variability include, but are not limited to, genetic and neurobiologic factors, associated medical conditions, rearing environment, and social and educational opportunities. Despite the variability, numerous studies have revealed certain developmental trends that appear to be characteristic of Down syndrome. For instance, a number of studies have demonstrated a nonlinear rate of cognitive development in children with Down syndrome during the first decade of life (Carr, 1988; Share, Koch, Webb, & Graliker, 1964). These investigators used declining developmental quotients (DQs and IQs) to argue for a slowing in the rate of cognitive development with age. These same studies reported a plateauing in the rate of cognitive development during the first decade. Another study found no evidence of decline in either DQ or IQ during the first 3 years of life (Schnell, 1984).

Factors that have been reported to correlate positively with enhanced cognitive outcome in Down syndrome include mosaicism for trisomy 21 (Fishler & Koch, 1991) and home rearing (Shipe & Shotwell, 1965; Shotwell & Shipe, 1964). Additional factors that are reported to influence cognitive outcome but that have been insufficiently proven in controlled studies include the effect of early intervention programs (Ludlow & Allen, 1979; Piper & Pless, 1980) and the parents' level of education and socioeconomic status (Bennett, Sells, & Brand, 1979; Libb, Myers, Graham, & Bell, 1983). Studies that have attempted to correlate cognitive outcome with the number or severity of physical stigmata of persons with trisomy 21 have shown no correlation (Baumeister & Williams, 1967). Factors noted to correlate negatively with cognitive outcome include the presence of severe CHD or hypotonia (Reed et al., 1984), seizures (Stafstrom & Konkol, 1994) and severe sensory impairments (Wisniewski, Miezejeski, & Hill, 1988). Reduced neuron number in the cerebral cortex and subcortical nuclei in conjunction with decreased synaptic number and density and altered spine morphology is thought to constitute the neurobiologic substrate of the cognitive impairments seen in children with Down syndrome.

Like cognitive development, it is difficult to define what constitutes "typical" speech and language development in the young child with Down syndrome. Studies have documented large individual differences in the onset and complexity of spoken language (LaVeck & Brehm, 1978). As a group, children with Down syndrome demonstrate greater deficits in verbal–linguistic skills relative to visual–spatial skills (Rohr & Burr, 1978; Wang & Bellugi, 1994). Many children demonstrate increasing deficits in verbal–linguistic skills with increasing chronologic age (Miller, 1985). There is also a tendency toward increasing deviance in language development beyond 4 or 5 years of life. Asynchrony of language development has been well documented in this population (Miller, 1988). Language comprehension and production skills often develop at significantly different rates, with production skills showing the greatest delays. Some of the factors that have been postulated to impact specifically on verbal–linguistic skills in children with Down syndrome include hearing loss, altered auditory perception, speech–motor control deficits, family and environmental variables, and specific neurobiologic impairments that impact on language-based learning. One study found a significant correlation between enhanced language production at 3 years of age and 1) higher cognitive level; 2) less severe hypotonia; and 3) gender, whereby girls generally performed better than boys (Strominger, Winkler, & Cohen, 1984).

There is a substantial literature dealing with many aspects of linguistic competency in Down syndrome; however, surprisingly little research has focused on the neurobiologic substrate of language-based learning in this condition. Elliott and Weeks proposed a neurologic model of "atypical cerebral specialization" in Down syndrome (Elliott & Weeks, 1993; Elliott, Weeks, & Gray, 1990; Weeks & Elliott, 1992). Their model proposes a disassociation between functional right hemispheric systems subserving speech perception and those left hemispheric systems associated with movement production, including speech sounds. They postulated that a breakdown in communication results from a partial loss of linguistic information secondary to the separation of speech perception and movement production systems.

Child and Family Needs Infant intervention programs for children from birth to 3 years are available in most areas (see Chapter 28, Volume I). Most research indicates that children with Down syndrome who participate in these programs exhibit higher intellectual and social quotients than children not enrolled in such programs. These intervention programs vary widely in the degree and type of parent participation, the composition of the disciplines of the professional staff, the balance between home-based and center-based activities, and the amount of intervention available. Individual families and children may benefit from different types of programs, and the pediatrician should help the parents find a program that meets their family's needs. These intervention programs can assist parents to become effective advocates for their child and to better use the information from different disciplines to become "experts" on their child.

Many public schools provide opportunities for inclusion, mainstreaming, and separate special education classes. Community activities are an important way to balance social and educational experience (see Chapter 25, Volume I). Parents have the added responsibility of being social facilitators in such positions as scout troop leaders, Sunday school teachers, and social function planners. Social activities remain extremely important for the optimal development of children with Down syndrome.

Adolescence

The care of the adolescent with Down syndrome is summarized in Table 7.

Medical Concerns A biannual examination is indicated to detect signs of hypothyroidism, obesity, and psychological problems. Vision and hearing screening is indicated yearly. Laboratory investigation should include thyroid screening with thyroid antibody level because of the increased risk for thyroiditis. Based on current information, repeated radiographs of the cervical spine to screen for atlantoaxial instability are indicated at the end of puberty.

In girls, a pelvic examination with a Pap test is indicated biannually. Because girls may occasionally be fertile, birth control options should be discussed with the family. Because of the difficulty in defining informed consent, sterilization procedures may be problematic. Referral to an obstetrician–gynecologist may help the family explore alternatives. Although boys are usually infertile, some families may request information about vasectomy. Many special education programs include sex education in the curriculum. If more information is needed, the family can be referred to a sex education unit in the school or local developmental disabilities unit (see Chapter 31, Volume I).

Psychiatric Disorders Disturbed behavior seen in the adolescent with Down syndrome may be due to a medical problem or a psychiatric disorder such as depression. One must rule out a medical etiology, such as hypothyroidism, cataracts, and impacted cerumen impairing hearing. Referral to a psychiatrist with a special interest in persons with developmental disabilitiy is indicated when a mental disorder is suspected (see Chapter 20, this volume).

Table 7. Management of the adolescent with Down syndrome

Screen for thyroid dysfunction.
Repeat cervical spine film.
Perform pelvic examination in girls.
Discuss issues involving sexuality.
Monitor prevocational training.
Continue annual physical and neurologic examination.
Discuss long-term financial plans with parents.
Discuss alternative community living resources available for individual when he or she becomes an adult.

Intervention Services The adolescent should participate in community programs to provide appropriate social and recreational stimulation. Leisure time activities should be appropriate. For too many adolescents leisure time activities consist of watching television and going to a shopping mall. Organized activities such as Special Olympics and church youth groups should be encouraged.

A vocational assessment involves a comprehensive evaluation of the individual's job-related skills. During midadolescence, the school curriculum shifts from academics to exploration of the individual's specific vocationally related skills and interests. A vocational evaluation should incite a review of an individual's progress in his or her special education program, an interview with the individual, a parent interview, and a formal intellectual assessment with standard instruments such as the Stanford-Binet. The parents can play an active role by encouraging the adolescent to try out different work experiences during summer vacations. Most communities have a wide spectrum of employment opportunities ranging from competitive employment, such as custodial work in a school building, to the traditional sheltered workshop where individuals are paid for piece work such as assembling and packaging.

Social skills training refers to methods to improve an individual's interpersonal interaction. This subject has gained increasing attention because children with mental retardation often are mainstreamed; that is, they have an opportunity to spend time in classes with students of the same age without disabilities. Techniques for training social or interpersonal skills include modeling, role playing, and positive reinforcement techniques for specific prosocial behaviors such as eye contact or initiation of social conversation. However, there may be difficulty with new social skills generalizing from the trained situation to natural settings.

Legal and Financial Issues Long-term financial, estate, and community living planning is critical for families with a child with Down syndrome. A will is needed to address the issue of custody in the event of the parents' death. It is helpful to have an attorney with experience in working with families with a child with Down syndrome or other developmental disabilities because laws governing trusts and other funds are complicated and vary from state to state. Families face additional problems in obtaining insurance coverage as well as finding an appropriate community living facility for an adult with Down syndrome. Parents may need to talk to a financial planner with experience in assisting families who have children with special needs. The local Arc and its members may be able to suggest experienced professionals in the community who can offer such financial planning and legal assistance. Many adults with Down syndrome move into community residential facilities such as group homes, assisted living apartments, or an intermediate care facility. Often, there are long waiting lists for community residential facilities, so parents need to investigate these living options 3–5 years before the anticipated need.

Young Adulthood

The care of young adults with Down syndrome is summarized in Table 8.

Medical Concerns The annual physical examination in the young adult (ages 20–35 years) should include a Pap smear and breast exam in women. Because of the increased risk for hearing and visual problems, auditory and vision screening must be included in the routine health examination. The adult requires a diphtheria–tetanus immunization every 10 years. Adults with CHD or recurrent, severe respiratory infections require an annual influenza vaccine and one pneumococcal vaccine. A PPD (tuberculin purified protein derivative) should be considered in adults placed in a workshop where they may be exposed to previously institutionalized patients at higher risk for tuberculosis infection. Monitoring of weight and exercise may help prevent obesity.

Table 8. Care of the young adult with Down syndrome

Perform annual physical and neurologic examination.
Screen vision and hearing annually.
Monitor vocational activities.
Screen thyroid dysfunction.
Monitor exposure to individuals with hepatitis, tuberculosis, and *Shigella* gastroenteritis.
Monitor for behavior changes and loss of skills.

Thyroid screening must continue in the adult because of the continued risk for thyroid dysfunction. Such screening should include a T_4 (thyroxine) and TSH with a thyroid antibody level because of thyroiditis seen in the adult.

The recently deinstitutionalized person with Down syndrome may present additional medical problems. Frequently, medical information is scanty, especially the immunization history. When an immunization history is not available, the clinician should consider a rubella or polio antibody screen to evaluate immune status. Alternatively, in selected cases, it may be more efficient to give the immunizations because administration of MMR (mumps–measles–rubella) vaccine or polio vaccine to an already immune individual is probably harmless. The individual living in an institution is at higher risk for tuberculosis, hepatitis, and *Shigella* gastroenteritis. A PPD, a chest radiograph, a stool culture, and hepatitis screening are clinically indicated before an individual enters the community.

People with Down syndrome are predisposed to develop chronic hepatitis B infection following exposure. Vaccination with hepatitis B vaccine is indicated following the standard guidelines.

The adult with Down syndrome must be monitored for cardiac disease even if CHD problems are not present because 57% of adults develop mitral valve prolapse and 11% develop aortic regurgitation.

Psychiatric Disorders The prevalence of psychiatric disorders in individuals with Down syndrome is not known. In one study, 13% of children with Down syndrome had a psychiatric disorder. The range of reported psychiatric disorders in individuals with Down syndrome includes depression, schizophrenia, and anorexia nervosa (see Chapter 20, this volume).

The diagnostic approach to an adult with Down syndrome and a possible psychiatric disorder calls for some general modifications. Some factors of mental retardation that affect the diagnostic process include the person's limited vocabulary, which decreases the ability to report feelings and behavior; mental disorganization that occurs under stress; and the increase of a variety of maladaptive behaviors (e.g., rocking) under stress.

Some general clinical guidelines for the care of a person with Down syndrome with serious behavior problems include

1.   Rule out medical problems that may precipitate a severe behavior problem (e.g., social isolation and withdrawal may be the presenting problem in a patient with an acquired hearing loss, cataracts, thyroid dysfunction, cardiac disease, or early Alzheimer's disease).

2.   Perform a simplified mental status examination, which consists of evaluating the patient's ability to complete simple tasks and follow directions. Rely on caregivers, teachers, or workshop staff for description of significant behaviors. Inquire about a history of loss of a significant person or an important change in living arrangements.

3.   Refer to an experienced psychiatrist for further evaluation and treatment when medications are considered.

Alzheimer-Type Dementia   The *Diagnostic and Statistical Manual of Mental Disorders* (4th ed.) characterizes dementia as an impairment of memory associated with impairment of higher cortical function (American Psychiatric Association, 1994). The disturbance is severe enough to affect social and occupational activities. A dementing disorder may be particularly difficult to diagnose during life in persons with mental retardation. In one retrospective review of 16 studies in which both postmortem brain tissue and clinical data were available to support the diagnosis of Alzheimer-type dementia, Dalton and Crapper described the behavioral and neurologic manifestations in 33 persons with Down syndrome who ranged in age from 35 to 60 years at the time of death. All individuals showed evidence of senile plaques or neurofibrillary tangles at autopsy (Dalton & Crapper-McLachlan, 1986). One or more clinical manifestations were found in 75% of these individuals. In decreasing frequency, these features included seizures (58%), change in personality (46%), focal neurologic signs (46%), apathy (36%), loss of conversational skills (36%), incontinence (36%), electroencephalographic abnormalities (33%), loss of self-help skills (30%), tremors or myoclonus (24%), visual or auditory deficits (24%), gait or mobility

problems (21%), stubborn or uncooperative behavior (21%), depression (18%), memory loss (18%), increased muscle tone (12%), disorientation (12%), and delusions or hallucinations (3%). Prospective studies reveal a different clinical picture of Alzheimer-related changes. One study reported memory loss, temporal disorientation, and reduced verbal skills as the earliest signs of Alzheimer-type dementia (Lai & Williams, 1989). Those individuals who functioned in the severe or profound range of mental retardation more often manifested apathy, inattention, and decreased social interaction early on. Loss of self-help skills, motor impairments, and new onset of seizures also were reported. In describing the natural history of Alzheimer-type dementia in Down syndrome, Evenhuis (1990) reported the mean age of onset to be 51.3 years in individuals with moderate retardation and 52.6 years in individuals with severe retardation. Once recognized, the clinical signs of dementia progressed rapidly in all subjects.

The assessment of dementia should include a through medical history, physical examination and laboratory testing, quantitative examination of mental status, neuropsychological testing, and reports by family members or other caregivers. Dalton (1992) developed a specific test battery for evaluating early psychological changes associated with Alzheimer-type dementia in Down syndrome. Improvements in the early diagnosis of dementia in this population should allow family members and service care providers an opportunity to plan changes in programs, adult day care, and other services to maintain a reasonably high quality of life for aged persons with Down syndrome. All families will require education and support. Community support groups may be helpful to some families. Getting in-home nursing care or assistance is usually necessary in the more advanced stages of dementia as the individual becomes more dependent.

Major affective disorders such as depression are relatively common in adult persons with Down syndrome and may be difficult for clinicians to distinguish from early changes of dementia (Warren, Holroyd, & Folstein, 1989). Failing to distinguish between the two entities may result in an incorrect diagnosis of dementia, for which no adequate medical treatment currently exists. Depression, in comparison, often responds to a combination of pharmacologic treatment, changes in the social and environmental milieu, and supportive counseling. A number of treatable medical conditions that may be associated with behavioral change also must be ruled out prior to arriving at a diagnosis of either depression or dementia, including visual or hearing loss; cardiovascular decompensation secondary to uncorrected CHD, mitral valve prolapse, or aortic regurgitation; hypothyroidism; obstructive sleep apnea with hypoxemia and multiple drug interactions (Dalton, Seltzer, Adlin, & Wisniewski, 1992).

CONCLUSIONS

The child with Down syndrome challenges the pediatrician in two ways. First, the pediatrician must be aware of the child's important medical problems, which require detection and management (see Chapter 23, Volume I). Second, he or she must be sensitive to the special education needs and support required by the family.

In the newborn period, the pitfall for the pediatrician managing a child with Down syndrome is failing to inform and educate the parents in a sensitive manner. This can be avoided by holding several informative meetings with the family, providing current educational material, and referring the family to a support group.

The pitfall in managing a child in the first year of life is the failure to detect and monitor critical medical problems, such as CHD, chronic ear infections, and gastrointestinal malformations. A rather benign clinical problem in a normal infant (e.g., constipation) can be an early sign of an extremely serious problem (e.g., Hirschsprung disease) in a child with Down syndrome.

The pitfall in managing a school-age child is the failure to identify medical problems that impair the acquisition of developmental skills. Chronic serous otitis media with a moderate conductive hearing loss, hypothyroidism, and severely impaired visual acuity are medical conditions that have devastating effects on classroom learning.

Pediatricians probably err most in managing children with Down syndrome during the transition from adolescence to adulthood. Medical problems such as Alzheimer's disease and mitral valve prolapse may be unfamiliar to a pediatrician. Management is further complicated by the lack of community resources to provide the young adult with appropriate vocational training, social skill development, recreational opportunities, or a facility for community living.

The pediatrician can carefully negotiate around these pitfalls by maintaining a high index of suspicion for medical problems, being sensitive to the needs of the families, being familiar with community resources, and advocating for community services that are not available.

REFERENCES

American Academy of Pediatrics Committee on Nutrition. (1993). *The pediatric nutrition handbook* (3rd ed.). Elk Grove Village, IL: Author.

American Psychiatric Association. (1994). *Diagnostic and statistical manual of mental disorders* (4th ed.). Washington, DC: American Psychiatric Press.

Anwar, F. (1981). Motor function in Down's syndrome. In *International Review of Research in Mental Retardation* (pp. 107–139). New York: Academic Press.

Baumeister, A., & Williams, J. (1967). Relationship of physical stigmata to intellectual functioning in mongolism. *American Journal of Mental Deficiency, 71*, 586–592.

Becker, L.E., Armstrong, D.L., & Chan, F. (1986). Dendritic atrophy in children with Down's syndrome. *Annals of Neurology, 20*, 520–526.

Bendotti, C., Forloni, G., Morgan, R., O'Hara, B., Oster-Granite, M., Reeves, R., Gearhart, J., & Coyle, J. (1988). Neuroanatomical localization and quantification of amyloid precursor protein mRNA by in situ hybridization in the brains of normal, aneuploid and lesioned mice. *Proceedings of the National Academy of Sciences of the United States of America, 85*, 3628–3632.

Bennett, F.C., Sells, C.J., & Brand, C. (1979). Influences on measured intelligence in Down's syndrome. *American Journal of Diseases in Children, 133*, 700–703.

Brooksbank, B.W.L., & Balazs, R. (1984). Superoxide dismutase, glutathione peroxidase and lipoperoxidation in Down's syndrome fetal brain. *Developmental Brain Research, 16*, 37–44.

Burger, P.C., & Vogel, S. (1973). The development of the pathologic changes of Alzheimer's disease in patients with Down's syndrome. *American Journal of Pathology, 73*, 457–476.

Capone, G., Bendotti, C., Oster-Granite, M., & Coyle, J. (1991). Developmental expression of the gene encoding growth-associated protein 43 (GAP43) in the brains of normal and aneuploid mice. *Journal of Neuroscience Research, 29*, 449–460.

Carr, J. (1988). Six weeks to twenty-one years old: A longitudinal study of children with Down's syndrome and their families. *Journal of Child Psychology and Psychiatry, 29*, 407–431.

Casey, D. (1993). Brookhaven National Laboratory researchers achieve sequencing advance. *Human Genome News, 4*(5), 1–16.

Centerwall, S., & Centerwall, W. (1960). A study of children with mongolism reared in the home compared to those reared away from home. *Pediatrics, 25*, 678–685.

Chumakov, I., Rigault, P., Guillou, S., Ougen, P., Billaut, A., Guasconi, G., Gervy, P., LeGall, I., Soularue, P., Grinas, L., Bougueleret, L., Bellanne-Chantelot, C., Lacroix, B., Barillot, E., Gesnouin, P., Pook, S., Vaysseix, G., Frelat, G., Schmitz, A., Sambucy, J., Bosch, A., Estivill, X., Weissenbach, J., Vignal, A., Riethman, H., Cox, D., Patterson, D., Gardiner, K., Hattori, M., Sakaki, Y., Ichikawa, H., Ohki, M., Le Paslier, D., Heilig, R., Antonarakis, S., & Cohen, D. (1992). Continuum of overlapping clones spanning the entire human chromosome 21q. *Nature, 359*, 380–387.

Clark, R.F., & Goate, A.M. (1993). Molecular genetics of Alzheimer's disease. *Archives of Neurology, 50*, 1164–1172.

Coyle, J., Oster-Granite, M., Reeves, R., Hohmann, C., Corsi, P., & Gearhart, J. (1991). Down syndrome and the trisomy 16 mouse: Impact of gene imbalance on brain development and aging. In P. McHugh & V. McKusick (Eds.), *Genes, brain and behavior* (pp. 85–99). New York: Raven Press.

Crome, L., Cowie, V., & Slater, E. (1966). A statistical note on cerebellar and brain-stem weight in mongolism. *Journal of Mental Deficiency Research, 10*, 69–72.

Cronk, C., Crocker, A., & Pueschel, S. (1988). Growth charts for children with Down syndrome: 1 month to 18 years of life. *Pediatrics, 81*, 102–110.

Dalton, A. (1992). Dementia in Down syndrome: Methods of evaluation. In L. Nadel & C. Epstein (Eds.), *Down syndrome and Alzheimer's disease* (pp. 51–76). New York: Wiley-Liss.

Dalton, A., & Crapper-McLachlan, D. (1986). Clinical expression of Alzheimer's disease in Down syndrome. *Psychiatric Clinics of North America, 9*, 659–670.

Dalton, AJ., Seltzer, G.B., Adlin, M.S., & Wisniewski, H.M. (1992). Association between Alzheimer's disease and Down's syndrome: Clinical observations. In J.M. Berg, A.J. Holland, & H. Karlinsky (Eds.), *Alzheimer's disease and Down's syndrome* (pp. 1–17). London: Oxford University Press.

Davidoff, L. (1928). The brain in mongolian idiocy. *Archives of Neurology and Psychiatry, 20*, 1229–1257.

Davisson, M., Schmidt, C., Reeves, R., Irving, N., Akeson, E., Harris, B., & Bronson, R. (1993). Segmental trisomy as a mouse model for Down syndrome. In C. Epstein (Ed.), *The phenotypic mapping of Down syndrome and other aneuploid conditions* (pp. 117–133). New York: Wiley-Liss.

Deng, H., Hentati, A., Tainer, J.A., Iqbal, Z., Cayabyab, A., Hung, W., Getzoff, E.D., Hu, P., Herzfeldt, B., Roos, R.P., Warner, C., Deng, G., Soriano, E., Smyth, C.P., Parge, H.E., Ahmed, A., Roses, A.D., Hallewell, R.A., Pericak-Vance, M.A., & Siddique, T. (1993). Amyotrophic lateral sclerosis and structural defects in Cu, Zn superoxide dismutase. *Science, 261*, 1047–1051.

Dickinson, J.J., & Singh, I. (1993). Down's syndrome, dementia, and superoxide dismutase. *British Journal of Psychiatry, 162*, 811–817.

Down, J.C.H. (1866). Observations on an ethnic classification of idiots. *London Hospital Clinical Lectures and Reports 3*, 259–262.

Elliott, D., & Weeks, D.J. (1993). Cerebral specialization for speech perception and movement organization in adults with Down's syndrome. *Cortex, 29*, 103–113.

Elliott, D., Weeks, D.J., & Gray, S. (1990). Manual and oral praxis in adults with Down's syndrome. *Neuropsychologia, 28*, 1307–1315.

Ellis, W. G., McCulloch, J.R., & Corely, C.L. (1974). Presenile dementia in Down's syndrome. *Neurology, 24*, 101–106.

Epstein, C.J. (1990). The consequences of chromosome imbalance. *American Journal of Medical Genetics, 7*(Suppl.), 31–37.

Evenhuis, H. (1990). The natural history of dementia in Down syndrome. *Archives of Neurology, 47*, 263–267.

Fishler, K., & Koch, R. (1991). Mental development in Down syndrome mosaicism. *American Journal of Mental Retardation, 96*, 345–351.

Gardiner, K. (1990). Physical mapping of the long arm of chromosome 21. In D. Patterson & C. Epstein (Eds.), *Molecular genetics of chromosome 21 and Down syndrome* (pp. 1–14). New York: Wiley-Liss.

Gaynon, M.W., & Schimek, R.A. (1977). Down's syndrome: A ten-year group study. *Annals of Opthalmology, 9*, 1495–1497.

Godridge, H., Renyolds, G.P., Czudek, C., Calcutt, N.A., & Benton, M. (1987). Alzheimer-like neurotransmitter deficits in adult Down's syndrome brain tissue. *Journal of Neurology, Neurosurgery, and Psychiatry, 50*, 775–778.

Griffin, W.S.T., Stanley, L.T., Ling, C., White, L., MacLeod, V., Perrot, L.J., White, C.L., III, & Araoz, C. (1989). Brain interleukin 1 and S-100 immunoreactivity are elevated in Down syndrome and Alzheimer disease. *Proceedings of the National Academy of Sciences of the United States of America, 86*, 7611–7615.

Haines, J.L., Guillemette, W., Rosen, D., Brown, R., Donaldson, D., & Patterson, D. (1993). A genetic linkage map of chromosome 21: A look at meiotic phenomena. In C. Epstein (Ed.), *The phenotypic mapping of Down syndrome and other aneuploid conditions* (pp. 51–61). New York: Wiley-Liss.

Hall, B. (1966). Mongolism in newborn infants. *Clinical Pediatrics, 5*, 4–8.

Hardy, J., & Allsop, D. (1991). Amyloid deposition as the central event in the aetiology of Alzheimer's disease. *Trends in Pharmacological Sciences, 12*, 383–388.

Hook, E. (1981). Down syndrome: Its frequency in human populations and some factors pertinent to variations in rates. In F. de la Cruz & P. Gerald (Eds.), *Trisomy 21 (Down syndrome): Research perspectives* (pp. 3–68). Baltimore: University Park Press.

Jaeger, E.A. (1980). Ocular findings in Down's syndrome. *Transactions of the American Ophthalmological Society, 158*, 808–845.

Jorgensen, O.S., Brooksbank, B.W.L., & Balazs, R. (1990). Neuronal plasticity and astrocytic reaction in Down syndrome and Alzheimer disease. *Journal of the Neurological Sciences, 98*, 63–79.

Kligman, D., & Hilt, D.C. (1988). The S100 protein family. *Trends in Biological Sciences, 13*, 437–443.

Kligman, D., & Hsieh, L. (1987). Neurite extension factor induces rapid morphological differentiation of mouse neuroblastoma cells in defined medium. *Developmental Brain Research, 33*, 296–300.

Korenberg, J.R. (1993). Toward a molecular understanding of Down syndrome. In C. Epstein (Ed.), *The phenotypic mapping of Down syndrome and other aneuploid conditions* (pp. 87–115). New York: Wiley-Liss.

Korenberg, J.R., Kawashima, H., Pullst, S.M., Allen, L., Magenis, E., & Epstein, C. (1990). Down sydrome: Toward a molecular definition of the phenotype. *American Journal of Medical Genetics, 7*(Suppl.), 91–97.

Lai, F., & Williams, R. (1989). A prospective study of Alzheimer's disease in Down's syndrome. *Archives of Neurology, 46*, 849–853.

LaVeck, B., & Brehm, S. (1978). Individual variability among children with Down syndrome. *Mental Retardation, 2*, 135–137.

Lejeune, J., Gautier, M., & Turpin, R. (1959). Etude des chromosomes somatique de neuf enfants mongoliens. *Comptes Rendus Academy de Sciences (Paris), 248*, 1721–1722.

Lemperlie, G. (1985). Plastic surgery. In D. Lane & B. Statford (Eds.), *Current approaches to Down's syndrome* (pp. 131–145). Sydney: Holt, Rinehart & Winston.

Libb, J.W., Myers, G.J., Graham, E., & Bell, B. (1983). Correlates of intelligence and adaptive behaviour in Down's syndrome. *Journal of Mental Deficiency Research, 27*, 205–210.

Lowe, R. (1949). The eyes in Mongolism. *British Journal of Ophthalmology, 33*, 131–154.

Ludlow, J., & Allen, L. (1979). The effect of early intervention and preschool stimulus on the development of Down syndrome children. *Journal of Mental Deficiency Research, 23*, 29.

Mann, D.M.A., Yates, P.O., & Marcyniuk, B. (1984). Alzheimer's presenile dementia, senile dementia of Alzheimer's type and Down's syndrome in the middle aged form an age related continuum of pathological changes. *Neuropathology and Applied Neurobiology, 10*, 185–207.

Marin-Padilla, M. (1972). Structural abnormalities of the cerebral cortex in human chromosomal aberrations: A Golgi study. *Brain Research, 44*, 625–629.

Marin-Padilla, M. (1976). Pyramidal cell abnormalities in the motor cortex of a child with Down's syndrome. *Journal of Comparative Neurology, 167*, 63–82.

McKusick, V. (1994). *Mendelian inheritance in man: A catalogue of human genes and genetic disorders* (11th ed.). Baltimore: Johns Hopkins University Press.

McLaren, J., & Bryson, S. (1987). Review of recent epidemiological studies of mental retardation: Prevalence, associated disorders and etiology. *American Journal of Mental Retardation, 92*, 243–254.

Miller, J.F. (1985). Language and communication characteristics of children with Down syndrome. In S.M. Pueschel, C. Tingey, J.E. Rynders, A.C. Crocker, & D.M. Crutcher (Eds.), *New perspectives on Down syndrome* (pp. 233–262). Baltimore: Paul H. Brookes Publishing Co.

Miller, J.F. (1988). The developmental asynchrony of language development in children with Down syndrome. In L. Nadel (Ed.), *The psychobiology of Down syndrome* (pp. 167–198). Cambridge, MA: MIT Press.

Mito, T., & Becker, L. (1993). Developmental changes of S-100 protein and glial fibrillary acidic protein in the brain in Down syndrome. *Experimental Neurology, 120*, 170–176.

Neve, R., Finch, E., & Dawes, E. (1988). Expression of the Alzheimer's amyloid precursor gene transcripts in the human brain. *Neuron, 1*, 669–677.

Palmer, C., Cronk, C., Pueschel, S., Wisniewski, K., Laxova, R., Crocker, A., & Pauli, R. (1992). Head circumference of children with Down syndrome (0–36 months). *American Journal of Medical Genetics, 42*, 61–67.

Percy, M.E., Dalton, A.J., Markovic, V.D., McLachlan, D.R.C., Hummel, J.T., Rusk, A.C.M., & Andrews, D.F. (1990). Red cell superoxide dismutase, glutathione peroxidase and catalase in Down syndrome patients with and without manifestations of Alzheimer disease. *American Journal of Medical Genetics, 35*, 459–467.

Piper, M.C., & Pless, I.B. (1980). Early intervention for infants with Down syndrome: A controlled trial. *Pediatrics, 65*, 463–468.

Reed, R.B., Pueschel, S.M., Schnell, R.R., & Cronk, C.E. (1984). Interrelationships of biological, environmental and competency variables. In S.M. Pueschel (Ed.), *The young child with Down syndrome* (pp. 285–297). New York: Human Sciences Press.

Reeves, R., Gearhart, J., & Littlefield, J. (1986). Genetic basis for a mouse model of Down syndrome. *Brain Research Bulletin, 16*, 803–814.

Rohr, A., & Burr, D.B. (1978). Etiological differences in patterns of psycholinguistic development of children of IQ 30 to 60. *American Journal of Mental Deficiency, 82*, 549–553.

Roizen, N.J., Mets, M.B., & Blondis, T.A. (1994). Ophthalmic disorders in children with Down syndrome. *Developmental Medicine and Child Neurology, 36*, 594–600.

Ross, M., Galaburda, A., & Kemper, T. (1984). Down's syndrome: Is there a decreased population of neurons? *Neurology, 34*, 909–916.

Rumble, B., Retallack, R., Hilbich, C., Simms, G., Multhaup, G., Martins, R., Hockey, A., Montgomery, P., Beyreuther, K., & Masters, C. (1989). Amyloid A4 protein and its precursor in Down's syndrome and Alzheimer's disease. *New England Journal of Medicine, 320*, 1446–1452.

Schmidt-Sidor, B., Wisniewski, K.E., Shepard, T.H., & Sersen, E.A. (1990). Brain growth in Down syndrome subjects 15 to 22 weeks of gestational age and birth to 60 months. *Clinical Neuropathology, 9*, 181–190.

Schnell, R. (1984). Psychomotor development. In S. Pueschel (Ed.), *The young child with Down syndrome* (pp. 207–225). New York: Human Sciences Press.

Selby, K.A., Newton, R.W., & Gupta, S., et al. (1991). Clinical predictors and radiological reliability in atlanto axial subluxation in Down's syndrome. *Archives of Diseases in Children, 66*, 876–878.

Share, J., Koch, R., Webb, A., & Graliker, B. (1964). The longitudinal development of infants and young children with Down's syndrome (mongolism). *American Journal of Mental Deficiency, 68*, 685–692.

Shipe, D., & Shotwell, A. (1965). Effect of out-of-home care on mongoloid children: A continuation study. *American Journal of Mental Deficiency, 69*, 649–652.

Shotwell, A., & Shipe, D. (1964). Effect of out-of-home care on the intellectual and social development of mongoloid children. *American Journal of Mental Deficiency, 68*, 693–699.

Sinet, P.M. (1982). Metabolism of oxygen derivatives in Down's syndrome. *Annals of the New York Academy of Sciences, 396*, 83–94.

Stafstrom, C. E. (1993). Epilepsy in Down syndrome: Clinical aspects and possible mechanisms. *American Journal of Mental Retardation, 98*(Suppl.), 12–26.

Stafstrom, C., & Konkol, R. (1994). Infantile spasms in children with Down syndrome. *Developmental Medicine and Child Neurology, 36*, 576–585.

Strominger, A., Winkler, M., & Cohen, L. (1984). Speech and language evaluation. In S.M. Pueschel (Ed.), *The young child with Down syndrome* (pp. 253–261). New York: Human Sciences Press.

Suetsugu, M., & Mehraein, P. (1980). Spine distribution along the apical dendrites of the pyramidal neurons in Down's syndrome. *Acta Neuropathologica, 50*, 207–210.

Takashima, S., & Becker, L. (1985). Basal ganglia calcification in Down's syndrome. *Journal of Neurology, Neurosurgery, and Psychiatry, 48*, 61–64.

Takashima, S., Duruta, H., Mito, T., Houdou, S., Konomi, H., Yao, R., & Onodera, K. (1990). Immunohistochemistry of superoxide dismutase-1 in developing human brain. *Brain Development, 12*, 211–213.

Tanzi, R.E., Haines, J.L., & Gusella, J.F. (1990). Detailed genetic linkage map of human chromosome 21: Patterns of recombination according to age and sex. In D. Patterson & C. Epstein (Eds.), *Molecular genetics of chromosome 21 and Down syndrome* (pp. 15–26). New York: Wiley-Liss.

Waardenburg, P.J. (1932). *Das Menschliche Auge und seine Erbanlagen.* Nijhoff den Haag: Martinus.

Wang, P.P., & Bellugi, U. (1994). Evidence from two genetic syndromes for a dissociation between verbal and visual-spatial short-term memory. *Journal of Clinical and Experimental Neuropsychology, 16*, 317–322.

Warren, A.C., Holroyd, S., & Folstein, F.M. (1989). Major depression in Down's syndrome. *British Journal of Psychiatry, 155*, 202–205.

Warren, A.C., Slaugenhaupt, S.A., Lewis, J.G., Chakravarti, A., & Antonarakis, S.E. (1989). A genetic linkage map of 17 markers on human chromosome 21. *Genomics, 4,* 579–591.

Watkins, P.C., Tanzi, R.E., Cheng, S., & Gosella, J. (1987). Molecular genetics of human chromosome 21. *Journal of Medical Genetics, 24,* 257.

Weeks, D.J., & Elliott, D. (1992). Atypical cerebral dominance in Down's syndrome. *Bulletin of the Psychonomic Society, 30*(1), 23–25.

Wisniewski, K., French, J., Rosen, J., Kozlowski, P., Tenner, M., & Wisniewski, H. (1982). Basal ganglia calcification (BGC) in Down's syndrome (DS)—Another manifestation of premature aging. *Annals of the New York Academy of Sciences, 396,* 179–189.

Wisniewski, K.E., Laure-Kamionowska, M., Connell, F., & Wen, G.Y. (1986). Neuronal density and synaptogenesis in the postnatal stage of brain maturation in Down syndrome. In C.J. Epstein (Ed.), *The neurobiology of Down syndrome* (pp. 29–45). New York: Raven Press.

Wisniewski, K.E., Miezejeski, C., & Hill, A. (1988). Neurological and psychological status of individuals with Down syndrome. In L. Nadel (Ed.), *The psychobiology of Down syndrome* (pp. 315–343). Cambridge, MA: MIT Press.

Wisniewski, K.E., & Schmidt-Sidor, B. (1989). Postnatal delay of myelin formation in brains from Down syndrome infants and children. *Clinical Neuropathology, 8,* 55–62.

Wisniewski, K.E., Wisniewski, H., & Wen, G. (1985). Occurrence of neuropathological changes and dementia of Alzheimer's disease in Down's syndrome. *Annals of Neurology, 17,* 278–282.

Yates, M., Simpson, J., Maloney, A.F.J., Allison, Y., Ritchie, I.M., & Urquhart, A. (1983). Catecholamines and cholinergic enzymes in pre-senile and senile Alzheimer-type dementia and Down's syndrome. *Brain Research, 280,* 119–126.

Yessayan, L., & Pueschel, S.M. (1984). Neurological investigations. In S.M. Pueschel (Ed.), *The young child with Down syndrome* (pp. 263–283). New York: Human Sciences Press.

Zausmer, E., & Shea, A. (1984). Motor development. In S.M. Pueschel (Ed.), *The young child with Down syndrome* (pp. 143–206). New York: Human Sciences Press.

Zuckerman, J.E., Herschman, H.R., & Levine, L. (1970). Appearance of a brain specific antigen (the S-100 protein) during human foetal development. *Journal of Neurochemistry, 17,* 247–251.

Appendix

Education and Support Groups for Parents of Children with Down Syndrome

The Arc
2501 Avenue J
Arlington, TX 76011
817-640-0204

National Down Syndrome Congress
1605 Chantilly Drive, Suite 250
Atlanta, GA 30324
800-232-NDSC

National Down Syndrome Society
66 Broadway
New York, NY 10012
800-221-4602

Siblings for Significant Change
105 East 22nd Street
New York, NY 10010
212-420-0776

Sibling Information Network
CUAP
Main Street East
Hartford, CT 06108
203-282-7050

Chapter 16

Prader-Willi Syndrome

Vanja A. Holm, M.D.

The multisystem disorder now known as Prader-Willi syndrome was first described in 1956. Still underdiagnosed, Prader-Willi syndrome has an estimated prevalence of 1:15,000 and is one of the more common of many "rare disorders" causing developmental disabilities in infants and children. The syndrome occurs with the same frequency in both sexes, although in young children it is easier to make a clinical diagnosis in boys. The condition has been described worldwide and probably affects all races.

HISTORY

Before Drs. Prader, Labhart, Willi, and Fanconi described Prader-Willi syndrome to the attendees of the VIIIth International Congress on Pediatrics held in Copenhagen in 1956, patients with this disorder were probably thought to have Frölich syndrome. The latter is a condition of obesity and sexual infantilism caused by trauma and other acquired lesions in the hypothalamus and surrounding regions. As detailed by Prader, Labhart, and Willi (1956), Prader-Willi syndrome is a congenital syndrome with additional physical, neurologic, and behavioral symptoms. Some of the issues discussed under nutrition and behavior management in this chapter are applicable to acquired Prader-Willi syndrome and also to other organic obesity syndromes (e.g., Bardet-Biedl and Cohen syndromes). However, these management techniques are not appropriate for treatment of common, nonorganic obesity.

Genetics

From the original description in 1956 until the early 1980s, the diagnosis of Prader-Willi syndrome was strictly a clinical one (Cassidy,

1984). Several researchers had observed chromosomal translocations in some patients with Prader-Willi syndrome, and it became apparent that chromosome 15 always was one of the chromosomes involved. With the advent of high-resolution chromosome studies chromosome 15 could be examined in more detail, and in 1981 Ledbetter and colleagues demonstrated a deletion of the proximal part of the long arm of chromosome 15 in Prader-Willi syndrome (Ledbetter et al., 1981). It soon became evident that some 60%–70% of patients with Prader-Willi syndrome had the deletion in the 15q1.1–1.3 region, which became known as the Prader-Willi Chromosome Region (PWCR). No significant clinical differences were noticed between the patients who did and those who did not have the deletion. The observation that the chromosome 15 with the deletion in the offspring had been donated by the father followed. A more accurate determination of the presence of the 15q deletion by studies using fluorescent in situ hybridization (FISH) was developed a few years later.

The next observation—that children with Angelman syndrome, an entirely different malformation syndrome, had an apparently similar deletion in the PWCR—came as a surprise. Eventually it was discovered that a number of persons with clinical classic Prader-Willi syndrome but no deletion had maternal disomy on chromosome 15; that is, both PWCRs of chromosome 15, often the whole chromosome, came from the egg (Mascari et al., 1992). Thus, the absence of a paternal genetic contribution to the proximal part of the long arm of chromosome 15 seemed to be the etiology for Prader-Willi syndrome. Subsequently, it was shown that in Angelman syndrome the deletion occurred in the chromosome 15 donated by the mother and that disomy of the paternal chromosome also could cause the syndrome. This was the first case of genomic imprinting, previously known to occur in animals, to be demonstrated in a human disorder (Hall, 1992).

A small percentage of persons with clinical Prader-Willi syndrome appeared to have neither the deletion nor the disomy. As molecular genetic research of the PWCR has expanded, most of these cases might now be explained. A candidate gene for Prader-Willi syndrome—the SNRPN gene—has been identified in the PWSR. Methylation studies of DNA in this most critical region are able to detect if the genetic material methylates, which indicates that it comes from the mother, or does not methylate, which means that it comes from the father. Two methylated regions indicates Prader-Willi syndrome; two unmethylated ones, Angelman syndrome. This technology is now contributing to the understanding of genomic imprinting. Most important for the clinician, methylation studies are fast becoming a comparatively inexpensive and accurate laboratory screen to confirm the diagnosis of Prader-Willi syndrome. An additional bonus is that this procedure does not require blood samples from biological parents, which are not always available. The present diagnostic challenge is to sort out the medical diagnoses in patients with Prader-Willi syndromes without laboratory confirmation, who usually present with atypical clinical findings.

CLINICAL DIAGNOSIS

The symptoms in Prader-Willi syndrome are listed in Table 1 roughly in the order of frequency of occurrence. The list was developed by consensus (Holm et al., 1993). A scoring system weighs the major criteria at 1 point each and minor criteria at ½ point each. In children 3 years of age or less, five points are required for diagnosis, four of which should come from the major group. In children 3 years of age up to adulthood, a total score of eight is necessary, with major criteria comprising five or more points. The supportive findings increase the certainty of the diagnosis but are not scored. The clinical picture of this syndrome changes throughout the life stages.

Table 1.   Diagnostic criteria for Prader-Willi syndrome

Major criteria

 Neonatal and infantile hypotonia

 Feeding problems in infancy and poor weight gain or failure to thrive

 Excessive or rapid weight gain after 12 months but before 6 years of age

 Characteristic facial features

 Hypogonadism

 Global developmental delay, mental retardation, or learning problems

 Hyperphagia, food foraging, obsession with food

 Cytogenetic or molecular abnormality of the Prader-Willi chromosome region (PWCR) on chromosome 15

Minor criteria

 Decreased fetal movement, infantile lethargy, or weak cry in infancy

 Characteristic behavior problems

 Sleep disturbances

 Short stature for genetic background

 Hypopigmentation

 Small hands and feet

 Narrow hands with straight ulnar border

 Eye abnormalities

 Thick, viscous saliva

 Speech articulation defects

 Skin picking

Supportive findings

 High pain threshold

 Decreased vomiting

 Temperature instability in infancy or altered temperature sensitivity in older children and adults

 Scoliosis, kyphosis

 Early adrenarche

 Osteoporosis

 Unusual skill with jigsaw puzzles

 Normal neuromuscular studies

Adapted from Holm et al. (1993).

Infancy

The mother of a child with Prader-Willi syndrome often notices less fetal activity than she had experienced during previous pregnancies. Breech presentations and cesarean sections are common. The infant is typically markedly hypotonic. If a neurologic evaluation is done, the conclusion after negative laboratory studies commonly is benign congenital hypotonia. The infant usually needs assisted feedings by tube or bottles with large-hole nipples. Breast feeding is only successful by manual expression. The infant is lethargic and has a weak cry. The head might be dolicocephalic but the facial features are not always characteristic. The astute clinician looking in the mouth might note strings of saliva. When thick and viscous saliva is present in a person with Prader-Willi syndrome, it is noticeable from the beginning. Drooling is then characteristically absent. An occasional child will manifest temperature instability. Hands and feet are *not* small at this age. If Prader-Willi syndrome is considered a clinical diagnosis can easily be made in the newborn period in a boy with a small penis and undescended testes. Diagnosis can also be made in girls if the syndrome is considered in the differential diagnosis in all cases of marked, unexplained infantile hypotonia.

The duration of the initial phase of failure to thrive varies but the condition usually lasts a few weeks. The hypotonia improves and the infant becomes more alert and sociable. Gross motor landmarks are typically mildly delayed, with sitting unsupported occurring around 1 year of age and walking independently occurring in the early to middle part of the third year.

Toddler and Preschool Age

Some time after their first birthday but before 6 years of age—most commonly by the end of the second year—children with Prader-Willi syndrome start gaining excessive weight. If the diagnosis of Prader-Willi syndrome has not been recognized up to this point, the parents are usually delighted with their thriving child until obesity becomes manifest in the preschooler. The great advantage of early diagnosis is that it allows the opportunity to prevent obesity. Weight gain in the child with Prader-Willi syndrome should be monitored on weight-for-length (or height) charts. As soon as this parameter has crossed two or more centiles, the child has fulfilled the third major clinical criteria for the syndrome and nutritional management is appropriate. Life-limiting obesity is *not* inevitable in this syndrome, as was previously believed.

Characteristic facial features become obvious in the preschool child with this syndrome (Figure 1) but are not present in all persons with this disorder. Other physical characteristics that might be present in some patients (minor criteria in Table 1) include lighter hair and eye coloring than family members, straight ulnar bor-

der, and small hands (less than 25th percentile) and feet (less than 10th percentile) for height age (the age of a hypothetical child, the same height as the patient, plotted at the 50th percentile). Eye problems such as strabismus and myopia are also common.

During the end of the second year, delays in language acquisition and play skills are added to the concerns of slow gross motor progress, and the child usually appears mildly globally delayed. Behavior is usually not a major problem to parents of the preschooler with Prader-Willi syndrome, but they might begin to complain that the child is stubborn and headstrong.

School Age

The future cognitive development of the young child with Prader-Willi syndrome typically is a concern for the parents, who are aware that mental retardation is a possibility. The average IQ in the school-age child with this disorder is in the upper end of the mild retardation range, with many youngsters testing out in the borderline and occasionally in the normal range. Rarely, a child with Prader-Willi syndrome will have moderate or severe retardation. Commonly, these children have a learning profile with strength in visual–perceptual areas—an uncanny skill with jigsaw puzzles frequently is observed—but this is not universal. Even though most children with Prader-Willi syn-

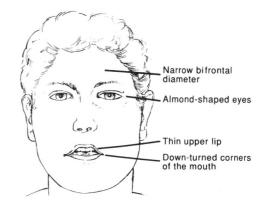

Figure 1. Facial features in Prader-Willi syndrome. (From Holm, V.A., Cassidy, S.B., Butler, M.G., Hanchett, J.M., Greenswag, L.R., Whitman, B.Y., & Greenberg, F. [1993]. Prader-Willi syndrome: Consensus diagnostic criteria. *Pediatrics, 91,* 400; reprinted by permission.)

drome eventually become quite verbal, an occasional youngster might have severe language difficulties, particularly expressive dyspraxia. Behavior difficulties tend to surpass learning as a problem as the child moves up in the grades in school.

As the child with Prader-Willi syndrome gets older, combating obesity becomes increasingly more difficult. Even though foraging for and preoccupation with food might have been noticed at home during the preschool years, it takes on new dimensions as the child gets increasingly more capable of obtaining food and spends time away from home. School lunches might need to be locked up. The child might get into neighbors' garbage or food storage areas. The older child procures money to buy food or shoplifts.

In addition to the hyperphagia, rated as a major criterion (Table 1) because it is both common and seemingly specific for the syndrome, the child with Prader-Willi syndrome usually exhibits many other behavior characteristics (minor criteria in Table 1). The stubbornness of the early years escalates to rigidity. Temper tantrums can become violent outbursts. Children with Prader-Willi syndrome tend to perseverate, especially verbally, with a tiresome habit of coming back to the same subject over and over again long after the conversation has changed to other topics. Often they are argumentative and possessive of their belongings. They can be quite oppositional and manipulative and often lie, especially about food and eating. Five of these behavioral characteristics must be present to count in the scoring system.

Adolescence

In addition to struggling with obesity and learning and behavioral difficulties, the child with Prader-Willi syndrome in the teenage years faces new challenges. Short stature and hypogonadism were described as typical features of the syndrome from the outset (Prader et al., 1956). These endocrinologic aberrations come to the forefront in adolescence.

Stature Length growth in utero is probably unremarkable, but the young child with Prader-Willi syndrome tends to drift down on the regular growth curve to the extent that the average

child with this syndrome grows between the 5th and the 10th percentile during childhood (Figures 2 and 3). As can be seen in these figures, the expected adolescent growth spurt usually is inadequate, and adolescents with Prader-Willi syndrome find themselves increasingly shorter than their age-mates.

Hypogonadism The hypogonadism in Prader-Willi syndrome is usually found to be hypogonadotrophic. The manifestation varies in boys and girls. However, pubic hair might appear early in either sex, because premature adrenarche is not uncommon in Prader-Willi syndrome.

In boys, the hypogonadism is variable but usually apparent during childhood. Virilization is usually incomplete in adolescence. In addition to contending with markedly short stature, the boy with Prader-Willi syndrome frequently does not have a voice change and has little facial and body hair, making him appear younger than his age and setting him further apart from his peers.

The manifestations of hypogonadism in girls with Prader-Willi syndrome are subtle when present before pubertal age. Sometimes the labia minora are absent or barely discernible and sometimes the clitoris is exceedingly small. However, appearance of the external genitals in

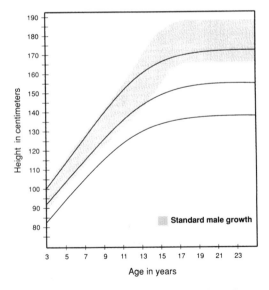

Figure 2. Height growth in boys with Prader-Willi syndrome age 3 to adulthood compared to boys without developmental disabilities.

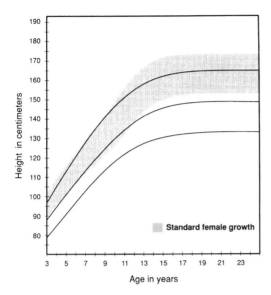

Figure 3. Height growth in girls with Prader-Willi syndrome age 3 to adulthood compared to girls without developmental disabilities.

prepubertal girls shows wide normal variations, and interpretation of hypogonadism should be made cautiously. Development of breasts might be apparent, especially in overweight girls, but on palpation little true breast tissue is present. The degree of feminization is variable. Eventually, approximately 50% of girls will menstruate, but the periods tend to be late in onset, infrequent, and sparse.

Adulthood

Young adults with Prader-Willi syndrome might appear younger than their chronologic age. No case of proven fertility has been recorded. Medical complications are numerous. In the overweight adult, lymphedema and poor circulation in the lower extremities can be debilitating, especially if aggravated by skin picking. Cardiopulmonary complications of obesity might become life threatening. Osteoporosis might be present at a young age, with the threat of fractures. In persons with this syndrome who have a combination of low pain sensitivity and decreased vomiting ability (supportive criteria in Table 1), there is a real danger that lack of normal physiologic response will mask the presence of potentially deadly disorders such as a perforated ulcer or appendicitis. With better management of obesity, adults with this disor-

der live longer; the oldest known survivor died in her early 60s. Observations of possible premature aging in surviving older adults are intriguing, but no studies have been made to assess this issue.

MANAGEMENT

Prader-Willi syndrome is a multisystem disorder, and management of the medical, nutritional, behavioral, educational, and social aspects is needed over the lifetime of affected individuals. A clinic staffed by an interdisciplinary team is the ideal setting for the management of this complex developmental disability. Aspects of management of Prader-Willi syndrome for the developmental pediatrician are covered here. A good source for more detailed information and ideas for a variety of professionals encountering persons with Prader-Willi syndrome is available in the text by Greenswag and Alexander (1995). Families find it invaluable.

Medical Management

Many medical problems encountered in Prader-Willi syndrome are managed the same way they are in individuals without the syndrome. Some physical complications that might require intervention include obstructive and central apnea; eye abnormalities, including esotropia and nonfamilial myopia; and scoliosis and kyphosis. Other symptoms are resistant to medical intervention, such as excessive daytime sleeping, skin picking, and crusting of the thick, viscous saliva in the corners of the mouth.

Hypogonadism The first issues in medical management specific to Prader-Willi syndrome tend to be urologic. The small penile size in boys with Prader-Willi syndrome usually concerns parents, but they might not bring it up as a problem. They should be informed that a few small doses of testosterone can be used, if needed, during the second or third year of life, to increase penile size enough to enable the boy to stand up to urinate. Surgery for undescended testes can wait in the Prader-Willi syndrome when the diagnosis is certain and the parents comfortable with it. Surgery for undescended testes is performed in young boys primarily to preserve fertility. However, as infertility is inevitable in this syndrome, this is not a valid indication for an operation. Instead it has been shown that the testes often descend spontaneously during childhood in boys with Prader-Willi syndrome. The difficulties of detecting possible development of cancer in the undescended testes is another indication for surgery. This issue must be discussed in adolescence. The rarity of the latter condition versus the possible risk of surgery must be considered by the young man and the family.

Sex hormone replacement and plastic surgery can be offered to normalize the virilization process and thereby the physical appearance of the young boy, but, as of yet, not enough experience has been accumulated to judge the effect of such treatment on behavior and well-being. The need for endocrinologic intervention for hypogonadism is less acute in adolescent girls, who frequently are satisfied with their appearance. Hormone replacement is available and can be used when indicated to enhance breast development. It will also initiate menstrual periods.

Short Stature Growth rate becomes an important parameter to monitor during the early childhood years. Growth hormone deficiency had been demonstrated in some early endocrinology studies of children with Prader-Willi syndrome. However, it was argued that this deficit was secondary to the increased weight, because it is well known that obese children have inadequate response to growth hormone stimulation tests. It has since been shown that many nonobese children with Prader-Willi syndrome also demonstrate growth hormone deficiency, and that children with Prader-Willi syndrome and such deficits respond to treatment with growth hormone replacement.

Length and height growth therefore must be carefully monitored during childhood. Two growth parameters must be watched during childhood: height for midparental height and the child's height growth plotted on the syndrome-specific growth charts. Such growth charts have been developed from Figures 2 and 3 and are available from the Prader-Willi Syndrome Association (USA). Referral for endocrine assessment of possible growth hormone

deficiency should be entertained in a child with Prader-Willi syndrome who is significantly shorter than expected for family height or whose growth is falling off in the height scale on the syndrome-specific growth charts. In the author's experience, such children typically have growth hormone deficiency and respond to growth hormone supplementation if offered. The age at which time such referral is made will depend on many factors: the degree of the child's and the family's concern about short stature, the child's sex (in boys, shortness of stature is more pronounced and typically more of a psychologic disability than in girls), and the willingness of the child and family to put up with daily shots. Growth hormone increases lean body mass. Persons with Prader-Willi syndrome have less muscle mass than age-mates and benefit from the administration of growth hormone not just with an increase in stature. They also seem to become stronger, with increased stamina.

Medication Psychotropic medications are frequently tried to control difficult behaviors in persons with Prader-Willi syndrome. No single medication has been shown to be consistently helpful. Medications must be individualized and should be reserved for older patients. Depression, obsessive–compulsive tendencies, or paranoia might be present and should be considered in the choice of drugs.

Nutrition

For a physician practicing in interdisciplinary settings, access to a nutritionist knowledgeable about the specific needs of patients with Prader-Willi syndrome is essential for management of such individuals. A typical diet prescribed for weight loss in most people will result in weight gain in this condition. For reasons that have not been elucidated adequately, persons with Prader-Willi syndrome must consume fewer calories than peers of the same age or size in order to maintain an appropriate weight gain (Holm & Pipes, 1976).

The typical child with Prader-Willi syndrome will maintain an appropriate weight gain on a daily intake of approximately 10–11 cal/cm/day. If a static weight is desired over a period of time to allow the child to "grow into" the weight, about 9 cal/cm will accomplish the goal. When weight loss is needed, one should not advise a daily caloric intake of less than 8 cal/cm, in order to assure a diet that is nutritionally adequate for a growing child. The average short, comparatively inactive adult with Prader-Willi syndrome usually maintains an appropriate weight on a diet of 1,000–1,200 cal/day and will lose weight on 800–1,000 cal/day. These are rough guidelines. Caloric intake must be individualized by an initial period of record keeping of food intake and monthly weight checks. Adjustments might be necessary to accomplish the goal of slow weight loss (more than 1 kg/month is seldom desirable), weight maintenance, or appropriately slow weight gain. The periods of record keeping and weight checks might occasionally need to be repeated.

The diet should be compatible with family and cultural eating patterns. An exchange system similar to the one used in the dietary management of diabetes is helpful. A daily vitamin supplement should be prescribed. No appetite-suppressing medication or special diets (e.g., low sugar diet) have proven to be helpful. The patient and the family must understand that a low-calorie diet is a lifetime commitment for survival in Prader-Willi syndrome.

Education

Birth-to-3 and preschool education programs are appropriate for most children with Prader-Willi syndrome. The severe infantile hypotonia and slow motor development will qualify infants with Prader-Willi syndrome for physical and occupational therapy services in such early intervention programs. Onset of language is typically mildly delayed, and speech and language services usually become appropriate. The most consistent finding in children with Prader-Willi syndrome is nasal speech, but other articulation difficulties might need intervention. The occasional child with severe language difficulties because of dyspraxia will need speech and language services, such as signing and other forms of augmented communication, over a long period of time.

In general, children with Prader-Willi syndrome function well in inclusive educational settings with access to resource rooms and other support services. Obviously each child's program needs will vary and must be individualized. An overriding educational issue for teachers of children with Prader-Willi syndrome is the management of food in the classroom (e.g., lunch pails brought by other children and treats for parties). The school cafeteria is a constant temptation. The goal for the child with Prader-Willi syndrome in the cafeteria is to eat only what the parents have provided in the lunch pail or a specially prescribed meal providing 300 calories or less. This goal requires monitoring. No food swapping and no eating from other children's plates can be allowed. The principal might also need to consider placement of garbage cans; the child with Prader-Willi syndrome might be tempted when walking by on legitimate errands. Everyone in the child's educational program needs to understand the importance of external control of food in the environment for a child with Prader-Willi syndrome. Physicians often need to assist parents by explaining the medical aspect of this disorder to educators and therapists who deal with the child on a regular basis.

Home economics is not a good subject for high school students with Prader-Willi syndrome. Too many temptations are nearby. The food-related behavior problems also must be considered when planning vocational training for persons with Prader-Willi syndrome. The food industry is a good working environment for populations with the cognitive level typical in this syndrome. However, for persons with Prader-Willi syndrome, working in restaurants or other places where food is abundantly available is catastrophic, even though the dream of many persons with the syndrome is to do just that.

Behavior Management

Behavior modification techniques are powerful tools in the management of behavior problems in Prader-Willi syndrome. However, many of the behavioral characteristics common in these children will test the ingenuity of even the experienced behavior management specialist. Examples are skin picking, verbal perseveration, violent rages, and repeated running away.

Behavior management specific to Prader-Willi syndrome centers around the need to control availability of unauthorized food. Caregivers learn not to leave unsupervised a room where food is being prepared or cleared away. Locks on cupboards and refrigerators, or locking the door to the kitchen, might become necessary. The problem is often not just the home where the child lives but neighborhood houses and stores and the homes of relatives and friends. Parents should be advised to enlist the cooperation of family, neighbors, store managers, and sometimes the local police. Parties and restaurant visits pose another challenge. Small treats of food that is usually off limits (later to be compensated for in the regular diet) is often useful.

Food is a powerful motivator in Prader-Willi syndrome. Foods can be used as primary reinforcers in therapy and educational programs but they must be low in calories. Conversely, withholding of special treats can be effective as a consequence of misbehaviors such as tantrums. Calmly pouring part of a can of low-calorie soda down the sink might more clearly than words depict the effect of an action to a child with Prader-Willi syndrome.

Social Service Support

The most helpful resource for parents of children with Prader-Willi syndrome is a parent support network, the Prader-Willi Syndrome Association (USA) (2510 Brentwood Boulevard, Suite 220, St. Louis, MO 63144 [1-800-926-4797]). The association was founded in 1975 and has met annually since 1979. This 4-day annual meeting combines a 1-day multidisciplinary scientific meeting with parent information and support services and also has a youth program attended by people of all ages with Prader-Willi syndrome and their siblings. Similar organizations now exist in many countries in Europe, in Australia, and elsewhere. The first meeting with an international scope was held in 1992 in Holland, and a second one was held in Norway in 1995. Efforts to keep these regular events are underway.

Local chapters of the Prader-Willi Syndrome Association (USA) are active in many parts of the country and provide friendship, informal exchange of experiences, and support for families. Parents should be given information about local chapters as well as the national association as soon as the diagnosis has been made. Parents also should be made aware at an early stage of community resources that might be helpful, such as the department of developmental disability. Unfortunately, some people with Prader-Willi syndrome are too high functioning on formal testing to be eligible for disability services. The physician must be an advocate for such persons. Individuals with Prader-Willi syndrome have severe physical and behavioral disabilities, even if some do not meet IQ requirements for many services available to populations with disabilities. Many service system authorities must have this fact explained to them.

Options for Living Situations

Most children with Prader-Willi syndrome live in the home of their biological parent(s). Some reside in foster homes. Most caregivers are comfortable with such arrangements when the children are young. However, the care of some children can become overwhelming as early as middle school age because of uncontrollable obesity and severe behavior problems. Rehabilitative service facilities are available for short-term habilitation (a few months) for such children. Thoughtful parents start preparing for the future when their children approach adolescence. Most recognize the need for their charges to grow up, leave the nest, and establish themselves in a living situation of their own.

Parents of all children with developmental disabilities face the question of the best long-term placement of their children. In Prader-Willi syndrome, the situation is complicated by the fact that these individuals have a medical condition that impels them to literally eat themselves to death. The present emphasis on inclusion and the least restrictive environment poses a dilemma in planning for young adults with Prader-Willi syndrome. The only living situation that has been proven to enable these individuals to live in the community and maintain a lifesaving weight is the dedicated group home. Kitchens can be locked, the diet can be kept low in calories for everyone, an emphasis on physical activity can be pursued, and appropriate work activities can be arranged. Anybody familiar with Prader-Willi syndrome will attest to the fact that the "least restrictive environment" for adults with Prader-Willi syndrome is one that is not inclusive but rather is geared to their very special medical needs.

CONCLUSIONS

Prader-Willi syndrome is a comparatively common developmental disability with profound medical, behavioral, and social implications. The clinical picture changes dramatically over the life span of affected individuals. An interdisciplinary team with knowledge of the varied aspect of Prader-Willi syndrome is the ideal setting for management of this multisystem disorder. The recent unraveling of the genetics of Prader-Willi syndrome has contributed to knowledge of genomic imprinting and provided new perspectives on molecular genetics.

REFERENCES

Cassidy, S.B. (1984). Prader-Willi syndrome. *Current Problems in Pediatrics, 14,* 1–55.

Greenswag, L.R., & Alexander, R.C. (Eds.). (1995). *Management of Prader-Willi syndrome* (2nd ed.). New York: Springer-Verlag.

Hall, J.G. (1992). Genomic imprinting and its clinical implications. *New England Journal of Medicine, 326,* 827–829.

Holm, V.A., Cassidy, S.B., Butler, M.G., Hanchett, J.M., Greenswag, L.R., Whitman, B.Y., & Greenberg, F. (1993). Prader-Willi syndrome: Consensus diagnostic criteria. *Pediatrics, 91,* 398–402.

Holm, V.A., & Pipes, P.L. (1976). Food and children with Prader-Willi syndrome. *American Journal of Diseases of Children, 130,* 1063–1067.

Ledbetter, D.H., Riccardi, V.M., Airhart, S.D., Strobel, R.J., Keenan, B.S., & Crawford, J.D. (1981). Deletion of chromosome 15 as a cause of the Prader-Willi syndrome. *New England Journal of Medicine, 304,* 325–329.

Mascari, M.J., Gottlieb, W., Rogan, P.K., Butler, M.G., Waller, D.A., Armour, J.A.L., Jeffreys, A.J., Ladda, R.L., & Nicholls, R.D. (1992). The frequency of uniparental disomy in Prader-Willi syndrome: Implications for molecular diagnosis. *New England Journal of Medicine, 326,* 1599–1607.

Prader, A., Labhart, A., & Willi, H. (1956). Ein Syndrom von Adipositas, Kleinwuchs, Kryptochismus und Oligophrenie nach myatonieartigem Zustand im Neugeborenenalter. *Schweizerische Medizinische Wochenschrift, 86,* 1260–1261.

Chapter 17

Fragile X Syndrome

Andrew Robert Adesman, M.D.

Fragile X syndrome was first described 25 years ago and now is recognized as the most common inherited form of mental retardation. This syndrome is of great importance not only because of its relative prevalence, but also because of the wide array of associated developmental disorders and its distinct mode of genetic transmission. It is estimated that 1 in 1,000 females are carriers of fragile X syndrome and that approximately 1 in 1,300 males are affected. Unlike Down syndrome—the only genetic cause of mental retardation more common than fragile X— the clinical diagnosis of fragile X syndrome is rarely made during infancy. Because the phenotypic appearance of individuals with fragile X syndrome is more variable and less obvious in prepubertal children, professionals must be familiar with the myriad clinical presentations for which this diagnosis must be considered. Early diagnosis of fragile X syndrome can have important implications not only with respect to the treatment of the child but also with respect to the counseling of the family.

HISTORICAL BACKGROUND

It has long been recognized that there is a predominance of men among people with mental retardation who live in institutions. However, a genetic basis for this imbalance was not suggested until 1943, when Martin and Bell described a family pedigree with 11 males with mental retardation within two generations; they postulated that mental retardation in this family might be transmitted on an X-linked basis. Herbert Lubbs provided the first laboratory evidence for X-linked mental retardation (XLMR); in 1969, he described a family with XLMR in association with dysmorphic features and a morphologic abnormality of the X chromosome. The "marker X" chromosome described by Lubs had a secondary constriction near the end of the long arm of the X chromosome (Figure 1).

During the 1970s, there were only sporadic reports of a marker X chromosome in families with XLMR. At that time, many cytogenetics laboratories had already switched from using Media 199 (which inherently is deficient in folate and thymidine) to a supplemented culture medium. It was not until 1977 that Sutherland reported that the marker X chromosome could be seen only under certain laboratory conditions. When Sutherland moved from Melbourne to Adelaide, Australia (upgrading his laboratory in the process), he found he was unable to replicate his own previous observation of the marker site. After further investigation, Sutherland realized that the marker was really a "fragile site" that could not be seen when the cells were cultured in an enriched growth medium.

Following the discovery that the expression of a fragile site on the X chromosome was media specific, the morphologic abnormality first described by Lubbs was subsequently noted by other laboratories in many families with pedigrees suggestive of XLMR, including the one originally reported by Martin and Bell. Other cytogenetic techniques for inducing expression of the fragile site have since been described. Given that folic acid is needed for thymidine metabolism, chemicals that inhibit other steps in the metabolism of thymidine (e.g., methotrexate, 5-fluorodeoxyuridine, trimethoprim) have also been shown to induce fragile site expression.

Fragile sites—points on a chromosome that tend to break nonrandomly when exposed to specific chemical agents or conditions of tissue culture—have been noted on several other chromosomes. At least 100 common or rare fragile

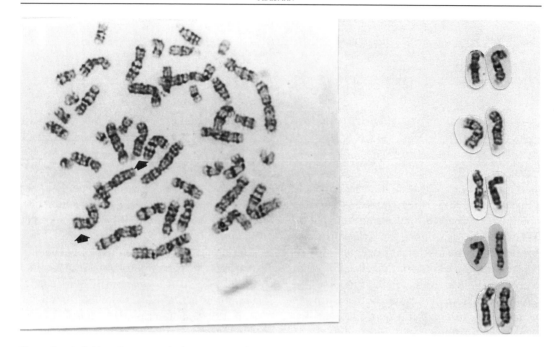

Figure 1. *Left,* Metaphase spread of a woman with a karyotype of 46, X, fra(X) (q27.3); fragile site is seen on one X chromosome (upper arrow) but not the other (lower arrow). *Right,* Partial karyotypes from five cells from the same woman; normal X chromosome is on the left and fragile X chromosome is on the right. (Courtesy of Ann-Leslie Zaslav, Ph.D., Division of Human Genetics, Schneider Children's Hospital, Long Island Jewish Medical Center, New Hyde Park, NY.)

sites have now been described. However, the rare fragile site on the long arm of the X chromosome described by Lubbs was the first to be consistently associated with a distinct clinical phenotype or with mental retardation (Nussbaum & Ledbetter, 1986). This fragile site, at position Xq27.3 near the end of the long arm of the X chromosome, is designated *FRAXA* (fragile site, X chromosome, A site). At least two other fragile sites (FRAXE, FRAXF) have since been noted on the X chromosome, one of which (FRAXE) represents mutational changes almost identical to FRAXA and is associated with mild mental retardation (Hirst et al., 1993; Knight et al., 1993; Sutherland & Baker, 1992).

GENETICS

It is now recognized that fragile X syndrome is an X-linked condition with an atypical pattern of inheritance, such that boys and girls can either be affected with the syndrome or be unaffected carriers. Although the syndrome segregates as an X-linked dominant disorder with reduced penetrance in females and nonpenetrance in males,

molecular genetics advances since the early 1990s have provided a new and fuller understanding of its mechanism of genetic transmission and variable clinical expression (Tarleton & Saul, 1993; Warren & Nelson, 1994).

Fragile X syndrome is due to a mutation of a specific gene on the X chromosome labeled *FMR-1* (fragile X mental retardation gene–1). In individuals without the syndrome, the *FMR-1* gene has a regulatory sequence (CpG island) and a repeated CGG_n sequence, where the number (n) of contiguous copies of the CGG trinucleotide varies from approximately 6 to 54 (average = 29 repeats). Although girls without the syndrome have two X chromosomes in each cell, only one of these is active; the other is inactivated early in fetal development. Methylation of a CpG island generally shuts off the expression of a gene. Thus, in these girls, the CpG island associated with *FMR-1* will be methylated in the inactive X chromosome but the *FMR-1* gene in the other normal X chromosome of each cell will be expressed fully.

Boys without the syndrome have only a single X chromosome, which is always "active";

that is, the genes on it are transcribed into mRNA and ultimately to protein. In these individuals, the *FMR-1* gene on the X chromosome has an unmethylated CpG island and is thus likewise expressed.

Through molecular genetic techniques, it has been established that fragile X syndrome is seen in those individuals with abnormally large (>200) CGG repeats and methylation of the CpG island. These techniques have also led to the identification of individuals with a "premutation"—individuals who have some amplification of the CGG repeat but do not have methylation of the CpG island. Instead of the 10–50 repeats seen in individuals without the syndrome, carriers with the premutation generally have an X chromosome with an expansion of 50–200 repeats, with 75–120 repeats being most typical. Gene expression does not seem affected by the amount of amplification. Men with the premutation are called "normal transmitting males"; they do not have any of the physical, developmental, or cytogenetic features of the fragile X syndrome.

If a female has the premutation, in addition to a normal X chromosome (<50 CGG repeats), she also has an allele with 50–200 repeats. As with transmitting males, these females have normal-appearing chromosomes cytogenetically, and generally do not have the more obvious physical or developmental features of fragile X syndrome.

Interestingly, whereas almost all boys with the full mutation will have mental retardation and the associated phenotype, this is not true for girls with the full mutation. Only some of these girls will have clinical or cytogenetic evidence of fragile X syndrome. The more variable clinical expression in girls with the full mutation is presumed to be due to lyonization—the random inactivation of one X chromosome in each cell in the body. Thus, in contrast to affected boys, girls with a full mutation may have a normal X chromosome expressed instead of the fragile X chromosome in at least a significant number of their body's cells.

Mosaicism for fragile X has been observed in both males and females with the full mutation. These individuals have some cells with alleles containing more than 200 CGG repeats but have other cells with repeats in the 50–200 range. Among individuals who carry the full mutation, mosaicism is more common among males than females (12% vs. 6%). Mosaic males have a larger CGG expansion than do mosaic females (Rousseau et al., 1994).

Geneticists describe fragile X syndrome as showing genetic "anticipation." This term refers to the increase in severity and progressively earlier age of onset of a genetic disease with each successive generation. Anticipation is also seen with myotonic dystrophy, one of the other common heritable disorders now recognized as being associated with a triplet repeat sequence (Caskey, Pizzuti, Fu, Fenwick, & Nelson, 1992; Warren & Nelson, 1994). When a female carrier for fragile X syndrome with the premutation passes the gene on, there is usually expansion (i.e., further amplication) of the CGG repeat. Interestingly, siblings who inherit this chromosome usually differ from each other and also their parent with regard to the length of their CGG rpeat. When a carrier (transmitting) male passes his mutated X chromosome to his daughter, it is usually only slightly expanded; thus, transmitting males generally have daughters that likewise have only the premutation for fragile X syndrome (Figure 2).

In carrier women, the size of the CGG repeat affects the likelihood that their male offspring will have the full mutation. For example, mothers with only 65 repeats have a 9% probability of having an affected male child with the full mutation (50% chance of inheriting the fragile X chromosome × 18% risk of expansion), whereas mothers with more than 100 repeats have a 50% chance of having a son with fragile X syndrome (50% chance of inheriting the fragile X chromosome × 100% likelihood of expansion) (Warren & Nelson, 1994). To a lesser extent, the maternal repeat size also influences the extent to which a woman's daughters will be affected. Fragile X syndrome is the first human disorder in which premutation DNA sequences in the parent predict substantial disease risk to progeny (Caskey et al., 1992).

Because daughters with the full mutation also have a normal X chromosome, approximately half (53%–59%) will have mental impairment. Unfortunately, at this time, there is no way of

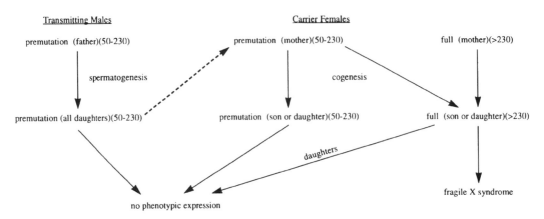

Figure 2.   Inheritance of premutations and full mutations in the fragile X syndrome. Numbers represent the approximate number of trinucleotide (CGG) repeats. Broken arrow indicates that the daughter of a transmitting male is a premutation carrier female. Premutation carrier females also may be the offspring of premutation carrier females. An initial estimate is that 53% of girls who inherit a full mutation from their mothers have mental retardation. (From Tarleton, J.C., & Saul, R.A. [1993]. Molecular genetic advances in fragile X syndrome. *Journal of Pediatrics, 122,* 169–185; reprinted by permission.)

predicting exactly which girls inheriting the full mutation will be clinically affected; however, girls with a relatively large mutation (>2,000 bp) are known to be at significantly increased risk for mental retardation (Rousseau et al., 1994). With mosaic men and women, it is also difficult to predict whether their offspring will have the full mutation.

LABORATORY DIAGNOSIS

Until the 1990s, diagnosis of fragile X syndrome relied on identification of the morphologic finding of the rare folate-sensitive fragile site (Xq27.3) by cytogenetic testing. Advances in molecular genetics, however, have enhanced significantly our ability to identify carrier status and distinguish between individuals with the full mutation and those with just the premutation. The advantages and limitations of each of these laboratory approaches to diagnosis are reviewed briefly here.

Cytogenetic Testing

Chromosomal karyotyping (using special laboratory techniques to induce fragility) was the original method for diagnosing fragile X syndrome. This approach relies on the identification by microscopy of the characteristic mor-

pholpologic abnormality, which is seen most consistently in affected males. Cytogenetic testing for fragile X is labor intensive and thus quite expensive (usually $500 or more). This is partly because the cytogeneticist must carefully examine a greater number of cells to accurately determine what percentage of cells, if any, have a rare fragile site at Xq27.3. There are two reasons why additional cells must be analyzed. Rare fragile sites at Xq27.3 have also been noted in a small percentage ($\leq$3%) of cells of normal individuals. Conversely, affected males with the full mutation do not have a fragile site evident on most of their X chromosomes. These individuals have a constriction visible at Xq27.3 in less than 50% of their cells (typically 10%–15%), even though the abnormal CGG sequence is present in every cell. These percentages are even lower in females with the full mutation; some have no fragile sites and others have no more than 10% of their cells with a morphologically abnormal X chromosome. In females, the percentage of cytogenetically visible fragile X chromosomes may decrease with age. If the cytogeneticist examined the chromosomes of only a small number of cells, sampling error could lead to missed (false-negative) or mistaken (false-positive) diagnoses. The diagnosis of fragile X syndrome may also be wrongly made if one of the several proximate fragile sites (Xq27.2, Xq28.1) on the X chromosome were present and mistaken for the rare fragile site at Xq27.3. Cytogenetic testing for fragile X syndrome must be done by knowledgeable, experienced, and well-trained professionals.

Although it has long been recognized that cytogenetic testing will not identify transmitting boys and many carrier girls, it had been considered very accurate in diagnosing boys with the full mutation. Later reports suggest, however, that, even among affected boys with the full mutation, the chromosomal karyotype will be normal in 7% of cases (Rousseau et al., 1994). Although a sensitivity of 93% is considered acceptable for many screening tests, chromosomal karyotype testing cannot be considered a "screening test." For these reasons, cytogenetic testing for fragile X syndrome increasingly will assume a secondary role in the laboratory evaluation of the child with mental retardation.

Compared to molecular genetic techniques, cytogenetic testing does have one advantage in that it provides some information about the patient's other chromosomes. For example, major deletions, translocations, and ring chromosomes would also be detected as part of a chromosomal karyotype ordered to rule out fragile X syndrome. However, high-resolution banding analysis should be done if other genetic abnormalities are suspected.

Linkage Analysis

Until 1991, DNA linkage testing was the only technique available that could enable geneticists to determine whether or not unaffected individuals with normal karyotypes and a family history positive for fragile X syndrome were likely to be carriers. An individual's carrier status was inferred by looking at the inheritance pattern of specific DNA sequences (i.e., restriction fragment length polymorphisms [RFLPs]) on either side of the fragile site. When alleles of RFLPs above and below the fragile site were inherited together, it was very likely that the fragile X gene was passed along as well (Hagerman, 1987). Although linkage analysis was helpful in identifying transmitting men and women with the premutation who were thus at significant

risk of having developmentally affected offspring (especially boys), many factors limit its clinical worth. To the extent that linkage analysis is not looking at the mutation itself (but rather only at genes proximate to the mutation site), it only allows for a reasonable inference or estimate of the likelihood of whether an individual is a carrier or not, not a definitive conclusion. If there is recombination involving the DNA markers, linkage analysis could give either false-negative or false-positive results. Finally, linkage analysis cannot distinguish between an individual with a premutation and an individual with the full mutation.

Molecular Genetic Testing

Molecular techniques now enable geneticists to directly assess the *FMR-1* gene on the X chromosome in individuals suspected of having or being carriers for fragile X syndrome. This information can be determined with either of two techniques: direct analysis (using electrophoresis and Southern blotting) or polymerase chain reaction (PCR) analysis. Although each of these techniques has its respective limitations, they share many advantages over the two other diagnostic approaches already described. These molecular genetic techniques are not as labor intensive or expensive, and they can reliably distinguish between individuals who have the premutation, those who have the full mutation, and those who are mosaics (Figure 3).

Direct analysis assesses the size of the CGG region as well as its methylation status. This technique involves the use of endonucleases to cut the *FMR-1* gene into specific fragments and a DNA probe to determine their size. It requires more DNA and does not provide results as rapidly as PCR. Because the PCR technique makes a large number of copies of a short segment of the *FMR-1* gene, there is enough DNA to allow rapid analysis of the gene segment with even a very small sample from the patient. Although this technique provides information regarding CGG amplification, it does not provide information regarding methylation. Nonetheless, in 90% of individuals, PCR analysis proves sufficient. For those cases in which the PCR bands are not readily visible, Southern blot assay is performed.

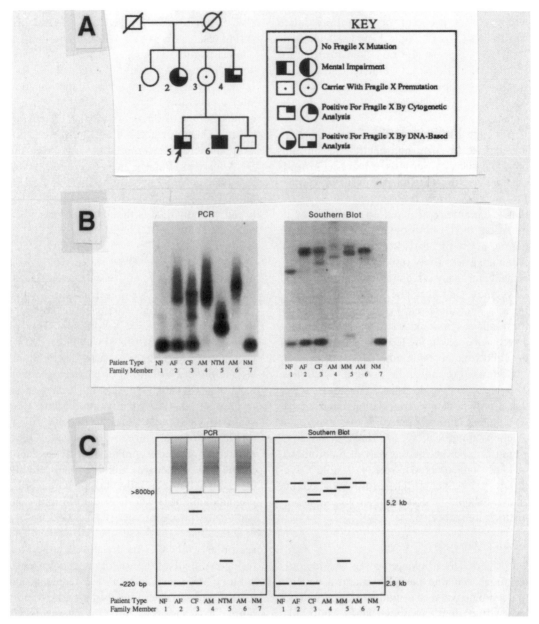

Figure 3. (A) Pedigree of case family. Individual 5 was referred for reevaluation of mental impairment. Family history is significant for fragile X syndrome in a sibling. (B) PCR and Southern blots of case family. PCR provides the fastest diagnostic results for affected, carrier, and unaffected individuals except when a male is mosaic for fragile X. In that case, Southern blotting can distinguish a male with a permutation from a male with somatic cell mosaicism. PCR results are reported in terms of fragment size rather than insert size. (C) Idiogram of the banding patterns seen in fragile X syndrome on PCR and Southern blot, respectively. (From Murphy, P.D. [1993]. Technical aspects of the diagnosis of fragile X syndrome. *Neurogenetic Advances, 2*(2), 2–3. [Worcester, MA: Genica Pharmaceuticals Corporation]; reprinted by permission.)

It should be noted that a small percentage of individuals with the full clinical phenotype of fragile X syndrome will have a negative cytogenetic analysis and will not have an expanded CGG region on the *FMR-1* gene. In some of these individuals, expression of the *FMR-1* gene is inhibited not because of methylation of the CpG island but because of other alterations to that gene (e.g., deletions, substitutions). It should be noted that, whereas all males with the full mutation (>200 repeats) have been shown to have inherited it from their mothers (who have either the premutation or the full mutation), there are de novo mutations involving the *FMR-1* gene that will lead to the classic fragile X phenotype both developmentally and on physical examination.

At this time, molecular genetic testing is significantly less expensive than cytogenetic analysis; moreover, these newer technologies lend themselves potentially to mass screening programs at even lower cost. Although not yet imminent, it is conceivable that screening for fragile X carrier status could be offered as part of routine family planning or prenatal testing. It is anticipated that, in the future, other diagnostic techniques such as enzyme-linked immunosorbent assay may also be developed to directly quantitate the mRNA or protein coded for by the *FMR-1* gene.

CLINICAL FEATURES IN AFFECTED MALES

Physical Examination

Table 1 lists the physical findings most commonly seen in males with fragile X syndrome. In adolescents and adult men, the three most common physical findings are long or prominent ears, a long face ($\pm$ prominent jaw), and large testicles. In adults, ear length greater than 7 cm is considered abnormal; typical measurement ranges are illustrated in Figure 4. Unfortunately for the pediatrician, the most consistent and reliable physical finding—macroorchidism—is not very common or striking among preadolescent boys. In the prepubertal boy, prominent ears, a relatively large head ($\geq$75%), a long face, a prominent forehead (with flattening of the nasal bridge), or a high-arched palate may be the only facial findings present to suggest fragile X syndrome (Simko, Hornstein, Soukup, & Bagamery, 1989).

In an adolescent or adult, the upper limit of normal for testicular volume is 25–30 ml, with the average being approximately 17 ml (Figure 5). Postpubertal males with fragile X syndrome typically have testicles that measure 40 ml or more in volume. Testicular volume can be assessed using an orchidometer (a set of ellipsoid shapes of known volume that are compared directly with the testicle) or calculated using the formula

$$\text{Testicular volume} = \pi/6 \times \text{length} \times \text{width}^2$$

In the prepubertal boy (ages 8 and under), the testicle generally has a volume less than 2 ml and should measure less than 1 inch in length. Whereas macroorchidism is present in 70%–90% of postpubertal males with fragile X syndrome, only 15%–40% of prepubertal boys will have testicular enlargement (Simko et al., 1989). Boys with fragile X syndrome who are less than

Table 1. Common physical findings in males with fragile X syndrome

Head	Usually large (>75%)
Facies	Large/prominent ears, long face, prominent jaw,[a] high-arched palate, flattened nasal bridge,[a] epicanthic folds, coarse facial features, (mild)[a] strabismus
Genitalia	Macroorchidism[a] (>2 ml prepubertal; >30 ml postpubertal), macrophallus[a]
Musculoskeletal system	Hyperextensible fingers (>90 degrees at metacarpophalangeal joints),[b] pes planus
Skin	Soft, smooth skin (especially on hands); simian crease (palms), hallucal crease (soles); calluses on hand (from self-injury)[a]
Central nervous system	Hypotonia, coordination problems, abnormal gait

[a]More commonly seen in postpubertal age groups.
[b]More commonly seen in prepubertal children.

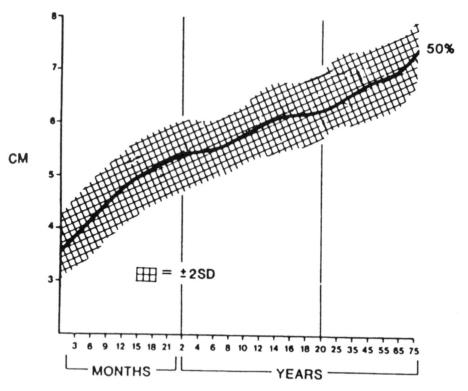

Figure 4. Normal values for mean ear length ± 2 standard deviations (*SD*). (From Hagerman, R.J. [1987]. Fragile X syndrome. *Current Problems in Pediatrics, 17,* 635; reprinted by permission.)

8 years of age have significantly larger mean testicular volumes than boys without fragile X syndrome; however, they seldom have true macroorchidism (≥ 4.0 ml, or two or more times normal) (Lachiewicz & Dawson, 1994).

A variety of other physical findings have frequently been noted in males with fragile X syndrome that suggest a connective tissue defect; these include hyperextensible finger joints (especially in prepubertal boys), flat feet, pectus excavatum, high-arched palate, velvetlike skin, and mitral valve prolapse with aortic root dilation. Ophthalmologic problems include strabismus (40%–56% of cases); refractive errors; and, less commonly, ptosis or nystagmus (Hagerman, 1991b).

Apart from flexible flat feet, common orthopedic findings include excessive joint laxity and scoliosis. Ligamentous laxity appears to decrease with age; metacarpal extension of greater than 90 degrees was noted in 73% of children with fragile X syndrome younger than 11, 56% of those 11–19, and only 30% of those 20 years

or older. Double-jointed thumbs are common in affected boys and girls, although dislocation is rare. Scoliosis and pectus excavatum are associated less commonly (Hagerman, 1991b).

In addition to having soft, smooth skin, examination of the hands also may reveal calluses from biting. Characteristic dermatoglyphics have been described, although most pediatricians do not have the clinical training and experience to assess these. A single palmar crease and Sydney lines have also been noted in affected individuals.

Although any of the other signs listed in Table 1 may be noted in young children with fragile X syndrome, none are specific to this syndrome. For example, on neurologic examination, children with fragile X syndrome may have mildly decreased muscle tone, hyperextensible joints, or problems with coordination or abnormal gait (Vieregge & Froster-Iskenius, 1989), yet each of these findings is fairly common in pediatric populations with developmental disabilities.

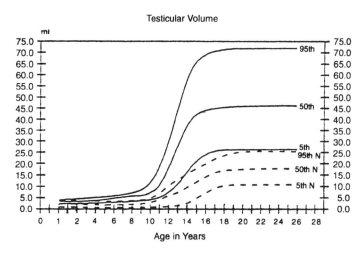

Figure 5. Testicular volume: standardized curves for males with fragile X syndrome (solid line) and males without developmental disabilities (broken line). (From Butler, M.G., Brunschwig, A., Miller, L.K., & Hagerman, R.J. [1992]. Standards for anthropometric measurements in males with the fragile X syndrome. *Pediatrics, 89,* 1059–1062; reprinted by permission.)

Developmental History

In addition to the physical findings described above, the diagnosis of fragile X syndrome also may be suggested by the developmental history. Almost all affected boys who express the fragile X site will manifest some degree of mental retardation. Although IQ is a relatively stable measure in most populations, boys with fragile X syndrome experience approximately a 10-point drop in IQ as they mature (Borghgraef, Fryns, Dielkens, Pyck, & VanDenBerghe, 1987). Thus, whereas most boys with fragile X syndrome will function in the mild to moderate range of mental retardation during their preschool years, adolescents and adults with fragile X syndrome more typically function in the moderate to severely retardation range. For some older children or adolescents with mental retardation, the diagnosis of fragile X syndrome will be established only on medical referral for evaluation of IQ decline (Figure 6). Several cases have also been described in which boys with fragile X syndrome have average intelligence but underachieve academically because of a learning disability (Hagerman, Kemper & Hudson, 1985). Also, some (but not all) studies

have suggested that males who are mosaic for fragile X syndrome may have less severe cognitive impairment, with some functioning in the borderline range (Rousseau et al., 1994).

Children with fragile X syndrome frequently have developmental deficits in two other spheres: speech–language and behavior/social skills (Bregman, Dykens, Watson, Ort, & Leckman, 1987). Boys with less severe retardation may have "cluttered" speech—speech that is characterized by a rapid rate, erratic rhythm, and a disorganized, repetitive style (Hansen, Jackson, & Hagerman, 1986). Other, less specific speech-language characteristics noted in children with fragile X syndrome are dysfluency, dyspraxia, poor articulation, and echolalia.

Approximately two thirds of prepubertal boys with fragile X syndrome are described as being hyperactive or inattentive (Simko et al., 1989). With respect to other interpersonal skills, individuals with fragile X syndrome are significantly less social when compared to IQ-matched individuals with Down syndrome (Wolff, Gardner, Paccia, & Lappen, 1989). Affected boys may exhibit only mild features of social withdrawal (such as shyness or gaze aversion), or they may present with the full clin-

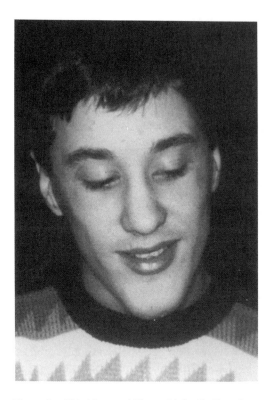

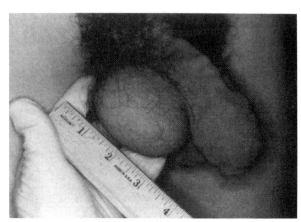

Figure 6. This 16-year-old boy with fragile X syndrome was referred for neurodevelopmental evaluation of IQ decline; routine chromosomal karyotype at age 3 years was normal. Fragile X syndrome was suggested by his long face, prominent chin, and gaze aversion (left) as well as by his orchidomegaly and macrophallus (right). Note that this boy does not have large or prominent ears.

ical picture of autism—including stereotypic hand movements and self-injurious behavior. Based on data pooled from multiple studies of autistic populations, it is estimated that only 6.5% (0%–16%) of autistic males have fragile X syndrome. Conversely, approximately 16%–17% of males with fragile X syndrome are thought to be autistic (Hagerman, 1991b).

CLINICAL FEATURES IN GIRLS

Because fragile X syndrome is an X-linked disorder, girls with a fragile site on one of their X chromosomes are heterozygous carriers; thus, they generally have less severe developmental disabilities and less frequently have the facial stigmata noted in affected boys. In the multicenter collaborative study by Rousseau et al. (1994), the majority (87%) of older males with the full fragile X mutation functioned in the moderate to profound range of mental retarda-

tion, whereas only 21% of females with the full mutation had an equivalent degree of retardation. Of the 170 females in this study with the full mutation, 100 (59%) presented with some mental impairment, 64 of whom had only mild cognitive impairment.

Female carriers of fragile X syndrome are also less likely to have physical stigmata than males with the full mutation. Whereas at least 85% of affected postpubertal males will have some of the physical features described above, only 28% of female carriers will have facial stigmata. Girls with the full mutation who have cognitive impairment are most likely to have such stigmata. Fifty-five percent of female carriers with mental retardation will have at least some characteristic facial features, but only 14% of all unaffected carrier females (with IQs >80) will have stigmata (Fryns, 1986). It is unclear whether there is a phenotypic impact of the *FMR-1* gene in cytogenetically negative females who have the premutation only. In a recent study comparing these women to controls without the *FMR-1* gene, women with the premutation had more prominent ears (based on anthropometric measurement) and had higher scores on a more subjective index of 10 physical findings associated with fragile X syndrome (Hull & Hagerman, 1993). In contrast, the multicenter study by Rousseau et al. (1994) found no difference; the girls with the premutation did not differ from women without the *FMR-1* gene with respect to presence or absence of dysmorphic facial features.

Female carriers also have a more variable developmental picture. With regard to neurocognitive functioning of cytogenetically positive females, several studies of adult women with the full mutation have demonstrated lower overall IQ scores and lower achievement scores in arithmetic. Whereas almost all males with the full mutation will have mental retardation, only 50% of females with the full mutation will have retardation. Twenty-five percent will have borderline intelligence and/or learning disabilities; mathematics and auditory processing are areas of particular weakness (Kemper, Hagerman, Ahmad, & Mariner, 1986). Performance on tasks reflecting frontal lobe functioning also appears to be compromised in these women (Mazzocco, Hagerman, Cronister-Silverman, & Pennington, 1992). Several recent studies have looked at whether there is any correlation in carrier females between the laboratory findings (cytogenetic and molecular genetics) and the clinical findings. Women with the premutation (50–200 CGG repeats) have a significantly higher median IQ than women with the full mutation (104 vs. 81). However, within each mutation group, there is no correlation between IQ and the size of the CGG repeat or the methylation status (Taylor et al., 1994). Thus, molecular genetics test results predict cognitive status only to the extent that they predict mutation status.

In adult female carriers, it is thought that there is a higher incidence of mental illness; approximately 10% of intellectually intact female carriers may have psychiatric conditions, most typically affective or schizoid disorders (Reiss, Hagerman, Vinogradov, Abrams, & King, 1988).

"OBSTACLES" TO THE DIAGNOSIS OF FRAGILE X SYNDROME

Molecular genetics testing represents a significant advance in the evaluation of children and adults with suspected fragile X syndrome. However, these studies may not be ordered (and the diagnosis missed) if the clinician believes the diagnosis has previously been ruled out or is not suggested clinically. Conversely, family history and physical examination each can suggest fragile X syndrome in children with other conditions.

Physical Examination

Although many physical findings have been described in fragile X syndrome, they lack sufficient specificity and sensitivity to enable a physician to make the diagnosis on clinical grounds alone. Many of the physical findings typical of fragile X syndrome are also frequently seen in persons with mental retardation and a normal chromosomal karyotype. In a study in which 267 males with mental retardation who lived in institutions were screened cytogenetically, 76% (13 of 17) of those with large ears as well as large testicles tested negative for fragile X syndrome (Hagerman et al., 1988). Conversely, many of the younger boys with fragile X syndrome will not have any of the classic phenotypic features. (Also, as noted above, almost half of the girls with mental retardation secondary to fragile X syndrome will not have phenotypic features [Fryns, 1986].)

Family History

Although a history of mental retardation in maternal relatives (uncles, first cousins) is strongly suggestive of XLMR, it is estimated that fragile X syndrome accounts for only 50% of all cases of XLMR. Moreover, in one recent study looking at young children with fragile X syndrome, only 65% of the cases had a family history positive for mental retardation (Simko et al., 1989). A family history that is negative for mental retardation is of even less predictive value if the mother herself has few brothers, nephews, or maternal uncles. Although the mother of any affected boy is assumed to be an obligate carrier, one cannot assume that she likewise inherited the fragile X gene from her mother; she may have acquired the mutation or premutation from her father, a nonpenetrant transmitting male (Sherman et al., 1985). Given that either the maternal grandfather or the maternal grandmother may have passed the gene for the fragile X syndrome to the mother of an affected boy, one must ask about cognitive impairment and emotional disturbance on both sides of the mother's family when evaluating a boy with mental retardation. When evaluating similarly affected girls with the full mutation, genetic evaluation should likewise generally focus on the maternal family history, because unaffected transmitting males never have affected daughters.

Laboratory Testing

Given that a karyotype for fragile X syndrome requires special culture media and involves additional time and expense, cytogenetic laboratories generally test for fragile X syndrome only when it is clinically suspected or the test is specifically requested. With "routine" chromosome testing, fragile X syndrome will be missed. Thus when taking a history, if a parent of a child with mental retardation states that the child's chromosomes were "normal" when previously tested (perhaps even by amniocentesis), the physician cannot assume that cytogenetic testing was done for fragile X syndrome. Of course, a chromosome karyotype, even when properly ordered and performed, will fail to identify some male and female carriers of the fragile X syndrome. Whereas chromosomal karyotype studies for fragile X are approximately 93% reliable in identifying affected males, it is estimated that 24% of males who carry the gene for fragile X have normal karyotypes and are phenotypically normal (the "transmitting males" described above). Similarly, with respect to females, 40% of obligate carrier women also have a normal karyotype.

GENETIC COUNSELING

All families with a child with fragile X syndrome should be referred to a clinical geneticist for further evaluation and testing of the immedi-

ate and extended family. Once other carriers with the premutation are identified, genetic counseling can be offered to assist with family planning and prenatal testing. To the extent that antepartum testing can be done using chorionic villus cells (9–12 weeks' gestation), amniocytes (14–18 weeks) or fetal blood cells (19+ weeks), one should be able to identify whether a fetus has normal chromosomes, the premutation, or the full mutation. However, knowing an individual's karyotype and carrier status can create as many clinical dilemmas as it solves. For example, what should a family do if prenatal testing reveals the premutation in a female fetus? As noted previously, although this baby will not have clinical problems because of the premutation, her offspring have a significant risk of "inheriting" the full mutation.

TREATMENT CONSIDERATIONS

Nonmedical Interventions

All of the mainstream therapeutic interventions for children with developmental disorders should be considered for the child with fragile X syndrome. Affected preschool children should be referred to local early intervention programs for comprehensive services at no expense to the family. In addition to special education services, speech-language therapy may also prove useful. Behavior modification techniques may be needed to improve problems such as hyperactivity and impulsivity, or to reduce autistic features such as self-injurious behavior or stereotypic movements (see Chapter 21, this volume). Physical or occupational therapy or both may be recommended if a child has decreased muscle tone, delays in gross or fine motor skills, or both; however, pediatricians must remember that the efficacy of these latter therapies is not well established.

Medical Interventions

As with the nonmedical interventions, the conventional medical therapies for children with other developmental disorders are likewise effective in children with fragile X syndrome. Medication may often be necessary for the treatment of seizures or hyperactivity in individuals with mental retardation or autism. Methylphenidate has been shown to be effective in the majority of children with fragile X syndrome who are hyperactive (Hagerman, Murphy, & Wittenberger, 1988); however, treatment with neuroleptics may prove necessary if the hyperactivity is not responsive to stimulant medication or if aggressive behavior compounds the clinical picture.

Several studies have shown that children with fragile X syndrome have a history of more frequent middle ear disease when compared to siblings or controls with mental retardation. Although the reason for this is unclear, it has been suggested that eustachian tube drainage may be compromised by craniofacial changes, connective tissue abnormalities, or both. Given that recurrent otitis media can lead to a fluctuating conductive hearing loss and is associated with slower language development, lower verbal IQ, and possibly impaired attentional skills, physicians must monitor middle ear functioning regularly so that these associated problems do not further compromise development.

If patients have evidence of mitral valve prolapse or aortic root dilatation, prophylaxis for subacute bacterial endocarditis is indicated.

Given that the fragile site on the X chromosome is expressed in vitro when grown in a folate-deficient culture medium, clinical trials of folic acid supplementation have been repeatedly attempted with mixed results (Aman & Kern, 1990/1991). Treatment with folate clearly does not improve behavior or cognition in postpubertal adolescents or adults with fragile X syndrome. However, several studies have shown improvement in the cognition, behavior, or both of prepubertal children (Gillberg, Wahlström, Johansson, Törnblom, & Albertsson-Wikland, 1986; Hagerman et al., 1986). Although various doses have been used experimentally, a regimen of 5 mg twice a day appears most reasonable for a clinical trial in affected prepubertal children. Because it typically takes several weeks to see clinical benefit, folic acid should be given for 3 months before assessing its efficacy (Hagerman, 1991a). This medication can be given in association with stimulants if necessary. A 10-mg/day dose is generally well toler-

ated, although loose stools have been noted in some children. To avoid a vitamin B_6 deficiency, which has also been reported, children should be given daily a multivitamin containing vitamin B_6. Uncontrolled studies have suggested that folic acid may exacerbate seizures in children whose seizures are not fully under control. Patients treated with folic acid should be examined periodically and should have urinalysis and blood work (including a complete blood count; levels of serum glutamic oxaloacetic transaminase, blood urea nitrogen, and creatinine; red blood cell folate levels; and serum levels of zinc, vitamin B_6, and folate) at least annually (Hagerman, 1991a). Interestingly, there is one report of trimethoprim (a folate antagonist) causing deterioration in behavior and cognitive skills when given as part of an antibiotic preparation to a child with fragile X syndrome (Lejeune et al., 1982).

CONCLUSIONS

Fragile X syndrome is the most common inherited cause of mental retardation. Unfortunately, even the most detailed developmental history, family pedigree, and physical examination can only suggest, not confirm, the diagnosis. Many young persons with mental retardation may have a family history negative for mental retardation and a physical examination unremarkable with respect to facial stigmata or other associated features. For this reason, physicians must consider the diagnosis of fragile X syndrome in any child (male or female) with mental retardation or autism of unknown etiology. Fragile X syndrome also should be considered in children with less severe developmental disorders (learning disabilities, attention-deficit/hyperactivity disorder) if the child's physical examination, social relatedness, or family history are otherwise suggestive of this diagnosis.

Pediatricians play an important role not only with respect to the diagnosis of fragile X syndrome but also in its treatment. Physicians should direct families to the various appropriate educational and therapeutic resources in their community. The National Fragile X Foundation

(1441 York Street, Suite 303, Denver, CO 80206; 303-333-6155, 800-688-8765) has many local and regional chapters and may be a useful resource for parents as well as professionals. Every family with a child with fragile X syndrome should be referred for further genetic evaluation and counseling. Even if the parents are not interested in having additional children, it is important that the carrier status of siblings, cousins, and other relatives be determined so that they may receive genetic counseling as indicated.

Stimulant and neuroleptic medications are frequently helpful in treating hyperactivity and aggression. At this time, the only medical treatment specific to patients with fragile X syndrome is folate supplementation, which appears to be helpful for only some affected preadolescents.

It is widely accepted that we cannot cure mental retardation in any form; accordingly, clinical and research efforts must continue to focus on its prevention. To the extent that pediatricians are generally the first child-care professional with whom parents discuss developmental concerns, they play a critical role in the evaluation, identification, treatment, and possible prevention of fragile X syndrome.

REFERENCES

Aman, M., & Kern, R. (1990/1991). The efficacy of folic acid in fragile X syndrome and other developmental disabilities. *Journal of Child and Adolescent Psychopharmacology, 1,* 285–295.

Borghgraef, M., Fryns, J.P., Dielkens, A., Pyck, K., & VanDenBerghe, H. (1987). Fragile X syndrome: A study of the psychological profile in 23 prepubertal patients. *Clinical Genetics, 32,* 179–186.

Bregman, J.D., Dykens, E., Watson, M., Ort, S.I., & Leckman, J.F. (1987). Fragile X syndrome: Variability of phenotypic expression. *Journal of the American Academy of Child and Adolescent Psychiatry, 26,* 463–471.

Butler, M.G., Brunschwig, A., Miller, L.K., & Hagerman, R.J. (1992). Standards for anthropometric measurements in males with the fragile X syndrome. *Pediatrics, 89,* 1059–1062.

Caskey, C.T., Pizzuti, A., Fu, Y.-H., Fenwick, R.G., Jr., & Nelson, D.L. (1992). Triplet repeat mutations in human disease. *Science, 256,* 784–789.

Fryns, J.P. (1986). The female and the fragile X. *American Journal of Medical Genetics, 23,* 157–169.

Gillberg, C., Wahlström, J., Johansson, R., Törnblom, M., & Albertsson-Wikland, K. (1986). Folic acid as an adjunct in the treatment of children with the autism fragile-X syndrome (AFRAX). *Developmental Medicine and Child Neurology, 28,* 624–627.

Hagerman, R.J. (1987). Fragile X syndrome. *Current Problems in Pediatrics, 17,* 621–674.

Hagerman, R.J. (1991a). Medical follow-up and pharmacotherapy. In R.J. Hagerman & A. Cronister-Silverman (Eds.), *Fragile X syndrome: Diagnosis, treatment, and research* (pp. 282–310). Baltimore: Johns Hopkins University Press.

Hagerman, R.J. (1991b). Physical and behavioral phenotype. In R.J. Hagerman & A. Cronister-Silverman (Eds.), *Fragile X syndrome: Diagnosis,* *treatment, and research* (pp. 3–68). Baltimore: Johns Hopkins University Press.

Hagerman, R., Berry, R., Jackson, A.W., III, Campbell, J., Smith, A.C., & McGavran, L. (1988). Institutional screening for the fragile X syndrome. *American Journal of Diseases of Children, 142,* 1216–1221.

Hagerman, R.J., Jackson, A.W., Levitas, A., Braden, M., McBogg, P., Kemper, M., McGavran, L., Berry, R., Matus, I., & Hagerman, P.J. (1986). Oral folic acid versus placebo in the treatment of males with fragile X syndrome. *American Journal of Medical Genetics, 23,* 241–262.

Hagerman, R., Kemper, M., & Hudson, M. (1985). Learning disabilities and attentional problems in boys with the fragile X syndrome. *American Journal of Diseases of Children, 139,* 674–678.

Hagerman, R.J., Murphy, M.A., & Wittenberger, M.D. (1988). A controlled trial of stimulant medication. *American Journal of Medical Genetics, 30,* 377–392.

Hansen, D.M., Jackson, A.W., III, & Hagerman, R.J. (1986). Speech disturbances (cluttering) in mildly impaired males with the Martin-Bell/ fragile X syndrome. *American Journal of Medical Genetics, 23,* 195–206.

Hirst, M.C., Barnicoat, A., Flynn, G., Wang, Q., Daker, M., Buckle, V.J., Davies, K.E., & Bobrow, M. (1993). The identification of a third fragile site, FRAXF, in Xq27–q28 distal to both FRAXA and FRAXE. *Human Molecular Genetics, 2,* 197–200.

Hull, C., & Hagerman, R. (1993). A study of the physical, behavioral, and medical phenotype, including anthropometric measures of females with fragile X syndrome. *American Journal of Diseases of Children, 147,* 1236–1241.

Kemper, M.B., Hagerman, R.J., Ahmad, R.S., & Mariner, R. (1986). Cognitive profiles and the spectrum of clinical manifestations in heterozyous fra(X) females. *American Journal of Medical Genetics, 23,* 139–156.

Knight, S., Flannery, A., Hirst, M., Campbell, L., Christodoulou, Z., Phelps, S., Pointon, J., Middleton-Price, H., Barnicoat, A., Pembrey, M., Holland, J., Oostra, B., Bobrow, M., & Davies, K. (1993). Trinucleotide repeat amplification and hypermethylation of a CpG island in FRAXE mental retardation. *Cell, 74,* 127–134.

Lachiewicz, A.M., & Dawson, D.V. (1994). Do young boys with fragile X syndrome have macroorchidism? *Pediatrics, 94,* 992–995.

Lejeune, J., Legrand, N., Lafourcade, J., Rethore, M.O., Raoul, O., & Maunoury, C. (1982). Fragilite du chromosome X et effets de la trimethoprime [X chromosome fragility and effects of trimethprim]. *Annales de Genetique (Paris), 25,* 149–151.

Lubbs, H.A. (1969). A marker X chromosome. *American Journal of Human Genetics, 21,* 231–244.

Martin, J.P., & Bell, J. (1943). A pedigree of mental defect showing sex-linkage. *Journal of Neurology, Neurosurgery and Psychiatry, 6,* 154–157.

Mazzocco, M., Hagerman, R., Cronister-Silverman, A., & Pennington, B. (1992). Specific frontal lobe deficits among women with the fragile X gene. *Journal of American Academy of Child and Adolescent Psychiatry, 31,* 1141–1148.

Murphy, P.D. (1993). Technical aspects of the diagnosis of fragile X syndrome. *Neurogenetic Advances, 2*(2), 2–3. (Worcester, MA: Genica Pharmaceuticals Corporation)

Nussbaum, R.L., & Ledbetter, D.H. (1986). Fragile X syndrome: A unique mutation in man. *Annual Review of Genetics, 20,* 109–145.

Reiss, A.L., Hagerman, R.J., Vinogradov, S., Abrams, M., & King, R.J. (1988). Psychiatric disability in female carriers of the fragile X chromosome. *Archives of General Psychiatry, 45,* 25–30.

Rousseau, F., Heitz, D., Tarleton, J., MacPherson, J., Malmgren, H., Dahl, N., Barnicoat, A., Mathew, C., Mornet, E., Tejada, I., Maddalena, A., Spiegel, R., Schinzel, A., Marcos, J.A.G., Schorderet, D.F., Schaap, T., Maccioni, L., Russo, S., Jacobs, P.A., Schwartz, C., & Mandel, J.L. (1994). A multicenter study on genotype-phenotype correlations in the fragile X syndrome, using direct diagnosis with probe StB12.3: The first 2,253 cases. *American Journal of Human Genetics, 55,* 225–237.

Sherman, S.L., Jacobs, P.A., Morton, N.E., Froster-Iskenius, U., Howard-Peebles, P.N., Nielsen, K.B., Partington, M.W., Sutherland, G.R., Turner, G., & Watson, M. (1985). Further segregation analysis of the fragile X syndrome with special reference to transmitting males. *Human Genetics, 69,* 289–299.

Simko, A., Hornstein, L., Soukup, S., & Bagamery, N. (1989). Fragile X syndrome: Recognition in young children. *Pediatrics, 83,* 547–552.

Sutherland, G.R. (1977). Fragile sites on human chromosomes: Demonstration of their dependence on the type of tissue culture medium. *Science, 197,* 265–266.

Sutherland, G.R., & Baker, E. (1992). Characterisation of a new rare fragile site easily confused with the fragile X. *Human Molecular Genetics, 1,* 111–113.

Tarleton, J.C., & Saul, R.A. (1993). Molecular genetic advances in fragile X syndrome. *Journal of Pediatrics, 122,* 169–185.

Taylor, A.K., Safanda, J.F., Fall, M.Z., Quince, C., Lang, K.A., Hull, C.E., Carpenter, I., Staley, L.W., & Hagerman, R.J. (1994). Molecular predictors of cognitive involvement in female carriers of fragile X syndrome. *JAMA, 271,* 507–514.

Vieregge, P., & Froster-Iskenius, U. (1989). Clinico-neurological investigations in the fra(X) form of mental retardation. *Journal of Neurology, 236,* 85–92.

Warren, S.T., & Nelson, D.L. (1994). Advances in molecular analysis of fragile X syndrome. *JAMA, 271,* 536–542.

Wolff, P.H., Gardner, J., Paccia, J., & Lappen, J. (1989). The greeting behavior of fragile X males. *American Journal of Mental Retardation, 93,* 406–411.

Chapter 18

Williams Syndrome

Barbara R. Pober, M.D.

Williams syndrome is a well-characterized clinical entity that produces a unique constellation of problems, including a distinctive facial appearance, vascular stenoses (especially supravalvar aortic stenosis), hypercalcemia, developmental delay, and "mental retardation." The etiology of Williams syndrome had been a mystery until 1993, when a microdeletion involving the elastin gene on the long arm of chromosome 7 was discovered. The loss of one copy of the elastin gene presumably results in decreased production of the elastin protein. This exciting discovery confirms that Williams syndrome has a genetic basis and not a maternal or teratologic basis, as had been previously hypothesized. Although Williams syndrome is rare, affecting only approximately 1 in 20,000 individuals, accurate recognition and diagnosis are important because of its medical, developmental, and genetic implications.

HISTORICAL ASPECTS

Scattered throughout the medical literature dating back to the late 1800s are isolated case reports describing new or unusual medical problems in patients now recognized as having Williams syndrome. Williams syndrome was first recognized as a separate clinical syndrome in 1961, with a report on four unrelated patients all with supravalvar aortic stenosis, "unusual" facial features, growth retardation, and mental "subnormality" (Williams, Barratt-Boyes, & Lowe, 1961). Shortly thereafter, several more patients were reported who, in addition to the above findings, also had other vascular stenoses, dental anomalies, and a friendly personality (Beuren, Apitz, & Harmjanz, 1962). In recognition of Beuren's contribution to the delineation of the phenotype, this condition is

sometimes referred to as Williams-Beuren syndrome, especially in the European literature.

A certain amount of confusion surrounds recognition that infantile hypercalcemia is a key feature of Williams syndrome. So-called idiopathic infantile hypercalcemia was a relatively common occurrence in the 1950s, especially in Great Britain. In the majority of cases, transient hypercalcemia occurred in conjunction with poor feeding and slow physical growth; these infants were diagnosed as having "mild" infantile hypercalcemia and ultimately did well following dietary restriction of calcium. However, in a minority of cases, the hypercalcemia was associated with other medical problems. Even after resolution of the hypercalcemia, these patients had persistent medical and developmental problems and were typically diagnosed as having "severe" infantile hypercalcemia (Fraser, Kidd, Kooh, & Paunier, 1966). In retrospect, it is likely that the vast majority of patients with "severe" hypercalcemia actually had Williams syndrome, whereas those with "mild" hypercalcemia had hypercalcemia on some other basis, such as excess vitamin D supplementation in milk.

Based on the accumulated clinical experience since the 1960s, our knowledge of the phenotypic spectrum of Williams syndrome has expanded. Given the recent discovery of the genetic basis of Williams syndrome, the "typical" Williams syndrome profile may change as studies correlating the underlying genetic mutation with specific physical and cognitive manifestations are completed.

DIAGNOSIS AND GENETICS OF WILLIAMS SYNDROME

The 1993 discovery of an elastin gene deletion in Williams syndrome currently is being used to provide confirmation of the clinical diagnosis. Prior to this discovery, the diagnosis of Williams syndrome was solely a clinical one, and, given the difficulty in clinical diagnosis, scoring systems were devised. Unfortunately, they have been of limited utility, being both subjective and cumbersome to use (Preus, 1984). Although diagnostic confirmation of Williams syndrome may soon be relegated to a laboratory test, suspicion about the diagnosis will always begin with the astute clinician. Accordingly, the Williams Syndrome Association Medical Advisory Board has generated a list of screening criteria that should alert physicians to the possibility of this diagnosis (Figure 1).

The discovery that Williams syndrome is a genetic microdeletion syndrome comes from the study of dozens of persons with the syndrome, over 95% of whom are hemizygous for the elastin gene (Ewart et al., 1993). Normally, each individual has two copies of the elastin gene, one on each of their No. 7 chromosomes. Patients with Williams syndrome are hemizygous for the elastin gene because their second copy of this gene has been deleted. This elastin gene deletion occurs as a sporadic event during either maternal or paternal gamete formation. Accordingly, the recurrence risk for healthy parents is negligible because the deletion was a chance event occurring in either the egg or the sperm that went into the affected individual's formation. However, individuals with Williams syndrome have a 50% chance that each of their own children will have the syndrome because half of their germ cells contain a chromosome 7 deleted for elastin.

The technique of fluorescent in situ hybridization (FISH) is being used as a laboratory test to confirm the clinical diagnosis of Williams syndrome. This technique works by fluorescently labeling a probe for the elastin gene. This probe is then hybridized to a chromosome preparation derived from a patient's blood sample. Normally, the probe will hybridize to two elastin genes, one on each copy of chromosome 7. In patients with Williams syndrome, the probe only hybridizes to one elastin gene because the second copy is missing. So far, FISH has confirmed the clinical diagnosis of Williams syndrome in over 95% of cases. The remaining cases may represent very small deletions that cannot be detected by currently used probes or, alternatively, phenocopies of Williams syndrome.

Elastin is an important protein that contributes to blood vessel wall and general connective tissue strength and elasticity. We speculate that a single copy of the elastin gene results in a decreased amount of elastin protein at a critical time in fetal development; this, in turn, produces a variety of problems, such as vascular stenoses, hernias, and diverticuli. The size of this genetic deletion is submicroscopic; that is, below the limits of detection by even high-resolution chromosome analysis. However, current analysis at the DNA level suggests that the deletions in persons with Williams syndrome are sufficiently large to encompass additional genes flanking the elastin locus. The size and extent of the deleted segments may vary between individuals, which, in turn, may account for the broad phenotypic variability seen.

MEDICAL PROFILE IN WILLIAMS SYNDROME

Williams syndrome is a multisystem disorder that may involve many organ systems. Certain problems may be present at birth, whereas others are more likely to develop later, to progress over time, or both.

Common Medical Problems/Physical Features

The following medical problems and physical features are common to over 50% of individuals with Williams syndrome:

Characteristic facial appearance
Cardiovascular disease
Physical growth along the lower percentiles
Musculoskeletal abnormalities
Oral abnormalities
Prolonged infantile "colic"/poor feeding/disturbed sleep patterns
Hyperacusis

Characteristic Facial Appearance The presence of the typical Williams syndrome facies is a prerequisite for the clinical diagnosis of this condition. Much has been written about the Williams syndrome facial appearance, but the

Williams syndrome is more common than most physicians realize, and can present a diagnostic dilemma. It is important to establish a diagnosis of Williams syndrome because some medical problems can worsen over time and because it is a heritable disorder.

This flier highlights *key features* that could alert a primary physician to suspect Williams syndrome.

1. Characteristic facial appearance (as demonstrated in photographs below)

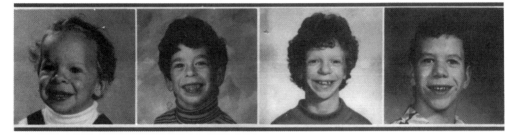

2. Cardiovascular problems; especially, but not limited to supravalvular aortic stenosis and/or peripheral pulmonary artery stenosis

3. Early feeding difficulties; prolonged irritability

4. Mild developmental delays/learning difficulties

5. Small for age

6. Hypercalcemia

7. Overly friendly/excessively social personality

8. Small or missing teeth/malocclusion

9. Low-pitched voice

We suggest that any child or adult who has suspicious facial appearance and one other feature be referred for diagnostic evaluation. Please be aware that Williams syndrome can occur without cardiovascular disease, hypercalcemia or "significant" mental retardation.

Figure 1. Key features of Williams syndrome. (Published by the Williams Syndrome Association, Clawson, MI; reprinted by permission.)

features can be subtle and difficult to recognize. No single feature is pathognomonic for Williams syndrome; rather, the constellation of features is highly characteristic so that instantaneous recognition of the "face" often occurs.

The facial appearance of the infant or young child with Williams syndrome has been described as "pixie" or "elfinlike." The most common facial features include bitemporal narrowing, stellate irides (occurring in approximately 50% of blue-eyed children with Williams syndrome but difficult to appreciate in those with dark eyes), epicanthal folds, flat nasal bridge, short upturned nose with anteverted nostrils, long philtrum, full lips, macrostomia that is most notable when laughing or crying, full

lower cheeks, and a small delicate chin (Burn, 1986).

The Williams syndrome facial appearance changes gradually over time. Overall, some coarsening of features occurs; the nose and lips become more prominent and the macrostomia more pronounced (Morris, Demsey, Leonard, Dilts, & Blackburn, 1988). Mild facial asymmetry can develop. Because most clinicians are less familiar with the characteristic Williams syndrome facial appearance in adolescents or adults, review of photographs taken at a younger age can be useful.

Cardiovascular Disease Cardiovascular disease occurs in approximately 80% of individuals with Williams syndrome. The most common lesion is supravalvar aortic stenosis (narrowing of the aorta directly above the aortic valve), which occurs alone or in combination with other vascular stenoses in approximately 60% of persons with Williams syndrome. Stenosis of the pulmonary arteries (involving central or peripheral stenoses or both) is the next most common type of involvement (Hallidie-Smith & Karas, 1988; Zalzstein, Moes, Musewe, & Freedom, 1991). Stenoses of other arteries, including the renal, mesenteric, and coronary arteries, also have been reported but their incidence is unknown (Conway, Noonan, Mario, & Steeg, 1990; Daniels, Loggie, Schwartz, Strife, & Kaplan, 1985). These vascular stenoses can be congenital or can develop later in life. In many individuals the degree of stenosis is stable, but in approximately one third progressive supravalvic aortic stenosis develops, requiring surgical intervention. The etiology and pathophysiology of the stenoses is unknown but they may represent a response to the genetic deletion of elastin, as discussed previously.

Children and adults with Williams syndrome are at increased risk for developing hypertension, even in the absence of significant vascular stenoses (Morris et al., 1988). The frequency of hypertension appears to be increased at all ages.

Physical Growth Along the Lower Percentiles   Typical Williams syndrome growth patterns include low-normal birth weight followed by slow, steady linear growth and weight gain along the 5th–10th percentiles. Failure to thrive complicates the postnatal course of a minority of infants with Williams syndrome (Morris et al., 1988; Pankau, Partsch, Gosch, Oppermann, & Wessel, 1992). Sometimes, catch-up in linear growth occurs in late childhood. Average or above-average growth parameters are not exclusionary criteria for the diagnosis of Williams syndrome.

Growth curves based on samples of persons with Williams syndrome have been published (Morris et al., 1988; Pankau et al., 1992). These curves are helpful in monitoring growth in young children with Williams syndrome and in predicting adult height. Adult stature in Williams syndrome typically falls in the low range of normal adult height.

Musculoskeletal Abnormalities   Infants and young children with Williams syndrome are generally hypotonic, with mild joint hyperextensibility. With advancing age, the hypotonia resolves and progressive joint limitation, resulting in contractures, often develops. Contractures are most common in the legs (especially the heel cords), affecting up to 80% of persons with Williams syndrome (Chapman, DePlessis, & Pober, in press; Kaplan, Kirschner, Watters, & Costa, 1989). Other musculoskeletal problems are lordosis, scoliosis, proximal muscle weakness, and radioulnar synostosis (Chapman et al., in press; Kaplan et al., 1989). Physical therapy can prevent or ameliorate many of these problems.

Oral Abnormalities   The majority of individuals with Williams syndrome have one or more of the following abnormalities in dentition: microdontia, excess interdental spacing, horizontal malocclusions (usually anterior crossbite), vertical malocclusions (either deep or open bite), and hypodontia (absence of one or more teeth). Class II or III skeletal malocclusions occur more often in persons with Williams syndrome than in the general population but affect only a small percentage of individuals. Delayed dental eruption and extensive caries are *not* typical of Williams syndrome. Most of the common oral problems found in Williams syndrome are readily amenable to orthodontic treatment (Hertzberg, Nakisbendi, Needleman, & Pober, 1994).

Prolonged Infantile "Colic"/Poor Feeding/Disturbed Sleep Patterns   Parental reports indicate that at least 50% of infants with Williams syndrome have marked irritability of unknown etiology (often diagnosed as "colic") that persists for up to 6–8 months of age (Morris et al., 1988). Many infants with Williams syndrome also have difficulty with coordinated sucking and swallowing; this presents with spitting, gagging, choking, vomiting, and/or difficulty with transition to solid foods.

Many infants with Williams syndrome have difficulty establishing normal sleep routines. A consistent pattern of sleeping through the night is rarely achieved before 6 months of age.

Hyperacusis   In several parent surveys, over 90% of children with Williams syndrome have been reported to have hyperacusis (heightened sensitivity) to certain sounds, which interferes with the ability to function in the presence of those sounds. Common offending sounds include vacuum cleaners, thunder, and sirens (Klein, Armstrong, Greer, & Brown, 1990). The biologic basis for hyperacusis is unknown; audiologic testing does *not* demonstrate a lower than normal hearing threshold. Older children and adults appear to "outgrow" (or adapt to) their hyperacusis.

Less Common Medical Problems/Physical Features

Additional medical problems and physical features that are found less commonly in Williams syndrome include

Documented hypercalcemia
Ophthalmologic abnormalities
Gastrointestinal abnormalities
Renal anomalies
Neurologic abnormalities
Recurrent otitis media
Anxiety

Documented Hypercalcemia The true frequency of hypercalcemia in Williams syndrome remains unknown. Hypercalcemia is most often found in infancy. Because the diagnosis of Williams syndrome generally is established after infancy, laboratory testing that documents infantile hypercalcemia may never have been obtained.

The etiology of hypercalcemia in Williams syndrome also is unclear. No consistent abnormalities in calcium or vitamin D regulatory hormones, or both, have been documented (Kruse, Pankau, Gosch, & Wohlfahrt, 1992; Martin, Snodgrass, & Cohen, 1984). Among those individuals found to have hypercalcemia, blood calcium levels are generally mildly elevated and the condition requires minimal or no treatment because the hypercalcemia usually resolves on its own. The occasional person found to have more significant elevations in blood calcium level (>12.0 mg/dl) may require short-term treatment with special low-calcium formulas, glucocorticoids, or both. Again, lengthy treatment is generally not needed because calcium levels return to normal within several months.

Discovery of hypercalcemia should prompt a more thorough search for systemic evidence of hypercalcemia, such as nephrocalcinosis or blood vessel wall calcification.

Ophthalmologic Abnormalities The most common abnormalities reported in persons with Williams syndrome include strabismus (affecting approximately 30%–60%) and hypermetropia (found in 85%) (Granet, Markowitz, & Schaffer, 1994; Greenberg & Lewis, 1988).

Gastrointestinal Abnormalities A broad variety of both "functional" and structural gastrointestinal abnormalities have been observed. Reported abnormalities include infantile colic, gastroesophageal reflux, inguinal hernias, rectal prolapse, and colonic diverticulosis with or without diverticulitis (occurring in young adults) (Martin et al., 1984; Morris et al., 1988). Some of these abnormalities are likely attributable to the elastin gene deletion (i.e., prolapse, diverticulosis), whereas the etiology of others is unknown.

Renal Anomalies Abnormalities of the kidneys and collecting system are reported to occur in 15%–50% of individuals with Williams syndrome. Common findings include nephrocalcinosis, solitary kidney, hypoplastic kidneys, and bladder diverticuli as well as diminished renal function (Ingelfinger & Newburger, 1991; Pober, Lacro, Rice, Mandell, & Teele, 1993). Decline in renal function is more likely to occur with advancing age. Toilet training is accomplished successfully by all children with Williams syndrome, although at a somewhat delayed age, especially for nighttime training. Multiple bladder diverticuli as well as bladder wall/detrusor muscle incoordination may contribute to urinary frequency and continence problems.

Neurologic Abnormalities Selected neurologic abnormalities commonly occur in Williams syndrome, although they have received scant mention in the published literature. Most individuals have lifelong abnormalities of fine and gross motor skills, balance, and gait coordination. Infants with Williams syndrome tend to be hypotonic and normoreflexic, whereas older children and adults progress to be hypertonic and hyperreflexic (Chapman et al., in press; Trauner, Bellugi, & Chase, 1989). Structural abnormalities of the brain rarely are documented on magnetic resonance imaging, although Chiari malformation type I appears to be more common in persons with Williams syndrome than in the general population (Pober & Filiano, 1995; Wang, Hesselink, Jernigan, Doherty, & Bellugi, 1992).

Recurrent Otitis Media   Recurrent otitis media can be a troubling problem, especially during the early childhood years. Surgical placement of ventilation ("PE") tubes may be necessary for treatment of infections and middle ear fluid. A formal audiologic evaluation, especially in the setting of recurrent ear infections, is necessary.

Anxiety   Although the typical personality of a person with Williams syndrome is reported as friendly, if not over-friendly, there is a pervasive anxious quality to the personality as well. Most children with Williams syndrome are described by both parents and teachers as worrying a great deal; obsessing over upcoming events; and having difficulty with transitions, new situations, or both (Arnold, Yule, & Martin, 1985; Bradley & Udwin, 1989). Many individuals develop good coping mechanisms as they mature, but, in our experience, a subset of individuals develop worsening anxiety and new-onset depression as adolescents and adults. In a survey of adults with Williams syndrome, the majority were receiving ongoing counseling/ therapy of some sort and a minority were receiving antianxiety or antidepressive medication, or both, under the supervision of a psychiatrist (B.R. Pober, personal observations).

General Considerations

Many of the medical problems described above are general pediatric problems common to infancy or early childhood and, by themselves, do not suggest the diagnosis of Williams syndrome. Accordingly, most children with Williams syndrome have had multiple pediatric visits during their first year of life for seemingly "nonspecific" medical problems *before* the diagnosis is ever considered or confirmed (Morris et al., 1988). The pediatrician must maintain a high index of suspicion about a possible underlying syndrome or condition when multiple ("nonspecific") medical problems occur in the same infant.

In spite of the lengthy list of potential medical complications described above, most individuals with Williams syndrome are quite healthy. Although there is the potential for multisystem involvement, no single individual will have all the problems listed. Lifelong medical monitoring is required to obtain periodic screening studies and to begin prompt treatment for any complications that do arise.

COGNITIVE PROFILE IN WILLIAMS SYNDROME

"Mental retardation has been generally considered as representing a uniform impairment in all domains of cognitive functioning. Williams syndrome appears to be a dramatic exception to this broad generalization" (Bellugi, Marks, Bihrle, & Sabo, 1988, p. 177). The overall level of cognitive functioning in Williams syndrome is reviewed here first, followed by presentation of evidence that Williams syndrome appears to be an exception among developmental disability conditions.

Developmental Milestones/IQ Testing

Acquisition of early language and motor milestones is mildly to moderately delayed in most children with Williams syndrome. Typically, first words are uttered between 12 and 15 months, stylized two-word combinations are produced at approximately 24 months, and independent walking is achieved at approximately 24 months. Social/interpersonal skills are usually age appropriate, so that the presence of delays in other areas often is overlooked or minimized. Data from standardized IQ testing shows that the average full-scale IQ in children and adults with Williams syndrome falls between 50 and 60 (Bennett, LaVeck, & Sells, 1978; Kataria, Goldstein, & Kushnick, 1984; Levine, 1993). Although there is considerable range in full-scale scores, the majority of individuals test in the range of mild mental retardation. However, published data (plus unpublished observations from testing in our Williams syndrome program) show that 5%–20% of individuals with Williams syndrome have a full-scale IQ score greater than 70. In this subset, most have borderline full-scale IQs and a few have low-average or average full-scale IQs. In our experience, profound mental retardation is uncommon.

Cognitive Strengths and Weaknesses

Persons with Williams syndrome do *not* demonstrate "uniform impairment" across cognitive domains. In selected cognitive areas, an individual with Williams syndrome can function normally or near-normally, whereas in other areas the same individual can have marked limitations (Crisco, Dobbs, & Mulhern, 1988; Wang & Bellugi, 1993). A full-scale IQ score, which averages scores across all cognitive domains tested, can be misleading and can obscure relative strengths and weaknesses. The typical cognitive profile, which seems to occur relatively independently of full-scale IQ, is the following:

Areas of relative intellectual strength: language and communications skills (syntax, vocabulary, prosody); long-term memory for general information; processing of "meaningful" information (memory for faces, interpretation of illustrations)

Areas of more significant intellectual deficiency: visual–spatial skills (spatial memory, spatial organization, left–right perception); fine motor skills; visual–motor integration (writing, puzzles); word retrieval skills

Given these strengths and weaknesses, an individual may appear almost age appropriate or markedly delayed, depending on the task at hand.

Another important and common feature of the Williams syndrome cognitive profile is a short attention span and easy distractibility (Wang & Bellugi, 1993). Some individuals are diagnosed as having attention-deficit/hyperactivity disorder. Common medications used to treat attention problems in school-age children without Williams syndrome, such as Ritalin, may be effective treatment in some individuals with the syndrome as well.

Bellugi has described individuals with Williams syndrome as "verbal high, spatial low"; this generalization fails to convey that the "typical" pattern is common but not universal and that all verbal abilities are not equally well preserved. The Williams syndrome profile is more accurately viewed as a "learning disability" pattern, which may or may not be accompanied by mental retardation and attention problems. Even among the highest functioning individuals with full-scale IQ scores greater than 80, a learning disability pattern and short attention span are likely to be present; thus, an individual with Williams syndrome may have mild disabilities but is never cognitively "normal."

Educational/Vocational Implications

The complexity of the Williams syndrome cognitive profile has significant educational implications. Young children should be monitored in early intervention programs and receive direct therapies (such as speech and language therapy or occupational therapy) as needed. Once enrolled in school, each child's education program must be individually tailored because he or she may have markedly different ability levels. Most children eventually require the benefits of special education classes, especially for reading and math. The majority of individuals with Williams syndrome learn to read; comprehension skills typically cluster between the second- and sixth-grade levels. Math skills are more significantly impaired and generally remain below the second-grade level. A computer with special education software can be of enormous benefit, especially to assist with written output.

WILLIAMS SYNDROME AND THE FAMILY

A child with Williams syndrome brings much joy and satisfaction into a family. However, many additional stresses are placed on family members, especially parents, given the developmental problems and the potential for medical problems.

During infancy, the common problems of irritability and poor feeding and sleeping interfere with the establishment of family routines and the incorporation of an infant with Williams syndrome into normal household routines. During childhood, the rate of developmental progress is gratifying, but the creation of an appropriate educational environment (given the unusual intellectual profile in Williams syndrome) becomes a major challenge for most parents. In adulthood, the focus shifts to finding appropriate vocational and living situations. Currently, most adults with Williams syndrome work in supervised settings, such as sheltered workshops, and live with their parents or other family members. Throughout all these periods, concerns that significant medical problems are present or may develop, plus concerns about the long-term future when the adult outlives the parents, are ever present.

A national volunteer parent organization, the Williams Syndrome Association (P.O. Box 297, Clawson, MI 48017-0297; 1-810-541-3630), provides information to parents and physicians regarding the diagnosis, prognosis, and genetics of Williams syndrome. This organization is equally important in providing emotional support for families dealing with the complexities of raising a child with Williams syndrome.

REFERENCES

Arnold R., Yule, W., & Martin, N. (1985). The psychological characteristics of infantile hypercalcaemia: A preliminary investigation. *Developmental Medicine and Child Neurology, 27*, 49–59.

Bellugi, U., Marks, S., Bihrle, A., & Sabo, H. (1988). Dissociation between language and cognitive functions in Williams syndrome. In D. Bishop & K. Mogford, (Eds.), *Language development in exceptional circumstances* (pp. 177–189). London: Churchill Livingstone.

Bennett, F.C., LaVeck, B., & Sells, C.J. (1978). The Williams elfin facies syndrome: The psychological profile as an aid in syndrome identification. *Pediatrics, 61*, 303–305.

Beuren, A.J., Apitz, J., & Harmjanz, D. (1962). Supravalvular aortic stenosis in association with mental retardation and a certain facial appearance. *Circulation, 26*,1235–1240.

Bradley, E.A., & Udwin, O. (1989). Williams' syndrome in adulthood: A case study focusing on psychological and psychiatric aspects. *Journal of Mental Deficiency Research, 33*, 175–184.

Burn, J. (1986). Williams syndrome. *Journal of Medical Genetics, 23*, 389–395.

Chapman, C., DePlessis, A., & Pober, B. (in press). Survey of neurologic findings in Williams syndrome. *Journal of Child Neurology.*

Conway, E.E., Jr., Noonan, J., Marion, R.W., & Steeg, C.N. Myocardial infarction leading to sudden death in the Williams syndrome: Report of 3 cases. (1990). *Journal of Pediatrics, 117*, 593–595.

Crisco, J.J., Dobbs, J.M., & Mulhern, R.K. (1988). Cognitive processing of children with Williams syndrome. *Developmental Medicine and Child Neurology, 30*, 650–656.

Daniels, S.R., Loggie, J.M.H., Schwartz, D.C., Strife, J.L., & Kaplan, S. (1985). Systemic hypertension secondary to peripheral vascular anomalies in patients with Williams syndrome. *Journal of Pediatrics, 106*, 249–251.

Ewart, A.K., Morris, C.A., Atkinson, D., Jin, W., Sternes, K., Spallone, P., Stock, A.D., Leppert, M., & Keating, M.T. (1993). Hemizygosity at the elastin locus in a developmental disorder, Williams syndrome. *Nature Genetics, 5*, 11–16.

Fraser, D., Kidd, B.S.L., Kooh, S.W., & Paunier, L. (1966). A new look at infantile hypercalcemia. *Pediatric Clinics of North America, 13*, 503–525.

Granet, D., Markowitz, G., & Schaffer, D. (1994, July 26–28). *Ocular examination in children with Williams syndrome*. Abstract presented at the Sixth International Professional Conference, Williams Syndrome Association, University of California, San Diego.

Greenberg, F., & Lewis, R.A. (1988). The Williams syndrome: Spectrum and significance of ocular features. *Ophthalmology, 95*, 1608–1612.

Hallidie-Smith, K.A., & Karas, S. (1988). Cardiac anomalies in Williams-Beuren syndrome. *Archives of Disease in Childhood 63*, 809–813.

Hertzberg, J., Nakisbendi, L., Needleman, H.L., & Pober, B. (1994). Williams syndrome—oral presentation of 45 cases. *Pediatric Dentistry, 16*, 262–267.

Ingelfinger, J., & Newburger, J. (1991). Spectrum of renal anomalies in patients with Williams syndrome. *Journal of Pediatrics, 119*, 771–773.

Kaplan, P., Kirschner, M., Watters, G., & Costa, M.T. (1989). Contractures in patients with Williams syndrome. *Pediatrics, 84*, 895–899.

Kataria, S., Goldstein, D.J., & Kushnick, T. (1984). Developmental delays in Williams ("elfin facies") syndrome. *Applied Research in Mental Retardation, 5*, 419–423.

Klein, A.J., Armstrong, B.L., Greer, M.K., & Brown, F.R. III. (1990). Hyperacusis and otitis media in individuals with Williams syndrome. *Journal of Speech and Hearing Disorders, 55*, 339–344.

Kruse, K., Pankau, R., Gosch, A., & Wohlfahrt, K. (1992). Calcium metabolism in Williams-Beuren syndrome. *Journal of Pediatrics, 121*, 902–907.

Levine, K. (1993.) *Williams syndrome: Information for teachers*. Clawson, MI: Williams Syndrome Association.

Martin, N.D.T., Snodgrass, G.J.A.I., & Cohen, R.D. (1984). Idiopathic infantile hypercalcaemia—a continuing enigma. *Archives of Disease in Childhood, 59*, 605–613.

Morris, C.A., Demsey, S.A., Leonard, C.O., Dilts, C., & Blackburn, B.L. (1988). Natural history of Williams syndrome: Physical characteristics. *Journal of Pediatrics, 113*, 318–326.

Pankau, R., Partsch, C.J., Gosch, A., Oppermann, H.C., & Wessel, A. (1992). Statural growth in Williams syndrome. *European Journal of Pediatrics, 151*, 751–755.

Pober, B.R., & Filiano, J.J. (1995). Association of Chiari I malformation in Williams syndrome. *Pediatric Neurology, 12*, 84–88.

Pober, B.R., Lacro, R.V., Rice, C., Mandell, V., & Teele, R.L. (1993). Renal findings in 40 individuals with Williams syndrome. *American Journal of Medical Genetics, 46*, 271–274.

Preus, M. (1984). The Williams syndrome: Objective definition and diagnosis. *Clinical Genetics, 25*, 422–428.

Trauner, D.A., Bellugi, U., & Chase, C. (1989). Neurologic features of Williams and Down syndromes. *Pediatric Neurology, 5*, 166–168.

Wang, P.P., & Bellugi, U. (1993). Williams syndrome, Down syndrome, and cognitive neuroscience. *American Journal of Diseases of Children, 147*, 1246–1251.

Wang, P.P., Hesselink, J.R., Jernigan, T.L., Doherty, S., & Bellugi, U. (1992). Specific neurobehavioral profile of Williams syndrome is associated with neocerebellar hemispheric preservation. *Neurology, 42*, 1999–2002.

Williams, J.C.P., Barratt-Boyes, B.G., & Lowe, J.B. (1961). Supravalvular aortic stenosis. *Circulation, 24*, 1311–1318.

Zalzstein, E., Moes, C.A.F., Musewe, N.N., & Freedom, R.M. (1991). Spectrum of cardiovascular anomalies in Williams-Beuren syndrome. *Pediatric Cardiology, 12*, 219–223.

Chapter 19

Fetal Alcohol Syndrome

Mary Leppert, M.D., and Karen Hofman, M.D.

The deleterious effects of alcohol on the developing fetus have been presumed for centuries. Use of alcohol by a bridal couple was prohibited in Carthage for fear of bringing about a "defective" child. Aristotle also warned that "drunken and hairbrained women most often bring forth children like unto themselves." Medical literature over the last four centuries has produced a range of theories on the nature and extent of alcohol effects on pregnancy and fetal development. The facts remained obscure until the work of Lemoine in France in 1968 (as cited in Streissguth, Landesman-Dwyer, Martin, & Smith, 1980), and that of Jones, Smith, Ulleland, and Streissguth in the United States in 1973, in which they described distinct patterns of dysmorphism, growth delays, and central nervous system dysfunctions associated with maternal alcohol use. Since Jones and colleagues described the fetal alcohol syndrome, there have been extensive investigations of the validity and extent to which abnormal fetal development can be ascribed to maternal alcohol ingestion (Brien & Smith, 1991; Burd & Martsolf, 1989; Russell, Czarnecki, Cowan, McPherson, & Mudar, 1991; Schenker et al., 1990; and West & Goodlett, 1990).

DEFINITION AND PREVALENCE

There is a wide range of expression of the teratogenic effects of alcohol. The spectrum ranges from the fetal alcohol syndrome (FAS) to fetal alcohol effect (FAE) to isolated deficits in growth or subtle central nervous system dysfunctions. Criteria for the diagnosis of fetal alcohol syndrome include a history of maternal alcohol ingestion and some component in each of the following three areas: craniofacial dysmorphism, growth retardation, and central nervous system dysfunction. The diagnosis of fetal alcohol effect requires components from only two of these areas and a history of maternal alcohol use. The most common findings in the three major categories of abnormalities include, respectively

1. Morphology: Microphthalmia, short palpebral fissures, poorly developed philtrum, thin vermillion border, and/or flattening of the maxillary area
2. Growth retardation: Prenatal and postnatal growth deficiency
3. Central nervous system effects: Mental retardation, learning disabilities, and behavioral difficulties

The variables that may influence the expression of alcohol use on the fetus include a probable maternal genetic predisposition to alcohol's teratogenicity, the timing of alcohol exposure during gestation, the amount of alcohol consumed (mild, moderate, and heavy consumption), and the pattern of alcohol use (binge versus chronic consumption). One drink is generally defined as 0.5 ounces of absolute alcohol; the exact amount will vary depending on the type of liquor consumed. Heavy drinking is defined as two or more drinks per day. Binge drinking is defined as five or more drinks per occasion.

The risk of fetal alcohol syndrome in the U.S. general population varies but is estimated at 1.9 in 1,000 live births. The incidence of fetal alcohol effect is unknown, but approximately 8% of mild mental retardation is thought to be attributable to alcohol exposure. These rates may vary in different populations because of differences in reporting. Rates may be increased in the offspring of women of different socioeconomic and ethnic backgrounds.

PATHOGENESIS

That alcohol is a teratogen is now certain, but the mechanism of teratogenesis is unclear. The first metabolite produced by the degradation of alcohol is acetaldehyde; the enzyme involved is alcohol dehydrogenase. Acetaldehyde has been shown in embryonic cell cultures to be toxic. In animal models, even in low doses, it appears to cause migrational abnormalities. Ethanol itself appears to be teratogenic, and its effects are seen even after its metabolism has been inhibited. Whether ethanol or acetaldehyde is the primary toxin is still under debate. It seems that both of these substances cross the placenta.

When discussing the mechanisms of teratogenesis in fetal alcohol syndrome, compounding factors must be considered. Malnutrition alone can cause growth deficits. Folate deficiencies are not uncommon in alcoholics, and folate is required for DNA synthesis and therefore growth. Other vitamins required for growth may also be deficient or have altered functions in the presence of alcohol, as might trace metals such as zinc (Schenker et al., 1990). Other factors often associated with alcoholism, such as tobacco, caffeine, and illegal drug use may also influence the outcomes of these alcohol-exposed fetuses (see Chapter 10, Volume I). The extent to which these factors contribute to growth impairment in particular is unclear.

CENTRAL NERVOUS SYSTEM PATHOLOGY

Not long after the description of fetal alcohol syndrome, structural brain anomalies were described in four infants exposed to significant amounts of alcohol in utero, all of whom had neural or glial migration effects (Clarren, Alvoid, Sumi, Streissguth, & Smith, 1978).

Some further neuropathologic investigations have been done but are quite limited and show a wide spectrum of lesions. The more common anomalies include cerebellar hypoplasia, neuroglial heterotopias (particularly leptomeningeal and periventricular), hydrocephalus, and reduced cerebral white matter. Other gross brain anomalies that have been reported include schizencephaly, porencephaly, agenesis of the corpus callosum, hydrocephalus, syringomyelia, and Dandy-Walker malformation. There is even less information on the changes that may take place in long-term survivors who have neuropsychological or behavioral disturbances. Postmortem information on fetuses and infants with fetal alcohol syndrome is limited. Animal model studies of to the syndrome have generated a plethora of very diverse findings.

Morphology

Jones and co-workers (1973) initially described eight unrelated children of different ethnic backgrounds who shared similar facial characteristics and were born to women who were known to consume alcohol chronically. Key features included short palpebral fissures, a hypoplastic upper lip, and a hypoplastic philtrum. There frequently was also midfacial hypoplasia.

Skeletal manifestations included joint anomalies, abnormal palmar creases and hypoplastic fifth fingernails, camptodactyly, and distal phalangeal anomalies (Table 1). The most common cardiac anomalies were ventriculoseptal defects, followed by atrial septal defects. Occasional minor anomalies were ptosis, strabismus, epicanthal folds, micrognathia, cleft lip or palate, renal anomalies, posterior rotation of the helix or protruding auricles of the ear, and hearing loss.

There is a relative paucity of literature on the natural history of the fetal alcohol syndrome, but existing studies suggest that the characteristic facial features of alcohol teratogenesis become less evident in adolescence and adulthood. Short palpebral fissures and anomalies of the eye, philtrum, and lip persist. The midfacial hypoplasia becomes less noticeable as children with fetal alcohol syndrome mature (Figure 1) (Streissguth et al., 1991).

Table 1. Associated features of the fetal alcohol syndrome observed in 245 persons affected

Area	Frequent[a]	Occasional[b]
Eyes	Ptosis, strabismus, epicanthal folds	Myopia, clinical microphthalmia, blepharophimosis
Ears	Posterior rotation	Poorly formed concha
Mouth	Prominent lateral palatine ridges	Cleft lip or cleft palate, small teeth with faulty enamel
Cardiac	Murmurs, especially in early childhood, usually atrial septal defect	Ventricular septal defect, great-vessel anomalies, tetralogy of Fallot
Renogenital	Labial hypoplasia	Hypospadias, small rotated kidneys, hydronephrosis
Cutaneous	Hemangiomas	Hirsutism in infancy
Skeletal	Aberrant palmar creases, pectus excavatum	Limited joint movements, especially fingers & elbows, nail hypoplasia, especially 5th, polydactyly, radioulnar synostosis, pectus carinatum, bifid xiphoid, Klippel-Feil anomaly, scoliosis
Muscular		Hernias of diaphragm, umbilicus or groin, diastasis recti

From Clarren, S.K., & Smith, D.W. (1978). The fetal alcohol syndrome. *New England Journal of Medicine, 298,* 1064; reprinted by permission.

[a]Reported in between 26% and 50% of patients.

[b]Reported in between 1% and 25% of patients.

Growth Retardation

The relationship between alcohol exposure and fetal growth varies depending on the timing and pattern of alcohol use. However, it is clear that pre- and postnatal growth deficiencies are a relatively constant finding in fetal alcohol syndrone, with affected children usually less than 2 standard deviations from the mean for both height and weight. Head circumference varies from the 10th percentile to frank microcephaly. The patterns of alcohol ingestion that predict growth deficiency also vary widely across studies.

Prospective studies have been done to assess growth patterns of children who were known to

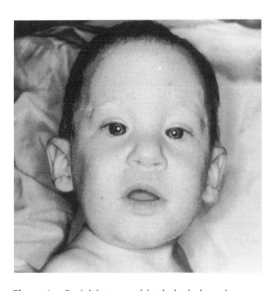 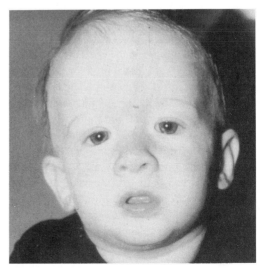

Figure 1. Facial features of fetal alcohol syndrome are most evident in infancy (left) and become less noticeable with age (right).

have prenatal alcohol exposure. A correlation was shown between the pattern (binge versus chronic) and timing (exposure to alcohol at a specific gestational age) and the growth patterns at 18 months. Binge drinking in the first and third trimester had significant effects on height, weight, and head circumference (Day et al., 1991; Day & Richardson, 1991). The effect of heavy drinking in the first trimester on head circumference was noticeable only when drinking continued throughout pregnancy. The average daily volume of alcohol (total amount of ethanol/average number of drinks per day) ingested during pregnancy was a consistent predictor of decreased size at 18 months. This suggests that chronic ethanol exposure is more influential on growth parameters than is binge drinking.

The question of catch-up growth is also somewhat controversial. In a study of adolescents and adults reported to have fetal alcohol syndrome/effect, the majority had height and head circumference measurements 2 standard deviations below the mean but approached the mean in weight, exhibiting catch-up growth in this parameter (Streissguth et al., 1991).

Central Nervous System Effects

The deleterious influence of alcohol on the developing brain varies with age. Studies of alcohol-exposed infants at 8 months of age show decreased Bayley Motor and Mental Developmental indexes (Streissguth, Barr, Marhm, & Herman, 1980). Studies of toddlers and preschool children show similar findings.

In school-age children with known prenatal alcohol exposure, there is diminished intellectual functioning, poorer academic performance, and increased behavioral problems. Follow-up studies of children with fetal alcohol exposure into the early school years reveal that these children exhibit diminished overall IQ, including mental retardation in full fetal alcohol syndrome expression, and a higher frequency of learning disabilities and attention deficits. The severity of cognitive deficits appears to be proportional to the severity of physical abnormalities. Children with fetal alcohol syndrome differ significantly from controls in neuropsychological and intellectual measures, whereas children

with fetal alcohol effect are not significantly different from controls (Conry, 1990).

A longitudinal study designed to determine the effects of moderate alcohol exposure on intelligence and learning concluded that an average of two or more alcoholic drinks per day corresponded with a 7-point IQ decrement in children when measured at 7 years of age (Streissguth, Barr, & Sampson, 1990). The same study also looked at the pattern of drinking with respect to IQ, achievement, and behavior. Full-scale, performance and verbal intelligence scores measured by the Wechsler Intelligence Scale for Children–Revised (WISC-R) were about 7 points lower in the alcohol-exposed children (1 oz. absolute alcohol/day) than in children with less alcohol exposure (Streissguth et al., 1990) (Figure 2).

The majority of children with fetal alcohol syndrome and fetal alcohol effect have significant academic difficulties, usually necessitating special education services and vocational or sheltered programs. Streissguth's study reevaluated children known to have fetal alcohol syndrome/effect as adolescents or adults at an average age of 17 years, and found that overall academic abilities were at second- to fourth-grade equivalents. The adaptive skills of this cohort averaged 7 years on the Vineland Adaptive Behavior Scale (Streissguth et al., 1991).

The best predictor of IQ deficit appears to be the number of ounces of absolute alcohol consumed per day (AAD) during pregnancy (Table 2). By comparison, the best prediction of academic achievement as assessed by the Wide-Range Achievement Test (WRAT) is binge drinking (Table 3) (Streissguth et al., 1990).

Neurobehavioral Outcome

There is a broad spectrum of neurobehavioral deviation in children with fetal alcohol syndrome and fetal alcohol effect. A number of reports that use the Brazelton Neonatal Behavioral Assessment Scales (NBAS) show that many alcohol-exposed infants have reduced ability to habituate to stimuli, increased instability, and disturbed reflexes and motor behaviors. These neurobehavioral abnormalities

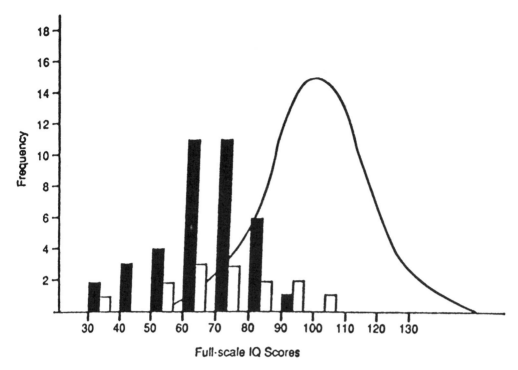

Figure 2. Frequency distribution of IQ scores from the Wechsler Adult Intelligence Scale–Revised and the Wechsler Intelligence Scale for Children–Revised, whichever was age appropriate. Mean chronologic age was 18 years. The bell-shaped curve represents the normal distribution. Solid bars indicate fetal alcohol syndrome ($N = 38$, mean IQ = 66); open bars, fetal alcohol effects ($N = 14$, mean IQ = 73). (From Streissguth, A.P., Aase, J.M., Clarren, S.K., Randels, S.P., LaDue, R.A., & Smith, D.A. [1991]. Fetal alcohol syndrome in adolescents and adults. *JAMA, 265,* 1964; reprinted by permission.)

have been studied in an attempt to tease out the differences between withdrawal symptoms and more persistent central nervous system consequences resulting from alcohol exposure. A 1-month follow-up in the neonatal period showed that alcohol-exposed children have more persistent NBAS aberrations than controls (Coles, Smith, Lancaster, & Falek,

1987). It is difficult to predict whether these neurobehavioral alterations would diminish over time as a result of brain plasticity and maturation.

Behavioral effects of prenatal alcohol exposure are evident in school-age populations. Difficulties with attention, hyperactivity, and impulsivi.y are more frequent in children with

Table 2. Multiple regression: IQ at age 7 years by ADD ($N = 482$)[a]

WISC IQ	R	Partial F (df)[b]	(p)	IQ decrement ≥ 1 oz/day[c]
Full Scale	.63	$F(3,462) = 7.18$	(.0001)	-6.7
Verbal	.62	$F(3,463) = 6.10$	(.0004)	-6.6
Performance	.51	$F(3,463) = 4.92$	(.0022)	-5.1

From Streissguth, A.P., Barr, H.M., & Sampson, P.D. (1990). Moderate prenatal alcohol exposure: Effects on child IQ and learning problems at age 7 1/2 years. *Alcoholism: Clinical and Experimental Research, 14,* 665; reprinted by permission.

[a]Covariates include maternal and paternal education; number of children in the household; household stress; prenatal nutrition; breast feeding and child's nutrition at 7 years; sex and race of child; prenatal exposure to aspirin, cigarettes, and caffeine; and exam conditions.

[b]The 3-*df* F-statistic is for a step function at 1 ounce midpregnancy, and the interactions of this alcohol measure with father's education and with number of children in the household.

[c]The IQ decrement is evaluated for families with father's education equal to 14 years, and with two children (the approximate means for this cohort).

Table 3. Multiple regression: Achievement at age 7 by binge drinking ($N = 482$)[a]

WRAT	R	Partial $F (df)$[b]	(p)	Achievement decrement: BINGE P
Reading	.55	$F(1,467) = 4.34$	(.038)	−3.3
Spelling	.58	$F(1,467) = 1.46$	(.227)	−1.8
Arithmetic	.62	$F(1,467) = 12.60$	(.000)	−3.3

From Streissguth, A.P., Barr, H.M., & Sampson, P.D. (1990). Moderate prenatal alcohol exposure: Effects on child IQ and learning problems at age 7 1/2 years. *Alcoholism: Clinical and Experimental Research, 14,* 665; reprinted by permission.

[a]Covariates include maternal and paternal education; number of children in the household; household stress; prenatal nutrition; sex, race, and grade of child; prenatal exposure to aspirin, cigarettes, and caffeine; and exam conditions.

[b]The 1-*df* F-statistic is for a binary indicator of binge drinking (any use of ≥5 drinks on an occasion) in early pregnancy.

fetal alcohol syndrome/effect than they are in controls without alcohol exposure in utero. Children with fetal alcohol syndrome/effect have been compared to children with attention-deficit/hyperactivity disorder (ADHD) and to controls without alcohol exposure or ADHD. The alcohol-affected children had lower mean IQ scores but similar Conner's scales and Child Behavior Checklist scores in comparison to the ADHD group (Nanson & Hiscock, 1990) (Table 4). The alcohol-exposed group also was more likely to be receiving special education services than either the ADHD or the control group. Behavior difficulties were present in children both with and without mental retardation who had been exposed to alcohol in utero. Evaluations of school-age children with fetal alcohol syndrome/effect and children exposed to moderate amounts of alcohol in utero show poor performance on vigilance tasks, with slower reaction times and more errors from impulsivity.

CONCLUSIONS

Since Clarren and Smith (1978) and Lemoine (as cited in Streissguth, Landesman-Dwyer, et al., 1980) have described the clinical constellation comprising the fetal alcohol syndrome, the debate about the teratogenicity of alcohol has abated. There is very strong evidence that growth deficiency, dysmorphology, and central nervous system effects relate to alcohol use. However, the specific deficits in all these parameters as well as the dose, frequency pattern, or timing of alcohol use in different periods of gestation remain unclear.

Additional questions arise concerning the effects of compounding variables such as malnutrition, tobacco, and multiple drug use. It is pos-

Table 4. Mean ages, sex ratios, educational placement, mean questionnaire scores, and IQ by groups

	Normal		FAS/FAE		ADD		
	Younger	Older	Younger	Older	Younger	Older	F value
Mean age (years)	7.3	11.2	7.4	10.3	8.6	10.5	
No. of males/10	7	5	2	4	10	8	
No. in special education	0	0	6	4	0	0	
Mean ATPQ	5	2	14*	14.1*	16*	16*	30.08
Mean SNAP	15	7	30*	33*	32*	32*	22.12
CBC hyperactivity	60	51	76*	72*	70*	70*	22.02
CBC total	51	49	67*	66*	69*	66*	15.81
Mean IQ	108	103	78*	78*	110	104	23.34

From Nanson, J.L., & Hiscock, M. (1990). Attention deficits in children exposed to alcohol prenatally. *Alcoholism: Clinical and Experimental Research, 14,* 658; reprinted by permission.

Note: ADD, attention-deficit disorder; ATPQ, Abbreviated Teacher Parent Questionnaire; CBS, Child Behavior Checklist; FAS/FAE, fetal alcohol syndrome/fetal alcohol effect.

*Different from normal $p < 0.001$.

sible that alcohol may interact with other agents, such as tobacco, in exerting teratogenic effects to produce the anomalies characterized in the fetal alcohol syndrome. Likewise, the mechanism and pathogenesis of alcohol as a teratogen remain under investigation.

Research in the area of fetal alcohol syndrome since the 1970s has brought the issue into the public arena. Thus, while the intricacies of the pathology are being worked out, there is a new responsibility to educate the public about this very preventable form of disability.

REFERENCES

Brien, J.F., & Smith, G.N. (1991). Effects of alcohol (ethanol) on the fetus. *Journal of Developmental Physiology*, *15*, 21–32.

Burd, L., & Martsolf, J.T. (1989). Fetal alcohol syndrome: Diagnosis and syndromal variability. *Physiology and Behavior*, *46*, 39–43.

Clarren, S.K., Alvoid, E.C., Jr., Sumi, M., Streissguth, A.P., & Smith, D.W. (1978). Brain malformation related to prenatal exposure to ethanol. *The Journal of Pediatrics*, *92*, 64–67.

Clarren, S.K., & Smith, D.W. (1978). The fetal alcohol syndrome. *New England Journal of Medicine*, *298*, 1063–1067.

Coles, C.D., Smith, I.E., Lancaster, J.S., & Falek, A. (1987). Persistence over the first month of neurobehavioral differences in infants exposed to alcohol prenatally. *Infant Behavior and Development*, *10*, 23–37.

Conry, J. (1990). Neuropsychological deficits in fetal alcohol syndrome and fetal alcohol effects. *Alcoholism: Clinical and Experimental Research*, *14*, 650–655.

Day, N.L., Goldschmidtt, L., Robles, N., Richardson, G., Cornelius, M., Taylor, P., & Geva, D. (1991). Prenatal alcohol exposure and offspring growth at 18 months of age: The predictive validity of two measures of drinking. *Alcoholism: Clinical and Experimental Research*, *15*, 914–918.

Day, N., & Richardson, G. (1991). Prenatal alcohol exposure: A continuum of effects. *Seminars in Perinatology*, *15*, 271–279.

Jones, K., Smith, D.W., Ulleland, C.N., & Streissguth, P.A. (1973). Patterns of malformation in offspring of chronic alcoholic mothers. *Lancet*, *1*, 1267–1271.

Nanson, J.L., & Hiscock, M. (1990). Attention deficits in children exposed to alcohol prenatally. *Alcoholism: Clinical and Experimental Research*, *14*, 656–661.

Russell, M., Czarnecki, D.M., Cowan, R., McPherson, E., & Mudar, P.J. (1991). Measures of maternal alcohol use as predictors of development in early childhood. *Alcoholism: Clinical and Experimental Research*, *15*, 1991–2000.

Schenker, S., Becker, H.C., Randall, C.L., Phillips, P.K., Baskin, G.S., & Henderson, G.I. (1990). Fetal alcohol syndrome: Current status of pathogenesis. *Alcoholism: Clinical and Experimental Research*, *14*, 635–647.

Streissguth, A.P., Aase, J.M., Clarren, S.K., Randels, S.P., LaDue, R.A., & Smith, D.A. (1991). Fetal alcohol syndrome in adolescents and adults. *JAMA*, *265*, 1961–1967.

Streissguth, A.P., Barr, H.M., Marhm, D.C., & Herman, C.S. (1980). Effects of maternal alcohol nicotine and caffeine use during pregnancy on infant mental and motor development at eight months. *Alcoholism: Clinical and Experimental Research*, *4*, 152–163.

Streissguth, A.P., Barr, H.M., & Sampson, P.D. (1990). Moderate prenatal alcohol exposure: Effects on child IQ and learning problems at age 7½ years. *Alcoholism: Clinical and Experimental Research*, *14*, 662–669.

Streissguth, A.P., Landesman-Dwyer, S., Martin, J.C., & Smith, D.W. (1980). Teratogenic effects of alcohol in humans and laboratory animals. *Science*, *209*, 353–361.

West, J.R., & Goodlett, C.R. (1990). Teratogenic effects of alcohol on brain development. *Annals of Medicine*, *22*, 319–325.

Chapter 20

Psychiatric Problems in People with Developmental Disabilities

Beverly A. Myers, M.D.

The psychiatric approach to disturbances of mood, thought, and behavior in people with mental retardation floundered in the 20th century until recently. The movement in the early 20th century away from psychiatric classification in the mode of Kraepelin toward the psychoanalytic approach led either to overinterpretation of the behavior of people with mental retardation and psychiatric disorders, or to loss of interest. A more fruitful approach has come with the recent return to a more medical approach, with operationally defined criteria for making diagnoses as specified in recent editions of the *Diagnostic and Statistical Manual of Mental Disorders* (DSM) of the American Psychiatric Association (1980, 1987, 1994) (see the appendix). The discovery of new psychopharmacologic agents in the last 30 years, in combination with the use of behavioral approaches, has improved the management of psychiatric disorders in people with mental retardation significantly and has reduced the use of antipsychotic drugs. This chapter aims to synthesize these systematic approaches to the diagnosis and management of psychiatric disorders in people with mental retardation.

APPROACHES TO PSYCHOPATHOLOGY

Psychiatric diagnoses are made by clinical history; examination of physical and mental status; and laboratory studies, including standardized scales of behavior. Recent editions of the DSM —the third (DSM-III, 1980), third revised (DSM-III-R, 1987), and fourth (DSM-IV, 1994)—have defined criteria for the diagnosis of psychiatric disorders in the general popula-

tion. These criteria can be applied, but with some difficulty, to the majority of people with mental retardation and disturbances of mood, thought, or behavior. However, unlike people of average to superior intelligence, who can describe their symptoms elaborately, people with mental retardation, who often cannot speak, are limited in describing their experiences. This necessitates reliance on observed behavior. The use of several approaches—multiaxial, developmental, etiologic, and categorical—enhances the understanding of the disturbances of mood, thought, and behavior of individuals with mental retardation.

Multiaxial Approach

The DSM-IV includes a multiaxial approach to be considered in each individual. Axis I includes the clinical syndromes. Axis II (see the appendix) includes lifelong patterns of behavior, both as developmental disorders and as personality disorders (e.g., mild mental retardation and histrionic personality). Axis III includes all physical or medical disorders (e.g., Down syndrome), and Axis IV includes the severity of psychosocial stressors, from none to catastrophic. Finally, Axis V is a global assessment of levels of functioning, including psychological, social, academic, and occupational. This allows the specific psychiatric diagnoses to be considered in a broader perspective, thus facilitating both clinical and research activities.

Developmental Approach

The developmental approach, an expansion of Axes II and V, in addition to changes in cognition and social abilities with age, recognizes that those psychiatric disorders occurring in childhood are different from those of adults, are often lifelong, and frequently are related to the intellectual and social levels of functioning. One must relate age to cognitive and social levels in all individuals with developmental and psychiatric disorders. One also must consider the lifetime history of a disorder. Autistic disorder, stereotyped behavior, hyperactivity, self-injurious behavior, and aggressive behavior tend to begin in childhood or adolescence and to be lifelong conditions. Thus, examining the onsets of these disorders and developing early interventions may prevent or reduce major problems occurring in adults with mental retardation that necessitate institutional placement.

Etiologic Approach

The nature of the psychiatric symptomatology, or its *form* (e.g., presence of hallucinations), often is linked to the biologic mechanism or etiology of the disorder (Axis III). Determination of the *function*, or the purpose for which this symptom or target behavior is used (e.g., attention seeking), is a more detailed approach to psychological and environmental etiologies. In order to understand the etiology of a disorder, one attempts to relate the form to the function. This expansion of Axis III can be combined with Axis IV (level of stressors) to clarify the sources of psychiatric disorders in persons with mental retardation. One must be clear about one's interpretation of mood, thought, and behavior and recognize the level of approach that one is using—form or function—in arriving at etiologic mechanisms. Misinterpretations of behavior may lead to grave errors in diagnosis and treatment of a psychiatric problem, particularly in a person with mental retardation. For example, tongue protrusion is the side effect of a phenothiazine, not a psychological response to stressful events (Myers, 1988).

Categorical Approach

McHugh and Slavney (1983) proposed that psychiatric problems be categorized into four complementary but discontinuous approaches to mental phenomena: *disease* (implying predominantly biologic etiologic mechanisms), *motivated behaviors* (involving both biologic and psychological mechanisms), *dimensions* of per-

sonality and behavior (involving both biologic and psychological mechanisms), and *life events* (implying psychological mechanisms). The use of these categories may enable the clinician to interpret the significance of a target behavior (e.g., aggressive behavior) as part of a disease (e.g., mania) or as part of a motivated behavior.

Summary

The diagnosis and management of psychiatric disorders in people with mental retardation includes all these approaches. From carefully taken psychiatric histories, including the behavioral observations of psychologists and others, and mental status examinations, one not only can specify the DSM-IV diagnosis but also can clarify etiologic factors and make therapeutic decisions involving both psychological and pharmacologic interventions in the majority of individuals. Using McHugh and Slavney's (1983) categories in combination with DSM-IV diagnoses and known etiologic factors, the following presentation includes the majority of psychiatric disorders seen in people with mental retardation.

CATEGORY I: DISEASE

Schizophrenia

Table 1 lists the DSM-IV criteria for schizophrenia. The key criteria include 6 months or more of a major change in social or occupa-

Table 1. DSM-IV (1994) criteria for schizophrenia

Characteristic symptoms (two or more for 1 month or less):
  Delusions
  Hallucinations
  Disorganized speech (derailment or incoherence)
  Disorganized or catatonic behavior
  Negative symptoms (affective flattening, alogia, or avolition)

Social/occupational dysfunction: one or more areas—work, interpersonal relations, self-care—below level previously achieved

Duration: continuous signs of the disturbance persist for at least 6 months (prodromal, active, and/or residual)

Schizoaffective and mood disorders excluded

Substance and general medical condition excluded

Adapted from American Psychiatric Association (1994).

tional functioning, or both, and at least two of the following symptoms: delusions, hallucinations, incoherent speech, disorganized or catatonic behavior, and negative symptoms (flat affect, alogia, or avolition).

Reid (1972b) clearly established that schizophrenia does occur in people with mental retardation. The DSM-IV emphasizes that low levels of social functioning, oddities of behavior, and impoverished affect and cognition may suggest schizophrenia, but it should not be diagnosed unless delusions and hallucinations are definitely present. Thought disorder alone is not schizophrenia. It may be impossible to diagnose schizophrenia in those persons with severe and profound mental retardation. There is no special mental retardation form of schizophrenia, or "pfropfschizophrenie," as once was suggested. The more acute psychotic disorders—acute schizophreniform disorder, brief psychotic disorder, delirium, and manic–depressive disorders—are alternate diagnoses to consider.

Schizophrenia is possibly more frequent in people with mental retardation than it is in the general population. The point prevalence rate of schizophrenia in the general population is 0.5%–0.8% (Regier & Burke, 1985); in persons with mental retardation, the point prevalence may be as high as 3%, but this value may be excessive (Turner, 1989). In admissions to a general psychiatric hospital, Myers (1986) found no differences in the number of cases of schizophrenia between persons with and without developmental disabilities, but those with developmental disabilities experienced more acute psychotic disorders. Schizophrenia is rare in children.

The current pharmacotherapy for schizophrenia in mental retardation is neuroleptic medication, which appears to have a specific action on dopamine receptor blockade (Menolascino, Wilson, Golden, & Ruedrich, 1986). The neuroleptics include phenothiazines, such as chlorpromazine and thioridazine, and butyrophenones, such as haloperidol, usually in low doses. The former are more sedating and the latter have more extrapyramidal side effects. The risk of tardive dyskinesia is significant with both groups and must be weighed against the potential benefits. Clozapine, a helpful but risky new antipsychotic, helps those who have not responded to the usual antipsychotics (Kane et al., 1988). Weekly blood level determinations are required with its use. No studies of clozapine in people with mental retardation have been reported. Risperidone is another new, less toxic antipsychotic.

Mood Disorders

Mood or affective disorders are classified as bipolar (both manic and depressive episodes occur periodically in a person along with periods of normality) or unipolar (only depressive episodes occur). A person who shows manic episodes invariably has depressed episodes: a bipolar or manic–depressive disorder. Bipolar disorder often begins in adolescence or young adulthood. The DSM-IV criteria for mania and depression are listed in Tables 2 and 3. A person with periods of both mania and non–mood-related hallucinations and delusions has a schizoaffective disorder.

Mania   Individuals with mental retardation can experience a manic disorder (Carlson, 1979; Kadambari, 1986; Reid, 1972a). The symptoms may be classic or truncated to periods of hyperactivity and sleep disorder, the latter being difficult to diagnose in persons with severe mental retardation. Symptoms that alone are not diagnostic—hyperactivity, assaultive behavior, and anger outbursts—may respond to lithium. Whether this represents a

Table 2.   DSM-IV (1994) criteria for manic episode

Abnormally persistently elevated, expansive, or irritable mood

Three of the following:
  Inflated self-esteem or grandiosity
  Decreased need for sleep
  Pressured talking
  Flight of ideas or subjective racing thoughts
  Distractibility
  Increase in goal: directed activity or psychomotor agitation
  Excessive involvement in pleasurable activities with high potential for painful consequences: unrestrained buying, business, sexual sprees

Marked impairment in occupational/social functioning

Not due to substance abuse or general medical condition

Adapted from American Psychiatric Association (1994).

Table 3. DSM-IV (1994) criteria for depressive disorders

Major depressive episode
  Five of the following for at least 2 weeks:
    Depressed mood
    Decreased interest or pleasure
    Weight loss or gain
    Insomnia or hypersomnia
    Psychomotor agitation or retardation
    Fatigue or loss of energy
    Feelings of worthlessness; guilt
    Impaired thinking and concentration, or
      indecisiveness
    Recurrent thoughts of death and/or suicide
  Clinically significant distress or impairment in
    social, occupational, or other areas of functioning
  Not due to substance abuse or general medical
    condition
Dysthymic disorder
  Depressed mood most of day for 2 years
    (1 year in children/adolescents)
  Two of the following:
    Poor appetite or overeating
    Insomnia or hypersomnia
    Low energy or fatigue
    Low self-esteem
    Poor concentration or indecisiveness
    Feelings of hopelessness

Adapted from American Psychiatric Association (1994).

manic disorder is unclear; the presence of episodes of depression as well is supportive. A family history of affective disorder is very helpful in diagnosis. The prevalence of manic disorders in persons with mental retardation is about 1%–3.5% in institutions (Reid, 1989), and is somewhat lower in the general population, at 0.4%–0.6% (Regier & Burke, 1985). The studies in persons with mental retardation are less precise, and thus the difference may not be significant.

Pharmacotherapy of mania in people with mental retardation is similar to that in the general population (Rivinus & Harmatz, 1979). Lithium alone at serum levels of 0.8–1.2 mEg/liter frequently brings a manic episode under control, but neuroleptics, particularly haloperidol, may be needed. Recently, the anticonvulsants, carbamazepine and valproic acid have been found useful in manic disorders in the general population (Lerer, Moore, Meyendorff, Cho, & Gershon, 1987; McElroy, Keck,

& Pope, 1981). In people with mental retardation, lithium, carbamazepine, and valproic acid, alone or in combination, are useful not only in mania but in atypical mood and behavior disorders; however, the studies are less rigorous (Reid, Naylor, & Kay, 1981; Sovner & Hurley, 1981). Long-term maintenance therapy with these medications, occasionally including antipsychotics, is needed to prevent both manic and depressive episodes.

Major Depression This most severe of the depressive disorders may occur alone or in combination with periods of mania. Features (Table 3) include depression or lack of pleasure, anorexia, insomnia, psychomotor retardation or agitation, social withdrawal, self-deprecation, pessimism, and possibly suicidal thoughts or acts. Psychotic symptoms of hallucinations or delusions may be present. The person with mental retardation may present with these characteristic features, but their most striking features may be marked social withdrawal, cessation of speech, inactivity, and sleep disorder.

Treatment of a major depressive disorder includes a combination of psychotherapy, antidepressants, antipsychotic drugs, and/or electroconvulsive therapy (ECT) (Frances & Hales, 1988). Those persons with average intelligence or mild mental retardation usually benefit from a combination of psychotherapy and antidepressants, which include tricyclic antidepressants such as amitriptyline and imipramine, secondary antidepressants such as trazodone and amoxapine, serotonergic antidepressants such as fluoxetine and sertraline, or monoamine oxidase inhibitors such as phenelzine and tranylcypromine (Sovner, Fox, Lowry, & Lowry, 1993). A psychiatrist may have to try more than one antidepressant to obtain a therapeutic response. With blood levels available, the physician can establish whether a therapeutic level has been reached in the person with a poor response. Psychotic symptoms may require neuroleptics as well as antidepressants. ECT is used in severely depressed persons of average intelligence but infrequently in those with mental retardation. (See Category IV: Life Events and Stresses for information on other types of depression.)

Delirium

Delirium is an acutely occurring and usually temporary condition characterized by impaired consciousness and attention, change in cognition (decreased memory, disorientation, disorganized and confused thinking), or the development of perceptual disturbances that tend to fluctuate over the day. The DSM-IV criteria for diagnosing delirium are shown in Table 4. Delirium may occur in people with mental retardation and should be considered in those presenting with acute psychotic states. Etiologies include medications and toxins, metabolic disorders (hypoxia, hypercarbia, hypoglycemia, and electrolyte disturbances), hepatic and renal failure, thiamine deficiency, systemic infections, trauma, and postoperative states. The abuse of or withdrawal from psychoactive substances (alcohol, narcotics, sedatives, hallucinogens, stimulants, inhalants) and the use of psychoactive medications (antidepressants, anticholinergics, lithium, anticonvulsants, benzodiazepines) are probably the most frequent causes. Toxic screens and drug levels are critical in people with mental retardation who present in an acutely psychotic, confused state. A significant percentage of these cases of delirium will be related to psychoactive drug abuse or withdrawal (Myers, 1986).

The treatment of delirium primarily involves removal or adjustment of the etiologic agent. When the delirium is prolonged and the person is agitated, small doses of haloperidol (1–5 mg orally or intramuscularly every 4 hours as needed) may enable the individual to be more tractable. Lighting, orientation, and a calm but firm approach are important elements of nursing care. Withdrawal reactions from alcohol or benzodiazepines will require the use of a benzodiazepine and subsequent gradual withdrawal (Hales & Yudofsky, 1987).

Dementia

Dementia is a progressive deterioration of all cognitive functions and can occur in people with mental retardation at any age. The DSM-IV criteria for dementia are listed in Table 5. Dementia is not necessarily a nonreversible state. Treatable causes include major depressive disorders, hydrocephalus, subdural hematoma, central nervous system infections, intoxications (e.g., bromide), and even otic cerumen (Myers & Pueschel, 1987). Some dementias may be irreversible, including those of hereditary degenerative diseases (e.g., Alzheimer and Huntington diseases); multiple infarctions; multiple sclerosis; Parkinson's disease; Jakob-Creutzfeldt disease; and postanoxic, posttraumatic, and posthypoglycemic states. Down syndrome is noted to be associated with Alzheimer's disease.

The clinical approach to any person with a deterioration in level of cognitive functioning requires a careful diagnostic evaluation, including physical and mental status examinations, psychological and neuropsychological assessments, toxic and metabolic screens, and neurologic studies such as electroencephalography,

Table 4. DSM-IV (1994) criteria for delirium

Disturbance of consciousness with reduced ability to focus, sustain, or shift attention

Change in cognition (e.g., memory deficit, disorientation) or the development of a perceptual disturbance that is not better accounted for by preexisting dementia

Disturbance develops over short time (hours to days) and tends to fluctuate during the course of the day.

Clinical evidence of physiologic etiology (general medical condition or substance intoxication)

Adapted from American Psychiatric Association (1994).

Table 5. DSM-IV (1994) criteria for dementia

The development of multiple cognitive deficits:

Memory impairment (short-term and long-term memory)

One (or more) of the following:

Aphasia (language disturbance)

Apraxia (impaired ability to carry out motor activities despite intact motor function)

Agnosia (failure to identify/recognize objects despite intact sensory function)

Disturbance in executive functioning (planning, organizing, sequencing, abstracting)

Significant impairment in social or occupational functioning and a significant decline from a previous level

Gradual onset and continuing decline

Organic etiology

Adapted from American Psychiatric Association (1994).

computerized tomography, and magnetic resonance imaging, to detect treatable diseases. With respect to supportive therapy for persons with mental retardation and dementias, one must teach staff to lower expectations gradually to avoid unnecessary distress. Agitation, especially in the evening, may be helped by small doses of haloperidol.

Autistic Disorder and Pervasive Developmental Disorders

Infantile autism first was described by Kanner in 1943 as a condition appearing in the first 2 years of life and presenting with the following characteristics: extreme aloneness, delayed language development, failure to use language for communication purposes, good rote memory, delayed echolalia, pronominal reversal, preservation of sameness, preoccupation with mechanical objects, and bizarre repetitive mannerisms. The term *pervasive developmental disorders* (PDDs) is now used for autism and all similar disorders presenting with a lifelong qualitative impairment in three dimensions: 1) reciprocal social interaction, 2) verbal and nonverbal communication and imaginative activity, and 3) a markedly restricted repertoire of activities and interests (Table 6). Autistic disorder consists of the full syndrome of infantile autism with at least 4 of the 14 items of behavior listed in Table 6 (two from dimension 1, one from dimension 2, and one from dimension 3). All other types of PDD are less complete. These three dimensions of symptoms—the persistent social deficits of aloofness with gaze aversion and incapacity to appreciate the feelings of others; the verbal and nonverbal language disorder with echolalia, pronominal reversals, and poor use of speech for communication; and the markedly restricted repertoire of activities and interests, with stereotyped body movements, persistent preoccupation with parts of objects, marked distress over changes, and insistence on following routines—begin under the age of 30 months and are usually (in 70% of cases) associated with some degree of intellectual impairment or mental retardation that persists into adulthood.

The principal approach to intervention in people with autistic disorder and other PDDs is special education and behavior modification (see Chapter 23, this volume). These approaches may enable the child, adolescent, or adult to adapt as much as possible to his or her environment. Residual language, social, and repetitive behavioral deficits frequently remain.

Medications are sometimes helpful with difficult and dangerous behavior, but good research is limited. Neuroleptics long have been

Table 6. DSM-IV (1994) criteria for autistic disorder

1. Qualitative impairment in social interaction: *two of*
    a. marked impairment in use of multiple nonverbal behaviors such as eye-to-eye gaze, facial expression, body postures, and gestures to regulate social interaction
    b. failure to develop appropriate peer relationships
    c. lack of spontaneous seeking to share enjoyment, interests, or achievements with other people
    d. lack of social or emotional reciprocity
2. Qualitative impairment in verbal and nonverbal communication: *one of*
    a. delay in or total lack in development of spoken language without compensatory communication
    b. marked impairment in ability to initiate or sustain conversation with others
    c. stereotyped and repetitive use of language or idiosyncratic language
    d. lack of appropriate spontaneous make-believe play or social imitative play
3. Restricted repetitive and stereotyped patterns of behavior, interests, and activities: *one of*
    a. encompassing preoccupation with one or more stereotyped and restricted abnormal patterns of interest
    b. inflexible adherence to specific, nonfunctional routines or rituals
    c. stereotyped and repetitive motor mannerisms (e.g., hand flapping, whole-body movements)
    d. persistent preoccupation with parts of objects
4. Delays or abnormal functioning with onset prior to 3 years in at least one of 1) social interaction, 2) language, or 3) symbolic or imaginative play

Adapted from American Psychiatric Association (1994).

used with persons with autism, but carefully done research has shown questionable improvement and excessive sedation. Because of common serotonergic links (low serotonin in platelets and brains of persons with autism), fenfluramine has attracted recent interest, but its effects in autism have been equivocal (du Verglas, Banks, & Guyer, 1988; Groden et al., 1987). Antianxiety agents such as benzodiazepines (clonazepam) and β blockers (propranolol) may play a role in reducing extreme tension in some adults with autism (McDaniel, 1986; Ratey et al., 1987). Interventions in cases of aggressive and self-injurious behavior are discussed in the section on Category II: Motivated Behaviors (see also Chapter 21, this volume).

Obsessive–Compulsive Disorder

Obsessive–compulsive disorder (OCD) is characterized by repetitive involuntary thoughts that are recognized as unwanted and are associated with an intense need to carry out repetitive actions (e.g., checking, washing, aligning of objects), no matter how inappropriate (DSM-IV, 1994). OCD can occur in people with mental retardation of all levels and often is not resisted.

Two types of therapy have been demonstrated to be of significant help in this formerly very incapacitating disorder: behavior modification and serotonergic antidepressants (Marks, 1986). Fluoxetine (Fontaine & Chouinard, 1986), clomipramine (Ananth & Lin, 1986), fluvoxamine, and sertraline have been demonstrated to be effective in people of average intelligence. The OCD that occurs in persons with mental retardation has responded to fluoxetine and sertraline (Cook, Terry, Heller, & Leventhal, 1990; Vitiello, Spreat, & Behar, 1989; Wiener & Lamberti, 1993).

Anxiety Disorders

In adults without mental retardation, anxiety disorders in recent years have been differentiated into simple phobia, panic disorder with and without agoraphobia, social phobia, posttraumatic stress disorder, and generalized anxiety disorder (Frances & Hales, 1988). Treatment includes behavioral approaches and chemotherapy (tricyclic antidepressants and monoamine oxidase inhibitors), benzodiazepines (alprazolam [Xanax]) and β blockers (propranolol [Inderal]).

Very little is known about anxiety disorders in people with mental retardation (Ollendick & Ollendick, 1982). Clinicians caring for people with mental retardation have observed anxiety (Richardson, Katz, Koller, McLaren, & Rubenstein, 1979), phobia (Matson, 1981), and avoidance (Sternlicht, 1979). Those persons who are chronically tense may respond successfully to benzodiazepines (particularly clonazepam) or β blockers. Antidepressants (tricyclics) may have a place in treating separation anxiety or school/center avoidence in children, adolescents, and adults with mental retardation (McDaniel, 1986).

Attention-Deficit/Hyperactivity Disorder

In children and adults of average intelligence, attention-deficit/hyperactivity disorder (ADHD) consists of short attention span, difficulty following instructions, hyperactivity, restlessness, distractibility, poor persistence on task, forgetfulness, difficulty waiting, impulsivity, and disorganization. It may occur in both children and adults with all levels of mental retardation but may represent a different disorder biochemically. The prevalence is estimated to be 8%–15% in children with mental retardation (Taylor, 1986) and 17%–52% among adults with mental retardation (Gostasen, 1985). The diagnosis may be quantified in children with and without mental retardation using screening tests such as the Conners checklist (Conners, 1969) and in adults with mental retardation using the Aberrant Behavior Checklist (Aman, Singh, Stewart, & Field, 1985) (Table 7). These measures are useful for monitoring treatment (see Chapter 29, this volume).

The medication treatment of hyperactivity in children and adults with mental retardation has been poorly studied. It sometimes is similar to the treatment of ADHD in the general population (see Chapter 29, this volume), which includes psychostimulants such as methylphenidate (Ritalin) and dextroamphetamine (Dexedrine) and antidepressants such as desipramine, but treatment frequently is not re-

Table 7.   The Aberrant Behavior Checklist

Subscale I (Irritability)
1. Injures self
2. Aggressive to other patients and staff
3. Screams inappropriately
4. Temper tantrums
5. Irritable ("grizzly" or "whiny")
6. Yells at inappropriate times
7. Depressed mood
8. Demands must be met immediately
9. Cries over minor annoyances and hurts
10. Mood changes quickly
11. Cries and screams inappropriately
12. Stamps feet while banging object or slamming doors
13. Deliberately hurts self
14. Does physical violence to self
15. Throws temper tantrums when he/she does not get own way

Subscale II (Lethargy)
16. Listless, sluggish, inactive
17. Seeks isolation from others
18. Preoccupied; stares into space
19. Withdrawn; prefers solitary activities
20. Fixed facial expression; lacks emotional reactivity
21. Does nothing but sit and watch others
22. Resists any form of physical contact
23. Isolates self from others
24. Sits or stands in one position for a long time
25. Unresponsive toward activities (does not react)
26. Is difficult to reach or contact
27. Prefers to be alone
28. Does not try to communicate by word or gestures
29. Inactive, never moves spontaneously
30. Responds negatively to affection
31. Shows few social reactions to others

Subscale III (Stereotypy)
32. Meaningless, recurring body movements
33. Stereotyped, repetitive movements
34. Odd, bizzare behavior
35. Moves or rolls head back and forth
36. Repetitive hand, body, or head movements
37. Waves or shakes the extremities repeatedly
38. Rocks body back and forth

Subscale IV (Hyperactivity)
39. Excessively active on ward
40. Boisterous (inappropriately noisy and rough)
41. Impulsive (acts without thinking)
42. Restless, unable to sit still
43. Disobedient; difficult to control
44. Disturbs others
45. Uncooperative
46. Does not pay attention to instruction
47. Disrupts group activities
48. Does not stay in seat during lesson period
49. Will not sit still for any length of time
50. Easily distractible
51. Constantly runs or jumps around the room
52. Pays no attention when spoken to
53. Tends to be excessively active
54. Deliberately ignores directions

Subscale V (Excessive speech)
55. Talks excessively
56. Repetitive speech
57. Talks to self loudly
58. Repeats a word or phrase over and over

From Aman, M., Singh, W.N., Stewart, A.W., & Field, C.J. (1985). Psychometric characteristics of the Aberrant Behavior Checklist. *American Journal of Mental Deficiency, 89,* 492–502; reprinted by permission.

sponsive to these agents. Clonidine is sometimes useful. When hyperactivity is associated with assaultiveness that is dangerous to others, and when the above medications and behavior modification have been incompletely effective, neuroleptics may be necessary, despite the risk of side effects. Hyperactivity is sometimes part of a chronic manic syndrome and responds to lithium.

CATEGORY II: MOTIVATED BEHAVIORS

This approach implies that behavior has a motivation or purpose and is a construct that attempts to make sense out of observations of activity. Motivated behaviors are characterized by their specific adaptive function, by the influence of an external stimulus, and by their internal changes. Abnormal behaviors are characterized by abnormalities in the strength of the urge, the mode of their expression, and the nature of their object. Etiologic factors include both environmental (psychological or functional) and biologic influences. An exhaustive behavioral analysis is usually required to make such determinations.

Examples of abnormalities of motivated behavior include alcoholism, drug abuse, anorexia nervosa and bulimia, suicide, and delinquency, all of which may be observed in people with mental retardation. Alcoholism and drug abuse appear no more often in people with mental retardation and apparently are driven by the same factors as in the general population. Anorexia nervosa and bulimia may be less common in adolescents with mental retardation (Myers & Pueschel, 1987). Suicide occurs in people with mild and moderate mental retardation and has received very little study. Other abnormal and motivated behaviors common in people with mental retardation include self-injurious behavior, aggressive behavior, and other behaviors peculiar to mental retardation.

Self-Injurious Behavior

Self-injurious behavior (SIB) is a serious behavior problem in people with mental retardation (see Chapter 21, this volume), and includes a wide range of behaviors severe enough to lead to tissue damage. SIB includes head banging, face slapping, self-biting, eye poking and other eye injury, lip and finger chewing, and limb banging (Oliver, Murphy, & Corbett, 1987). Head banging is the most common SIB in children of average intelligence; the remainder are peculiar to people with mental retardation. The frequency depends on the population studied, with 3% occurrence among persons with mental retardation in the community and up to 15% in those residing in institutions (Oliver et al., 1987).

One disorder specifically associated with SIB is Lesch-Nyhan disease, with a disorder of the enzyme hypoxanthine-guanine-phosphoribosyltransferase and severe chewing and destruction of lips and digits (Lesch & Nyhan, 1964). It may respond temporarily to 5-hydroxytryptophan. Other etiologies of SIB in people with mental retardation are incompletely understood. It may be associated with major depression and respond to antidepressants. Environmental variables that increase SIB include decreased adult attention, increased academic demands, restricted access to tangibles, and unstructured settings (Durand & Crimmins, 1988).

The treatment or management of SIB in people with mental retardation is a major challenge. Careful behavioral analysis should be conducted before any intervention. Behavioral modalities include the use of positive reinforcement (differential reinforcement of other behaviors [DRO], overcorrection, time-out, air splints, and DRO plus overcorrection) or, rarely, aversive stimuli (lemon juice, ammonia, physical restraints, or electric shock) (Gorman-Smith & Matson, 1985). Aversive stimuli, sometimes

used in extreme problems, may lead to significant behavioral change, but their use requires careful supervision for protection against injuries and invasion of rights (Fedura, Lindsey, & Walker, 1987). Other interventions for SIB include goggles, coverings for hands, helmets, and wheelchairs, which also require careful supervision.

When behavioral approaches are incompletely successful, medications may be helpful. Neuroleptics often have been tried with some benefit. However, with the side effects of tardive dyskinesia, neuroleptic malignant syndrome, and cataracts, alternatives should be sought (Gualtieri, Lefler, Guimond, & Staye, 1982; Zimmerman & Heistad, 1982). Serotonergic antidepressants have recently been reported to be of value in SIB (Gedye, 1993; Sovner et al., 1993). Other medications include lithium, naltrexone, low-dose haloperidol, and benzodiazepines (Farber, 1987).

Aggressive and Assaultive Behavior

Aggressive and assaultive behavior is by no means peculiar to people with mental retardation. It is more common to people with brain damage or dysfunction (Silver & Yudofsky, 1987). When it is part of other delinquent behavior, it is included in conduct disorder or antisocial personality. Isolated aggression outbursts are known as intermittent explosive disorder. Aggressive behavior may be part of other psychiatric disorders such as mania or schizophrenia. Aggression and assaultive behavior in people with mental retardation is often a longstanding behavior problem. It is seen at all levels of mental retardation, but is more common in persons functioning at the severe and profound levels. It is more common in males, younger people, and those who reside in institutions, where it may be reinforced if not dealt with.

A careful analysis of the aggressive behavior in a person with mental retardation is essential to any therapeutic intervention or prevention (Mace, Page, & Ivancic, 1986). Environmental determinants in children with mental retardation include contingent social disappointment, the application of instructional demands, and the structuring of play. The primary intervention to interrupt and reduce aggressive behavior is behavior modification, both reinforcing and, rarely, aversive.

When behavior modification approaches have been utilized extensively and properly, but are incompletely effective, medication may be helpful when used in combination with behavioral interventions. Careful variation of one factor at a time is necessary to determine the value of a medication or behavioral intervention. Specific diagnoses (e.g., schizophrenia, mania) indicate specific medications (e.g., neuroleptics, lithium). With associated affective disturbances (hostility, mood lability) lithium, carbamazepine (Tegretol), and/or valproate (Depakene) have proven helpful (Rapport, Sonis, Fiaalkov, Matson, & Kazdin, 1982; Reid et al., 1981; Sovner & Hurley, 1981). Buspirone has been noted to be useful in those persons with mental retardation and anxiety (Ratey, Sovner, Parks, & Rogentine, 1991).

Propranolol and other β blockers have been found useful for aggressive behavior with schizophrenia, acute and chronic organic brain damage, and intermittent explosive disorder, as well as aggressive behavior, in those with mental retardation (Greendyke, Kauter, & Schuster, 1986; Ratey et al., 1986). The mechanism of action is not known but may be via reductions of anxiety or arousal because fear and panic are reduced. Doses of up to 600 mg/day may be used and are not usually associated with clinical symptomatology. Side effects of bradycardia and hypotension have not prevented the use of propranolol.

Although antipsychotic or neuroleptic drugs have been used frequently to treat aggression in persons with mental retardation, they are specifically indicated only in those individuals with psychotic symptoms (e.g., schizophrenia, mania). When aggressive behavior is significantly dangerous to others and behavior modification and nonneuroleptic medications have been unsuccessful, neuroleptics may become a necessary alternative. Risperadone, a new antipsychotic, may have fewer side effects. With vigorous attempts at behavior modification and/or the use of lithium, carbamazepine, valproate, clonazepam, and β blockers, and

systematic efforts to avoid or reduce the use of antipsychotics, the prevalence of the use of antipsychotics may continue to decrease.

Other Behaviors

One may identify other target or problem behaviors in people with mental retardation. These behaviors include rectal digging, stripping, crying, pica, hyperactivity, running off, agitation, uncooperativeness, stealing, self-stimulation, stereotypic behavior, and vocal disturbances. When the behavior is part of a psychiatric syndrome, appropriate medication should be used. For example, a recent onset of hyperactivity, hostility, hyperverbosity, and insomnia is likely to represent mania and require lithium, valproate, or carbamazepine. Tourette disease, a chronic motor and vocal tic disorder, should be distinguished from other behaviors and treated with low doses of haloperidol. The primary therapeutic approach to most of these behaviors is behavior modification after careful analysis of the target behavior. However, some severe behavior problems (e.g., rectal digging and smearing) may respond well to and be prevented by lithium. The relationship of rectal digging to bipolar disorder is unknown.

CATEGORY III: DIMENSIONS

The DSM-IV approach to diagnosis of behavior problems is a qualitative and categorical one whereby a diagnosis is arrived at by the fulfillment of various criteria. An alternative approach that is more quantitative examines the correlation of many behaviors to reveal various dimensions of behavior. This approach is useful in examining longstanding or lifelong dimensions or traits. In children these include conduct and developmental disorders; in adults, personality disorders.

Dimensions of Behavior in Children

Extensive research into the dimensional approach of behavior in children has been conducted by Quay, Peterson, Werry, Achenbach and others. A well-known standardized measure of children's behavior emerging from this dimensional approach is the Child Behavior Checklist by Achenbach & Edelbrock (1983). Its major categories are externalizing and internalizing behaviors or dimensions. Externalizing behaviors—for example, for boys 6–11 years of age—include hyperactive, aggressive, delinquent behaviors. Internalizing behaviors (for boys 6–11) include schizoid–anxious, depressed, uncommunicative, obsessive–compulsive, and somatic. These factors correlate somewhat with DSM-IV diagnoses but also allow for a recognition of problem behaviors that are not sufficient for a specific diagnosis. There is some evidence that problem dimensions noted in childhood may become lifelong traits. This is demonstrated by Robins' (1966) research (and that of many others since) showing good correlations of antisocial behavior in children followed into adulthood 20–25 years later.

Conduct Disorder   Delinquent behavioral disturbances known as conduct disorder invariably begin in childhood (DSM-IV, 1994). Conduct disorder includes the following delinquent behavior: stealing, lying, running away, fire setting, truancy, breaking and entering, destruction of property, cruelty to animals, forced sexual activity, use of weapons, mugging or robbery, and physical cruelty or injury. Patterns of conduct disorders in the general population have been recognized in individuals: aggression toward people or animals, destruction of property, deceitfulness or theft, and serious violation of rules. Conduct disorders are the most frequent behavior problem in children in the general population (Rutter, Tizard, & Whitmore, 1966). Children and adolescents with mental retardation are somewhat more prone to delinquent behavior than are children and adolescents in the general population (Rutter et al., 1966).

Behavior modification is the primary intervention in delinquent behaviors in children and adolescents with and without mental retardation. Psychotherapy is infrequently a primary treatment in a person with conduct disorder. It is only after careful trials of behavior modification and when conduct disorders become seriously aggressive and dangerous that one considers psychotropic medication (as for aggression).

Developmental Disorders   The Child Behavior Checklist has been utilized in children and adolescents with mild and moderate mental retardation, among whom a variety of problem dimensions may be noted. In children and adults with severe and profound mental retardation, among whom varieties of behavior are more limited, the Aberrant Behavior Checklist (ABC) (Table 7) with five dimensions of behavior is utilized (Aman et al., 1985).

In approaching intervention for behavior problems in children or adults with mental retardation, it may be useful to identify not only target behaviors but also those dimensions of behavior that are most problematic. This may assist in developing plans for behavioral and medication interventions. For example, those persons showing a new appearance of lethargic behaviors on ABC may be developing a depression. The ABC can also be used to measure responsiveness to behavioral and medication interventions.

Personality Disorders in Mental Retardation

This subject has been almost completely unstudied. Personality disorders as they are observed in the general population (Table 8) occur in persons with mild mental retardation and are no more prevalent than in persons without retardation (Gostasen, 1985). Antisocial and histrionic personality disorders are perhaps more readily recognized than other personality disorders. The dimensions seen in the ABC may represent the residua of personality disorders in severe and profound mental retardation.

CATEGORY IV: LIFE EVENTS AND STRESSES

The application of the life story approach to psychiatric disorders in people with mental retardation is both useful and difficult. The likely presence of both biologic and psychological factors influencing behavior and emotion in a person with mental retardation make interpretations of the source of a behavioral deviation a challenge. The impairments in brain physiology and

Table 8. Personality disorders as defined by DSM-IV (1994)

Cluster A	
Paranoid	Pervasive tendency to interpret people's actions as threatening or demeaning
Schizoid	Indifference to social relationships
Schizotypal	Peculiarities of ideation, appearance, and behavior, with impaired social relatedness
Cluster B	
Antisocial	Irresponsible antisocial/delinquent behavior from childhood
Borderline	Pervasive pattern of instability of mood, self-image, and interpersonal relationships
Histrionic	Excessive emotionality and attention seeking
Narcissistic	Excessive emotionality and lack of empathy
Cluster C	
Avoidant	Social discomfort and fear of negative evaluations
Dependent	Submissive behavior
Obsessive-compulsive	Perfectionism and inflexibility

Adapted from the American Psychiatric Association (1994).

the level of mental retardation may influence the form of these persons' psychopathology in response to a stressful event. Determining the relative importance of environmental influences is not as obvious as it may seem.

Nevertheless, discerning the meaning and function of disturbances of mood, thought, and behavior is possible, even in persons with severe mental retardation. With the help of other observers, one can understand the person's story and determine the connections between life events (e.g., loss of a close staff person) and behavior. Environmental events may work in a variety of ways to influence the behavior of a person with mental retardation. The meaning of the event (death of a parent) may in itself affect him or her. Environmental changes in routine may also work on a different level to produce disruptive behavior. New and inappropriate expectations may contribute to the problem behaviors. A careful examination of all changes in the life of a person with mental retardation may reveal the source of a new disturbance of mood, thought, or behavior.

However, one must be cautious in interpreting these changes as the source of the problem. It may in fact be a biologic influence that plays a major role. For example, an adolescent girl with spina bifida and moderate mental retardation who was very unhappy in a nursing home bit her tongue off in an emergency room after being told she was to return to the nursing home. A careful inquiry revealed that she had been on large doses of Compazine, a pheno-

thiazine, for the previous 5 days for nausea and vomiting. Acute dystonia with tongue protrusion secondary to the Compazine was the diagnosis. Her tongue biting was not solely due to her distress over the nursing home, and making a correct diagnosis and treating with intramuscular Benadryl would have saved her tongue (Myers, 1988).

There is some evidence that people with mental retardation may manifest their reactions to life events in ways that are different from those of people without retardation (Stack, Haldepur, & Thompson, 1987). One study has found more acute psychotic reactions unrelated to drugs, more self-destructive and aggressive behavior, and fewer depressive disorders in people with developmental disabilities who are hospitalized as compared to people of average intelligence (Myers, 1986). The person with mental retardation may have less ability to inhibit behavior in response to stress and thus may react in odd and dramatic manners that may be misinterpreted as psychotic. The dramatic response is often short lived and thus would carry a better prognosis than the inexperienced psychiatrist might think.

The prevalence of depression and anxiety appearing in response to stressful events in the life of a person with mental retardation is nevertheless high. Depression of mild degrees not requiring hospitalization is commonly observed in people with mental retardation (Kazdin, Matson, & Senatore, 1983). Environmental etiologies of great significance for the person with mental retardation include trauma and losses, the stigma of social rejection (Kazdin et al., 1983), the pattern of learned helplessness (Reynolds & Miller, 1985), the lack of social supports (Reiss & Benson, 1985), and poor social skills (Benson, Reiss, Smith, & Laman, 1985).

The interventions for these depressions are primarily environmental and preventive. Environmental changes are particularly important preventively to stop stigmatization, to improve pleasure from social interactions, to enhance self-esteem, and to provide support during stressful events. Psychotherapy, particularly of the supportive kind, may reduce the symptoms of mild or moderate depressions. Depression in people with mild mental retardation has been known to respond to behavior therapy. Antidepressants are sometimes needed, particularly in the moderate to severe depressions showing the symptoms of major depressive disorder (see Table 3).

Therapeutic interventions for environmental stresses in persons with mental retardation primarily should involve direct supports. Those in direct contact, whether family or staff, must provide empathy and support both verbally and nonverbally. However, there will come a time when excessive sympathy is not constructive and when painful memories must be left behind, rather than perseverated. Behavior modification to learn new behaviors instead of self-pity, or environmental change to facilitate adaptation, may be necessary. When this is not enough, cognitive or supportive psychotherapy to focus directly on the stresses (while the environment avoids them) may be helpful to those individuals with verbal communication. One must carefully select those who need and can benefit from this often limited resource.

EPIDEMIOLOGY

The epidemiology of psychiatric disorders among people with mental retardation has been variable. One reason is the multiplicity of populations: people with mild mental retardation blend with the general population; people with severe and profound mental retardation may live in various more restrictive settings. Psychiatric diagnoses are made with variable validity and reliability. Estimates of the prevalence of behavior problems in institutional settings among persons with moderate to profound mental retardation have been in the range of 10%–50% (Corbett, 1979; Gostasen, 1985; Jacobson, 1982; Lund, 1985b; Reiss, 1982). Studies of children yield figures in the same range. The best epidemiologic assessment of children is the Isle of Wight study, in which 6% of control children in the general population showed behavioral and emotional disorders and 11% of chronically ill children, 30% of children with mental retardation, and 36% of children with a neurologic disability showed psychiatric disorders (Rutter, Graham, & Yule, 1970).

Table 9 provides estimates of prevalences of the various psychiatric and developmental disorders in children. Adults with mild and moderate mental retardation exhibit similar types of psychopathology, as listed in the appendix, with significant numbers having PDD, SIB, aggressive behavior, and "other" behaviors as described above (Benson et al., 1985). Abnormal behaviors in people with severe and profound mental retardation may represent unrecognized diseases or personality disorders (Jacobson, 1982).

The development of standardized instruments for quantifying psychopathology among people with mental retardation may yield better estimates. The Psychopathology Instrument for Mentally Retarded Adults is useful for those who have mild mental retardation (Matson, Kazdin, & Senatore, 1984). The ABC (Table 7) is useful for adults with severe and profound mental retardation (Aman et al., 1985).

Presence of Other Developmental Disabilities

Children and adults with *epilepsy* are at greater risk for psychiatric disorders than is the general population, as are people with mental retardation and epilepsy. In the Isle of Wight study, 56% of children with epilepsy and mental retardation had psychiatric disorders, as compared with 6% of the controls (Rutter et

Table 9. Prevalence of psychiatric and developmental disorders arising in childhood

Disorder	Prevalence (percent) in general population
Disruptive behavior disorders	5–15
Attention-deficit/hyperactivity disorder	
Conduct disorder	
Oppositional defiant disorder	
Anxiety disorders	2–5
Separation anxiety disorder	
Avoidant disorder	
Overanxious disorder	
Eating disorders	<1.0
Anorexia nervosa	
Bulimia nervosa	
Pica	
Rumination disorder	
Gender identity disorders	<0.01
Tic disorders	<0.1
Elimination disorders	5-15
Other disorders	<1.0
Elective mutism	
Stereotypy/habit disorder	
Depression disorders	5–8
Developmental disorders	
Mental retardation	3
Pervasive developmental disorder	0.01
Specific developmental disorder	
Academic skill disorder	10–15
Language and speech disorder	10–15
Motor skills disorder	5–8

der. Given similar degrees of physical severity, a neurologic disorder such as *cerebral palsy* leads to a greater risk for a psychiatric disorder than does a nonneurologic orthopedic disorder (Seidel, Chadwick, & Rutter, 1975).

Children with *speech and language disorders* have been found to be at very high risk for behavioral and emotional disorders, with as many as 50% of such children found to have significant psychiatric problems (Baker & Cantwell, 1987).

Children in the general population with *dyslexia* are at greater risk for psychiatric disorders (Rutter et al., 1966). The strong correlation between conduct disorders and dyslexia is apparent in the one third of persons with dyslexia who have antisocial behavior and the one third of those with antisocial behavior who have dyslexia. Adults in prisons have a high risk for reading disorders.

Children and adults with *pervasive developmental disorder* are at greater risk for other psychiatric disorders than other children and adults with similar levels of mental retardation. Self-injurious and aggressive behaviors, hyperactivity, and anxiety are psychiatric problems that are likely to occur in these autistic disorders (Ratey et al., 1987).

al., 1970). In adults with mental retardation and epilepsy, the prevalence is 52%, compared to 26% in adults with mental retardation without epilepsy (Lund, 1985a). The risk is particularly high in people with temporal lobe seizure disorders, with a greater risk for a schizophrenic-like disorder or a viscous perseverative personality disorder after many years (Baer & Fedis, 1977; Slater & Beard, 1962). Preictal, ictal, and postictal events may present as a psychiatric disorder, calling for high diagnostic acumen.

Central nervous system damage, such as cerebrovascular accident, is associated with an increased risk for psychiatric disorder, but the severity of a *physical disability* does not correlate with an associated psychiatric disor-

TREATMENT OF PSYCHIATRIC DISORDERS IN PERSONS WITH MENTAL RETARDATION

Behavior Modification

Behavior modification is a major tool developed by psychologists that is used for the habilitation of children and adults with mental retardation, particularly those with disturbances of behavior (Rojahn & Schroeder, 1983); it is discussed in Chapter 30 (this volume). When these behavioral interventions are insufficient, psychopharmacologic agents can be used. The continued careful measurement of target behaviors with the help of psychologists is essential in the successful use of psychopharmacologic agents.

Psychopharmacologic Agents

Whereas phenothiazines such as thorazine had been the major psychopharmacologic intervention since their introduction in the 1950s, the psychoactive medication approach is changing. With increasing normalization and use of behavior modification in people with mental retardation, the need for antipsychotic or neuroleptic agents is being reduced. The range of other specific pharmacologic agents has greatly expanded in the past decade and will continue to expand (Aman & Singh, 1983; McDaniel, 1986; Ratey, 1991). Careful and meticulous reviews of family psychiatric histories as well as past and present disturbances of mood, thought, and behavior with all treatment responses; attentive mental status examinations; and behavioral measures of target behaviors will allow for specific use of these agents, which are listed in Table 10.

Psychotherapy

The ability to communicate verbally in some form, whether by speech, communication board, or sign language, is important in influencing mood and attitudes in people with mental retardation. Although such influences often occur in interactions in group home or classroom settings, psychotherapy can be helpful, particularly in individuals with mild or moderate mental retardation. Issues likely to be addressed include self-esteem, adjustment to disability, learning more adaptive behavior, accepting losses, adapting to sexuality, and relating to family and friends (Reiss, Levitan, & McNally, 1982) (see also Chapter 26, Volume I). The therapeutic modality may be individual, family, or group, and preferably should be supportive, cognitive, or interpersonal rather than psychoanalytic in approach. Concreteness in communication is essential. Directive approaches, such as social skills training, may be useful.

For children and adolescents, parental interventions are particularly important. These may include behavior training, education, and individual or group psychotherapy. Adjustment to one's child's disability can lead to improve-ment in the child's behavior (see Chapter 26, Volume I).

Residential Care and Psychiatric Hospitalization

When behavioral and emotional problems become more severe than a family can handle in spite of behavioral, medication, and psychotherapeutic interventions, substitute care may be considered. Sometimes short-term respite care or even foster care is an alternative when parents are overwhelmed. Group homes have developed extensively in the past decade and are valuable alternatives to institutional care. Behavior modification approaches are extensively employed in group homes and at workshop or other day facilities and are often successful in reducing behavior problems. More intensive treatment programs for severe behavior problems, particularly self-injurious and assaultive behavior, may be needed for some children, adolescents, and adults (Fedura, Lindsey, & Walker, 1987). Sophisticated psychopharmacologic consultations, provided by psychiatrists who are familiar with people with mental retardation, are useful adjuncts to the behavioral and other psychological interventions that are provided.

With mental health and mental retardation services often being separate in states, major conflicts over the financial responsibilities for psychiatric inpatient care may be problematic. Fortunately, some inpatient psychiatric facilities may be available for such acute short-term psychiatric disorders as mania, depression, schizophrenic relapse, delirium, and drug abuse (Myers, 1986), particularly in persons with mild to moderate mental retardation. Alternatively, with psychological and psychiatric consultations extensively available to staff in group homes, acute psychiatric problems may be handled by mental retardation professionals without the need for psychiatric hospitalization. Chronic behavior problems, especially antisocial, self-injurious, and aggressive behaviors in persons with severe mental retardation, are dealt with less successfully in acute psychiatric units and may require special behavioral residential or hospital units (Fedura et al., 1987).

Table 10. Psychopharmacologic agents

Category	Disorders	Dosage	Side effects	Comments
Neuroleptics				
Phenothiazines (e.g., Mellaril, Thorazine)	Schizophrenia, mania, psychotic depression, acute psychosis, agitation	25–500 mg/day	Constipation, sedation, cataracts, tardive dyskinesia	Large doses are required for a long time
Thioxanthines (e.g., Navane)	Same as above	5–60 mg/day	Constipation, sedation, cataracts, parkinsonism, akithesia, tardive dyskinesia	
Butyrophenones (e.g., Haldol)	Same as above	5–50 mg/day	Dystonia, constipation, parkinsonism, akithesia, tardive akithesia	Give IM Benedryl 50 mg; Cogentin 0.5–4.0 mg/day
Antimanics				
Lithium carbonate	Mania, depression, aggression	300–1,800 mg/day (0.8–1.2 mg/L)	Thirst, tremor Toxic: vomiting, severe tremor, confusion	Use for prophylaxis of maria and depression
Anticonvulsants	Same as above			
Tegretol		200–1,800 mg/day	Agranulocytosis	
Depacote		500–2,000 mg/day	hepatic damage	
Klonopin		1–9 mg/day	sedation	
Antidepressants	Depression, panic disorder			
Tricyclics (e.g., Tofranil)		50–250 mg/day	Dry mouth, constipation	
MAOIs Tyramine-free diet required (e.g., Nardil)		15–60 mg/day	Hypertensive episodes	
SSRIs (e.g., Prozac)	Self-injury	10–80 mg/day		
Others (e.g., Desyrel)		75–250 mg/day	Priapism	
Antianxiety	Panic disorder, agoraphobia		Drug dependence	
Benzodiazepines (e.g., Xanax)		0.5–4.0 mg/day	sedation, dizziness	
β Blockers (e.g., Inderal)	Aggression	10–500 mg/day	bradycardia	
Buspar	Aggression	10–60 mg/day		
Stimulants (e.g., Ritalin, Dexedrine)	Attention-deficit/ hyperactivity disorder	5–60 mg/day 2.5–40 mg/day	Anorexia, insomnia	
Antiobsessives (e.g., Prozac, Anafranil)	Obsessive–compulsive disorder	20–80 mg/day 75–200 mg/day	Anorexia constipation, dry mouth	

Note: MAOIs, monoamine oxidase inhibitors; SSRIs, selective serotonin reuptake inhibitors.

CONCLUSIONS

A careful diagnostic approach to the disorders of mood, thought, and behavior that occur in children, adolescents, and adults with mental retardation is an essential component to their ha-

bilitation. It allows one to arrive at appropriate diagnoses and their likely biologic and environmental etiologies and to develop specific interventions. Such interventions include behavioral and environmental tactics, psychotherapies, and sometimes psychopharmacologic treatments.

REFERENCES

Achenbach, T.M., & Edelbrock, C.S. (1983). *Manual for the Child Behavior Checklist and Revised Child Behavior Profile*. Burlington, VT: University Associates in Psychiatry.

Aman, M.C., & Singh, N.N. (1983). Pharmacological intervention. In J. Matson & J. Mulick (Eds.), *Handbook of mental retardation* (pp. 79–107). Elmsford, NY: Pergamon.

Aman, M.G., Singh, N.N., Stewart, A.W., & Field, C.J. (1985). Psychometric characteristics of the Aberrant Behavior Checklist. *American Journal of Mental Deficiency*, 89, 492–502.

American Psychiatric Association. (1980). *Diagnostic and statistical manual of mental disorders* (3rd ed.). Washington, DC: American Psychiatric Press.

American Psychiatric Association. (1987). *Diagnostic and statistical manual of mental disorders* (3rd ed., rev.). Washington, DC: American Psychiatric Press.

American Psychiatric Association. (1994). *Diagnostic and statistical manual of mental disorders* (4th ed.). Washington, DC: American Psychiatric Press.

Ananth, J. & Lin, K.M. (1986). Propranolol in psychiatry: Therapeutic uses and side effects. *Neuropsychobiology*, 15, 20–27.

Baer, D.M., & Fedis, P. (1977). Quantitative analysis of interictal behavior in temporal lobe epilepsy. *Archives of Neurology*, 34, 454–467.

Baker, L., & Cantwell, D.P. (1987). Factors associated with the development of psychiatric illness in children with early speech/language problems. *Journal of Autism and Developmental Disorders*, 17, 499–510.

Benson, B.A., Reiss, S., Smith, D.C., & Laman, D.S. (1985). Psychosocial correlates in mentally retarded adults: II. Poor social skills. *American Journal of Mental Deficiency*, 89, 657–659.

Carlson, G. (1979). Affective psychoses in mental retardates. *Psychiatric Clinics of North America*, 2, 499–510.

Conners, C.K. (1969). A teacher rating scale for drug studies with children. *American Journal of Psychiatry*, 126, 804–888.

Cook, E.H., Terry, E.J., Heller, W., & Leventhal, B.L. (1990). Fluoxetine treatment of borderline mentally retarded adults with obsessive-compulsive disorder [Letter]. *Journal of Clinical Psychopharmacology, 10*, 228–229.

Corbett, J.A. (1979). Psychiatric morbidity and mental retardation. In F.E. James & R.P. Snarth (Eds.), *Psychiatric illness and mental handicap* (pp. 11–25). London: Gaskell.

Durand, V.M., & Crimmins, D.B. (1988). Identifying the variables maintaining self-injurious behavior. *Journal of Autism and Developmental Disorders, 18*, 99–117.

du Verglas, G., Banks, S.R., & Guyer, K.E. (1988). Clinical effects of fenfluramine on children with autism: A review of the research. *Journal of Autism and Developmental Disorders, 18*, 297–308.

Farber, J.M. (1987). Psychopharmacology of self-injurious behavior in the mentally retarded. *Journal of the American Academy of Child and Adolescent Psychiatry, 26*, 296–302.

Fedura, J.C., Lindsey, E.R., & Walker, G.R. (1987). A special behavioral unit for treatment of persons who are mentally retarded. *Mental Retardation, 25*, 107–111.

Fontaine, R., & Choninard, G. (1986). An open clinical trial of fluoxetine in the treatment of obsessive-compulsive disorder. *Journal of Clinical Psychopharmacology, 6*, 908–910.

Frances, A.J., & Hales, R.E. (1988). *Review of Psychiatry—Vol. 7*. Washington, DC: American Psychiatric Press.

Gedye, A. (1993). Evidence of serotonergic reduction of self-injurious movements. *The Habilitative Mental Healthcare Newsletter, 12*, 53–56.

Gorman-Smith, D., & Matson, J.L. (1985). A review of treatment research for self-injurious and stereotyped responding. *Journal of Mental Deficiency Research, 29*, 295–308.

Gostasen, R. (1985). Psychiatric illness among the mentally retarded: A Swedish population study. *Acta Psychiatrica Scandinavica, 71*(Suppl. 318), 1–117.

Greendyke, R.M., Kauter, D.R., & Schuster, D.B. (1986). Propranolol treatment of assaultive patients with organic brain disease: A double blind crossover placebo-controlled study. *Journal of Nervous and Mental Disorders, 174*, 290–294.

Groden, G., Groden, J., Donley, M., Zana, T., Pueschel, S.M., & Veliceur, W. (1987). Effects of fenfluramine on the behavior of autistic individuals. *Research in Developmental Disabilities, 8*, 203–211.

Gualtieri, C.T., Lefler, W.H., Guimond, M., & Staye, J.L. (1982). Corneal and lenticular opacities in mentally retarded young adults treated with thioridazine and chlorpromazine. *American Journal of Psychiatry, 139,* 1178–1180.

Hales, E., & Yudofsky, S.C. (Eds.). (1987). *Textbook of neuropsychiatry.* Washington, DC: American Psychiatric Press.

Jacobson, J.W. (1982). Problem behavior and psychiatric impairment within a developmentally disabled population. II. Behavior severity. *Applied Research in Mental Retardation, 3,* 369–381.

Kadambari, S. (1986). Manic depressive psychosis in a mentally handicapped person: Diagnosis and management. *British Journal of Psychiatry, 148,* 595–596.

Kane, J., Honigfeld, G., Singer, J., Meltzer, H., & Clozaril Collaborative Study Group. (1988). Clozapine for the treatment resistant schizophrenic. *Archives of General Psychiatry, 45,* 789–796.

Kanner, L. (1943). Autistic disturbances of affective contact. *Nervous Child, 2,* 217–240.

Kazdin, A.E., Matson, J.L., & Senatore, V. (1983). Assessment of depression in mentally retarded adults. *American Journal of Psychiatry, 140,* 1040–1043.

Lerer, B., Moore, N., Meyendorff, E., Cho, S.R., & Gershon, S. (1987). Carbamazepine vs. lithium in acute mania. *Journal of Clinical Psychiatry, 48,* 89–93.

Lesch, M., & Nyhan, W.L.A. (1964). A familial disorder of uric acid metabolism and central nervous system function. *American Journal of Medicine, 36,* 561–565.

Lund, J. (1985a). Epilepsy and psychiatric morbidity in the mentally retarded adult. *Acta Psychiatrica Scandinavica, 72,* 557–562.

Lund, J. (1985b). The prevalence of psychiatric morbidity in mentally retarded adults. *Acta Psychiatrica Scandinavica, 72,* 563–570.

Mace, F.C., Page, T.J., & Ivancic, M.T. (1986). Analysis of environmental determinants of aggression and disruption in mentally retarded children. *Applied Research in Mental Retardation, 7,* 203–221.

Marks, I. (1986). Behavior and drug treatment of phobic and obsessive-compulsive disorders. *Psychotherapy and Psychosomatics, 46,* 35–44.

Matson, J.L. (1981). A controlled outcome study of phobias in mentally retarded adults. *Behavior Research and Therapy 19,* 101–107.

Matson, J.L., Kazdin, A.E., & Senatore, V. (1984). Psychometric properties of the psychopathology instrument for mentally retarded adults. *Applied Research in Mental Retardation, 5,* 81–89.

McDaniel, K.D. (1986). Pharmacologic treatment of psychiatric and neurodevelopmental disorders in children and adolescents *Clinical Pediatrics, 25,* 65–71, 143–146, 198–204.

McElroy, S.L., Keck, P.E., & Pope, H.G. (1981). Sodium valproate: Its uses in primary psychiatric disorders. *Journal of Clinical Psychopharmacology, 7,* 16–24.

McHugh, P.R., & Slavney, P.R. (1983). *The perspectives of psychiatry.* Baltimore: Johns Hopkins University Press.

Menolascino, F.J., Wilson, J., Golden, C.J., & Ruedrich, S.L. (1986). Medication and treatment of schizophrenia in persons with mental retardation. *Mental Retardation, 24,* 277–283.

Myers, B.A. (1986). Psychopathology in hospitalized developmentally disabled individuals. *Comprehensive Psychiatry, 27,* 115–126.

Myers, B.A. (1988). Psychological misinterpretations in the diagnosis of acute dystonia. *Psychosomatics, 29,* 224–226.

Myers, B.A., & Pueschel, S. (1987). Pseudodementia in the mentally retarded: A case report and review of possible etiologies. *Clinical Pediatrics, 26,* 275–277.

Oliver, C., Murphy, G.H., & Corbett, J. (1987). Self-injurious behavior in people with mental handicap: A total population study. *Journal of Mental Deficiency Research, 31,* 147–162.

Ollendick, T.H., & Ollendick, D.G. (1982). Anxiety disorders. In J.L. Matson & R.F. Barrett (Eds.), *Psychopathology in the mentally retarded* (pp. 77–119). New York: Grune & Stratton.

Rapport, M.D., Sonis, W.A., Fiaalkov, M.J., Matson, J.L., & Kazdin, A.E. (1982). Carbamazepine and behavior therapy for aggressive behavior treatment of a mentally retarded postencephalitic adolescent with seizure disorder. *Behavior Modification, 7,* 255–265.

Ratey, J.J. (Ed.). (1991). *Mental retardation: Developing pharmacotherapies.* Washington, DC: American Psychiatric Press.

Ratey, J.J., Mikkelson, E.J., Smith, G.B., Upadhyaya, A., Zuckerman, S., Martell, D., Sorgi, P., Polakoff, S., & Bemporad, J. (1986). Beta-blockers in the severely and profoundly mentally retarded. *International Clinical Psychopharmacology, 6,* 103–107.

Ratey, J.J., Mikkelson, E., Sorgi, P., Zuckerman, S., Polakoff, S., Bemporad, J., Bick, P., & Kadiah, W.L. (1987). Autism: The treatment of aggressive behaviors. *Journal of Clinical Psychopharmacology, 7,* 35–41.

Ratey, J.J., Sovner, R., Parks, A., & Rogentine, K. (1991). Buspirone treatment of aggression and anxiety in mentally retarded patients: A multiple-baseline, placebo lead-in study. *Journal of Clinical Psychiatry, 52,* 159–162.

Regier, D.A., & Burke, J.D. (1985). Epidemiology. In B.J. Sadock (Ed.), *Comprehensive textbook of psychiatry* (4th ed., pp. 295–312). Baltimore: Williams & Wilkins.

Reid, A.H. (1972a). Psychoses in adult mental defectives: I. Manic depressive psychosis. *British Journal of Psychiatry, 120,* 205–212.

Reid, A.H. (1972b). Psychosis in adult mental defectives: II. Schizophrenic and paranoia psychosis. *British Journal of Psychiatry, 120,* 213–218.

Reid, A.H. (1989). Schizophrenia in mental retardation: Clinical features. *Research in Developmental Disabilities, 10,* 241–249.

Reid, A.H., Naylor, G.J., & Kay, D.S.G. (1981). A double-blind placebo controlled crossover trial of carbamazepine in overactive severely mentally handicapped patients. *Psychological Medicine, 11,* 109–113.

Reiss, S. (1982). Psychopathology and mental retardation: Survey of a developmental disabilities mental health program. *Mental Retardation, 20,* 128–132.

Reiss, S., & Benson, B. (1985). Psychosocial correlates of depression in mentally retarded adults. I. Minimal social support. *American Journal of Mental Deficiency, 89,* 331–337.

Reiss, S., Levitan, G.W., & McNally, R.J. (1982). Emotionally disturbed mentally retarded people— an underserved population. *American Psychologist, 37,* 361–367.

Reynolds, W.M., & Miller, K.L. (1985). Depression and learned helplessness in mentally retarded and nonmentally retarded adolescents: An initial investigation. *Applied Research in Mental Retardation, 6,* 295–306.

Richardson, S.A., Katz, M., Koller, H., McLaren, L., & Rubenstein, B. (1979). Some characteristics of a population of mentally retarded young adults in a British city: A basis for making some service needs. *Journal of Mental Deficiency Research, 23,* 275–283.

Rivinus, T.M., & Harmatz, J.S. (1979). Diagnosis and lithium treatment of affective disorders in the retarded: Five case studies. *American Journal of Psychiatry, 136,* 551–554.

Robins, L. (1966). *Deviant children grown up: A sociological and psychological study of psychopathological persons.* Baltimore: Williams & Wilkins.

Rojahn, J., & Schroeder, S.R. (1983). Behavioral assessment. In J. Matson & J. Mulick (Eds.), *Handbook of mental retardation* (pp. 227–243). Elmsford, NY: Pergamon.

Rutter, M., Graham, P., & Yule, W.A. (1970). *A neuropsychiatric study in childhood (Clinics in Developmental Medicine, No. 35/36).* London: Spastics International Medical Publications in association with William Heinemann Medical Books, Ltd.

Rutter, M., Tizard, J., & Whitmore, K. (1966). *Education, health, and behaviour.* London: Longman.

Seidel, U.P., Chadwick, D., & Rutter, M. (1975). Psychological disorders in crippled children: A comparative study of children with and without brain damage. *Developmental Medicine and Child Neurology, 7,* 563–573.

Silver, J.M., & Yudofsky, A.C. (1987). Aggressive behavior in patients with neuropsychiatric disorders. *Psychiatric Annals, 17,* 367–384.

Slater, E., & Beard, A.W. (1962). The schizophrenia-like psychosis of epilepsy. *British Journal of Psychiatry, 109,* 95–150.

Sovner, R., Fox, C.J., Lowry, M.J., & Lowry, M.A. (1993). Fluoxetine treatment of depression and associated self-injury in two adults with mental retardation. *Journal of Intellectual Disability Research, 37,* 301–311.

Sovner, R., & Hurley, A. (1981). The management of chronic behaviors in mentally retarded adults with lithium carbonate. *Journal of Nervous and Mental Disease, 161,* 191–195.

Stack, L.S., Haldepur, E.V., & Thompson, M. (1987). Stressful events and psychiatric hospitalization of mentally retarded patients. *American Journal of Psychiatry, 144,* 661–663.

Sternlicht, M. (1979). Fears of institutionalized mentally retarded adults. *Journal of Psychology, 101,* 67–71.

Taylor, E. (1986). *The overactive child (Clinics in Developmental Medicine, No. 97).* Philadelphia: J.B. Lippincott.

Turner, T.H. (1989). Schizophrenia and mental handicap: An historical review, with implications for further research. *Psychological Medicine, 19,* 301–314.

Vitiello, B., Spreat, S., & Behar, D. (1989). Obsessive-compulsive disorder in mentally retarded patients. *Journal of Nervous and Mental Disease, 177,* 232–236.

Wiener, K., & Lamberti, J.S. (1993). Sertraline and mental retardation with obsessive-compulsive disorder [Letter]. *American Journal of Psychiatry, 150,* 1270.

Zimmerman, R.L., & Heistad, G.T. (1982). Studies of the long term efficacy of antipsychotic drugs in controlling the behavior of institutionalized retardates. *Journal of the American Academy of Child Psychiatry, 21,* 136–143.

DSM Diagnostic Codes for Clinical Syndromes

Some diagnoses have the same code number to maintain compatibility with the International Classification of Diseases, 9th Revision, Clinical Modification. NOS, not otherwise specified.

Disorders Usually First Diagnosed in Infancy, Childhood, or Adolescence

Mental Retardation (Axis II)
- 317 Mild Mental Retardation
- 318.0 Moderate Mental Retardation
- 318.1 Severe Mental Retardation
- 318.2 Profound Mental Retardation

Learning Disorders
- 315.00 Reading Disorder
- 315.1 Mathematics Disorder
- 315.2 Disorder of Written Expression

Motor Skills Disorder
- 315.4 Developmental Coordination Disorder

Communication Disorders
- 315.31 Expressive Language Disorder
- 315.31 Mixed Receptive-Expressive Language Disorder
- 315.39 Phonological Disorder
- 307.0 Stuttering

Pervasive Development Disorder
- 299.00 Autistic Disorder
- 299.80 Rett's Disorder
- 299.10 Childhood Disintegrative Disorder
- 299.80 Asperger's Disorder
- 299.80 Pervasive Developmental Disorder NOS

Attention-Deficit and Disruptive Behavior Disorders
- 314. Attention-Deficit/Hyperactivity Disorder
  - .01 Combined Type
  - .00 Predominantly Inattentive Type
  - .01 Predominantly Hyperactive-Impulsive Type
- 312.8 Conduct Disorder
- 313.81 Oppositional Defiant Disorder

Feeding and Eating Disorders of Infancy or Early Childhood
- 307.52 Pica
- 307.53 Rumination Disorder

307.59   Feeding Disorder of Infancy or Early Childhood

Tic Disorders
307.21   Transient Tic Disorder
307.22   Chronic Motor or Vocal Tic Disorder
307.23   Tourette's Disorder

Elimination Disorders
787.6   Encopresis, With Constipation and Overflow Incontinence
307.7   Encopresis, Without Constipation and Overflow Incontinence
307.6   Enuresis (Not Due to a General Medical Condition)

Other Disorders of Infancy, Childhood, or Adolescence
309.21   Separation Anxiety Disorder
313.23   Selective Mutism
313.89   Reactive Attachment Disorder of Infancy or Early Childhood
307.3   Stereotypic Movement Disorder
              Specify if: With Self-Injurious Behavior

Delirium, Dementia, and Amnestic and Other Cognitive Disorders

Delirium
293.0   Delirium Due to . . . *[Indicate the General Medical Condition]*
              Substance Intoxication Delirium
              Substance Withdrawal Delirium
              Delirium Due to Multiple Etiologies

Dementias
290.   Dementia of the Alzheimer's Type, With Early Onset
    .10   Uncomplicated
    .11   With Delirium
    .12   With Delusions
    .13   With Depressed Mood
290.40   Vascular Dementia, Uncomplicated
294.9   Dementia Due to HIV Disease
294.1   Dementia Due to Head Trauma
294.1   Dementia Due to Parkinson's Disease
294.1   Dementia Due to Huntington's Disease
290.10   Dementia Due to Pick's Disease
290.10   Dementia Due to Creutzfeldt-Jakob Disease
294.1   Dementia Due to . . . *[Indicate the General Medical Condition Not Listed Above]*
              Substance-Induced Persisting Dementia
              Dementia Due to Multiple Etiologies

Mental Disorders Due to a General Medical Condition Not Elsewhere Classified

293.89   Catatonic Disorder Due to . . . *[Indicate the General Medical Condition]*
310.1   Personality Change Due to . . . *[Indicate the General Medical Condition]*

Substance-Related Disorders

Alcohol-Related Disorders
Alcohol Use Disorders
303.90   Alcohol Dependence
305.00   Alcohol Abuse

Alcohol-Induced Disorders
   303.00   Alcohol Intoxication
   291.8   Alcohol Withdrawal
   291.0   Alcohol Intoxication Delirium
   291.2   Alcohol-Induced Persisting Dementia
   291.1   Alcohol-Induced Persisting Amnestic Disorder
   291.   Alcohol-Induced Psychotic Disorder
     .5   With Delusions
     .3   With Hallucinations
   291.8   Alcohol-Induced Mood Disorder
   291.8   Alcohol-Induced Anxiety Disorder
   291.8   Alcohol-Induced Sexual Dysfunction
   291.8   Alcohol-Induced Sleep Disorder

Amphetamine-Related Disorders

  Amphetamine Use Disorders
   304.40   Amphetamine Dependence
   305.70   Amphetamine Abuse

  Amphetamine-Induced Disorders
   292.89   Amphetamine Intoxication
   292.0   Amphetamine Withdrawal
   292.81   Amphetamine Intoxication Delirium
   292.   Amphetamine-Induced Psychotic Disorder
   292.84   Amphetamine-Induced Mood Disorder
   292.89   Amphetamine-Induced Anxiety Disorder
   292.89   Amphetamine-Induced Sexual Dysfunction
   292.89   Amphetamine-Induced Sleep Disorder

Caffeine-Related Disorders
  Caffeine-Induced Disorders
   305.90   Caffeine Intoxication
   292.89   Caffeine-Induced Anxiety Disorder
   292.89   Caffeine-Induced Sleep Disorder

Cannabis-Related Disorders
  Cannabis Use Disorders
   304.30   Cannabis Dependency
   305.20   Cannabis Abuse

  Cannabis-Induced Disorders
   292.89   Cannabis Intoxication
   292.81   Cannabis Intoxication Delirium
   292.   Cannabis-Induced Psychotic Disorder
   292.89   Cannabis-Induced Anxiety Disorder

Cocaine-Related Disorders
  Cocaine Use Disorder
   304.20   Cocaine Dependence
   305.60   Cocaine Abuse

  Cocaine-Induced Disorders
   292.89   Cocaine Intoxication

292.0   Cocaine Withdrawal
292.81   Cocaine Intoxication Delirium
292.   Cocaine-Induced Psychotic Disorder
292.84   Cocaine-Induced Mood Disorder
292.89   Cocaine-Induced Anxiety Disorder
292.89   Cocaine-Induced Sexual Dysfunction
292.89   Cocaine-Induced Sleep Disorder

Hallucinogen-Related Disorders
  Hallucinogen Use Disorders
    304.50   Hallucinogen Dependence
    305.30   Hallucinogen Abuse

  Hallucinogen-Induced Disorders
    292.89   Hallucinogen Intoxication
    292.89   Hallucinogen Persisting Perception Disorder
    292.81   Hallucinogen Intoxication Delirium
    292.   Hallucinogen-Induced Psychotic Disorder
    292.84   Hallucinogen-Induced Mood Disorder
    292.89   Hallucinogen-Induced Anxiety Disorder

Inhalant-Related Disorders
  Inhalant Use Disorders
    304.60   Inhalant Dependence
    305.90   Inhalant Abuse

  Inhalant-Induced Disorders
    292.89   Inhalant Intoxication
    292.81   Inhalant Intoxication Delirium
    292.82   Inhalant-Induced Persisting Dementia
    292.   Inhalant-Induced Psychotic Disorder
    292.84   Inhalant-Induced Mood Disorder
    292.89   Inhalant-Induced Anxiety Disorder

Nicotine-Related Disorders
  Nicotine Use Disorder
    305.10   Nicotine Dependence

  Nicotine-Induced Disorder
    292.0   Nicotine Withdrawal

Opioid-Related Disorders
  Opioid Use Disorders
    304.00   Opioid Dependence
    305.50   Opioid Abuse

  Opioid-Induced Disorders
    292.89   Opioid Intoxication
    292.0   Opioid Withdrawal
    292.81   Opioid Intoxication Delirium
    292.   Opioid-Induced Psychotic Disorder
    292.84   Opioid-Induced Mood Disorder
    292.89   Opioid-Induced Sexual Dysfunction

292.89   Opioid-Induced Sleep Disorder

Phencyclidine-Related Disorders
  Phencyclidine Use Disorders
    304.90   Phencyclidine Dependence
    305.90   Phencyclidine Abuse

  Phencyclidine-Induced Disorders
    292.89   Phencyclidine Intoxication
    292.81   Phencyclidine Intoxication Delirium
    292.   Phencyclidine-Induced Psychotic Disorder
    292.84   Phencyclidine-Induced Mood Disorder
    292.89   Phencyclidine-Induced Anxiety Disorder

Sedative-, Hypnotic-, or Anxiolytic-Related Disorders
  Sedative, Hypnotic, or Anxiolytic Use Disorders
    304.10   Sedative, Hypnotic, or Anxiolytic Dependence
    305.40   Sedative, Hypnotic, or Anxiolytic Abuse

  Sedative-, Hypnotic-, or Anxiolytic-Induced Disorders
    292.89   Sedative-, Hypnotic-, or Anxiolytic Intoxication
    292.0   Sedative-, Hypnotic-, or Anxiolytic Withdrawal
    292.81   Sedative-, Hypnotic-, or Anxiolytic Delirium
    292.81   Sedative-, Hypnotic-, or Anxiolytic Withdrawal Delirium
    292.82   Sedative-, Hypnotic-, or Anxiolytic-Induced Persisting Dementia
    292.83   Sedative-, Hypnotic-, or Anxiolytic-Induced Persisting Amnestic Disorder
    292.   Sedative-, Hypnotic-, or Anxiolytic-Induced Psychotic Disorder
    292.84   Sedative-, Hypnotic-, or Anxiolytic-Induced Mood Disorder
    292.89   Sedative-, Hypnotic-, or Anxiolytic-Induced Anxiety Disorder
    292.89   Sedative-, Hypnotic-, or Anxiolytic-Induced Sexual Dysfunction
    292.89   Sedative-, Hypnotic-, or Anxiolytic-Induced Sleep Disorder

Polysubstance-Related Disorder
  304.80   Polysubstance Dependence

Schizophrenia and Other Psychotic Disorders

  295.   Schizophrenia
    .30   Paranoid Type
    .10   Disorganized Type
    .20   Catatonic Type
    .90   Undifferentiated Type
    .60   Residual Type
  295.40   Schizophreniform Disorder
  295.70   Schizoaffective Disorder
  297.1   Delusional Disorder
  298.8   Brief Psychotic Disorder
  297.3   Shared Psychotic Disorder
  293.   Psychotic Disorder Due to . . . *[Indicate the General Medical Condition]*
           Substance-Induced Psychotic Disorder *(Refer to Substance-Related Disorders)*

Mood Disorders

Depressive Disorders
  296.   Major Depressive Disorder

300.4   Dysthymic Disorder
311.   Depressive Disorder NOS

Bipolar Disorders
296.   Bipolar I Disorder
296.89   Bipolar II Disorder
301.13   Cyclothymic Disorder
293.83   Mood Disorder Due to . . . *[Indicate the General Medical Condition]*
           Substance-Induced Mood Disorder *(Refer to Substance-Related Disorders)*

Anxiety Disorders

300.01   Panic Disorder Without Agoraphobia
300.21   Panic Disorder With Agoraphobia
300.22   Agoraphobia Without History of Panic Disorder
300.29   Specific Phobia
300.23   Social Phobia
300.3   Obsessive-Compulsive Disorder
309.81   Posttraumatic Stress Disorder
308.3   Acute Stress Disorder
300.02   Generalized Anxiety Disorder
293.89   Anxiety Disorder Due to . . . *[Indicate the General Medical Condition]*
           Substance-Induced Anxiety Disorder *(Refer to Substance-Related Disorders)*

Dissociative Disorders

300.12   Dissociative Amnesia
300.13   Dissociative Fugue
300.14   Dissociative Identity Disorder
300.6   Depersonalization Disorder

Sexual and Gender Identity Disorders

Sexual Dysfunctions
Sexual Desire Disorders
    302.71   Hypoactive Sexual Desire Disorder
    301.79   Sexual Aversion Disorder

Sexual Arousal Disorders
    302.72   Female Sexual Arousal Disorder
    302.72   Male Erectile Disorder

Orgasmic Disorders
    302.73   Female Orgasmic Disorder
    302.74   Male Orgasmic Disorder
    302.75   Premature Ejaculation

Sexual Pain Disorders
    302.76   Dyspareunia (Not Due to a General Medical Condition)
    306.51   Vaginismus (Not Due to a General Medical Condition)

Sexual Dysfunction Due to General Medical Condition
    625.8   Female Hypoactive Sexual Desire Disorder Due to . . . *[Indicate the General Medical
               Condition]*

608.89   Male Hypoactive Sexual Desire Disorder Due to . . . *[Indicate the General Medical Condition]*

607.84   Male Erectile Disorder Due to . . . *[Indicate the General Medical Condition]*

625.0   Female Dyspareunia Due to . . . *[Indicate the General Medical Condition]*

608.89   Male Dyspareunia Due to . . . *[Indicate the General Medical Condition]*

608.89   Other Male Sexual Function Due to . . . *[Indicate the General Medical Condition]*
         Substance-Induced Sexual Dysfunction *(Refer to Substance-Related Disorders)*

Paraphilias
  302.4   Exhibitionism
  302.81   Fetishism
  302.89   Frotteurism
  302.2   Pedophilia
  302.83   Sexual Masochism
  302.3   Transvestic Fetishism
  302.82   Voyeurism

Gender Identity Disorders
  302.   Gender Identity Disorder
    .6   in Children
    .85   in Adolescents or Adults

Eating Disorders
  307.1   Anorexia Nervosa
  307.51   Bulimia Nervosa

Sleep Disorders

Primary Sleep Disorders
  Dyssomnias
    307.42   Primary Insomnia
    307.44   Primary Hypersomnia
    347   Narcolepsy
    780.59   Breathing-Related Sleep Disorder
    307.45   Circadian Rhythm Sleep Disorder

  Parasomnias
    307.47   Nightmare Disorder
    307.46   Sleep Terror Disorder
    307.46   Sleepwalking Disorder

Sleep Disorders Related to Another Mental Disorder
  307.42   Insomnia Related to . . . *[Indicate the Disorder]*
  307.44   Hypersomnia Related . . . *[Indicate the Disorder]*

Other Sleep Disorders
  780   Sleep Disorder Due to . . . *[Indicate the General Medical Condition]*
           Substance-Induced Sleep Disorder *(Refer to Substance-Related Disorders)*

Impulse Control Disorders Not Elsewhere Classified

  312.34   Intermittent Explosive Disorder
  312.32   Kleptomania

312.33   Pyromania
312.31   Pathological Gambling
312.39   Trichotillomania

Adjustment Disorders

309.   Adjustment Disorder
309.0   With Depressed Mood
309.24   With Anxiety
309.28   With Mixed Anxiety and Depressed Mood
309.3   With Disturbance of Conduct
309.4   With Mixed Disturbance of Emotions and Conduct
309.9   Unspecified

Personality Disorders (Axis II)

301.0   Paranoid Personality Disorder
301.20   Schizoid Personality Disorder
301.22   Schizotypal Personality Disorder
301.7   Antisocial Personality Disorder
301.83   Borderline Personality Disorder
301.50   Histrionic Personality Disorder
301.81   Narcissistic Personality Disorder
301.6   Dependent Personality Disorder
301.4   Obsessive-Compulsive Personality Disorder

Other Conditions That May Be a Focus of Clinical Attention

Medication-Induced Movement Disorders
332.1   Neuroleptic-Induced Parkinsonism
333.92   Neuroleptic Malignant Syndrome
333.7   Neuroleptic-Induced Acute Dystonia
333.99   Neuroleptic-Induced Acute Akathisia
333.82   Neuroleptic-Induced Tardive Dyskinesia
333.1   Medication-Induced Postural Tremor
333.90   Medication-Induced Movement Disorder NOS

Relational Problems
V61.9   Relational Problem Related to a Mental Disorder or General Medical Condition
V61.20   Parent-Child Relational Problem
V61.1   Partner Relational Problem
V61.8   Sibling Relational Problem
V62.81   Relational Problem NOS

Problems Related to Abuse or Neglect
V61.21   Physical Abuse of Child
V61.21   Sexual Abuse of Child
V61.21   Neglect of Child
V61.1   Physical Abuse of Adult
V61.1   Sexual Abuse of Adult

Additional Conditions That May Be a Focus of Clinical Attention
V15.81 Noncompliance with Treatment
V65.2   Malingering
V71.01 Adult Antisocial Behavior
V71.02 Child or Adolescent Antisocial Behavior
V62.89 Borderline Intellectual Functioning
780.9   Age-Related Cognitive Decline
V62.82 Bereavement
V62.3   Academic Problem
V62.2   Occupational Problem

Chapter 21

A Transdisciplinary Approach to Self-Injurious Behavior

Susan L. Hyman, M.D.

Repetitious and chronic behaviors that can cause physical harm are termed self-injurious behavior. The most common forms are 1) self-striking (face slapping, head banging); 2) self-biting; 3) pinching, scratching, gouging, or pulling body parts; 4) repeated vomiting or rumination; and 5) severe pica (eating nonedible substances) and coprophagia (Favell et al., 1982).

Most practitioners who care for persons with developmental disabilities deal with people who engage in self-injury. The prevalence of self-injurious behavior among residents of facilities for people with mental retardation is 5.3%–37.1% (Singh, 1981); among people with mental retardation living in the community it has been surveyed to be 1.7%–2.6% (Griffin et al., 1987; Rojahn, 1986). The study and treatment of severe behavioral disorders such as self-injurious behavior requires appreciation of relevant biologic and behavioral components.

EPIDEMIOLOGY

Self-Injurious Behavior in Children Without Developmental Disabilities

Self-injurious behavior can be seen in the course of typical development in up to 20% of infants and preschool children (Singh, 1981). Body rocking, head rolling, and head banging first appear around 8–9 months of age and disappear under normal circumstances before 4 years of age. A 3:1 male–female predominance has been noted. The onset of self-injurious behavior has been correlated with episodes of otitis media and with tooth eruption. The rhythmic activity may soothe the infant to sleep, serve as a distraction from a painful condition, or communicate a need to the parent. Children may engage in infrequent self-injurious behavior during tantrums as well (Sallustro & Atwell, 1978). Self-injurious behavior in children without disabilities rarely requires specific treatment. As the child grows and develops more sophisticated means of communication and stimulation, the behavior almost always disappears. However, there are reports of individuals who continue to bang their head, especially during the latency period before sleep (Sormann, 1982).

Self-Injurious Behavior in Persons with Developmental Disabilities

Unlike the self-injurious behavior often seen in young children without developmental disabilities, that in people with developmental disabilities may persist for long periods and may result in serious tissue damage. Among people with mental retardation, a positive relationship between age up to adulthood and self-injurious behavior has been described (Oliver, Murphy, & Corbett, 1987). Self-injurious behavior that causes tissue damage may be found in 3%–4% of children with developmental disabilities under age 10 and in 12% of people with developmental disabilities over 15 years of age.

It is most common in people with severe or profound mental retardation (Griffin, Williams, Stark, Altmeyer, & Mason, 1984; Hyman, Fisher, Mercugliano, & Cataldo, 1990). People with more severe cognitive disabilities may be more likely to be placed in residential facilities, thus accounting for the increased prevalence of self-injurious behavior in people with mental retardation who reside in institutions. It has been reported that persons living in institutions who engage in self-injurious behavior have been in residential placement longer. This may reflect the difficulty families have in dealing with this behavior, or the effect of the institutional environment on the development and maintenance of behavioral dysfunction (Singh, 1981).

ETIOLOGY

Severe behavior problems in people with mental retardation most frequently are managed with techniques of behavior modification, and most research on self-injurious behavior has examined it as a behavioral phenomenon. With greater understanding of neurobehavioral systems, however, more comprehensive explanations of the biobehavioral interaction that results in self-injurious behavior are being sought. Self-injurious behavior seems to occur in response to many different neurologic and environmental insults and is likely to be due to more than one etiologic factor (Carr, 1977; King, 1993).

Behavioral Etiologies

Positive Reinforcement   Self-injurious behavior may be learned when a maladaptive act is reinforced with attention, thus encouraging its recurrence. An example of this would be the young child who bangs his or her head and receives social attention, sympathy, or cuddling. Another example is a person with mental retardation residing in an institution who receives the greatest amount of social attention for the most aberrant behavior. This would suggest that, if attention to self-injurious behavior was removed, the behavior would decrease in frequency. Extinction—the behavioral treatment in which an undesired behavior is ignored while desired behaviors are reinforced—can result in decreased occurrence of self-injurious behavior, indicating that positive reinforcement may maintain, if not cause, some cases (Rincover, 1986).

Negative Reinforcement   Self-injurious and other maladaptive behaviors may be learned under conditions in which the individual can terminate or avoid undesired activities by engag-

ing in the behavior. If self-injurious behavior is escape motivated, an individual might engage in the behavior and have an academic or daily living demand removed as a result, thus reinforcing the continuation of that behavior.

Communication   People who have delayed or deviant language development often use other means of communicating their needs. Self-injurious behavior and other maladaptive behaviors, such as aggression, may serve as a generalized sign for attention or to make wants known (Prizant & Wetherby, 1987). This is supported by the observation that training in appropriate communication has been associated with decreases in the behavior in some cases (Durand & Carr, 1991).

Self-Stimulation   It has been hypothesized that self-injurious behavior may serve to provide increased tactile, kinesthetic, vestibular, or other sensory stimulation in some people (Cataldo & Harris, 1982). It has been suggested that stereotypic behavior occurs at three levels: as rhythmic behaviors as seen in typically developing infants, as an adaptive response to modulate the level of arousal, and as a learned response that is used to obtain responses from others (Guess & Carr, 1991). Using this three-level approach may help the clinician determine appropriate interventions, such as substitution of other stimuli, environmental alterations, desensitization, or enhancement of communication or compliance.

Psychiatric Etiologies

Psychodynamic etiologies of self-injurious behavior have been theorized. Chronic self-injury has been described in persons without developmental disabilities who attempt to alleviate guilt or who modulate agitation and arousal through self-harm (Carr, 1977). It is likely that some individuals with mental retardation do engage in self-injurious behavior for similar reasons, although the techniques involved in assessment and treatment of these factors may not be easily applicable to patients without speech or with limited insight.

Because people with mental retardation suffer from the same psychiatric illnesses as the rest of the population, self-injurious behavior might be expected occasionally to represent a symptom of psychiatric illness. Self-mutilation has been reported in patients with acute psychoses in which delusional instruction directs such behavior. People with appropriate language abilities must be interviewed in a standard fashion to diagnose such thought disorders. Diagnostic interviews designed for populations with cognitive limitations, questionnaires for caregivers, and observational assessments can all provide useful information (Loschen & Osman, 1992). 1992).

There is much evidence that psychiatric disorders in people with mental retardation can be diagnosed and can respond to appropriate pharmacologic treatment. In people with more severe retardation, the thought disorder is less emphasized in making the diagnosis, and the diagnosis may be based on abnormal psychomotor and constitutional findings (Carlson, 1979). In depressed people, alterations in sleep and appetite, loss of interest in activities, and psychomotor slowing may be present. In manic episodes, sleep and appetite may be decreased and motor activity and distractibility increased. It is necessary to document alterations from previous behavior and episodic or cyclic exacerbations that may be present.

Other psychiatric illnesses, such as schizophrenia, obsessive–compulsive disorder, and panic/anxiety, may result in the symptom of self-injurious behavior. Objective observation, review of data from caregivers, consideration of family history, and observation or interview of the patient may permit diagnosis of these and other disorders.

Self-injurious and stereotypic behaviors are frequently encountered in people with pervasive developmental disorders. In one study, 23% of 97 patients less than 21 years of age treated on an inpatient basis for self-injurious behavior were diagnosed as having pervasive developmental disorders (Hyman et al., 1990). Although stereotypic behaviors, including self-injurious behavior, may be neurologically mediated in some patients with autism, the isolation from interpersonal communication that is the hallmark of the disorder may function to isolate a child from stimulation in a way similar to that in which sensory impairment works. Thus self-injurious behavior in a person with autism also may represent an aberrant attempt to communicate or a compulsive act.

Organic Etiologies

Self-injury may be a physiologic response that occurs in a characteristic fashion in a person with known biologic abnormalities. The presence of a maladaptive behavior in a group of individuals with a common disorder provides an opportunity to study the biologic factors that could produce self-injurious behavior (Table 1). However, it must be remembered that the majority of people with mental retardation and self-injurious behavior do not have a syndrome that is associated with such behavior; it is the cognitive disability that predisposes them to the development of the behavior.

Lesch-Nyhan Syndrome The Lesch-Nyhan syndrome was first described in 1964 in two males with choreoathetoid cerebral palsy, mental retardation, hyperuricemia, and severe self-mutilation. They bit their lips, tongue, and fingers, causing severe tissue destruction. The Lesch-Nyhan syndrome has a prevalence of 1 in 10,000 male births. The molecular basis of the disease has been attributed to a mutation in the structural gene for the enzyme hypoxanthine–guanine phophoribosyltransferase (HGPRT) (Baumeister & Frye, 1985). The gene is inherited in an X-linked recessive fashion, so that only male children who have complete absence of the enzyme are affected. Spontaneous mutations in girls have been reported. Patients with partial enzyme deficiency and the female heterozygotes may have hyperuricemia without the neurologic or behavioral dysfunction.

Table 1. Disorders associated with self-injurious behavior

Autistic spectrum disorders
de Lange syndrome
Fragile X syndrome
Hereditary sensory neuropathy
Lesch-Nyhan syndrome
Rett syndrome
Severe and profound mental retardation
Tourette syndrome
Visual impairment

Children with the Lesch-Nyhan syndrome have irritability and oral–motor dysfunction in infancy. The parents may note orange uric acid crystals in the child's diaper. On neurologic examination, children have choreoathetoid cerebral palsy, usually accompanied by the progression from hypotonicity to hypertonicity with dystonic posturing. Dysphagia and dysarthria are present. The onset of self-biting is between 6 months and 16 years of age. Cognitive skills in the mild to moderate ranges of mental retardation are often reported; however, the dysarthria and impaired motor abilities common in these children may impair testing significantly. In a recent survey of 42 patients, only one family described their child as having significant cognitive impairment (Anderson, Ernst, & Davis, 1992).

Because uric acid accumulates secondary to the absence of HGPRT, all patients are treated with allopurinol to prevent renal calculi. Elevated levels of serum or urine uric acid, or both, are present prior to therapy.

The presence of a known biochemical disturbance has led to investigation of a neurochemical etiology of self-injurious behavior in these children. Elevations of uric acid or hypoxanthine do not produce such behavior in animals or in heterozygous girls. The use of histochemical techniques in the examination of two autopsy specimens documented a decreased amount of dopamine in the basal ganglia and striatum (Lloyd, Hornykiewicz, Davidson, Shannak, & Fox, 1981). This was corroborated by the finding that boys with the Lesch-Nyhan syndrome have decreased levels of homovanillic acid, a dopamine metabolite, in their spinal fluid (Silverstein, Johnston, Hutchinson, & Edwards, 1985). Because the absence of the enzyme HGPRT makes it necessary for the brain to engage in de novo purine synthesis to meet its needs, neurochemical processes dependent on enzymes such as adenylcyclase could be affected. It has been suggested that the reduced adenosine in these individuals may contribute to the self-biting (Breese, Criswell, Duncan, & Mueller, 1989). Although the Lesch-Nyhan syndrome is a relatively infrequent cause of self-injurious behavior, identification of the specific neurochemical changes in these children may provide a neurochemical etiology of this behavior that is common to other groups.

De Lange Syndrome The de Lange syndrome is a rare disorder characterized by severe to profound mental retardation, failure to thrive, microcephaly, synophrys (a single eyebrow), small anteverted nares, and hand and limb malformations. No enzymatic, chromosomal, or neurochemical abnormalities have been identified. An association with autistic features has been described (Johnson, Ekman, Freisen, Nyhan, & Shear, 1976). Multiple topographies of self-injurious behavior occur in these patients, and it has been suggested that the behavior may be secondary to the pathologic events that result in this behavior in other people with mental retardation (Singh & Pulman, 1979). People with de Lange syndrome can respond to behavioral modification techniques and pharmacologic therapies that are prescribed for their individual behavioral characteristics.

Congenital Sensory Neuropathy Congenital sensory neuropathy, also known as congenital insensitivity to pain, includes several heritable disorders of autonomic nervous system dysfunction (Axelrod & Pearson, 1984). Affected patients fail to respond with an axon flare to intradermal histamine. They are then classified by their degree of sensory loss; the presence or absence of visceral pain; their deep tendon reflexes; their ability to perspire; their ability to tear; their blood pressure control, muscle tone, and gastrointestinal motility dysfunction; the results of a methacholine chloride test; and the degree of cognitive impairment. Skeletal abnormalities are sometimes present. Peripheral nerve biopsy may demonstrate specific changes, as may electromyography and nerve conduction velocities. Familial dysautonomia (the Riley-Day syndrome) has been the most extensively studied of these disorders.

Children with these disorders often present with severe mutilation of the tongue, fingers, and lips. Because pain does not limit the extent of the self-injurious behavior, there is no natural contingency for the behavior; that is, discomfort does not terminate it. Assessment of one child determined that he engaged in head banging and finger biting during tantrums, which responded to a behavioral intervention. His cheek biting and autoextraction of teeth was determined not to occur in response to environmental stimuli and did not respond to behavioral treatment. Incomplete insensitivity to pain, such as with denervation injury with paresthesia, may result in a patient engaging in self-injurious behavior for stimulation purposes.

Fragile X Syndrome   X-linked mental retardation may be responsible for 2%–6% of severe mental retardation in boys and men (see Chapter 17, this volume). The abnormality is found in 1 in 2,000 male births and the carrier state is found in 1 in 1,000 girls (Chudley & Hagerman, 1987). The chromosomal abnormality is a fragile site on the distal arm of the X chromosome that requires incubation of the sample in folate-deficient media to be detected on chromosome analysis. A specific diagnosis may be made by direct DNA analysis (Rousseau et al., 1991). Physical features may include a large head, large ears, a prominent jaw, increased testicular volume, and joint hypermobility. Boys are usually more cognitively affected than the heterozygous girls. These children are reported to have specific behavioral characteristics, including language-based learning difficulties and autistic features. Hand biting productive of callus formation is commonly reported.

Rett Syndrome   Rett syndrome is characterized by normal birth history, normal head circumference at birth, and normal acquisition of milestones until 6–18 months of age, followed by a degeneration of fine motor and language skills (see Chapter 25, this volume). Female sex is not a diagnostic criteria, although male cases are controversial. Currently, the disorder has no diagnostic chromosomal, biochemical, or neurochemical findings. Classic midline hand-wringing, hand-waving, and hand-sucking behaviors eventually preclude purposeful hand use. Hand biting, and less frequently head banging, is reported. Behavioral treatment of the hand wringing has not demonstrated long-term success, but clinically significant decreases in self-injurious hand biting and hand mouthing are possible (Iwata, Pace, Willus, Gamache, & Hyman, 1986).

Other Syndromes   Although not characteristic of most persons with these disorders, self-

injurious behavior has been described in the Tourette syndrome (Robertson, Trimble, & Lees, 1989), and in the 47XYY and 49XXXXY chromosomal anomalies (Singh, 1981). It has been observed in patients with Down syndrome, cri-du-chat syndrome (5p−), congenital rubella, prematurity, fetal alcohol syndrome, and postnatal brain injury. It can be found in patients with any disorder that results in mental retardation. Whether specific neurochemical abnormalities exist that predispose the individual to self-injurious behavior requires further study.

Neurochemical Abnormalities

The biologic basis of self-injurious behavior is being investigated in the laboratory using both animal models and human pathologic samples. Mice with experimentally induced otitis media have been observed to bang their heads, giving credence to the hypothesis that masking painful stimuli may play a role in some forms of self-injurious behavior (Carr, 1977). Primates will autogroom to the point of self-injury when placed in situations of social deprivation, thus validating the hypothesis that some stereotypical self-injurious behavior may occur as a form of self-stimulation (Jones, 1982). When primates in isolation are prevented from aggressing toward an intruder, their heightened arousal has been observed to be modulated by self-directed biting and aggression that may serve as a model for tantrum-related self-injurious behavior. The neurochemical responses of animals in these situations must be studied to identify the actual mechanisms that result in self-injurious behavior.

Dopamine Hypothesis   Specific biochemical abnormalities have been produced that cause animals to engage in self-injurious behavior. Administration of amphetamine and pemoline in high doses causes rodents to engage in self-mutilation. Behavioral effects of the stimulant drugs are thought to be due to decreased dopamine reuptake in the brain. Pemoline-induced self-injurious behavior is stereotypic and is reversed by the dopamine blocker haloperidol (Mueller, Saboda, Palmour, & Nyhan, 1982). Toxic destruction of dopaminergic neurons in the neonatal period causes animals to self-bite with the later administration of the dopamine precursor L-dopa, secondary to stimulation of the dopamine-1 (D_1) receptor (Breese et al., 1989; Criswell, Mueller, & Breese, 1992). Denervation of nigrostriatal dopamine neurons by surgical lesioning will also result in self-injurious behavior when the animal is treated with dopamine agonists, particularly those that stimulate the D_1 receptor subtype (Goldstein, 1989). These findings are consistent with the decreased levels of dopamine metabolites found in the brains of boys with the Lesch-Nyhan syndrome. It is also compatible with the decrease in self-injurious behavior a minority of people with mental retardation experience as a result of neuroleptic medications. A dopaminergic hypothesis cannot be a singular explanation, however, because boys with the Lesch-Nyhan syndrome as well as most other persons with self-injurious behavior do not inhibit such behavior when treated with neuroleptics. Further investigations into the effects of manipulation of specific dopamine receptors are ongoing.

Self-injurious behavior can be induced in rodents given clonidine, an antihypertensive medication that is an α adrenergic agonist that also inhibits catecholamine reuptake. Theophylline and caffeine also produce self-biting in high doses, perhaps through blockade of adenosine receptors (Katsuragi, Ushijima, & Furukawa, 1984).

Injection of muscimol, a γ aminobutyric acid (GABA) antagonist, into the substantia nigra resulted in self-biting in mice (Frye, Baumeister, Crotty, Newman, & Kotrla, 1985) and aggravated self-injurious behavior in mice who had dopaminergic neurons lesioned neonatally (Breese et al., 1989). This is supported by the observation that baclofen, a GABA agonist, resulted in a decrease in self-injurious behavior in a small clinical series (Primrose, 1979).

Serotonin Hypothesis   The neurotransmitter serotonin plays a role in pain sensation. Potentiation of serotonin production in the brain by increased availability of its precursor, the amino acid tryptophan, was initially reported to decrease self-injurious behavior in several boys with the Lesch-Nyhan syndrome, but this finding could not be sustained (Baumeister & Frye, 1985). Increased serotonin production does not result in self-injurious behavior in animal mod-

els. The utility of serotonergic agents in patients with compulsive behaviors, including self-injurious behaviors, has been documented (King, 1993).

Opiate Hypothesis   The hypothesis that a decreased sensitivity to pain or a need to self-stimulate opiate receptors with naturally occurring opioids has resulted in clinical trials in which opiate antagonists were administered and the rate of self-injurious behavior was measured (Sandman, Barron, & Colman, 1990). The levels of endorphin measured in plasma of people with self-injurious behavior and stereotypy were found to be higher than those of controls with developmental disabilities (Sandman, Barron, Chicz-DeMet, & DeMet, 1990), but the relationship of this finding to what is found at the receptor level in the brain is unclear. Elevated levels of endorphin in cerebrospinal fluid have been reported in autistic children (Gillberg, Terenius, & Lonnerholm, 1985). In a sample of 10 children with self-injurious behavior and mental retardation, only 2 had elevated levels of β-endorphin in cerebrospinal fluid (Ragheb, Hyman, Coyle, & Batshaw, 1989). The neuroendocrine function of neuropeptides may be another potential association with self-injurious behavior. The decreased release of adrenocorticotrophic hormone, pituitary β-endorphin, and cortisol in people with such behavior may be secondary to hypersecretion of pineal melatonin (Osman & Loschen, 1992).

Biobehavioral research in both basic and clinical areas is necessary to define the multiple neurochemical etiologies of self-injurious behavior and to identify the most appropriate treatment strategies for particular patient groups.

TREATMENT

Behavioral Therapy

Behavior management strategies have been the mainstay of treatment for self-injurious behavior among people with mental retardation. They are used in conjunction with educational, ecologic, and pharmacologic interventions. A functional analysis should determine which, if any, environmental factors influence the occurrence of the behavior. The factors that initially caused the behavior may no longer be present, but the behavior may persist (be maintained) because of the environmental responses it produces (Iwata, Dorsey, Slifer, Bauman, & Richman, 1982). A data-based system to monitor the effect the treatment plan has on decreasing the undesired behaviors and increasing desired behaviors is crucial in determining if the treatment is successful. Behavioral treatments are relatively labor intensive and require ongoing data collection and analysis by trained personnel.

Schools, residential facilities for people with mental retardation, and specialized inpatient units must have human rights committees to oversee application of treatment protocols for maladaptive behavior. Such groups review both behavioral and pharmacologic interventions to make certain the treatment is humane, logical, and appropriately monitored.

Behavior Enhancement Techniques Critical to any behavior program is positive reinforcement for desired behaviors. Reinforcement increases the likelihood that these behaviors will occur and thus may decrease the likelihood of maladaptive behaviors. Differential reinforcement of other behavior (DRO) is a commonly used technique that provides reinforcement for a response other than self-injurious behavior. Reinforcement can be delayed by the institution of a token program in which tokens that can be traded at some later time for reinforcement are awarded for appropriate behavior. A variation on this approach is differential reinforcement of an incompatible behavior (DRI), in which the reinforcement is provided for behaviors that cannot be performed at the same time as the self-injurious behavior. An example would be a person learning to keep his or her hands in the pockets instead of engaging in face hitting. A third variation is differential reinforcement of communication (DRC), which is used when self-injurious behavior is thought to serve a communicative function. In this circumstance, a more appropriate method of communication, such as signing, is reinforced. Functional independence training also may result in the decrease of inappropriate behaviors by increasing compliance and teaching adaptive and

leisure skills (National Institutes of Health, 1989).

Because these treatment strategies require a period of learning, they cannot be used to treat acute problems. Factors that may decrease the success of this class of interventions include the potential that the person will lose interest in the reinforcer, that a behavior not currently in the person's repertoire may need to be learned, that no reinforcer can be identified, and the possibility that the behavior occurs so frequently that no other behavior occurs that can be reinforced (National Institutes of Health, 1989). Interventions that teach appropriate behaviors were found to be preferable to reductive treatments among staff who work with people with mental retardation, and acceptability of accelerative treatments was not affected by severity of self-injurious behavior (Tarnowski, Mulick, & Rasnake, 1990).

Ecologic Treatments It has been demonstrated that self-injurious behavior can vary according to the stimuli provided by the environment (Touchette, MacDonald, & Langer, 1985). A treatment strategy may increase the time a person spends in activities or environments that are correlated with low rates of self-injurious behavior. Less desired activities then could be faded into that situation.

Behavior-Reduction Techniques Behavioral treatments in which an environmental change occurring after a behavior decreases the likelihood of occurrence of that behavior are known as behavior-reduction techniques (National Institutes of Health, 1989). Behavior-reduction techniques do not teach appropriate behaviors that can replace the self-injurious behavior, so behavioral enhancement strategies must also be in effect. Overcorrection and positive practice involve rehearsal of a desired behavior on the occurrence of an undesired behavior. An example would be repetitively performing a personal hygiene routine as a consequence for fecal smearing. Time-out is a procedure in which a person is removed from a reinforcing situation for a brief period after a maladaptive behavior occurs. Response cost involves the removal of tokens earned for appropriate behavior on the occurrence of an inappropriate behavior. Other behavior-reduction strategies for reducing self-injurious behavior include verbal reprimand and extinction or the removal of attention for the behavior.

Application of aversive stimuli such as bitter substances, a spray of water mist, an ammonia inhalant, or mild electric shock to the skin have all been reported as treatments for self-injurious behavior. Proponents of such therapy believe that it is justified in situations in which the behavior has not responded to other conventional treatments and the individual is at high risk for morbidity (National Institutes of Health, 1989). Advocacy groups for people with developmental disabilities have taken the position that any treatment that inflicts pain, results in injury, or is perceived as dehumanizing or degrading by people without developmental disabilities is unacceptable.

Protective Equipment   Protective equipment is sometimes necessary to prevent a person with self-injurious behavior from sustaining further injury. Protective equipment should be used only as part of a program that is designed to increase adaptive behavior. Helmets are used to decrease the likelihood of soft tissue injuries from head banging or hitting. Arm extension splints prevent head hitting, eye gouging, and hand biting. Gloves, padded clothing, and goggles are also used. These devices may prevent self-injurious behavior for mechanical reasons, because the stimulatory response is blunted, or because the presence of the restraint becomes a stimulus that is associated with the inability to self-injure. Techniques such as gradually fading out the presence of the restraint may permit enhancement of functional activities.

Pharmacotherapy

Pharmacologic treatment of self-injurious behavior is used to ameliorate acute situations, as part of a treatment plan that includes educational and behavioral objectives, or to address specific disorders (National Institutes of Health, 1989). Because self-injury itself is a symptom rather than a disease, the underlying disorder should be the focus of treatment. Initially, psychotropic medications were used to decrease severe maladaptive behaviors in people with mental retardation on the assumption that the underlying pathology was similar to the psychi-

atric conditions that cause bizarre behaviors in the general population. Up to 40%–50% of people with mental retardation living in institutions in the United States are treated with behavior-modifying drugs (Lapierre & Reesal, 1986). Drugs that are used in the treatment of self-injurious behavior are listed in Table 2. Many psychopharmacologic agents have been reported to decrease self-injury in single cases or among small groups of patients. However, most studies have been flawed by vague outcome measures, confounding medications, design difficulties, and heterogeneous patient groups. Clearly, a better understanding of the behavioral and organic pathology leading to self-injurious behavior is necessary so that drugs can be used in a more directed manner.

Neuroleptic Medications   The drugs most frequently used to diminish self-injurious behavior are neuroleptics (Farber, 1987; Lapierre & Reesal, 1986). The sedating side effects of these agents may produce a reduction in self-injurious behavior, or the effect may be due to the primary antiagitation and antipsychotic actions. Thioridazine and chlorpromazine are the drugs most commonly used to treat severe behavioral dysfunction in persons with mental retardation, with desired results seen in 10%–15% of treated individuals (Lapierre & Reesal, 1986). Butyrophenones such as haloperidol have been demonstrated to decrease aggression and self-injurious behavior at relatively low doses in people with mental retardation (Mikkelson, 1986). Because stereotypic movements are mediated through dopaminergic pathways, stereotypic self-injurious behavior might be expected to diminish with drugs in this class that block dopamine receptors. Other neuroleptic drugs tested in small populations to control aggression and self-injurious behavior include mesoridazine, pipamperone, and milenperone. The latter two did no better than behavior management or placebo (Lapiere & Reesal, 1986).

Because sedation accompanies neuroleptic use in most cases, the effect of treatment with these drugs on learning is of concern. Treatment with drugs in this class has been demonstrated to interfere with performance of workshop tasks and with the response to reinforcement protocols (Lapierre & Reesal, 1986). Single case reports, however, describe people in whom behavior management strategies act synergistically with neuroleptic drugs to decrease self-injurious behavior when neither therapy alone was sufficient (Durand, 1982).

Alternatives to long-term neuroleptic therapy are desirable because of the risk of tardive dyskinesia, which develops in approximately 15% of patients (Lapierre & Reesal, 1986). This risk may be higher in patients with preexisting brain pathology. Transient withdrawal dyskinesias and worsening of target behaviors in the 4 weeks after discontinuing a neuroleptic drug may occur.

In a systematic attempt to discontinue behavior-modifying drugs in one state institution, it was determined that the medications could be decreased or discontinued in the majority of people with mental retardation studied without a change in behavior control (D. E. Williams, Weir, Hargrave, & Parker, 1984).

Antidepressants Antidepressant medications are being used with greater frequency for behavior control in people with mental retardation, largely because of the newer agents with serotonergic properties. Treatment with imipramine increased attention and decreased maladaptive behavior at doses of 10–75 mg/day in an institutional setting (Huessy & Ruoff, 1984). One report in the literature describes an individual whose family history of depression, cyclic occurrence of the behavioral disturbance,

Table 2. Drugs used in the treatment of self-injurious behavior (SIB)

Class	Examples	Indications	Other uses
Anticonvulsants	Carbamazepine	Seizures, neuralgias	Bipolar illness, mood disorder, aggression/SIB
	Valproic acid	Seizures	Mood disorders ± SIB
Antidepressants	Trazedone	Depression	SIB
	Tricyclics	Depression, enuresis	ADHD, OCD, SIB/aggression
	Clomipramine	OCD, depression	SIB/aggression, ADHD
	Fluoxetine	Depression, OCD	SIB/aggression
Benzodiazepines	Diazepam	Anxiety, sleep disorders, spasticity, seizures	
β-Blockers	Propranolol, nadolol	Hypertension, anxiety	Rage, SIB, aggression
Clonidine		Hypertension	Anxiety, ADHD Tourette syndrome
Lithium		Mania	SIB/aggression
Neuroleptics	Butyrophenones Phenothiazines Fluphenazine	Psychosis	SIB/aggression, ADHD, Tourette syndrome
Opiate antagonist	Naltrexone	Opiate withdrawal	SIB, PDD
Serotonin reuptake inhibitors	Buspirone	Anxiety	SIB/aggression, PDD
	Clomipramine (see antidepressants)		
	Fluoxetine (see antidepressants)		

Note: ADHD, attention-deficit/hyperactivity disorder; OCD, obsessive–compulsive disorder; PPD, pervasive personality disorder.

and positive dexamethasone challenge test suggested affective illness; successful management of symptoms occurred with desipramine (Hardy, Waters, & Cohen, 1984). Careful analysis of family history; episodic occurrence of behaviors; and constitutional symptoms such as changes in sleep, appetite, and activity level can help identify depression in people with mental retardation that then can be treated appropriately.

The efficacy of serotonin reuptake inhibitors in decreasing symptoms of obsessive–compulsive behavior has led to their use in people with mental retardation with perseverative behaviors, including self-injurious behavior. Although clomipramine is used in the treatment of depression and attention-deficit/hyperactivity disorder, it has primary antiobsessive effects (Green, 1991). Self-injurious behavior decreased by 50% or more in 10 of 11 patients with developmental disabilities treated with clomipramine in one series (Garber, McGonigle, Slomka, & Monteverde, 1992). Doses used ranged from 25 to 125 mg/day. Fluoxetine, an antidepressant that blocks serotonin reuptake, has been reported to significantly diminish self-injurious behavior and aggression thought to be compulsive in nature. In one report, 7 of 10 people with mental retardation responded to fluoxetine versus none of six comparison subjects with similar maladaptive behaviors not thought to be compulsive in origin (Bodfish & Madison, 1993). Fluoxetine also has been successful in the treatment of skin picking in the Prader-Willi syndrome (Warnock & Kestenbaum, 1992). Of the 45 reported cases of self-injurious behavior treated with fluoxetine, 43 had a positive response to the drug, suggesting that further scientifically sound evaluation is indicated (Ricketts, Goza, Ellis, Singh, & Cooke, 1993).

Buspirone, an anxiolytic agent with few side effects, diminished aggressive and self-injurious behaviors in 9 of 14 individuals with developmental disabilities when treated with doses of 15–45 mg/day (Ratey, Sovner, Mikkelson, & Chmielinski, 1989). Treatment success with this serotonin reuptake inhibitor has been described in other populations, such as children with autism, and may be due to the anxiolytic action (Osman & Loschen, 1992).

Lithium Agitation, aggression, and autoaggression in people with mental retardation have been treated with lithium because of similarities to mania. When self-injurious behavior occurs in a cyclic pattern, with constitutional symptoms of affective illness, and especially with a family history, lithium may be an effective therapy. Lithium at blood levels between 0.5 and 1.0 mEq/L may decrease self-injurious behavior and aggression in patients with a consistent history, agitation, or mood lability. Some other patients with stereotyped self-injury and autistic features may respond to lithium as well, although aggression is the most solid indication (Lapierre & Reesal, 1986; Pary, 1991). In one retrospective study, the 31 patients of 74 treated who demonstrated a response to lithium were older and had psychotic symptomatology (Langee, 1990).

Identification of mood symptomatology accompanying self-injurious behavior might suggest treatment with the anticonvulsant valproic acid (Kastner, Friedman, Plummer, Ruiz, & Henning, 1990). This agent potentiates GABA function and decreases dopaminergic transmission, and has utility in the treatment of manic–depressive illness.

Carbamazepine Carbamazepine, a drug often used to treat bipolar affective disorders, is used for intermittent agitation and aggression in episodic discontrol as well as for affective illness in the general population. As an anticonvulsant, it is the drug of choice for seizure foci in the temporal or limbic lobes of the brain. Its utility in the treatment of behavioral dysfunction in people with mental retardation may be through one or both of these mechanisms. The relatively low toxicity and multiple reports of success in reported cases suggest further controlled evaluations of this drug are warranted (Evans, Clay, & Gualtieri, 1987; Osman & Loschen, 1992).

β-Adrenergic Blockers β-Blockers such as propranolol are being used for treatment of aggression, akathisia, anxiety, panic, and organic psychosis in psychiatric practice. Doses of over 520 mg/day have been reported to be necessary, although other groups have reported successful behavior control of maladaptive behaviors in patients with mental retardation with doses of

40–240 mg/day (Ratey et al., 1986). There is some individual variation in the length of treatment required to obtain a response. The anxiolytic effects of β-blockers may occur through both peripheral and central mechanisms. Nonlipophilic drugs in this class, such as pindolol and nadolol, may also produce the behavioral response, presumably by the peripheral mechanism (Osman & Loschen, 1992).

Opiate Antagonists Opiate antagonists have theoretical interest because self-injurious behavior has been postulated to increase the production of endogenous opiates that the person then must continue to produce to maintain brain opiate receptors in a bound state. A second hypothesis suggests that persons with self-injurious behavior have altered sensation because of a developmental up-regulation of the opioid receptors (Osman & Loschen, 1992). The oral preparation naltrexone has nonspecific binding to all classes of opiate receptors and is approved for use in treatment of exogenous opiate addiction. Other clinical uses being evaluated include treatment of central apnea, precocious puberty, and obesity. Naltrexone, or the parenteral preparation naloxone, has been associated with a decrease in self-injurious behavior in controlled settings in most, but not all, published studies (Barrett, Feinstein, & Hole, 1989; Sandman, Barron, & Colman, 1990). When successful, the medication seems to have the greatest effect at doses of up to 1.5 mg/kg/day (Herman et al., 1987). Naltrexone does not seem to diminish stereotypy or have its effect through sedation (Sandman, Barron, & Colman, 1990).

Benzodiazepines Drugs in the benzodiazepine family frequently are used in chronic management of seizure disorders and sleep dysfunction. Their use specifically for decreasing self-injurious behavior is not generally supported. Diazepam is frequently used in controlling the spasticity of patients with Lesch-Nyhan syndrome; it does not alter the self-injurious behavior, however. The sedative and anxiolytic actions of these medications may have utility in individual cases.

Other Drugs Several other drugs have been investigated as a treatment of self-injurious behavior. The GABA analogue baclofen subjectively decreased self-injurious behavior in 22 of 28 institutionalized adults (Primrose, 1979). Stimulant medications, such as methylphenidate, generally have not proved effective for treatment of self-injurious behavior. In Lesch-Nyhan syndrome, hydroxytryptophan, the precursor of serotonin, was administered in an attempt to decrease autoaggression. Initially promising results could not be reproduced or sustained even with the addition of carbidopa (Farber, 1987). Dietary manipulations, including supplementation with large amounts of vitamin B_6 and magnesium, and purine-free diets have also been prescribed, although no data are available as to the behavioral outcome.

Choice of Drug Therapy The clinician must access available medical, behavioral, psychiatric, historical, and environmental information about an individual to determine if medication is a necessary part of the treatment plan. If so, there is no ready algorithm that substitutes for a knowledge of the literature and the patient, diagnosis of a specific psychiatric disorder, and a data-based system of assessing symptomatic relief.

PHYSICAL SEQUELAE

Topographies

Clinicians caring for people who engage in self-injurious behavior must be aware of the potential complications of the behavior so that appropriate monitoring can take place. More than one type of such behavior is usually demonstrated. In a population of school-age children with developmental disabilities, 18.6% engaged in one topography, 29.9% in two, 26.8% in three, 13.4% in four, and 11.3% in five or more. Studies of primarily adult populations report similar findings (Griffin et al., 1984).

The three most common forms of self-injurious behavior in a school-age population were head banging against objects, self-biting, and head hitting with fist or palm. Scratching, eye poking, ear poking, hair pulling, kicking, neck whipping, and body hitting were also common. Pica is a potentially self-injurious behavior that is normal for younger children but may persist in people with mental retardation (Figure 1). A more unusual topography, aerophagia (the excessive swallow-

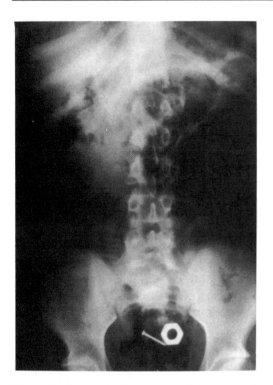

Figure 1. Foreign bodies seen on abdominal radiograph of an adolescent boy with profound mental retardation and severe pica.

ing of air), is generally a benign condition. It can result in chronic gastric and intestinal dilatation with resultant perforation in some individuals who engage in it in a perseverative manner.

Rumination is the volitional regurgitation and reswallowing of food. It places the individual at risk for esophagitis, esophageal rupture, stricture formation, malnutrition, anemia, tooth damage, and aspiration. Gastroesophageal reflux may predispose a child to the development of this form of self-injurious behavior. Medical and surgical treatment of rumination has not proved successful. Behavioral approaches enjoy limited success (Winton & Singh, 1983).

Injuries

Injuries produced by self-injurious behavior are most frequently to the soft tissues, with excoriations (scrapes, scratches, minor cuts, abrasions) being the most common result. Permanent scars and hypertrophic callus formation are also common, as is hematoma formation. Serious self-biting with alteration in physiognomy, such as

lip removal and autoamputation of digits, is seen primarily in patients with Lesch-Nyhan syndrome and hereditary sensory neuropathies. The Self-Injury Trauma Scale has been developed as a standardized way of measuring type and severity of self-inflicted injury (Iwata, Pace, Kissel, Nau, & Farber, 1990).

Therapy for local infections (e.g., cellulitis, impetigo, abscesses) was required by 16.5% of the individuals treated by the author and her colleagues (Hyman et al., 1990). Chronically open wounds can lead to systemic infection and osteomyelitis.

Dental injuries occurred in 11.3% of children in one sample who were treated as inpatients for self-injurious behavior. Head hitting and banging can result in tooth loosening and fracture. Gum picking can lead to tooth-threatening gingival disease. Inadequate dental hygiene and prophylaxis may place a child at greater risk for dental injury. The author and her colleagues have observed autoextraction of teeth in two patients with hereditary sensory neuropathies.

Head injuries are the complication most feared by the caregivers of self-injurious persons. Repeated subconcussive injury results in a syndrome of dementia and motor impairment in boxers, a group who also suffer repeated blows to the head. Pyramidal tract findings and deterioration were noted but not quantified or followed longitudinally in a group of persons with self-injurious behavior whose roentgenographic findings were reported (J.P. Williams, Fowler, Pribram, Delaney, & Fish, 1972). There is a reference in the literature to a fatal subdural hematoma attributed to head banging in a patient with Tourette syndrome (Robertson et al., 1989). Much more commonly seen are the chronic changes of thickening of the skull secondary to periosteal hematoma formation, cauliflower ears, and hematomas and lacerations of the scalp.

Permanent eye damage is one of the most serious sequelae of head banging and head hitting. Repeated subconcussive blows to the head can result in cataract formation, glaucoma, and retinal detachment (Figure 2) (Robertson et al., 1989). Decreased visual acuity may cause a

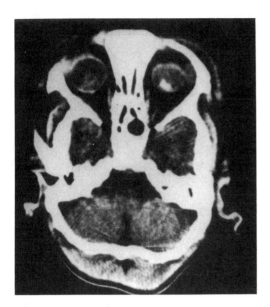

Figure 2. Total retinal detachment with calcification in area of old hemorrhage is seen on this cranial computerized tomography scan of a young adult man with profound mental retardation and a 20-year history of head banging.

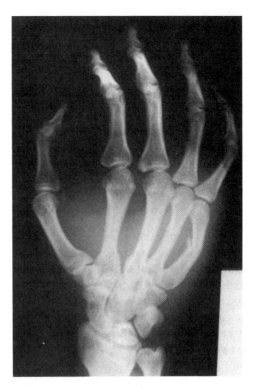

Figure 3. Fracture of the fifth metacarpal bone is seen on this hand radiograph taken for assessment of swelling and tenderness in an adolescent boy with profound mental retardation and a long history of head hitting.

child to engage in eye-gouging behavior as a form of self-stimulation. Direct eye poking can result in corneal abrasions, perforation of the globe, and even enucleation. Mild pressure on a closed lid, however, is not likely to lead to injury.

"March hematuria" is a well-known phenomenon of hemoglobinuria that results from repeated trauma. Hemoglobinuria is generally benign and can be managed with increased fluid intake. Head banging in a child with hyperviscosity secondary to a congenital heart lesion has been associated with renal failure, however (Blaser & Macknin, 1983).

The bone most likely to be damaged in head hitting may be not the skull but the hand (Figure 3). Sequelae of vigorous and repetitive self-injurious behavior can include fractures of the ribs, tibia, humerus, and foot.

Medical Evaluation of the Self-Injurious Patient

The patient and caregivers must be interviewed to obtain an accurate history relating to the self-injurious behavior. Information regarding the onset, duration, frequency, and severity of the behavior should be gathered. Special emphasis should be given to changes in the behavior over time and cyclic variation. Association with other maladaptive behaviors, such as tantrums, should be documented. Family history of psychiatric and medical illness should also be obtained, and the patient's cognitive and language functioning levels should be assessed. Potential psychiatric and behavioral etiologies should be considered.

Review of systems and physical examination should rule out any medical conditions that could lead to an acute exacerbation of the behavior. Otitis media, migraine headaches, sinusitis, dental abscess, dysmenorrhea, visual loss, constipation, and abdominal pain have all been implicated in worsening behavior in individual cases. Other painful conditions, such as pathologic fractures, increased intracranial pressure with hydrocephalus, and reflux esophagitis, should be considered.

Medical evaluations should be determined by the findings of the history and physical with two exceptions. Patients who engage in repetitive subconcussive head injury should be followed by an ophthalmologist to monitor for retinal detachment. Patients with open wounds or aggression should be screened for human immunodeficiency virus and hepatitis and be considered for hepatitis B immunization. In the initial evaluation, specific syndromes associated with self-injurious behavior should be considered and the appropriate workup performed when indicated. Routine electroencephalographic and neuroimaging studies are not likely to demonstrate findings that would alter treatment plans. These studies should be performed when specific symptoms suggest they are indicated.

CONCLUSIONS

Self-injurious behavior is a maladaptive behavior engaged in for operant or organic reasons by people with developmental disabilities. It causes physical injury, compromises educational and habilitation programs, and may prevent home or community placement. Many different types of medications and behavioral interventions have been used to decrease self-injury. Most of them are used without critical assessment by controlled studies with objective outcome measures over an adequate period of follow-up. Patients are often not assessed for physiologic markers or symptoms of underlying pathology that might respond to specific management. An analysis of the etiology of the behavior would help target which patients require combinations of behavioral and pharmacologic therapy, and would also help explain the lack of response to pharmacologic management in specific cases. Many clinicians put up artificial barriers and view the treatment of self-injurious behavior as either behavioral or medical. In fact, no medication can succeed without a plan for acquisition of appropriate behaviors, and behavioral treatment may be enhanced by diminishing agitation or other organic pathology present.

REFERENCES

Anderson, L.T., Ernst, M., & Davis, S. V. (1992). Cognitive abilities in patients with Lesch-Nyhan disease. *Journal of Autism and Developmental Disorders, 22,* 189–203.

Axelrod, F.B., & Pearson, J. (1984). Congenital sensory neuropathies. *American Journal of Diseases of Children, 138,* 947–954.

Barrett R.P., Feinstein, C., & Hole, W. T. (1989) Effects of naloxone and naltrexone on self-injury: A double-blind, placebo-controlled analysis. *American Journal of Mental Retardation, 93,* 644–651

Baumeister, A.A., & Frye, G.D. (1985). The biochemical basis of the behavioral disorder in the Lesch-Nyhan syndrome. *Neuroscience and Biobehavioral Reviews, 9,* 169–178.

Blaser, S., & Macknin, M.L. (1983). Head-banging with subsequent hemoglobinuria and acute renal failure. *Cleveland Clinic Quarterly, 50,* 347–350.

Bodfish, J.W., & Madison, J.T. (1993). Diagnosis and fluoxetine treatment of compulsive behavior disorder of adults with mental retardation. *American Journal of Mental Retardation, 98,* 360–367.

Breese, G.R., Criswell, H.E., Duncan, G.E., & Mueller, R.A. (1989). Dopamine deficiency in self-injurious behavior. *Psychopharmacology Bulletin, 25,* 353–357.

Carlson, G. (1979). Affective psychoses in mental retardates. *Psychiatric Clinics of North America, 2,* 499–510.

Carr, E.G. (1977). The motivation of self-injurious behavior: A review of some hypotheses. *Psychological Bulletin, 64,* 800–816.

Cataldo, M.F., & Harris, J. (1982). The biologic basis for self-injury in the mentally retarded. *Analysis and Intervention in Developmental Disabilities, 2,* 21–39.

Chudley, A.E., & Hagerman, R.J. (1987). Fragile X syndrome. *Journal of Pediatrics, 110,* 821–831.

Criswell, H.E., Mueller, R.A., & Breese, G.R. (1992). Pharmacologic evaluation of SCH-39166, A69024, NO-0756 and SCH-23390 in neonatal 6-OHDA lesioned rats: Further evidence that self-mutilatory behavior induced by L-dopa is related to D1 dopamine receptors. *Neuropsychopharmacology, 7,* 95–103.

Durand, V.M. (1982). A behavioral/pharmacological intervention for the treatment of self-injurious behavior. *Journal of Autism and Developmental Disorders, 12,* 243–251.

Durand, V.M., & Carr, E.G. (1991). Functional communication training to reduce challenging behavior: Maintenance and application in new settings.

Journal of Applied Behavior Analysis, 24, 251–264.

Evans, R.W., Clay T.H., & Gualtieri, C.T. (1987). Carbamazepine in pediatric psychiatry. *Journal of the American Academy of Child and Adolescent Psychiatry, 26,* 2–8.

Farber, J.M. (1987). Psychopharmacology of self-injurious behavior in the mentally retarded. *Journal of the American Academy of Child and Adolescent Psychiatry, 26,* 296–302.

Favell, J.E., Azrin, N.H, Baumeister, A.A., Carr, E.G., Dorsey M.F., Forehand, R., Foxx, R.M., Lovaas, O.I., Rincover, A., Risley, T.R., Romanczyk, R.G., Russo, D.C., Schroeder, S.R., & Solnick, J.V. (1982). The treatment of self-injurious behavior. *Behavior Therapy, 13,* 529–554.

Frye, G.D., Baumeister, A.A., Crotty, K., Newman, K.D., & Kotrla, K.J. (1985). Evaluation of the role of antinociception in self-injurious behavior following intranigral injection of muscimol. *Neuropharmacology, 25,* 717–726.

Garber, H.J., McGonigle J.J., Slomka, G.T., & Monteverde, E. (1992). Clomipramine treatment of stereotypic behaviors and self-injury in patients with developmental disabilities. *Journal of the American Academy of Child and Adolescent Psychiatry, 31,* 1157–1160.

Gillberg, C., Terenius, L., & Lonnerholm, G. (1985). Endorphin activity in childhood psychosis. *Archives of General Psychiatry, 42,* 780–783.

Goldstein, M. (1989). Dopaminergic mechanisms in self-inflicting biting behavior. *Psychopharmacology Bulletin, 25,* 349–352.

Green, W.H. (1991). *Child and adolescent clinical psychopharmacology.* Baltimore: Williams & Wilkins.

Griffin, J.C., Ricketts, R.W., Williams, D.E., Locke, B.J., Altmeyer, B.K., & Stark, M.T. (1987). A community survey of self-injurious behavior among developmentally disabled children and adolescents. *Hospital and Community Psychiatry, 38,* 959–963.

Griffin, J.C., Williams, D.E., Stark, M.T., Altmeyer, B.K., & Mason, M. (1984). Self-injurious behavior: A state-wide prevalence survey of the extent and circumstances. In J.C. Griffin, M.T. Stark, D.E. Williams, B. K. Altmeyer, & H.K. Griffin (Eds.), *Advances in the treatment of self-injurious behavior* (pp. 1–25). Austin: Texas Planning Council for Developmental Disabilities.

Guess, D., & Carr, E. (1991). Emergence and maintenance of stereotypy and self injury. *American Journal of Mental Retardation, 96,* 299–319.

Hardy, P.M., Waters, J.M., & Cohen, M.S. (1984). A biomedical basis for self-injury. In J.C. Griffin, M.T. Stark, D.E. Williams, B.K. Altmeyer, & H.K. Griffin (Eds.), *Advances in the treatment of self-injurious behavior* (pp. 153–164). Austin: Texas Planning Council for Developmental Disabilities.

Herman, B.H., Hammock, M.K., Arthur-Smith, A., Egan, J., Chatoor, I., Werner, A., & Zelnick, N. (1987). Naltrexone decreases self-injurious behavior. *Annals of Neurology, 22,* 550–552.

Huessy, H.R., & Ruoff, P.A. (1984). Towards a rational drug usage in a state institution for retarded individuals. *Psychiatric Journal of the University of Ottawa, 9,* 56–58.

Hyman, S.L., Fisher, W., Mercugliano, M., & Cataldo, M.F. (1990). Children with self-injurious behavior. *Pediatrics, 85,* 437–441.

Iwata, B.A., Dorsey, M.F., Slifer, K.J., Bauman, K.E., & Richman, G.S. (1982). Toward a functional analysis of self-injury. *Analysis and Intervention in Developmental Disabilities, 2,* 3–20.

Iwata, B.A., Pace G.M., Kissel, R.C., Nau, P.A., & Farber, J.M. (1990). The Self-Injury Trauma (SIT) scale: A method for quantifying surface tissue damage caused by self-injurious behavior. *Journal of Applied Behavior Analysis, 23,* 99–110.

Iwata, B.A., Pace, G.M., Willus, K.D., Gamache, T.B., & Hyman, S.L. (1986). Operant studies of self-injurious hand biting in the Rett syndrome. *American Journal of Medical Genetics, 24,* 157–166.

Johnson, H.G., Ekman, P., Freisen, W., Nyhan, W.L., & Shear, C. (1976). A behavioral phenotype in the de Lange syndrome. *Pediatric Research, 10,* 843–850.

Jones, I.H. (1982). Self-injury: Toward a biologic basis. *Perspectives in Biology and Medicine, 26,* 137–150.

Kastner, T., Friedman, D.L., Plummer, A.T., Ruiz, M.Q., & Henning, D. (1990). Valproic acid for the treatment of children with mental retardation and mood symptomatology. *Pediatrics, 86,* 467–472.

Katsuragi, T., Ushijima, I., & Furukawa, T. (1984). The clonidine-induced self-injurious behavior of mice involves purinergic mechanisms. *Pharmacology, Biochemistry, and Behavior, 20,* 943–946.

King, B.H. (1993). Self-injury by people with mental retardation: A compulsive behavior hypothesis. *American Journal of Mental Retardation, 98,* 93–112.

Langee, H.R. (1990). Retrospective study of lithium use for institutionalized mentally retarded individuals with behavior disorders. *American Journal of Mental Retardation, 94,* 448–452

Lapierre, Y.D., & Reesal, R. (1986). Pharmacologic management of aggressivity and self-mutilation in the mentally retarded. *Psychiatric Clinics of North America, 9,* 745–754.

Lloyd, K.G., Hornykiewicz, O., Davidson, L., Shannak, K., & Fox, I.H. (1981). Biochemical evidence of dysfunction of brain neurotransmitters in the Lesch-Nyhan syndrome. *New England Journal of Medicine, 305,* 1106–1111.

Loschen, E.L., & Osman, O. T. (1992). Self-injurious behavior in the developmentally disabled: Assessment techniques. *Psychopharmacology Bulletin*, *28*, 433–438.

Mikkelson, E. J. (1986). Low-dose haloperidol for stereotypic self-injurious behavior in the mentally retarded. *New England Journal of Medicine, 315*, 398–399.

Mueller, K., Saboda, S., Palmour, R., & Nyhan, W.L. (1982). Self-injurious behavior produced in rats by daily caffeine and continuous amphetamine. *Pharmacology, Biochemistry, and Behavior, 17*, 613–617.

National Institutes of Health Consensus Development Panel on Treatment of Destructive Behavior in Persons with Developmental Disabilities. (1989). Bethesda, MD: National Institutes of Health.

Oliver, C., Murphy, G.H., & Corbett, J.A. (1987). Self-injurious behavior in people with mental handicap: A total population study. *Journal of Mental Deficiency Research, 31*, 147–162.

Osman, O.T., & Loschen, E.L. (1992) Self-injurious behavior in the developmentally disabled: Pharmacologic treatment. *Psychopharmacologic Bulletin, 28*, 439–449.

Pary, R.J. (1991). Towards defining adequate lithium trials for individuals with mental retardation and mental illness. *American Journal of Mental Retardation, 95*, 681–691.

Primrose, D.A. (1979). Treatment of self-injurious behavior with a GABA (gamma-aminobutyric acid) analogue. *Journal of Mental Deficiency Research, 23*, 163–173.

Prizant, B.M., & Wetherby, A.M. (1987). Communicative intent: A framework for understanding social-communicative behavior in autism. *Journal of the American Academy of Child And Adolescent Psychiatry, 26*, 472–479.

Ragheb, J.A., Hyman, S.L., Coyle, J.T., & Batshaw, M.L. (1989). Neurochemical correlates of self-injurious behavior. *Pediatric Research, 25*, 359A.

Ratey, J.J., Mikkelsen, E.J., Smith, G.B., Upadhaya, A., Zuckerman, H.S., Martelli, D., Sorgi, P., Polakoff, S., & Bemporad, J. (1986). β-Blockers in the severely and profoundly mentally retarded. *Journal of Clinical Psychopharmacology, 6*, 103–107.

Ratey, J.J., Sovner, R., Mikkelson, E., & Chmielinski, H.E. (1989). Buspirone therapy for maladaptive behavior and anxiety in developmentally disabled persons. *Journal of Clinical Psychiatry, 50*, 382–384.

Ricketts, R.W., Goza, A.B., Ellis, C.R., Singh, Y.N., & Cooke, J.C. (1993). Fluoxetine treatment of severe self-injury in young adults with mental retardation. *Journal of the American Academy of Child and Adolescent Psychiatry, 32*, 865–869.

Rincover, A. (1986). Behavioral research in self-injury and self stimulation. *Psychiatric Clinics of North America, 9*, 755–766.

Robertson, M.M., Trimble, M.R., & Lees, A.J. (1989). Self-injurious behavior and the Gilles de la Tourette syndrome: A clinical study and review of the literature. *Psychological Medicine, 19*, 611–625.

Rojahn, J. (1986). Self-injurious and stereotypic behavior of noninstitutionalized mentally retarded people: Prevalence and classification. *American Journal of Mental Deficiency, 91*, 268–276.

Rousseau, F., Heitz, D., Biancalana, V., Blumenfeld, S., Kretz, C., Boue, J., Tommerup, N., Van Der Hagen, C., DeLozier-Blanchet, C., Croquette, M.F., Gilgenkrantz, S., Jalbert, P., Voelckel, M.A., Oberle, I., & Mandel, J.L. (1991). Direct diagnosis by DNA analysis of the fragile X syndrome of mental retardation. *New England Journal of Medicine, 325*, 1673–1681.

Sallustro, F., & Atwell, C.A. (1978). Body rocking, head banging, and head rolling in normal children. *Journal of Pediatrics, 93*, 704–708.

Sandman, C.A., Barron, J.L., Chicz-DeMet, A., & DeMet E.M. (1990). Plasma β-endorphin levels in patients with self-injurious behavior and stereotypy. *American Journal of Mental Retardation, 95*, 84–92.

Sandman, C.A., Barron, J.L., & Colman, H. (1990). An orally administered opiate blocker, naltrexone, attenuates self-injurious behavior. *American Journal of Mental Retardation, 95*, 93–102.

Silverstein, F.S., Johnston, M.V., Hutchinson, R.J., & Edwards, N.L. (1985). Lesch-Nyhan syndrome: CSF neurotransmitter abnormalities. *Neurology, 35*, 907–911.

Singh, N.N. (1981). Current trends in the treatment of self-injurious behavior. *Advances in Pediatrics, 28*, 377–440.

Singh, N.N., & Pulman, R. M. (1979). Self-injury in the de Lange syndrome. *Journal of Mental Deficiency Research, 23*, 79–84.

Sormann, G.W. (1982). The headbangers tumour. *British Journal of Plastic Surgery, 35*, 72–74.

Tarnowski, K.J., Mulick, J.A., & Rasnake, L.K. (1990) Acceptability of behavioral interventions for self-injurious behavior: Replication and interinstitutional comparison. *American Journal of Mental Retardation, 95*, 182–187.

Touchette, P.E., MacDonald, R.F., & Langer, S.N. (1985). A scatter plot for identifying stimulus control of problem behavior. *Journal of Applied Behavior Analysis, 18*, 343–351.

Warnock, J.K., & Kestenbaum, T. (1992). Pharmacologic treatment of severe skin-picking behaviors in Prader-Willi syndrome: Two case reports. *Archives of Dermatology, 128*, 1623–1625.

Williams, D.E., Weir, H.F., Hargrave, R.L., & Parker, C.M. (1984). Effects of a facility wide psychoactive drug evaluation-behavior management system. In J.C. Griffin, M.T. Stark, D.E.

Williams, B.K. Altmeyer, & H.K. Griffin (Eds.), *Advances in the treatment of self-injurious behavior* (pp. 135–151). Austin: Texas Planning Council on Developmental Disabilities.

Williams, J.P., Fowler, G.W., Pribram, H.F., Delaney, C.A., & Fish, C.H. (1972). Roentgeno-graphic changes in headbangers. *Acta Radiologica Diagnostica, 13*, 37–42.

Winton, A.S.W., & Singh, N.N. (1983). Rumination in pediatric populations: A behavioral analysis. *Journal of the American Academy of Child Psychiatry, 22*, 269–275.

PART V

THE SPECTRUM
OF LANGUAGE AND
COMMUNICATION DISORDERS

Chapter 22

The Child Who Does Not Speak

Rita Panoscha, M.D.

Communication skills are an important and cherished aspect of human life. In their varied forms, be they verbal, written, sign, Morse code, braille, or gestures, touch, and facial expression, these skills have been used to convey feelings, needs, and information for generations across cultures and throughout history. Socialization skills are strongly dependent on the ability to communicate with other members of the community in order to maintain this common thread that holds a group together. Thus, the stream of development encompassing communication skills, particularly verbal language, is a very important part of a child's development. Similar to the gross motor milestone stream and the first independent step, language milestones, particularly the first words, are much anticipated by families. If these are not met, this should raise some concern about the child and his or her ability to function effectively in such a strongly communication-based society.

The child who does not speak or does not start speaking at an age-appropriate time is not uncommon and is encountered at some time by almost anyone who works extensively with preschool children. Various studies have been done over the years, and the actual prevalence reported may vary somewhat depending on the exact definition or range of deficiency included under a language or speech delay or both. The prevalence is higher with a less stringent definition of speech delays or disorders. Silva in Dunedin, New Zealand, found that 8.4% of the children in his study were delayed in expressive or receptive language or both at 3 years of age, with a significantly larger proportion of boys being delayed. Three percent of the children had delays in both these areas of language (Silva, 1980). The London Prevalence Study by Stevenson and Richman (1976) found a ratio of 5.7 per 1,000 for expressive language delay without "general retardation," with higher rates (31.2 and 22.7 per 1,000) for various degrees of expressive delay in general.

The Isle Of Wight Study reported a language delay ratio of 0.8 per 1,000 in children of school age (Rutter, Graham, & Yule, 1970). Four percent of children defined by Fundudis and his group in the Newcastle Upon Tyne Study were described as "speech retarded" at the age of 36 months. The speech retardation was defined by a lack of "three or more words strung together to make some sort of sense by the age of 36 months" (Fundudis, Kolvin, & Garside, 1979, p. 3). On follow-up, one fifth of these children had significant disabilities, including cognitive and physical disabilities. Three percent of them had a continued speech disorder (Fundudis et al., 1979). Kindergartners at age 5 years in the Ottawa-Carleton region of Canada had a 19% prevalence of speech and language disorders. Of this group, 6.4% had speech impairment only, without a language disorder, and 8.04% had language problems only (Beitchman, Nair, Clegg, & Patel, 1986). In various studies, boys tended to outnumber girls in the language delay group, with a ratio of approximately 2 to 1 (Fundudis et al., 1979).

For some children, this language delay is not always a permanent disorder. Long-term studies as well as anecdotal histories show that there are some children who are "late talkers" but subsequently develop adequate language skills. The long-range studies done by Silva's group found that language delay between 3 and 7 years could be transitory, yet even 42.5% of these children, whose language delays subsequently showed improvement, were found later to have low IQ or reading difficulties. These researchers also noted that those children with a more stable language delay or whose delay was picked up at an early age seemed to be more likely to have these related problems (Silva, McGee, & Williams, 1983). Silva and his group continued following their cohort through 11 years of age and found that reading delays were more likely in children with previous history of language delays, as were lower IQ scores and increased incidence of behavioral problems. Those children showing a more global language delay were more likely to have problems than were children with isolated expressive language delay (Silva, Williams, & McGee, 1987).

Another 10-year follow-up study done in Cleveland followed preschoolers with language disorders and similarly found that these youngsters were more likely to have subsequent social or behavioral problems along with added special educational needs (Aram, Ekelman, & Nation, 1984). Cantwell and colleagues found psychiatric disorders to be more prevalent in their cohort of children with language disorders, and to a lesser degree in those children with speech or articulation problems. Included in the diagnoses of psychiatric disorders were attention-deficit/hyperactivity disorder and oppositional and anxiety disorders (Cantwell, Baker, & Mattison, 1981). Another study done by Cohen and her colleagues found that their group of preteenagers referred for psychiatric or behavior problems included approximately 28% who had a previously undiagnosed language disorder (Cohen, Davine, & Meloche-Kelly, 1989).

Twins, as a group, have been observed as having delays in their overall development of language. Likewise, much has been made of their cryptophasia, or "twin talk," whereby the twin pair jabber or seemingly communicate with each other but less so with others in their environment. Preschool twins have been found on average to be 6 months behind their single counterparts, with male twins more delayed (approximately 8 months) as compared to the female twin pairs (Hay, Prior, Collett, & Williams, 1987). This was found to be an overall immaturity of language rather than a specific language disorder (Mittler, 1970).

TYPICAL LANGUAGE DEVELOPMENT

Although we may often think of language development as starting with the first "dada" or "mama" or the first true word and taking place mainly in the preschool years, many key prelinguistic skills are already forming in earliest infancy. Progression in this developmental stream extends through the school years, with refinements throughout adulthood. These earliest language milestones may not receive as much attention by families because other streams of development, particularly gross motor skills, typically are progressing at a very dramatic rate during the first year of life. Nevertheless, these prelinguistic skills are an important foundation for further language development.

Even during these earliest years of language development, the developmental stream can be roughly divided into two parts: receptive and expressive language. Receptive language is the receiving or intake and understanding of messages. Expressive language is the expressing or relaying on of thoughts or information to others. Further subcategories of language also develop over time and gain much more emphasis during later childhood. Such substreams would include phonology, or the actual sound production of speech; pragmatics, or the appropriate usage of language, including the social context; and semantics, or the meaning of language and grammar.

Expressively, the earliest crying, alerting to sound, and cuddling of the infant can be construed as having a communicative effect that eventually advances to a more conscious communication, such as crying for attention or in protest (Martlew, 1987). Earlier guttural crying sounds progress to the long vowel sounds of cooing at approximately 3 months, with the gradual addition of such consonants as p, d, and m at approximately 6 months, which results in what we initially call a prebabble and eventually true babbling sounds (Fletcher, 1987). Natural gestures used in communication, such as pointing, start developing before the first birthday and continue to evolve with refinements as further fine motor skills develop, finally adding single words to the appropriate gesture (Martlew, 1987). These prelinguistic skills may well be an inherent part of development because some children with hearing impairment meet these early expressive milestones close to the expected time (Murphy, 1964). The later production of meaningful words in the appropriate language or dialect and the continued usage of language may also require some external reinforcement, along with the innate cognitive abilities needed to handle the linguistic symbols.

There is a very rapid development of language after the first word, which occurs near the first birthday. Particularly in preschoolers, vocabulary size increases dramatically, and, by the time a child reaches 21 months, he or she has a 20–25 single-word vocabulary and novel two-word combinations. Three-word sentences should be present by at least 36 months and four-word sentences by 48 months, which eventually leads to the more complex, more grammatically correct adult-type sentences. The length of utterances increases to the point of being able to relate simple stories by 4 years of age. Rutter and Bax (1972) described these early single words as more of a "reflex labelling" response that eventually transitions to a higher "symbolic naming" (p. 5). Thus, the concept of words emerges and the ability to think about and use language in novel ways to communicate evolves. Symbolism, pretending, or plays on words are results of these newly developing abilities.

During this time of rapid vocabulary increase, speech may not always be completely clear. In part this is due to continued development of phonologic skills, because not all speech sounds are mastered at the same time. This may result in children dropping or deleting syllables, reducing consonant clusters, or substituting letters for sounds that they are not yet able to produce. Some very mild dysfluences or stuttering also may occur but should not impede communication, nor should they persist in typically developing children (Ingram, 1972). Some mild echoing of words can be heard but generally should not continue beyond 30 months (Fay, 1967). This early repeating may in effect be a part of vocabulary learning and should not be confused with the persistent nonfunctional echoing or canned "cocktail chatter" of some language disorders, in which novel communica-

tion may be sparse or nonexistent. By the age of about 4 years, a child's speech should be mostly understandable even to strangers.

Likewise, receptive language abilities also are progressing, starting with the early prelinguistic skills of reciprocal exchanges, vocalizing, and eye contact (Martlew, 1987). Turning in response to sound, and the eventual understanding of simple words such as "no" occurs around 9 months, and following commands with gestures occurs just prior to a year. Overall, the comprehension of language begins before the first words are expressed. Like expressive language skills, the length and complexity of the commands and questions that a child can comprehend and follow improve as the child's overall language skills mature. By the time the child reaches 3 years of age, he or she is able to answer "Wh-" questions, such as "What is your name?" Likewise, at 3 years, the ability to differentiate various prepositions develops and children are then able to follow various prepositional commands.

Beyond 3 years, language acquisition becomes more complex, with the improvement and refinement of grammar, syntax, and pragmatics. Although receptive language skills and vocabulary continue to increase throughout the preschool years, the understanding of language, including more abstract concepts, continues to develop and may develop ahead of the actual utterances associated with these thoughts. Pragmatics, or the social appropriateness of language usage, also continues to improve with the ability to "read" emotional expression or use appropriate forms of speech. Phonetic skills likewise progress to the point that all sounds can be produced by 9 years of age at the latest. Sounds such as *s*, *z*, *ng*, or *s* clusters may be the last to be mastered (Smit, Hand, Freilinger, Bernthal, & Bird, 1990).

EVALUATION

There is always cause for concern when a child does not meet these early language milestones at appropriate times. This can occur in one or more of the various substreams of language development, including expressive or receptive language, or can manifest as specific problems in vocabulary, syntax, phonology, or pragmatics. Various terms are used to describe specific abnormal attainment of milestones. A child who is significantly behind age-appropriate language skills would be considered to have *language delay*. Some children meet milestones irregularly with scatter, thus skipping some earlier milestones while they learn other higher language skills. This is frequently called *deviancy* in language development. *Dissociation* is the term frequently used to describe those children who have variable rates of development within the different language streams, particularly in expressive and receptive language. For example, expressive language skills may be more delayed than receptive language skills. Also very concerning are those children who have lost previously mastered language skills, which is a *degeneration* of abilities. In evaluating a child with abnormal language or communication skills development, it is important to remember these definitions as well as the other specific substreams of language.

There are a number of methods available to the pediatrician or practitioner in assessing a child where there are concerns about language. The first and foremost of such methods would be a very careful history, paying particular attention to developmental milestones in all of the developmental streams, including gross motor, fine motor, and adaptive. Other information from the medical history would include any parental concerns regarding hearing status and any particular behavioral concerns, including how the child is able to interact with other people and the environment. Likewise, a family history looking for other family members with speech or language problems or learning disabilities, particularly in reading, which also is communication based, might provide important clues as to the etiology of the child's delay. A good physical examination, including the child's general behaviors and interactions, any dysmorphic features, the oral-motor structures, hearing status, and a good neurologic evaluation, is essential in assessing a child's language delays. Thus, a complete history and physical examination emphasizing the various streams of development as well as the child's overall ability to interact is very important because language is interrelated with other areas of the child's daily functioning.

For those children less than 3 years of age, there are various screens that can be done by the pediatrician or health care provider to assess more specifically a child's overall language development. Included in this group is the Clinical Linguistic and Auditory Milestone Scale (CLAMS) (Capute et al., 1986). Using this scale, developmental language quotients can be obtained in both the receptive and the expressive language streams. It covers the prelinguistic as well as the early linguistic milestones. Information to complete the CLAMS can be obtained either from direct observation and examination or from parent history and indicates the child's specific language level of functioning at that particular time (Capute, Shapiro, & Palmer, 1987).

When the other portion of the test instrument, the Clinical Adaptive Test (CAT), is used in conjunction, information can be obtained not just about the child's language abilities but also about his or her visual-motor skills. Thus with this combination the examiner gets a much better idea of the child's overall cognitive abilities. Developmental quotients (DQs) can be obtained in both cognitive streams by dividing the average age score obtained on the testing by the child's chronologic age. A disassociation between the CLAMS, or the language portion of the test, and the nonlanguage, or CAT, portion would indicate a potential communication or language disorder, if the language score is significantly lower. If both areas on this test show a significant delay—in other words, a global delay in overall cognitive function—other differential diagnoses, such as mental retardation, might be indicated. Thus in combination the CAT/CLAMS is a useful tool not only in determining the present language skill level but also as a first step in defining an etiology or differential diagnoses (Hoon, Pulsifer, Gopalan, Palmer, & Capute, 1993).

For older children, language development has become much more complex, and the various substreams of language are attaining ever greater prominence in the development of language. In the older child, it becomes much more difficult to tease out specific language disorders on one simple developmental screen. Very few screening tools available to the pediatrician or health care provider go beyond age 3. The aid of a good speech pathologist is always useful in differentiating speech and language delays or disorders but becomes much more critical in evaluating these much older children with suspected speech and language problems.

DIFFERENTIAL DIAGNOSES

A number of children may initially present to the clinician as having a "simple language delay," yet this is just a description of one area of a child's functioning. An etiology or a more specific diagnosis must be determined in any child undergoing a language assessment for delays. Making the appropriate diagnosis may have an impact on future treatment as well as overall prognosis for the child.

Hearing Impairment

First on the list of differential diagnoses that must be considered is the hearing status of the child with language delay. Some but not all children with hearing impairment already have noticeable signs prior to their first birthday. They may not respond to sounds, particularly those produced behind them and out of their line of vision, as would be expected. The quantity and quality of prelinguistic skills such as babbling and cooing may vary from typical to severely impaired. There is still a subpopulation of deaf children who can meet their early intrinsic language milestones either on target or close to the expected time. It is only once the external stimuli to learn particular words in a specific language play a factor in language development that the delays and the hearing impairment become more evident (Murphy, 1964). Children with a partial hearing loss may pick up some words. They may have difficulty producing those sounds that they have difficulty hearing, such as high-tone sounds in those children with a high-frequency hearing loss (Rutter, 1972). Often children with isolated hearing impairment will try to communicate by some other means besides verbally. They tend to make eye contact, may use gestures spontaneously, and are generally described as interactive and sociable.

The prevalence of sensory hearing loss ranges between 0.56 and 2.3 per 1,000 children, with genetic etiologies being responsible in about 30%–50% of these children (Davidson, Hyde, & Alberti, 1988; see also Chapter 32, this volume). Other causes of hearing impairment may include congenital infections, particularly rubella or cytomegalovirus, meningitis, and ototoxic medications. The prevalence of an unknown etiology for children with hearing impairment may range from 10% to 40% (Allen & Schubert-Sudia, 1990).

With modern technology, children of any age can now be tested for hearing status. These forms of testing include brainstem-evoked auditory response, otoacoustic emissions, testing in the sound field condition, and pure-tone testing under headphones. The latter often is done better in the older, somewhat more mature and cooperative child. With accurate testing, information is available as to the degree of hearing loss, the frequencies involved, and whether this is unilateral or bilateral in nature. Some hearing loss may be corrected or partially compensated for by hearing aids. Other adjustments, too, may need to be made in teaching of "language" and communication skills in an alternate fashion, such as the use of sign language.

Cognitive Disability

A common reason for not meeting language milestones is a more global developmental delay or mental retardation. Language as well as the other developmental streams, particularly the visual-motor stream and adaptive skills, are an important component of overall cognition. A delay in early language milestones may be the first indicator of the child's mental capacity, particularly to parents of the child with mild mental retardation, because early gross motor milestones may have been on target. Rather than a delay in an isolated area of language development or a disordered language, these children may show more of an immaturity of their overall language skills. Interest in communicating with others may be present, particularly in the milder forms of mental retardation, but may be delayed in its timing or expression.

Silva found that approximately 85% of the 3-year-old children in his longitudinal study who had delays in both receptive and expressive language also had low IQ scores. When only one area, either receptive or expressive language, was delayed, a much lesser percentage of children also had low IQ scores. When followed up 2 years later, as many as 75% of these children still were described as having an IQ of less than 77, showing a fairly high stability over time (Silva, 1980). The possibility of an overall cognitive delay should not be overlooked in any child with a language impairment, because it has implications for further education.

Autism

Autism, a disorder mainly descriptive in nature, can be thought of as the more severe end of the spectrum encompassed by the term *pervasive developmental disorder* (see Chapter 23, this volume). It is defined by three major categories as outlined by the *Diagnostic and Statistical Manual of Mental Disorders*, fourth edition (DSM-IV): language impairment, abnormal or deviant social development, and stereotypical behaviors with findings expressed in children prior to 3 years of age. Mental retardation is not a specific criterion for a diagnosis of autism but often is an associated finding with this condition (American Psychiatric Association, 1994). Kanner (1943), in originally describing autism, did not find his patients to have mental retardation (see also Chapter 24, this volume).

The language delay in these children may be so severe as to present as an *aphasia*; thus the children have no expressive language. Those children who do develop language skills often show impairments along the whole range of severity. Echolalia, both immediate and delayed, is commonly heard, giving the impression on casual observation that expressive skills are better than they functionally are. This finding is sometimes described as cocktail chatter talk. Requests by the child may be phrased as a question as if exactly echoed from a previously heard question. Difficulty with appropriate pronoun usage is a feature, with these children often referring to themselves by their given name or "you" instead of the appropriate "me" or "I." A subpopulation of about 37% of children with autism may develop some language, such as a small, single-word vocabulary, and lose these

skills around 18 months of age. The reason for this loss has not yet been determined (Kurita, 1985).

Language impairment is only one of the aspects of autism. A significant impairment in socialization skills, including poor eye contact and various degrees of unresponsiveness to other people in the immediate environment, is present. When this aspect of autism is combined with the language impairment, very poor pragmatic communication skills can result in the child. Kanner, in his early descriptions, used the term "extreme autistic aloneness" to describe these children (1944, p. 211). Frith's description was of a "beautiful child imprisoned in a glass shell" (1993, p. 108).

According to the Utah Epidemiologic Study by Ritvo and co-workers, the prevalence of autism is 4 per 10,000 in the general population, with a male-to-female ratio of 4:1. There is an increased recurrence risk in families who already have one autistic child of 8.6%, which increases to 14.5% if this first affected child is a female. The recurrence risk goes up to 35% if there are already two older affected children (Ritvo et al., 1989). The exact etiology of autism in general is not certain, but several other conditions can be reminiscent of autism, including fragile X syndrome (Goldson & Hagerman, 1992; see also Chapter 17, this volume) and Rett syndrome (American Psychiatric Association, 1994; see also Chapter 25, this volume).

Selective Mutism

Selective mutism is a much less common condition that often starts before the age of 5 or 6 years, around the time the child first leaves home to go to school. These children are otherwise healthy, without hearing impairment and generally with average intelligence. Speech and language milestones are usually met on time, and these children speak in a typical manner in certain situations, usually the home, yet do not speak in various other specific social environments, very frequently the school (American Psychiatric Association, 1994). Most commonly this is a transient condition, although it can persist at times (Wilkins, 1985). Some authors have alluded to these children as shy, anxious, or manipulative and have called selective mutism a neurosis. Sometimes this was believed to be a family problem involving an overattachment to a family member. There is generally a similar frequency in both sexes, although there might be a slightly increased prevalence in girls (American Psychiatric Association, 1994). Some studies, however, on careful evaluation of these children have found that some 33% may have an underlying speech problem (Wilkins, 1985).

Landau-Kleffner Syndrome

One other entity causing considerable language difficulties is seizures, very specifically the Landau-Kleffner syndrome. This is a rare disorder in which typically developing children in their late preschool to early school years develop severe aphasia associated with electroencephalographic changes and often overt seizure activity. The children remain socially interactive, unlike with autism, although some develop behavior problems. No further degeneration is noted (Landau & Kleffner, 1957).

The language disorder in Landau-Kleffner syndrome is more of a verbal–auditory *agnosia* (Rapin, Mattis, Rowan, & Golden, 1977), or difficulty understanding spoken language, with the expressive component thought to be secondary to the receptive disorder (Mantovani & Landau, 1980). Many children initially are perceived as deaf, yet hearing test results are normal. The exact pathology is uncertain because no structural defect has been noted on computerized tomography. It has been proposed that the disturbance involves cerebral integration (Gordon, 1990) or a high-level auditory processing disorder (Bishop, 1985). The exact etiology likewise is unclear. Gascon, Victor, Lombroso, and Goodglass (1973) suggested an encephalitis.

The seizures appear to be short lived, lasting a few years in those children who have been followed over the long term. Speech usually recovers, often after speech therapy and special education, although a number of children have residual language deficits, including difficulty understanding speech with background noise (Mantovani & Landau, 1980). The younger the child at onset of symptoms, the more likely he or she is to have residual difficulties (Bishop, 1985).

Speech Impediments

When a child is not speaking, he or she may be exhibiting speech difficulties because of an isolated speech impediment or phonologic delay. These difficulties may include delay in phonologic development, a true dysarthria, or stuttering, which is also called dysfluency. Dysfluency in particular may be heard in very young children as they are first learning vocabulary, but it usually does not cause an impediment to speech, nor does it persist. If these problems are prolonged or are found in association with other delays, this could be an indication of another diagnosis (Ingram, 1972).

Other considerations in a child with difficulty speaking may include anatomic or functional problems with sound production, as in a child with cleft palate or cerebral palsy. Speech delays in a child with cerebral palsy in particular may be multifactorial because a number of these children also have mental retardation in addition to their motor impairment, which may be affecting language development. Other multifactorial considerations would be hearing impairment in addition to the functional oral-motor or coordination difficulties. Particularly, those children with a choreoathetoid form of cerebral palsy seem to be more likely to have a dysarthric or slowed and labored speech. Other children with the hemiplegic form of cerebral palsy may be more likely to have a typical speech pattern (Ingram, 1964).

Developmental Language Disorders

When all other etiologies have been ruled out, the developmental language disorders remain. These usually occur in children with average IQs and normal hearing with no other neurologic deficits or loss of skills. No definite classification system has been established yet for these children, who frequently are categorized descriptively as having either a receptive or expressive language delay or disorder. Those children categorized as having a communication disorder usually have language skills that are significantly behind other nonlanguage cognitive skills, with a 15-point or greater IQ difference classically being given as the definition.

Rapin and her group have further classified these developmental language disorders, which she calls dysphasias. They have grouped these dysphasias roughly into three categories. The first group, which they call output disturbances, include disturbances of expressive language in which comprehension is normal. Phonologic disorders, including severe dysfluencies and more complex articulation problems, would also fall under this subcategory. The second category is a mixed disturbance in which expressive language is impaired but there also are difficulties with receptive language or comprehension of language. Included in this group would be verbal–auditory agnosia as an extreme example, in which the child develops no or minimal language skills. The third group is the higher order of processing disorders. The clarity of speech is usually good in this group, but the content and composition of the speech may be abnormal (Klein & Rapin, 1990).

CONCLUSIONS

Language skills are one portion of the stream of development making up overall cognition. Needless to say, it is a very important portion because language and communication abilities have a very strong impact on overall functioning in day-to-day life, particularly in regard to socialization skills. Any child who is showing delays or abnormalities in the development of speech and language skills warrants an evaluation and appropriate further intervention.

REFERENCES

Allen, M.C., & Schubert-Sudia, S.E. (1990). Prevention of prelingual hearing impairment. *Seminars in Hearing, 11,* 134–149.

American Psychiatric Association. (1994). *Diagnostic and statistical manual of mental disorders* (4th ed.). Washington, DC: American Psychiatric Press.

Aram, D.M., Ekelman, B.L., & Nation, J.E. (1984). Preschoolers with language disorders: 10 years later. *Journal of Speech and Hearing Research, 27,* 232–244.

Beitchman, J.H., Nair, R., Clegg, M., & Patel, P.G. (1986). Prevalence of speech and language disorders in 5-year-old kindergarten children in the Ottawa-Carleton region. *Journal of Speech and Hearing Disorders, 51,* 98–110.

Bishop, D.V.M. (1985). Age of onset and outcome in "acquired aphasia with convulsive disorder" (Landau-Kleffner syndrome). *Developmental Medicine and Child Neurology, 27,* 705–712.

Cantwell, D.P., Baker, L., & Mattison, R. (1981). Prevalence, type, and correlates of psychiatric diagnoses in 200 children with communication disorder. *Developmental and Behavioral Pediatrics, 2,* 131–136.

Capute, A.J., Palmer, F.B., Shapiro, B.K., Wachtel, R.C., Schmidt, S., & Ross, A. (1986). Clinical linguistic and auditory milestone scale: Prediction of cognition in infancy. *Developmental Medicine and Child Neurology, 28,* 762–771.

Capute, A.J., Shapiro, B.K., & Palmer, F.B. (1987). Marking the milestones of language development. *Contemporary Pediatrics, 4,* 24–41.

Cohen, N.J., Davine, M., & Meloche-Kelly, M. (1989). Prevalence of unsuspected language disorders in a child psychiatric population. *Journal of the American Academy of Child and Adolescent Psychiatry, 28,* 107–111.

Davidson, J., Hyde, M.L., & Alberti, P.W. (1988). Epidemiology of hearing impairment in childhood. *Scandinavian Audiology Supplementum, 30,* 13–20.

Fay, W.H. (1967). Childhood echolalia: A group study of late abatement. *Folia Phoniatrica, 19,* 297–306.

Fletcher, P. (1987). Aspects of language development in the preschool years. In W. Yule & M. Rutter (Eds.), *Language development and disorders (Clinics in Developmental Medicine, No. 101/102)* (pp. 70–89). Oxford, England: Blackwell Scientific Publications Ltd.

Frith, U. (1993, June). Autism. *Scientific American, 268*(6), 108–114.

Fundudis, T., Kolvin, I., & Garside, R.F. (1979). *Speech retarded and deaf children: Their psychological development.* London: Academic Press.

Gascon, G., Victor, D., Lombroso, C.T., & Goodglass, H. (1973). Language disorder, convulsive disorder, and electroencephalographic abnormalities. *Archives of Neurology, 28,* 156–162.

Goldson, E., & Hagerman, R.J. (1992). The fragile X syndrome. *Developmental Medicine and Child Neurology, 34,* 822–832.

Gordon, N. (1990). Acquired aphasia in childhood: The Landau-Kleffner syndrome. *Developmental Medicine and Child Neurology, 32,* 267–274.

Hay, D.A., Prior, M., Collett, S., & Williams, M. (1987). Speech and language development in preschool twins. *Acta Geneticae Medicae et Gemellologiae (Roma), 36,* 213–223.

Hoon, A., Pulsifer, M., Gopalan, R., Palmer, F., & Capute, A. (1993). Clinical Adaptive Test/Clinical Linguistic Auditory Milestone Scale in early cognitive assessment. *The Journal of Pediatrics, 123,* 81–88.

Ingram, T.T.S. (1964). The complex speech disorders of cerebral palsied children. In C. Renfrew & K. Murphy (Eds.), *The child who does not talk* (*Clinics in Developmental Medicine, No. 13*) (pp. 163–170). London: The Spastics Society Medical Education and Information Unit in Association with William Heinemann Medical Books Ltd.

Ingram, T.T.S. (1972). The classification of speech and language disorders in young children. In M. Rutter & J.A.M. Martin (Eds.), *The child with delayed speech* (*Clinics in Developmental Medicine, No. 43*) (pp. 13–32). London: William Heinemann Medical Books Ltd.

Kanner, L. (1943). Autistic disturbances of affective contact. *Nervous Child, 2*, 217–250.

Kanner, L. (1944). Early infantile autism. *Journal of Pediatrics, 25*, 211–217.

Klein, S.K., & Rapin, I. (1990). Clinical assessment of pediatric disorders of higher cerebral function. *Current Problems in Pediatrics, 20*(1), 7–60.

Kurita, H. (1985). Infantile autism with speech loss before the age of thirty months. *Journal of the American Academy of Child Psychiatry, 24*, 191–196.

Landau, W.M., & Kleffner, F.R. (1957). Syndrome of acquired aphasia with convulsive disorder in children. *Neurology, 7*, 523–530.

Mantovani, J.F., & Landau, W.M. (1980). Acquired aphasia with convulsive disorder: Course and progress. *Neurology, 30*, 524–529.

Martlew, M. (1987). Prelinguistic communication. In W. Yule & M. Rutter (Eds.), *Language development and disorders* (*Clinics in Developmental Medicine, No. 101/102*) (pp. 53–69). Oxford, England: Blackwell Scientific Publications Ltd.

Mittler, P. (1970). Biological and social aspects of language development in twins. *Developmental Medicine and Child Neurology, 12*, 741–757.

Murphy, K. (1964). Development of normal vocalisation and speech. In C. Renfrew & K. Murphy (Eds.), *The child who does not talk* (*Clinics in Developmental Medicine, No. 13*) (pp. 11–15). London: The Spastics Society Medical Education and Information Unit in Association with William Heinemann Medical Books, Ltd.

Rapin, I., Mattis, S., Rowan, A.J., & Golden, G.G. (1977). Verbal auditory agnosia in children. *Developmental Medicine and Child Neurology, 19*, 192–207.

Ritvo, E.R., Jorde, L.B., Mason-Brothers, A., Freeman, B.J., Pingree, C., Jones, M.B., McMahon, W.M., Petersen, P.B., Jenson, W.R., & Mo, A. (1989). The UCLA-University of Utah Epidemiologic Survey of Autism: Recurrence risk estimates and genetic counseling. *American Journal of Psychiatry, 146*, 1032–1036.

Rutter, M. (1972). Clinical assessment of language disorders in the young child. In M. Rutter & J.A.M. Martin (Eds.), *The child with delayed speech* (*Clinics in Developmental Medicine, No. 43*) (pp. 33–47). London: William Heinemann Medical Books Ltd.

Rutter, M., & Bax, M. (1972). The normal development of speech and language. In M. Rutter & J.A.M. Martin (Eds.), *The child with delayed speech* (*Clinics in Developmental Medicine, No. 43*) (pp. 1–12). London: William Heinemann Medical Books Ltd.

Rutter, M., Graham, P., & Yule, W. (1970). *A neuropsychiatric study in childhood* (*Clinics in Developmental Medicine, No. 35/36*). London: Spastics International Medical Publications in association with William Heinemann Medical Books Ltd.

Silva, P.A. (1980). The prevalence, stability and significance of developmental language delay in preschool children. *Developmental Medicine and Child Neurology, 22*, 768–777.

Silva, P.A., McGee, R., & Williams, S.M. (1983). Developmental language delay from three to seven years and its significance for low intelligence and reading diffculties at age seven. *Developmental Medicine and Child Neurology, 25*, 783–793.

Silva, P.A., Williams, S., & McGee, R. (1987). A longitudinal study of children with developmental language delay at age three: Later intelligence, reading and behavior problems. *Developmental Medicine and Child Neurology, 29*, 630–640.

Smit, A.B., Hand, L., Freilinger, J.J., Bernthal, J.E., & Bird, A. (1990). The Iowa Articulation Norms Project and its Nebraska replication. *Journal of Speech and Hearing Disorders, 55*, 779–798.

Stevenson, J., & Richman, N. (1976). The prevalence of language delay in a population of three-year-old children and its association with general retardation. *Developmental Medicine and Child Neurology, 18*, 431–441.

Wilkins, R. (1985). A comparison of elective mutism and emotional disorders in children. *British Journal of Psychiatry, 146*, 198–203.

Chapter 23

Autism and Other Communication Disorders

Jon Matthew Farber, M.D.

Communication disorders, along with mental retardation and cerebral palsy, constitute the "big three" of early childhood developmental disabilities. Of the communication disorders, autism is the most extreme form; it is also the most researched and has been the most confusing since it was first described by Kanner and Asperger over 50 years ago (e.g., Kanner, 1943). With an estimated incidence on the order of 4 per 10,000 for autism, and a higher incidence for the less severe forms, the communication disorders are common enough that it is necessary for the pediatrician working in the field of developmental disabilities to have a good understanding of them. This chapter emphasizes a clinical approach to the child with a communication disorder, focusing primarily on autism as a prototype.

DIAGNOSIS OF AUTISM

The diagnostic process begins when the child is referred for evaluation. Although most referrals are initiated by the child's pediatrician, many also originate either with the parents themselves (when the child's primary physician has advocated a "wait-and-see" approach) or with early childhood education specialists who have been working with the child because of developmental delays. Perhaps surprisingly, autism is not often raised as a possibility by either the parents or the professionals. Most often the chief complaint is delayed speech; other possibilities include generalized delays, behavioral problems, or possible deafness.

Given the complaint, the practitioner then proceeds along traditional pathways toward a diagnosis. History is primary, physical examina-

tion secondary, and laboratory tests ancillary. The data generated are next compared to the diagnostic criteria for autism to determine degree of fit. Multiple criteria have been proposed to establish a diagnosis. The most commonly used are those of the *Diagnostic and Statistical Manual of Mental Disorders*, fourth edition (DSM-IV) (American Psychiatric Association, 1994). The DSM-IV represents an attempt to provide objective criteria (e.g., 1 out of 4 behavioral criteria are required), although it is clear that subjective features remain (as in the emphasis on "qualitative" impairments). The reality is that autism is a descriptive diagnosis rather than a physiologic, biochemical, genetic, or other such diagnosis, encompassing heterogeneous entities; as such, exact objectivity is not possible, and it is usually not very productive to debate whether a given "borderline" child falls just within or without the diagnostic boundaries. The DSM-IV does contain a category for "autistic-like" conditions in children who do not quite meet criteria for autism, called *pervasive developmental disorder not otherwise specified* (PDD-NOS).

Although the DSM-IV can provide an approach to diagnosis, it is easier—and in a clinical (as opposed to research) setting, probably just as useful—to base a diagnosis on the following four criteria, proposed by Rutter (1971):

1. Serious impairment in the development of social skills
2. Delayed and deviant language development
3. Ritualistic and compulsive behavior
4. Onset before 30 months

Symptoms that truly begin after 30–36 months, as documented by detailed history, strongly argue against autism.

As previously stated, history is the most important part of making a diagnosis. Impairment in the development of social skills will be evidenced by such features as delayed smiling, aloofness/withdrawn behavior, using people as objects, lack of interest in playing with others, and so forth. Language milestone ascertainment allows determination of linguistic delay and deviancy. Frequently seen deviancies include pronominal reversal, echolalia, and the presence of "superior" expressive abilities as a result of rote verbal production. Common ritualistic and compulsive behaviors include a fascination with spinning objects, self-stimulation, lining up toys or other items in a repetitive fashion, and extreme perseveration.

The physical examination can help the diagnosis. For this purpose, the neurodevelopmental examination is central, with the emphasis on supporting the information obtained by history; searching for autistic features in the child's interactions, play, and language use; or both. Does the child respond to people as objects, exhibit awareness of his or her environment, or engage in stereotypy? What is the child's level of language? How is language used? What are the child's other developmental skills? For diagnostic purposes, these are the key features.

The traditional physical examination may provide clues to the cause of autism (Table 1), but will not assist in determining whether or not autism is present. Many organic conditions have been associated with autism (Gillberg & Coleman, 1993). Use of a Wood's lamp to detect signs of tuberous sclerosis or hypomelanosis of

Table 1. Organic conditions reported in association with autism

Phenylketonuria
Tuberous sclerosis
Hypomelanosis of Ito
Congenital rubella syndrome
de Lange syndrome
Goldenhar syndrome
Sotos syndrome
Thalidomide embryopathy
Lead poisoning
Down syndrome
Fetal alcohol syndrome
Fragile X syndrome

Ito should be incorporated into the examination. It should be noted that, of the organic conditions associated with autism, none are fully specific or sensitive for this condition, but rather simply reflect that brain damage (from whatever cause) and autism go together.

The laboratory neither confirms nor denies the diagnosis: Autism is a clinical diagnosis. The laboratory is therefore used as an adjunct to explore etiology. Routinely, testing for the fragile X chromosome anomaly should be obtained in boys, because this appears to be present in 2%–5% of cases of autism (Wright, Young, Edwards, Abramson, & Duncan, 1986), and the absence of the full clinical phenotype is not sufficient to rule out the entity, particularly in younger children (see Chapter 17, this volume). There are insufficient data to indicate the value of testing girls, although some authorities advocate this as well. Phenylketonuria should be assessed in children with profound retardation because, even with universal screening, some cases are missed. Other laboratory tests can be ordered based on suspicions raised by the history and physical (e.g., a computerized tomography scan if tuberous sclerosis is suspected). It should be noted that routine neuroimaging studies are not indicated in the evaluation of autism. Although some subtle abnormalities, such as cerebellar hypoplasia or forebrain defects, have been reported, they are inconsistent at best and add nothing to the diagnosis or treatment of the individual child. It should also be noted that, in the large majority of cases, establishing a specific etiology is not of benefit in guiding treatment, but is primarily of use in giving parents a "cause" for their child's condition.

One last test that should be performed in all children with autism is a formal hearing assessment. Although one can usually determine on examination that a child is not profoundly deaf, an accurate audiologic evaluation is necessary to rule out lesser degrees of hearing loss.

It must be noted that an exploration of parenting skills is not part of the diagnostic process (although such information will be helpful in providing treatment advice). Early theories that autism is induced by abnormal parenting have been refuted, although unfortunately this perception still persists among some professionals and lay people. There is a plethora of data indicating that specific personality traits or nurturing deficits are not seen in the parents of autistic children (McAdoo & DeMyer, 1978). Conversely, the organic basis of autism is positively indicated from several different avenues, including its association with genetic defects (Baumgardner & Reiss, 1994) and embryopathies (Chess, 1971), increased incidence of neuro-anatomic abnormalities on imaging studies (Courchesne, Press, & Yeung-Courchesne, 1993; Courchesne et al., 1994), abnormal central spinal fluid neurotransmitter concentrations (Martineau, Barthélémy, Jouve, Muh, & Lelord, 1992), and the presence of language/cognitive delays in "unaffected" siblings (Minton, Campbell, Green, Jennings, & Samit, 1982).

What sorts of errors are made when considering the diagnosis of autism? Of what pitfalls must the practitioner beware? False-positive diagnoses are rare, unless a hearing test is not performed on a deaf child. Although physicians may disagree in some cases as to whether a child is autistic or autistic-like, for practical purposes, this is of little importance. Similarly, whether, for example, Asperger syndrome represents a subgroup of high-functioning individuals with autism or is a completely separate entity may be of importance in a research setting, but clinically it does not impact on the approach to the individual child (see Chapter 24, this volume).

There are some cases of autism in which development is close to typical during the first year or so, following which there is a stage of regression before the child reaches a new plateau and then resumes forward development, albeit slowly, from there. This can raise some diagnostic confusion between autism and a degenerative condition. However, the latter usually will be accompanied by "hard" neurologic signs such as hyperreflexia, spasticity, retinal changes, and seizures. If doubts persist after an appropriate evaluation, an observation period of a few months will confirm whether there is further regression or attainment of a plateau. Another possible source of a false-positive diagnosis is Rett syndrome, which shares some behavioral overlap with autism. However, once the possibility of the former is ascertained, it is straightforward to distinguish between the two (Olsson & Rett, 1987; see also Chapter 25, this volume).

One pitfall that can result in a false diagnosis is an overreliance on questionnaires. Several have been proposed, and they are reliable at distinguishing the autistic from the developmentally normal population. However, they have not been shown to be sufficiently accurate at separating autism from severe to profound mental retardation.

The more common diagnostic error is the false negative. One cause of this is professional reluctance to use the word "autism" for fear of labeling a child. It does no good to avoid the diagnostic term when appropriate. Short-term gains (e.g., not upsetting parents) are more than offset by long-term losses (e.g., parental resentment when the truth is finally revealed). A second reason for missing the diagnosis results from overinterpreting inflated language skills in deciding that a child does not have delayed and deviant language. Echolalia combined with excellent verbal memory may enable a child to talk in long sentences. The key here is to realize the rote nature of the skill as distinct from any understanding of language per se, because the latter is the important feature of useful language. Thus, a child may ask, "What's your name?", "How are you?", "Where do you live?", and sound as though he or she is conversing. However, if the child goes through this litany without regard for the answers, his or her language skills are not typical.

Perhaps the most common error in making the diagnosis of autism, however, is that of incompleteness—omitting the consideration of mental retardation once autism is diagnosed. Many people, including professionals and parents, believe that a diagnosis of autism implies typical intellectual functioning, just waiting for some key to unlock it. In fact, most people with autism have mental retardation, usually moderate to profound (DeMyer et al., 1974). When autism and retardation coexist, it is essential to diagnose both entities; they are not mutually exclusive.

DIAGNOSIS OF COMMUNICATION DISORDERS

As previously noted, autism represents a subgroup on one end of the spectrum of communication disorders. The diagnostic confusion over autism is minor compared to that which exists for communication disorders, for which there are no well-accepted definitions. Various attempts have been made to standardize diagnoses, usually from one of two perspectives: neuroanatomic or specific processing features. Both are inherently flawed.

Neuroanatomic approaches tend to be based on concepts derived from adult neurology, in which such terms as *aphasia*, *dysphasia*, and *oromotor apraxia* are encountered. All of these proposed systems suffer from the same flaw. Communication disorders in children are developmental phenomena, whereas those in adults are not. Aphasia is a valid, reproducible phenomenon in adults, localizable in the brain following such injury as a stroke, and therefore adults with similar dominant hemisphere injuries present similar language impairments. In children, however, our understanding of the neuroanatomic underpinnings is still in its infancy; the site of brain damage in a communication disorder is typically not localizable. Thus, two children who appear "aphasic" may have two completely different sets of deficits, a finding obscured by a neuroanatomic categorization.

Another approach has been to try to sort communication disorders by processing features such as verbal retrieval, auditory memory, and the like. Communication disorders are therefore subtyped according to the presumed underlying processing deficits, as determined by neuropsychological testing. Although this approach offers a greater potential at present than the neuroanatomic one, it can only be as accurate as the measures employed. Unfortunately, pediatric neuropsychological tests are less well standardized than, for example, intelligence tests (Hooper & Tramontana, 1992). The processes they purportedly tap are often labels chosen by the creator of the test, and thus a child may have, for example, normal auditory sequencing abilities on one measure but not another. The result is that this approach to classifying communication disorders, although promising (particularly from a research aspect), is of unproven clinical utility.

At present, therefore, the concept of a communication disorder, like that of autism, should be viewed as primarily descriptive. Two broad categories can be defined: global communication disorders, in which language skills are significantly below performance skills, and expressive language disorders, in which expressive language skills are significantly below both receptive language and performance skills. In this definition, "significant" can be defined as a gap of 15 or more IQ or developmental quotient (DQ) points.

It should be noted that there is no entity for a receptive language disorder. True expressive skills cannot exceed receptive abilities. One cannot state a thought with meaning (expressive language) without understanding it (receptive language). In situations in which this at first appears to be the case, closer inspection will reveal that the expressive abilities are rote, without true usefulness. An apparent receptive language disorder thus indicates an actual global deficit.

Just as in autism, communication disorders and mental retardation are not mutually exclusive. A child with a performance IQ of 50 and a verbal IQ of 20 has mental retardation with a superimposed communication disorder. One should also not make the mistake of assuming a child is of average intelligence based solely on performance skills. A child with a performance IQ of 100 and a verbal IQ of 50 is not of average intelligence because language, a main (if not the main) determinant of intelligence, is impaired. This is a child with typical performance skills (not average intelligence) and a communication disorder. Furthermore, his or her typical performance skills do not imply that he or she therefore has the "potential" for typical verbal skills.

Communication disorders usually present in one of two ways. The more straightforward is the child who is not talking (see Chapter 22, this volume). The second presentation is that of behavioral concerns, including possible hyperactivity, aggression, disobedience, and difficulty toileting. Once the possibility of a communication disorder is established, the diagnostic process proceeds as with autism: history, physical examination, developmental evaluation, and laboratory tests. Some children will meet the full criteria for autism, some will have a "pure"

communication disorder without significant behavioral components, and others will fall in between, with autistic-like features.

One last point must be emphasized. A diagnosis of autism or other communication disorders can be made by the pediatrician. Input
from psychologists, special education specialists, and others is valuable, particularly for planning treatment, but is not required for making a
diagnosis. This is because autism and communication disorders represent descriptive, qualitative categories, and normed psychometric quantitative values are not part of the definition. The
developmental pediatrician can assess levels of
functioning in the various developmental
spheres with sufficient accuracy to allow for
what is, after all, a descriptive diagnosis.

OUTCOME IN
AUTISM AND OTHER
COMMUNICATION DISORDERS

Although treatment and outcome are usually analyzed in that order, in autism and communication disorders, it is more useful to consider outcome before treatment. This is because, without
a firm understanding of the natural history of
these conditions, it is not possible to analyze the
effects of therapy. This is compounded by the
fact that language disorders encompass a heterogeneous population of children, resulting in
a variety of possible outcomes.

Outcome in Autism

Because of the fascinating nature of autism,
most of the language disability literature is concentrated on this small subgroup. Early assumptions that autism would evolve into adult schizophrenia have been shown to be erroneous
(Howells & Guirguis, 1984), and accordingly
autism is not to be considered an example of
childhood psychosis. The most common outcome, rather, is that autism evolves into mental
retardation (see below).

Cognitive functioning is the most important
predictor of outcome, as has been documented
repeatedly (DeMyer et al., 1973; Lotter, 1974),
regardless of the measure of intelligence used
(e.g., the Leiter Performance Scale or the Wechsler Intelligence Scale for Children). It is partic-

ularly accurate for children above the age of 5.
For younger children, if they do not have severe
to profound mental retardation, there is often a
catch-up or acceleration in cognitive abilities
(particularly in language) between the ages of 3
and 5, although even here the preschool IQ remains the best predictor. The presence or absence of language before age 5 has also been reported to be of predictive value. However, its
use is probably due to its high correlation with
overall IQ, and thus it can be viewed as a short-
cut to estimating IQ.

In general, the higher the IQ, the better the
outcome. Approximately half of autistic children with average intelligence can achieve independent adult status, and several have attended
college (Szatmari, Bartolucci, Bremner, Bond,
& Rich, 1989). Despite this level of academic
and social success, these individuals can continue to exhibit qualitative difficulties in
language and socialization. They are often relatively isolated, adhering closely to the boundaries of family and gravitating to occupations
that do not require much personal interaction or
initiative. Close, enduring relationships (e.g.,
marriage) are rare at best. Social quotients are
on the order of 20 points below the verbal IQ
(Rumsey, Rapoport, & Sceery, 1985), a
reversal of the discrepancy found in other
disabilities.

At the other end of the spectrum are those
children with severe to profound mental retardation as part of their autism, a group that represents the largest subcategory. As they develop,
so too do their language and social skills, generally to an extent where they outgrow many of
their autistic features. Their eye contact improves and they spend less time perseverating,
but the more obvious features of profound mental retardation emerge: poor to absent self-
care skills, minimal vocabulary, possibly self-
injurious behavior, and the like. Hyperkinesis
often gives way to hypokinetic behavior (Rutter, Greenfeld, & Lockyer, 1967). Without taking a history, it is often not possible to tell from
examining an adult with profound mental retardation whether or not he or she was autistic as a
child.

In between these two extremes lies a range of
cognitive and social impairments, reflecting the

heterogeneous nature of autism. The better the language development, the better the outcome; behavior and socialization abilities often reflect these skills. However, in the autistic person with nontypical language skills, obvious language problems remain, above and beyond those seen in someone of comparable IQ without autism. Conversational topics are often circumscribed (a type of stereotypy), and dysprosody is common.

Epilepsy has been seen often in autism, with an incidence around 25% overall (Wolf & Goldberg, 1986). Seizures usually begin in adolescence and are associated with IQ scores below 70. Many adolescents will experience a deterioration in behavior for unclear reasons. This can be either permanent or temporary, and is more common in, but not confined to, those teenagers who do develop seizures (Gillberg, 1991).

Looking at overall numbers, approximately 5% of children with autism become self-sufficient adults. Half do not develop useful language, and a similar proportion have hyperactive, aggressive, and/or self-injurious behavior. As adults, some 60% are completely dependent on others for daily living needs (Gillberg, 1991).

The most important point in predicting an outcome for autism is to realize that, by itself, the diagnosis of autism conveys very little prognostic information. This will be of crucial importance when examining the results of treatment, and especially claims of cures. An adult with autism can have profound mental retardation with total dependency in self-care skills, can be cognitively typical and fully independent, or can fall anywhere in between. It is essential to assess global intelligence, considering both performance and language skills, to determine prognosis. The older the child, the more accurate the prediction, but reasonable prognostic statements also can be made for the child below 5, particularly for the more impaired subgroup.

Outcome in Communication Disorders

Less is known concerning the natural outcome of early communication disorders. As with autism, there can be either normal or abnormal cognitive functioning. In the child with persisting language disabilities, performance skills tend to decline (Paul, Cohen, & Caparulo, 1983), decreasing the discrepancy between performance and verbal skills, so that the older child or adult will function more as a person with uniform mental retardation. Although there are adults with delayed language skills and typical performance abilities, this pattern is less common.

The other outcome is, of course, that of typical language development. This is the classic "slow talker" who "did not start talking until he had something to say." An experienced pediatrician will have seen many such children going on to become adults without language impairment, indicating that this is a typical developmental variant. However, in other children the outcome will be less favorable, with continuing language problems and a high incidence of learning disabilities. Studies suggest that 50% or more of these children will have academic underachievement (Silva, Williams, & McGee, 1987; Weiner, 1985).

Behavior problems are also seen with increasing frequency in the follow-up of children with communication disorders. These include such findings as attention-deficit/hyperactivity disorder and anxiety.

In trying to determine the most likely outcome in an individual child with a communication disorder, the developmental evaluation is, as always, of primary importance. The family history may reveal a similar pattern, and having relatives who "outgrew" their delays fully is a positive predictor. However, care must be exercised in obtaining the history; if, for example, a parent reports that he or she did not talk until age 2, it will obviously be of importance to determine whether by talking is meant saying the first word, or first phrases. Of more predictive value is, as always, the neurodevelopmental examination. As with autism, overall DQ/IQ remains the best predictor. During the examination, it is necessary to distinguish between performance skills, receptive language, nonverbal expressive language (i.e., gestures), and verbal expressive language capabilities. The better the language skills, the better the prognosis. The same is true of performance skills, but their predictive validity is weaker. Also, in observing the child carrying out performance tasks, the examiner often can sense whether these skills are being performed in a mechanical or rote fashion, having been memorized without an understanding of what precisely is being accomplished. Such children often will perseverate on the task, or else demonstrate little pleasure or enthusiasm. This is a warning sign that performance DQ may be overestimated, and will decline when the child is older. Regarding language deficits, global delays are obviously more worrisome than expressive ones, and are more likely to persist (Silva et al., 1987). The slow learner who is most likely to outgrow his or her disability is the younger one with a suggestive family history and typical performance, receptive language, and nonverbal expressive language skills.

A thorough developmental evaluation can provide a wealth of diagnostic and prognostic information. Even greater accuracy is gained from multiple observations over time, allowing the rate of progress to be determined. Thus, the child who will ultimately function as an adult with mental retardation will exhibit a continued slow rate of language development and a steady decline in performance skills, as the rote nature of many of these becomes limiting. Conversely, the child who is going to outgrow a language impairment will show an acceleration of skills, usually between the ages of 2 and 3, during which time he or she will start to demonstrate gains at a faster than normal rate. Reliable predictions about subsequent academic functioning, however, usually remain problematic until the child actually enters school.

Thus, the ultimate outcomes for autism and other communication disorders vary from profound retardation to normal functioning, with the complete range of language and learning disorders in between. The best single predictor is current functioning in all cognitive developmental skills, with language abilities being of greatest importance. The best overall predictor is sequential developmental evaluation, emphasizing once again the importance of careful developmental follow-up.

TREATMENT OF AUTISM AND OTHER COMMUNICATION DISORDERS

The treatment of communication disorders, particularly autism, must be viewed from an ame-

liorative or palliative, as opposed to curative, context. These disabilities are neurologically based, at some level related to the hard-wiring of the brain. No neuroscience techniques are currently available for complete repair, nor are any likely to become available in the near future. Although there are frequent reports of promising treatments or even cures, these must be received skeptically, in light of the natural history of the condition. Despite this caveat, treatment approaches are not to be dismissed. A number of therapies can lead to improved outcome, even though the underlying neurologic deficit is unchanged. Even for the more impaired children, treatment can improve functioning in areas such as self-care and behavior, while for the higher-functioning child, communication and learning can be enhanced to maximize potential.

Language, behavioral, neurochemical (medical), and parent education approaches are reviewed here. Unproven methods of treatment are also examined. These are legion, and will continue to flourish. A few of the more popular ones are examined, along with methods for critiquing future nonmainstream therapies.

Language Therapy

Language therapy, conducted by speech and language therapists directly or by classroom teachers under their supervision, is the main treatment approach for children with language impairment. Despite its wide use, there are few well-designed studies demonstrating that it is of any value. Most reports do not use control groups; those that do tend to show no gains or gains of dubious clinical significance (Cooper, Moodley, & Reynell, 1979; Stevenson, Bax, & Stevenson, 1982). Intervention techniques include modeling appropriate language, labeling objects, behaviorally based linguistic reinforcement, vocabulary instruction, and augmented communication/sign language (Simonson, 1979). Many children's communication disorders do progress rapidly while in therapy. Infants tend to do less well, presumably because they are more impaired (and hence diagnosed at a younger age), as do older children. The best results thus are seen in children during the age period in which there is the greatest probability of spontaneous improvement. Studies have not teased out the influence of therapy versus the influence of the natural history, nor have they documented whether short-term gains result in long-term improvement.

In any case, language therapy does ensure that the teacher and parent are focusing on stimulating the child, and this is beneficial, even if the precise nature of how this works remains unclear. Language therapy should not be viewed in a curative context, however. Rather, it should be seen as maximizing potential. Educational approaches such as language therapy entail determining which skills are developing in a child and helping them to emerge; it does not involve creating new skills de novo, without a child having the underlying building blocks. Thus an understanding of developmental sequence is of key importance in planning an educational program. A child cannot talk in sentences until he or she uses phrases, phrases are not spoken until there is a sufficient single-word vocabulary, and so forth. For therapy, the child's level of language is determined and he or she is then assisted in reaching the next step. Not providing such assistance can certainly impede learning, but there is no evidence that providing such aid in some fashion alters the underlying neurologic deficits. Education thus should be seen as maximizing some fixed potential (perhaps indeterminate but fixed, finite, and often subnormal, nevertheless) rather than curing the child's disability.

Behavior Modification

Behavior modification is another key approach in the treatment of autism in particular. The inward-directed, self-stimulating nature of the condition often makes it difficult to teach the child, and behavioral techniques have much to offer here. Success rates (defined as placement in a regular school program) as high as 47% have been reported (McEachin, Smith, & Lovaas, 1993), albeit with a preselected population. Many nonstandard therapies owe much of their success to incorporating behavior modification components.

The main techniques used for behavior modification are positive reinforcement, shaping, differential reinforcement of other behaviors (DRO), and punishment (Bellack & Hersen, 1985). They are not mutually exclusive. Positive reinforcement entails rewarding a desired behavior in order to increase the likelihood of its recurrence, such as providing a candy treat for pointing to a named object. Shaping involves reinforcing closer and closer approximations to the desired behavior. For example, if a child does not imitate words, he or she can first be reinforced for any noise, then for making sounds in response to an adult's sounds, then for imitating consonants, and finally for achieving word imitation. Although positive reinforcement techniques are theoretically straightforward, in practice they often require much ingenuity and a great deal of time. Some studies base their results on 40 or more hours per week of therapy conducted over several years.

In children with autism, it is often necessary to eliminate negative behaviors (e.g., spinning, self-injury) as well as promote positive ones. Extinction (the ignoring of undesirable behavior) often does not work well because self-stimulatory behaviors are often reinforcing in and of themselves. DRO can be useful here. In DRO, rewards are given for behavior incompatible with the undesirable ones, thus combining reinforcement with extinction. For example, two-handed toy play can be differentially reinforced and is incompatible with self-hitting.

In some cases, even DRO is insufficient, and negative behaviors can only be diminished by aversive techniques (i.e., punishment). In behavioral terms, punishment is the application of an aversive stimulus contingent on a given activity to reduce its occurrence. It is often confused with negative reinforcement, which involves removal of an aversive stimulus contingent on a desired behavior to increase its frequency. Thus, if pressing a bar avoids a mild shock, bar pressing will be negatively reinforced and increase in frequency. If pressing a bar results in a shock, this is a punishment, and bar pressing will decrease in frequency. Negative reinforcement is not commonly used in working with children. Punishment, however, despite a poor press, can be effective if properly applied under careful guidelines. Mild aversives may include saying no, hand slapping, and spraying with water. Time-out (removing a child to a quiet area for misbehaving), a well-known technique, also has a punishment component. For more severe behavior, such as self-injury, stronger aversives may be necessary, such as the Self-Injurious Behavior Inhibiting System (SIBIS), which produces a mild shock contingent on head banging (Linscheid, Hartel, & Cooley, 1993). Of course, aversive conditioning only eliminates behavior; it must be combined with positive reinforcement to build up an acceptable behavioral repertoire.

The literature on the behavioral treatment of autism consists largely of case reports that are almost always successful (a recognized publication bias). Furthermore, in order to achieve the best results, intensive intervention is necessary. For example, in the study by McEachin et al. (1993), the experimental group received 40 or more hours of one-on-one treatment weekly for 2 years, with treatment assignment based on the availability of therapists. In conducting a behavior modification program, the proper training and supervision of personnel appears to be crucial. Of all the treatment approaches available so far, behavior modification techniques appear to have the best success rate. Unfortunately, because of the labor-intensive nature of the intervention, it is not always possible to find the necessary financial and personnel resources in the community, and the search continues for a more widely applicable approach.

Psychopharmacology

As the concept that "psychiatric" disorders are frequently neurochemical in nature has gained greater general acceptance, and as more and more psychopharmacologic agents are developed, physicians are considering the use of medication as a treatment for autism more and more often. This approach holds the greatest theoretical promise for correcting the underlying biochemical defects causing autism, although, in practice, attainment has fallen far short of the promise. Along these lines, almost every "psychiatric" medication known has been tried in the autistic population (e.g., Sloman, 1991).

Reflecting the early view of autism as a type of psychosis, the first medications tried were the antipsychotics (major tranquilizers). Of these, haloperidol in dosages of 0.5–4.0 mg daily has been used most often. Reports show behavioral benefits, particularly for fidgetiness, hyperactivity, and aggression; gains in learning or increased socialization are less apparent (Anderson et al., 1984). This suggests that it is the sedating aspects of the medication that are of most benefit. Side effects of major tranquilizers are of course of concern, particularly tardive dyskinesia with long-term use, so that for most children with autism these medications are contraindicated, although they still can be of benefit for the more uncontrollable child.

Children with autism and other communication disorders often have secondarily shortened attention spans, so stimulant medications have been tried. There are no well-conducted studies in this area, but anecdotal evidence suggests some benefits, again primarily in behavior. Because stimulants do not enhance communicative cognitive skills, it is not anticipated that they would have much impact on *learning* (i.e., the acquisition and long-term retention of new material), although they may improve school *performance* (i.e., the production of material already learned). Nevertheless, stimulants have a good safety record and most physicians are quite familiar with them, making them a reasonable first-line medicine, realizing that the likelihood of benefit is less than the 75% usually quoted for children with a primary attention deficit.

Fenfluramine, a serotonin antagonist, has been tried based on the observation that a subgroup of children with autism had elevated serotonin levels. Treatment doses are on the order of 0.75 mg/kg given twice daily. There was an original spate of studies reporting positive results (e.g., Geller, Ritvo, Freeman, & Yuwiler, 1982), although closer analysis of the data revealed that most children did not respond and that, of those who did, benefits were usually minor (Farber, 1986; Gualtieri, 1986). Because of this, fenfluramine has grown out of favor with most practitioners.

Antidepressants have been studied in children with autism. Because of some of the stereotypical features of the disorder, clomipramine, which is of benefit for obsessive–compulsive disorder, has been tried. At doses on the order of

4 mg/kg/day, improvements have been reported not only in obsessive–compulsive behaviors but also in ratings of anger and autism (Gordon, Rapoport, Hamburger, State, & Mannheim, 1992).

Endorphins, naturally occurring opiate receptor agonists that mediate much of the chemical functioning of the brain, are another important research area in psychopharmacology. The prototypical drug is naltrexone, an oral endorphin blocker (Deutsch, 1986). Elevated levels of endogenous opioid peptides have been reported in some studies of autism, offering a biochemical rationale for their use. At doses ranging from 0.5 to 2.0 mg/kg/day, some positive effects on self-injury (Richardson & Zaleski, 1983) and autistic features such as withdrawal and verbal production have been reported (Leboyer et al., 1992; Panksepp & Lensing, 1991). Studies remain in the preliminary stage.

As mentioned, the gamut of psychopharmacologic agents has been tried in dealing with autism (Table 2). These include clonidine (both oral and in patch form), fluoxetine, anxiolytics, β blockers (Ratey et al., 1987), anticonvulsants (for their behavioral, not antiepileptic, aspects), enzymes (Naruse et al., 1987), synthetic hormones, dopamine agonists, and dopamine antagonists. All of these studies of these medications tend to be either open or, if controlled, conducted with small numbers of children representing a heterogeneous population of autism. Therefore, none is even close to being definitive.

In general, neuropharmacologic agents have been able to benefit selected behavioral difficulties (e.g., self-injury, hyperactivity) in many

Table 2. Some medications used in treating autism

Methylphenidate
Haloperidol
Clonidine
Clomipramine
Fluoxetine
Buspirone
Naltrexone
Nadolol
Fenfluramine
ORG 2766 (a synthetic corticotropin analogue)
Tetrahydrobiopterin

cases (Farber, 1987), but have not influenced cognitive development. Based on current understanding of neurologic function, it is expected that better medicines for ameliorating problem behaviors will continue to be developed, but there is no reason to believe that any one drug will prove to be effective for all children with autism. Furthermore, there is no practical basis for anticipating the creation of drugs that improve intelligence anytime in the near future.

Nonstandard Therapies

In examining approaches to autism, it is necessary to consider the category of what has been termed nonstandard or "fringe" therapies. Autism is a field ripe for exploitation: It is a heterogeneous entity with a wide variety of possible manifestations and diverse outcomes, there is no known cure, and it is generally but not universally associated with a poor prognosis. The heterogeneity means that some children will have a relatively good outcome regardless of the treatment approach, so that improvement coincident with, rather than resulting from, a unique therapy is definitely possible. The poor prognosis leads parents to try unproven approaches and hope for a cure.

Nonstandard therapies share a number of common features (see Chapter 33, Volume I). Usually they are based on a quasi-scientific interpretation of the condition in question, but an interpretation that ignores much of what is known. They claim to treat a wide variety of conditions without causing harm. They are not well studied, usually relying on case reports, and often employ a strong emotional appeal. To this could be added that many are touted as "natural," and their proponents use the antiscientific stance of requiring critics to prove the treatments ineffective.

Some popular fringe therapies of the past include patterning, the Option Method, and holding therapy (Table 3). Patterning involves having adults move a child through various positions to retrain neurologic circuits, and is associated with the Institute for the Advancement of Human Potential in Philadelphia (Doman, Spitz, Zucman, Delacato, & Doman, 1960). The Option Method involves imitating everything a child does to "break through" to him or her (Kaufman, 1976). Holding therapy, as the name implies, includes much holding of the child (Tinbergen & Tinbergen, 1985). These methods have had their moments in the sun, but are now primarily of historical interest.

Other fringe therapies with greater staying power have included food allergy avoidance (often with antiyeast medications), and the use of megavitamins/trace minerals, with or without "supportive" hair analysis. Various vitamins and minerals have been tried. The most popular is probably a combination of vitamin B$_6$ (pyridoxine) and magnesium. Proponents claim that its value has been confirmed with double-blind studies, although, as with fenfluramine, the data are not as impressive as proponents would like. For example, one commonly quoted favorable study (Rimland, Callaway, & Dreyfus, 1978) did not actually demonstrate gains with pyridoxine; rather, children placed on pyridoxine did not improve but did worsen when it was withdrawn. Another popular nutritional supplement at present is dimethyl glycine. Again, data are lacking, although positive anecdotal reports are commonly found in family-oriented literature, such as the *Autism Research Review International* (San Diego, CA).

There are two newer popular fringe therapies at this time: auditory training and facilitated communication. Auditory training entails determining to what sound frequencies an autistic child is hypersensitive, then playing music for the child with those frequencies filtered out. It follows the typical pattern for a "breakthrough" in autism therapy: Namely, one patient with autism, who had a good prognosis regardless of therapy, underwent auditory training for unclear reasons and, not unexpectedly, subsequently went on to function in the "normal" world.

Table 3. Fringe therapies used in treating autism

Patterning
Option method
Holding therapy
Megavitamins/nutritional supplements
Antiallergy therapy
Anti-*Candida* therapy
Sensory integration therapy
Auditory training
Facilitated communication

Rather than attributing this to the natural history of her autism, however, it was hailed as a "miracle" brought about by the therapy. It should be noted, however, in an unusual approach for a fringe therapy, that scientific studies are actually being conducted. One report found some statistically significant findings (out of how many possible ones is not stated) of unclear clinical significance (Rimland & Edelson, 1994). However, for-profit centers that perform auditory training are springing up across the country, before the data are in. A course of therapy can cost over $1,000, and families have been advised that results may not be apparent for up to 6 months after the completion of therapy.

The other fringe therapy of the moment is facilitated communication (FC), originating in Australia and launched in this country by Biklen (1990). FC differs from the usual pattern of nonstandard therapies in that it has been reported to benefit hundreds of children rather than a handful, and has supposedly been successful with almost all autistic children, not just those who are high functioning. It is to be distinguished from augmented communication. In augmented communication, an assistive device, such as a computer with a keyboard, is provided to allow for communication by someone who has an expressive disability such as dysarthria or verbal dyspraxia. The child accesses the device by him or herself, and augmented communication is an accepted technique, clearly of benefit for many children. With FC, in contrast, a facilitator's hand is placed on the child's hand, to provide support in striking the keyboard. This hand-on-hand contact is what distinguishes FC from augmented communication. FC has received extensive publicity in television, newspapers, and parent information networks. Initial media reports were highly favorable, although more recent reports have shone a more negative light on FC.

Skeptics question whether, with FC, the facilitator is guiding the autistic child subconsciously, similar to what happens with a Ouija board. Proponents of FC believe that this does not happen and that the output is that of the child. It is also claimed that virtually all children can use FC successfully. It should be noted that this view implies that, in autism, language intelligence is essentially typical, and that part of the underlying problem is a verbal dyspraxia, along with a very specific fine motor dyspraxia, in which a child may be able to string beads, self-feed and self-dress, and perform similar fine motor tasks, yet be unable to touch a keyboard accurately. It also implies that autistic children have learned how to read and spell, even if they have never been taught to do so.

It would appear to be simple enough to test FC. One could, for example, show an object to an autistic child without the facilitator seeing it, then determine if the child can name that object by FC. However, proponents of FC have argued that faith is an essential ingredient in using FC; because testing implies some doubts about its validity, there would therefore be a lack of faith, so that FC could then be unsuccessful if tested. This argument logically implies that FC is unprovable.

This has not deterred people from trying. Studies have shown that almost no children, under test conditions, can use FC effectively, even when the facilitators are confident that it works (e.g., Prior & Cummins, 1992; Wheeler, Jacobson, Poglieri, & Schwartz, 1993). As another problem with FC, over 15 cases of unsubstantiated child sexual abuse have been reported. Parents have latched onto FC with great gusto in the belief that they are at last reaching their autistic children, but the evidence so far indicates that, for the overwhelming majority, in FC it is the facilitator, subconsciously, with whom one is communicating, and not the child.

Fringe therapies will rise up, and then, if unsuccessful, fade from view, to be replaced by others. All that is required to create a "cure" is an idea, an anecdotal success, a flair for publicity, and a disregard for the scientific method. A pediatrician will be hard pressed to keep abreast of every "theory" that comes along. When confronted with parents anxious to try a new approach, there are several ways to assist them. They will usually be able to provide written materials on the proposed therapies. An analysis will usually lead to readily discernible flaws in the theoretical underpinnings. The anecdotal, unscientific nature of the method can also be pointed out. Side effects can be explored; these are usually glossed over or ignored completely by proponents of the treatment. Common side effects of fringe therapies include financial costs, loss of time (many are very time consuming), and medical complications (even so-called natural compounds can be toxic in megadoses).

Despite all this, some parents will still wish to try a fringe therapy. After discussing the pros and cons with them, it is important not to try to win a rancorous debate with the parents. Not only will this be ineffective, it will also serve to alienate them, so that they will be reluctant to return when the therapy is ineffective. Exploring nonstandard options is a common approach at some point, often as part of a bargaining stage in coping with grief over the diagnosis of autism. Fortunately, almost all fringe therapies pose no serious risks of morbidity for the child. If the proposed treatment is relatively innocuous, and the family has been informed of its hidden side effects and still wishes to pursue it, the parents can be supported in their efforts while the physician expresses his or her doubts. If the proposed treatment is riskier, the physician should voice his or her disagreement while recognizing the parents' need to try, and their primary responsibility in caring for the child. The physician should remain available for follow-up. In this way, he or she can maintain the therapeutic alliance, and the family will continue to use him or her after the treatment has proven unsuccessful and is dropped.

PEDIATRIC MANAGEMENT

So far, it is apparent that the pediatrician often does not have a major role in treating autism in the traditional medical sense: Medications are usually not indicated, and the pediatrician is not responsible for conducting behavioral or educational therapy. Nevertheless, he or she can play a central role in the care of the child with autism by assisting in case management and educating the family (Table 4).

The physician is in a prime position for overseeing and coordinating services. By training, he or she has a good understanding of chronic disabling conditions (both physical and mental), as well as insight into the strengths and limitations of associated disciplines, even though he or she is not a practitioner of them. The pediatri-

Table 4.   Roles of the pediatrician in autism

Educating families
Making the diagnosis
Looking for possible etiologies
Handling medication
Overseeing the multidisciplinary care
Discussing fringe therapies

cian is therefore in the best professional position to assess the net effects of the various treatment regimens from the points of view of likely impact, time and energy constraints, and medical appropriateness. He or she can help mediate differences of opinion between disciplines, and assist in resolving conflicting suggestions over interventions. He or she can thus provide an overall professional perspective to supplement that of the family.

Another key strength of the pediatrician is that of continuity. The pediatrician is usually available for as long as the family wishes to continue the relationship. This is in contradistinction to therapists, who often change with the child's age, school, school program, and school year.

The pediatrician can also provide advice on behavior problems and discipline. Not all behavioral issues that arise require sustained counseling input. Many can be resolved by putting the problem into a developmental perspective and offering appropriate advice. This developmental perspective is among the pediatrician's skills. For example, a 4-year-old child may not put his toys away when asked, if his language skills are at 18 months and he does not understand the question. A more effective approach would therefore be for the parent to put away some toys as a game, relying on the child's parallel play tendencies to pitch in and help.

The last and perhaps most important function of the pediatrician is that of parental education (Farber & Capute, 1984). Members of the allied disciplines usually do not feel comfortable introducing emotion-laden terms to families or discussing their ramifications in detail, so that disabilities often are described to the family in educational terms (e.g., your child has delayed language skills; speech and language services are recommended). It thus falls to the pediatri-

cian to introduce the label autism and explore with parents the etiology of the disorder (paying particular attention to the fact that it is not caused by inadequate parenting), the child's current level of functioning, short-term needs, long-term prognosis, and parental reaction to the diagnosis.

A Model of Autism for Parents

The parents can be brought to understand the organic, cognitive nature of the deficit in autism, and steered away from the view of autism as an emotional disorder that they have in some fashion caused. However, it is still very often difficult for them to understand why their child has the behavioral features he or she does. This is not surprising in view of the difficulty professionals have in comprehending autism. A simple conceptual model depicting autism as primarily a communication disorder, social interaction as a communication skill, and behavior as being heavily inner language based can be used to provide a framework. The parents can be informed that interpersonal skills are, by their very nature, communication skills; relating to others is the basis of communication. Thus, because autism is a communication disorder, poor eye contact, use of others as objects, withdrawn behavior, and other aberrant social skills can all be viewed as flowing from the underlying deficit.

Similarly, much of how people control their own behavior appears to be based on internal language: At some level, people talk to themselves to organize their actions ("later today I need to go shopping for food") or to provide rules for making sense of life ("the food will be expensive; I had better bring along more cash"), rather than using an intuitive approach. In autism, one can view the communication disorder as also impairing the ability to talk to one's self. The child may be able to generate only simple rote concepts because of a lack of complexity and abstraction in language use. Thus, he or she may view wheels as "things that spin" and therefore perseverate on that, because he or she does not have the internal language to describe other features of wheels. Stereotypy, preservation of sameness, and so forth would naturally follow.

Because autism is primarily a communication disorder, nonverbal intelligence need not always be impaired. Thus, a child may have typical or even superior skills in these areas (e.g., doing puzzles) and still be autistic.

This model is, of course, too simple to explain all the features of autism. However, as an initial approach it is broadly accurate, readily adaptable to explain most autistic behaviors, and easily grasped and used by parents. Therefore, it can be beneficial in providing them with an explanation of why their child with autism does the things he or she does.

Parent Counseling

Educating the parents about autism is one of the major roles of the pediatrician. Some general guidelines for optimal counseling can be developed (Table 5). The importance of the initial discussion cannot be overemphasized. It lays the groundwork for the family to function and cope as best as possible. It is essential that the discussion take place in an unhurried, supportive atmosphere, after regular office hours if need be. Both parents should be present.

When parents receive the diagnosis, it represents the "death of the perfect child" that had been previously fantasized. The standard grief reactions can be anticipated: denial, anger, bargaining, depression, and acceptance (Kubler-Ross, 1969). To these can be added an early transient stage of shock and numbness. Parents need to hear the diagnosis and receive some general information about autism, but it is not necessary to convince them of the diagnosis. Denial will often be present, and trying to break this down by logical debating is not only impossible but counterproductive. Some parents (more often the mother) will react to the diagnosis by crying; others (more often the father) will

Table 5.   General guidelines for the initial parent counseling session

Provide ample time
Have both parents present if at all possible
Give specific diagnosis if known
Provide written material
Avoid professional jargon
Ask parents for their questions and thoughts
Arrange for follow-up discussion

become analytical and ask practical questions. Because of his or her own anxieties, the pediatrician will often want to focus on the latter parent, but he or she must be careful not to ignore the needs of the former. Neither style of parental reaction is superior, and in any case, because of the shock, much of the information will be forgotten. Having a parent cry does not mean a session has been poorly conducted; it does mean the diagnosis has been heard. Provision of tissues, judicious use of pausing, light touch (e.g., shoulder patting), and sometimes even offering to leave the room briefly during a crying spell can be helpful.

What parents remember most about the delivery of the diagnosis is the manner in which it was presented; details are not as well recalled (Cunningham, Morgan, & McGucken, 1984). Because this information will not be well retained at first, a written outline, summarizing the most salient information, can be given to the family. This can be helpful in giving them a tangible focus for the diagnosis and intervention plan. Subsequently, as adjustment begins, they can be provided with a full report.

It is important to remember the role of relatives. The parents should be informed that the physician will be willing to talk with any close relatives, should the family desire. Most parents will choose to break the news themselves, but some will take advantage of the offer.

No purpose is served in avoiding presenting a diagnosis once it has been established. It may seem as though one would be doing the parents a favor by not giving them bad news, but this is not so (Quine & Pahl, 1987). The news is bad no matter when it is presented; the earlier it is given, the sooner the parents can go through the necessary stages toward acceptance and plan for the future accordingly. If a diagnosis is hidden from parents, when told later, they are usually angry at the professionals who did so. Reluctance to give a diagnosis to parents almost always reflects a pediatrician's own anxiety; if he or she cannot do this, he or she is obligated to refer to a professional who can.

After the initial session is ended, the education of the parents has begun. Very little information will be retained in many cases. It is important to inform the family that you will follow up in 1–2 weeks, and then do so. It can also be useful, at the end of the session, to review with the family some reactions they may have to the diagnosis.

After the initial session, parent adjustment continues. Grief stages are often presented as occurring in orderly sequence, but in actuality they overlap and can go forward or backward from time to time. For example, feelings of stress and sadness often well up at key developmental periods (e.g., when a younger sibling surpasses the autistic child) (Zajicek-Farber, 1990). The practitioner should be cognizant of where parents are in their adjustment, realizing that both parents may not be at the same stage simultaneously. Referral for outside counseling to deal with grief should not be necessary, unless the parents express an interest, there is an inability to cope with daily activities, or there is excessively prolonged depression (e.g., greater than 3 months). Parents often benefit from knowing families with similarly involved children, and from having an opportunity to participate in a community group committed to helping people with autism. The Autism Society of America (7910 Woodmont Avenue, Bethesda, MD 20814-3015; 301-657-0881) is an excellent lay organization with regional chapters.

Acceptance of the diagnosis can take years. What is necessary is to enlist the parents in a therapeutic alliance, so that they will be willing and able to do what is needed to help the child (e.g., arranging for special education) even if they are actively denying the diagnosis. The role of the pediatrician in educating the parents is a long-term one, achieved over the course of years. During this time, he or she will assist with school programming, planning for the future, exploring fringe therapies, and other issues as they arise. It is in this role, as a supportive, informed, accessible professional with a long-term relationship with the child and family, that the pediatrician can best serve to treat not just the child, but the family as well.

A MODEL OF AUTISM FOR PROFESSIONALS

The preceding sections have discussed the conventional interpretation of autism and associated methods of diagnosis and treatment. A psychological model of autism has now been developed that, although not fully confirmed and not of immediate practical use to the professional dealing with the autistic child, is of sufficient importance and potential power that the practitioner should be aware of it for future understanding.

Expressed concisely, this theory postulates that the primary psychological disorder in autism is that of a deficit in the ability to form and use second-order and higher representations (i.e., representations of representations) (Frith, 1989). A first-order representation is a literal one; for example, a banana represents a banana. An example of a second-order representation would be that of pretending to use a banana as a telephone receiver.

It is readily apparent from such a theory how the features of autism, such as the concrete use of language and lack of imaginative play, would arise. However, the model can be extended further. Another example of a higher order representation is the attributing of mental states to others—that is, realizing that other people think and feel, have motivations behind their words and actions, and so forth. Autistic children, even after correcting for mental age, have a deficit in developing this "theory of mind." Accordingly, this would explain the abnormal socialization seen in autism, such as responding to others as if they were objects.

Autism may be associated with other disabilities (such as mental retardation), but this inability to make abstractions is central. Without this deficit, autism will not be seen.

Based on our current understanding of information-processing systems (such as brains and computers), it has been proposed that novel higher order representations arise not from a specific site within the system, but rather from the totality of the interconnections (Hofstadter, 1981). For the computer, these representations will not be programmed directly but will emerge indirectly from subprograms. For the brain, these representations will arise from the interconnections between various parts of the brain. Combining this with the "theory of mind" leads to the conclusion that a specific anatomic site of injury in autism will not be localizable.

It should be borne in mind that this framework is still theoretical, and experimental support is still being developed. However, as a model, it is already very powerful and can be very useful to the professional in helping to understand the mystery of autism.

CONCLUSIONS

Looking at cognitive outcome in the communication disorders, it is apparent that there is a great deal of variety, ranging from a typical outcome to learning disabilities to profound mental retardation. This no doubt reflects the heterogeneity of the conditions subsumed under the labels of autism and communication disorders. The natural history of these disorders has not been as well studied as one would like, but in general the finding, not unexpectedly, is that the better the functioning early on, the better the long-term outcome. Behavioral outcomes tend to follow cognitive functioning: Self-injurious behavior, hyperactivity, and poor self-care skills are common among children with severe to profound mental retardation; poor social awareness and being a loner accompany average intelligence.

The role of the developmental pediatrician is crucial. He or she usually makes the diagnosis, which also entails discussing short-term and long-term issues as they pertain to a given child. He or she will handle medication when indicated, and can serve as co-coordinator with the family for the multiple disciplines that will be working with the child.

To date, the value of the different available interventions remains unclear. With the exception of the occasional child who benefits from medication, therapy falls mostly into the special education/speech-language/behavioral psychology domain. In the community, this is most often provided by the public schools. There is nothing to suggest that the treatment approaches are curative in any sense of the word. Rather, they attempt to maximize whatever innate potential an affected child has. It is also not clear which components of a given therapeutic method are of value and which are a waste of time and effort. The need for carefully researched studies of all aspects of diagnosis, intervention, and outcome remains paramount.

REFERENCES

American Psychiatric Association. (1994). *Diagnostic and statistic manual of mental disorders* (4th ed.). Washington, DC: American Psychiatric Press.

Anderson, L.T., Campbell, M., Grega, D.M., Perry, R., Small, A.M., & Green, W.H. (1984). Haloperidol in the treatment of infantile autism: Effects on learning and behavioral symptoms. *American Journal of Psychiatry, 141,* 1195–1202.

Baumgardner, T., & Reiss, A.L. (1994). Fragile X syndrome: A behavioral genetics window into understanding social emotional learning disability. In A.J. Capute, P.J. Accardo, & B.K. Shapiro (Eds.), *Learning disabilities spectrum: Attention-deficit disorder, attention-deficit/hyperactivity disorder, and learning disability* (pp. 67–84). Baltimore: York Press.

Bellack, A.S., & Hersen, M. (1985). *Dictionary of behavior therapy techniques.* Elmsford, NY: Pergamon.

Biklen, D. (1990). Communication unbound: Autism and praxis. *Harvard Educational Review, 60,* 291–314.

Chess, S. (1971). Autism in children with congenital rubella. *Journal of Autism and Childhood Schizophrenia, 1,* 33–47.

Cooper, J., Moodley, M., & Reynell, J. (1979). The developmental language program: Results from a five year study. *British Journal of Disorders of Communication, 14,* 57–69.

Courchesne, E., Press, G.A., & Yeung-Courchesne, R. (1993). Parietal lobe abnormalities detected with mental retardation in patients with infantile autism. *American Journal of Radiology, 160,* 387–393.

Courchesne, E., Saitoh, O., Yeung-Courchesne, R., Press, G.A., Lincoln, A.J., Haas, R.H., & Schreibman, L. (1994). Abnormality of cerebellar vermian lobules VI and VII in patients with infantile autism. *American Journal of Radiology, 162,* 123–130.

Cunningham, C.C., Morgan, P.A., & McGucken, R.B. (1984). Down's syndrome: Is dissatisfaction with disclosure of diagnosis inevitable? *Developmental Medicine and Child Neurology, 26,* 33–39.

DeMyer, M.K., Barton, S., Alpern, G.D., Kimberlin, C., Allen, J., Yang, E., & Steele, R. (1974). The measured intelligence of autistic children. *Journal of Autism and Childhood Schizophrenia, 4,* 42–60.

DeMyer, M.K., Barton, S., DeMyer, W.E., Norton, J.A., Allen, J., & Steele, R. (1973). Prognosis in autism: A follow-up study. *Journal of Autism and Childhood Schizophrenia, 3,* 199–246.

Deutsch, S.I. (1986). Rationale for the administration of opiate antagonists in treating infantile autism. *American Journal of Mental Deficiency, 90,* 631–635.

Doman, R.J., Spitz, E.B., Zucman, E., Delacato, C.H., & Doman, G. (1960). Children with severe brain injuries. *JAMA, 174,* 119–124.

Farber, J.M. (1986). Fenfluramine and autism [Letter]. *Developmental Medicine and Child Neurology, 28,* 817–818.

Farber, J.M. (1987). Psychopharmacology of self-injurious behavior in the mentally retarded. *Journal of the American Academy of Child and Adolescent Psychiatry, 26,* 296–302.

Farber, J.M., & Capute, A.J. (1984). Understanding autism. *Clinical Pediatrics, 23,* 199–202.

Frith, U. (1989). A new look at language and communication in autism. *British Journal of Disorders of Communication, 24,* 123–150.

Geller, E., Ritvo, E.R., Freeman, B.J., & Yuwiler, A. (1982). Preliminary observations on the effect of fenfluramine on blood serotonin and symptoms in three autistic boys. *New England Journal of Medicine, 307,* 165–169.

Gillberg, C. (1991). Outcome in autism and autistic-like conditions. *Journal of the American Academy of Child and Adolescent Psychiatry, 30,* 375–382.

Gillberg, C., & Coleman, M. (1993). *The biology of the autistic syndromes.* Cambridge, England: Cambridge University Press.

Gordon, C.T., Rapoport, J.L., Hamburger, S.D., State, R.C., & Mannheim, G.B. (1992). Differential response of seven subjects with autistic disorder to clomipramine and desipramine. *American Journal of Psychiatry, 149,* 363–366.

Gualtieri, C.T. (1986). Fenfluramine and autism: Careful reappraisal is in order. *Journal of Pediatrics, 108,* 417–419.

Hofstadter, D.R. (1981). Prelude . . . and fugue. In D.R. Hofstadter & D.C. Dennett (Eds.), *The mind's I* (pp. 149–201). New York: Basic Books.

Hooper, S.R., & Tramontana, M.G. (1992). Neuropsychological assessment of children. In M.D. Levine, W.B. Carey, & A.C. Crocker (Eds.), *Developmental-behavioral pediatrics* (pp. 663–666). Philadelphia: W.B. Saunders.

Howells, J.G., & Guirguis, W.R. (1984). Childhood schizophrenia 20 years later. *Archives of General Psychiatry, 41,* 123–128.

Kanner, L. (1943). Autistic disturbances of affective contact. *Nervous Child, 2,* 217–250.

Kaufman, B.N. (1976). *Son-rise.* New York: Warner Books.

Kubler-Ross, E. (1969). *On death and dying.* New York: Macmillan.

Leboyer, M., Bouvard, M.P., Launay, J., Tabuteau, F., Waller, D., Dugas, M., Kergelhue, B., Lensing, P., & Panksepp, J. (1992). Brief report: A double-blind study of naltrexone in infantile autism. *Journal of Autism and Developmental Disorders, 22,* 309–319.

Linscheid, T.R., Hartel, F., & Cooley, N. (1993). Are aversive procedures durable? A five year follow-up of three individuals treated with contingent electric shock. *Child and Adolescent Mental Health Care, 3,* 67–76.

Lotter, V. (1974). Social adjustment and placement of autistic children in Middlesex: A follow-up study. *Journal of Autism and Childhood Schizophrenia, 4,* 11–32.

Martineau, J., Barthélémy, C., Jouve, J., Muh, J., & Lelord, G. (1992). Monoamines (serotonin and catecholamines) and their derivatives in infantile autism: Age-related changes and drug effects. *Developmental Medicine and Child Neurology, 34,* 593–603.

McAdoo, W.G., & DeMyer, M.K. (1978). Personality characteristics of parents. In M. Rutter & E. Schopler (Eds.), *Autism: A reappraisal of concepts and treatment* (pp. 251–267). New York: Plenum.

McEachin, J.J., Smith, T., & Lovaas, O.I. (1993). Long-term outcome for children with autism who received early intensive behavioral treatment. *American Journal of Mental Retardation, 97,* 359–372.

Minton, J., Campbell, M., Green, W.H., Jennings, S., & Samit, C. (1982). Cognitive assessment of siblings of autistic children. *Journal of the American Academy of Child Psychiatry, 21,* 256–261.

Naruse, H., Hayashi, T., Takesada, M., Nakane, A., Yamazaki, K., Noguchi, T., Watanabe, Y., & Hayaishi, O. (1987). Therapeutic effect of tetrahydrobiopterin in infantile autism. *Proceedings of the Japan Academy, 63,* 231–233.

Olsson, B., & Rett, A. (1987). Autism and Rett syndrome: Behavioural investigations and differential diagnosis. *Developmental Medicine and Child Neurology, 29,* 429–441.

Panksepp, J., & Lensing, P. (1991). Brief report: A synopsis of an open-trial of naltrexone treatment of autism with four children. *Journal of Autism and Developmental Disorders, 21,* 243–249.

Paul, R., Cohen, D.J., & Caparulo, B.K. (1983). A longitudinal study of patients with severe developmental disorders of language learning. *Journal of the American Academy of Child Psychiatry, 22,* 525–534.

Prior, M., & Cummins, R. (1992). Questions about facilitated communication and autism. *Journal of Autism and Developmental Disorders, 22,* 331–338.

Quine, L., & Pahl, J. (1987). First diagnosis of severe handicap: A study of parental reactions. *Developmental Medicine and Child Neurology, 29,* 232–242.

Ratey, J.J., Bemporad, J., Sorgi, P., Bick, P., Polakoff, S., O'Driscoll, G., & Mikklesen, E. (1987). Brief report: Open trial effects of beta-blockers on speech and social behaviors in 8 autistic adults. *Journal of Autism and Developmental Disorders, 17,* 439–446.

Richardson, J.S., & Zaleski, W.A. (1983). Naloxone and self-mutilation. *Biological Psychiatry, 18,* 99–101.

Rimland, B., Callaway, E., & Dreyfus, P. (1978). The effect of high doses of vitamin B6 on autistic children: A double-blind crossover study. *American Journal of Psychiatry, 135,* 472–475.

Rimland, B., & Edelson, S.M. (1994). The effects of auditory integration training on autism. *American Journal of Speech and Language Pathology, 3,* 16–24.

Rumsey, J.M., Rapoport, J.L., & Sceery, W.R. (1985). Autistic children as adults: Psychiatric, social, and behavioral outcomes. *Journal of the American Academy of Child Psychiatry, 24,* 465–473.

Rutter, M. (1971). The description and classification of infantile autism. In D.W. Churchill, G.D. Alpern, & M.K. DeMyer (Eds.), *Infantile autism: Proceedings of the Indiana University colloquium* (pp. 8–29). Springfield, IL: Charles C Thomas.

Rutter, M., Greenfeld, D., & Lockyer, L. (1967). A five to fifteen year follow-up study of infantile psychosis. II. Social and behavioural outcome. *British Journal of Psychiatry, 113,* 1183–1199.

Silva, P.A., Williams, S., & McGee, R. (1987). A longitudinal study of children with developmental language delay at age three: Later intelligence, reading and behaviour problems. *Developmental Medicine and Child Neurology, 29,* 630–640.

Simonson, L.R. (1979). *A curriculum model for individuals with severe learning and behavior disorders.* Baltimore: University Park Press.

Sloman, L. (1991). Use of medication in pervasive developmental disorders. *Psychiatric Clinics of North America, 14,* 165–182.

Stevenson, P., Bax, M., & Stevenson, J. (1982). The evaluation of home based speech therapy for language delayed pre-school children in an inner city area. *British Journal of Disorders of Communication, 17,* 141–148.

Szatmari, P., Bartolucci, G., Bremner, R., Bond, S., & Rich, S. (1989). A follow-up study of high-functioning autistic children. *Journal of Autism and Developmental Disorders, 19,* 213–225.

Tinbergen, N., & Tinbergen, A.E. (1985). *"Autistic" children: New hope for a cure.* Hemel Hempstead, England: George Allen & Unwin.

Wheeler, O.L., Jacobson, J.W., Paglieri, R.A., & Schwartz, A.A. (1993). An experimental assessment of facilitated communication. *Mental Retardation, 31,* 49–60.

Wolf, L., & Goldberg, B. (1986). Autistic children grow up: An eight to twenty-four year follow-up study. *Canadian Journal of Psychiatry, 31,* 550–556.

Wright, H.H., Young, S.R., Edwards, J.G., Abramson, R.K., & Duncan, J. (1986). Fragile X syndrome in a population of autistic children. *Journal of the American Acadeemy of Child Psychiatry, 25,* 641–644.

Zajicek-Farber, M.L. (1990). *Stress experience in parents raising a child with Down syndrome as related to the child's transitional developmental period, parents' appraisal of the child's handicapping condition, and their personal coping and social resources.* Unpublished doctoral dissertation, Catholic University of America, Washington, DC.

Chapter 24

The Continuum of High-Functioning Autism

Thomas A. Blondis, M.D., and Catherine Lord, Ph.D.

In 1995, it is generally recognized by both the medical and the psychology communities that autism is a developmental disability with an organic basis (Gillberg, & Coleman, 1992; Rutter, 1983). This topic has been covered thoroughly in Chapter 23 (this volume), which also reviewed the essential medical and scientific aspects of autism (Farber, 1991; Farber, & Capute, 1984). Since the first edition of *Developmental Disabilities in Infancy and Childhood*, high-functioning autism, which represents the minority of children diagnosed on the autistic continuum, has been an area of expanding clinical research. The accepted and controversial aspects of this continuum of children represent an area of which developmental pediatricians should be aware and investigating.

Asperger syndrome, which had been a separate condition accepted in Europe but in general viewed with uncertainty by the North American medical community, now appears as a separate psychiatric code in the *Diagnostic and Statistical Manual of Mental Disorders*, fourth edition (DSM-IV) (American Psychiatric Association [APA], 1994). The clinical research and controversies that surround the continuum of children who present with the characteristic neurodevelopmental deviance and dysfunction of autism, yet do not have mental retardation, regularly appears in journals representing the disciplines of psychiatry, psychology, and speech and language, as well as child neurology (Mesibov & Schopler, 1992; Lord, Mulloy, Wendelboe, & Schopler, 1991).

High-functioning autism is defined in this chapter as the condition in which an individual with the neuropsychological and behavioral deficits characteristic of autism has measured intelligence in the average or above-average range (Wolff & Barlow, 1979). The DSM-IV (APA, 1994) and the *International Classification of Diseases*, 10th edition (ICD-10) (World Health Organization [WHO], 1992) now agree that autistic subtypes should be considered as *pervasive developmental disorders* (PDDs). The DSM-IV refers to all PDD categories as disorders; thus the ICD-10 Asperger syndrome becomes Asperger's disorder in the DSM-IV. In this chapter, we refer to the high-functioning autistic continuum as *high-functioning PDD* and use WHO terminology for Childhood Autism and Asperger syndrome.

It is noteworthy that both the DSM-IV and the ICD-10 have deleted the category that encompasses communication dysfunction for those children with Asperger syndrome. Even though communication is not within the current diagnostic criteria delineated by the APA and the WHO, others disagree with this and have determined that communication dysfunctions are a characteristic feature among children with Asperger syndrome (Gillberg & Coleman, 1992). It is the goal of this chapter to present what is known, suspected, and raised as conjecture about differences that exist among high-functioning children with PDD and other disorders that must be considered and ruled out before a diagnosis can be made. The chapter also describes some of the teaching interventions and modifications that may be useful for habilitation. Clearly, the developmental pediatrician must understand the basic differences

The authors would like to thank Dr. Margaret Shaklee for her editorial assistance.

between what at this time are called Asperger syndrome and childhood autism to determine which is a better fit for describing a particular child. This differentiation has implications in the public health domain and may prove to have meaning from the habilitative and educational perspectives as well (Klin, 1994; Rutter & Schopler, 1987).

ASPERGER SYNDROME: DSM-IV VERSUS ICD-10

When Kanner (1943, 1971) and Asperger (1991; Frith, 1991) described cases of children characterized by a cluster of symptoms, the majority of the cases described were children estimated to be functioning above the level of mental retardation. This phenomenon in the population of children diagnosed with disorders on the autistic continuum has not held up over time, and today epidemiologic studies estimate that 70%–90% of children with PDD have an IQ below 70 (Rutter, 1983). Whether the child has Asperger syndrome or autism, high-functioning children with PDD pose a unique set of problems and require different management approaches than their peers with mental retardation. What is not clear at this time is whether children with the Asperger variant would require significantly different interventions from children with high-functioning childhood autism; the DSM-IV (APA, 1994) and the ICD-10 (WHO, in press) suggest that language function is a significant point of differentiation.

Recently the Committee on Childhood Disorders from the APA and a committee from the WHO have reached a consensus on the diagnostic criteria for each PDD subtype (APA, 1994; WHO, in press). Table 1 compares the wording that the different committees have used to describe the Asperger subtype. At this time there are essentially no differences in the description of what both committees consider the core features, nor are there significant differences with regard to secondary features.

This is a shift for the WHO committee, who earlier published a different set of criteria for Asperger syndrome (WHO, 1992). In the newer version, several controversial features are either not in the text at all or are mentioned briefly without the same certitude that existed when the ICD-10 criteria were published for the first time (WHO, 1992). It is a worthwhile exercise to review the changes that have taken place and how the criteria previously differed.

Under the first category, "qualitative impairments in reciprocal social interaction," the DSM-IV was more descriptive in describing criteria than the first publication of the ICD-10 criteria for Asperger syndrome, but the WHO, like the APA, did place a great deal of emphasis on the inability to read and to respond to visual signals. Criteria for both Asperger syndrome and Asperger's disorder describe poor nonverbal *communication*, as well as deficits in the formation of relationships (primarily with peers) and in social reciprocity, the affective understanding of the give and take of social interaction (Wing & Atwood, 1987). Under the second DSM-IV diagnostic category, "restricted, repetitive, and stereotyped patterns of behavior, interests, and activities," the criteria were from the onset virtually identical with those of the ICD-10.

Differences also previously existed between the DSM-IV and the ICD-10 with regard to Asperger syndrome in the areas of motor and adaptive functions. The DSM-IV criteria make no mention of motor function, but the initial publication of the ICD-10 criteria made "motor clumsiness" a separate criterion. In a revised text of ICD-10 criteria for Asperger syndrome, this is gone as a separate criterion, although the ICD-10 (WHO, in press) does choose to mention that many children with Asperger syndrome frequently do exhibit a deficit in motor function. Criteria V in the DSM-IV emphasizes that self-help skills for Asperger's disorder are age appropriate with the exception of those that require social interaction. In the original ICD-10 criteria, self-help skills were not addressed, but in the new revised criteria (WHO, in press) the WHO committee specifies that a difference in adaptive skills does not exist during the first 3 years of life as a part of the third diagnostic category (see Table 1). The DSM-IV excludes Asperger's disorder if the child meets criteria for another form of PDD or for schizo-

Table 1. Asperger criteria: ICD-10 versus DSM-IV

ICD-10 diagnostic criteria	DSM-IV diagnostic criteria
I. There are qualitative impairments in reciprocal interactions:	I. Qualitative impairments in social interaction (two or more) exist:
1. Failure to adequately use eye-to-eye gaze, facial expression, body posture, and gesture to regulate social interaction	1. Marked impairment in the use of multiple nonverbal behaviors such as eye-to-eye gaze, facial expression, body postures, and gestures to regulate social interaction
2. Failure to develop (in a manner appropriate to mental age, etc.) peer relationships that involve a mutual sharing of interests, activities, and emotions	2. Failure to develop peer relationships appropriate to developmental level
3. Lack of socio-emotional reciprocity as shown by an unpaired or deviant response to other people's emotions	3. A lack of spontaneous seeking to share enjoyment, interests, or achievements with other people
4. Lack of spontaneous seeking to share enjoyment, interests, or achievement with other people	4. Lack of social or emotional reciprocity
II. Restricted, repetitive, and stereotyped patterns of behavior, interests, and functional routines exist:	II. Restricted, repetitive, and stereotyped patterns of behavior, interests, and activities (one or more of the following behaviors) are present:
1. Encompassing preoccupation with one or more stereotyped and restricted patterns of interest that are abnormal in content or focus	1. Encompassing preoccupation with one or more stereotyped and restricted patterns of interest that is abnormal either in intensity or focus
2. Compulsive adherence to specific, nonfunctional routines or rituals	2. Apparently inflexible adherence to specific, nonfunctional routines or rituals
3. Stereotyped and repetitive motor mannerisms that involve either hand or finger flapping or twisting, or complex whole body movements	3. Stereotyped and repetitive motor mannerisms
4. Preoccupations with part-objects or nonfunctional elements of play materials (e.g., their odor, the feel of their surface, or the noise or vibration that they generate)	4. Persistent preoccupation with parts of objects
III. The following developmental pattern applies:	III. The disturbance causes clinically significant impairment in social, occupational, or other important areas of functioning.
1. No clinically significant delay in language or cognitive development	IV. There is no clinically significant general delay in language.
2. Single words developed by 2 years . . . and communicative phrases used by 3 years or earlier	V. There is no clinically significant delay in cognitive development or in the development of age-appropriate self-help skills, adaptive behavior (other than in social interaction), and curiosity about the environment in childhood.
3. Self-help skills, adaptive behavior, and curiosity about the environment during the first 3 years of age at levels consistent with normal intellectual development	VI. Criteria are not met for another specific pervasive developmental disorder or schizophrenia.
4. Motor milestones somewhat delayed and motor clumsiness a usual although not a necessary diagnostic feature	
5. Isolated special skills, often related to abnormal preoccupations, are common but are not required for diagnosis	
IV. The disorder is not attributable to the other varieties of pervasive developmental disorders, simple schizophrenia, schizotypal disorder, obsessive-compulsive disorder, reactive and disinhibited attachment disorders of childhood.	

Adapted from American Psychiatric Association (1994) and World Health Organization (1993).

phrenia, and, although not incorporated as exclusionary criteria in the first published draft of the ICD-10 criteria, the amended draft will exclude schizotypal disorder, obsessive-compulsive disorder, anankastic personality disorder, and reactive and disinhibited attachment disorders of childhood.

At this point in time, few clinical scientists studying PDD would argue that childhood autism and Asperger syndrome are separate conditions that are lifetime neurodevelopmental disabilities with several distinct clinical and developmental findings. Although for the moment the WHO and APA committees can accept recently agreed on diagnostic criteria, this is only a starting point for examining this newly described subtype of PDD. The original points of contention with regard to Asperger syndrome (communication, adaptive skills, and clumsiness) that existed between the ICD-10 (WHO, 1992) and the DSM-IV (APA, 1994) have not been cleared up. Medical science has yet to validate and thus define the exact neurodevelopmental deficits of Asperger syndrome.

CONTROVERSIAL AREAS OF DEVELOPMENT AND ASPERGER SYNDROME

Language and Communication

Prior to 1992, studies that compared the language of high-functioning children with PDD to controls generally lumped all of these intelligent children with PDD into one group. It was not hard to demonstrate significant differences between the subjects with PDD and the controls. Of interest to this discussion are notable findings of the use of neologisms and idiosyncratic language in the high-functioning PDD group (Volden & Lord, 1991). Neologisms are "nonwords" or words that are obviously peculiar (LeConteur et al., 1989). High-functioning children with PDD tend to converse in an overly formal manner, and their conversation is distinctive for its literalness, stereotypicity, peculiarity, and inappropriateness. LeConteur and his colleagues concluded that characterizing the idiosyncratic usage of language by both high- and low-functioning children with PDD would demand further research.

Another significant linguistic characteristic of children with PDD is that they make a high number of irrelevant comments in their discourse with others (Szatmari, Bartolucci, & Bremmer, 1989). What appears to be significant in the studies of Szatmari and his colleagues is the inability of children with PDD to expand on what another might say to them and thus to develop the capacity to conduct interrelated communication.

Szatmari and colleagues next studied only higher-functioning children with PDD (both childhood autism and Asperger syndrome) with regard to their semantic and social usage of language. They hypothesized that, in order to converse relevantly, a speaker must be able to anticipate what information will be needed by his or her interlocutor in order to understand the message he or she is trying to deliver. This capability is associated with *theory of mind* (Baron-Cohen, 1988), in that the speaker must perceive accurately what must be said in order to deliver the message coherently to the listener.

In further refining this idea of interlocutor reliability among high-functioning children with PDD, Fine, Bartolucci, Szatmari, and Ginsberg (1994) analyzed the semantics of audiotaped conversations between each subject and the interviewer. The data were measured for six variables, three of which showed significant differences between the Asperger syndrome and childhood autism groups (both of which were compared with an outpatient control group): 1) references to antecedent conversation with the listener, 2) references to external objects in the environment, and 3) unclear references. The reference components were measured as proportions of nominal clusters, a reliable approach to analysis (Bartolucci & Fine, 1987). Figure 1 shows the hierarchy of linguistic measures that are used as referents. In the Fine et al. study, differences among control, Asperger, and autism patients were compared in terms of *phoric* errors. Of significance is the fact that the childhood autism and Asperger syndrome groups were matched for intelligence, although the childhood autism group was appreciably older than the Asperger syndrome group.

The study demonstrated that children with childhood autism and Asperger syndrome and

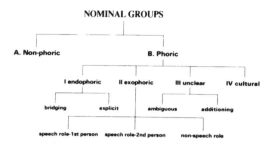

Figure 1. Hierarchy of linguistic measures used as referents. (From Fine, J., Bartolucci, G., Szatmari, P., & Ginsberg, G. [1994]. Cohesive discourse in pervasive developmental disorders. *Journal of Autism and Developmental Disabilities, 24*, 315–329; reprinted by permission of Plenum Publishing Company.)

without mental retardation have significant problems with cohesion of discourse; however, the errors in Asperger syndrome were markedly different from those of childhood autism, even opposite. For example, the children with Asperger syndrome were similar to the controls in frequency of references to earlier conversation (endophoric references) and in number of references to the external environment (exophoric references); in contrast, the childhood autism group made significantly *fewer* endophoric references than the control group and significantly *more* exophoric references. Furthermore, the Asperger syndrome group made significantly more unclear references (addition type) than both the control group and the childhood autism group. This suggests that high-functioning children with Asperger syndrome are able to make coherent links to prior conversation, unlike their childhood autism counterparts; however, they also add a significant amount of additional, unclear references that muddy their communication. High-functioning children with childhood autism, in contrast, make too few connections to prior conversation to be coherent and confuse their conversation with too many references to the setting and external stimuli. The speculations stemming from this study are that the Childhood Autism group has communication problems linked to both a verbal and a social language deficit. The Asperger syndrome group exhibits errors related to the inability to monitor what information is needed by the listener. If this is true, then the committees who have made Asperger syndrome distinct from childhood

autism, in part on the basis of the presence of typical language abilities in children with Asperger syndrome, are correct.

Is there a way that cohesive language can be evaluated by the clinician? There are a number of standardized tests that speech and language pathologists administer in their analysis of pragmatic language. These standardized instruments include the Test of Language Competence (Wiig & Secord, 1989), Evaluating Communicative Competence (Simon, 1986), and the Test of Problem Solving (Zachman, Jorgensen, Huisingh, & Barrett, 1984). Although these tests are not as precise in measuring the components of cohesive language, they do give age equivalents and standard scores concerning areas related to semantic usage in conversation.

Other areas of communicative incompetence in high-functioning children with PDD include dysprosody, abnormalities in the content of speech, and marked abnormal nonverbal communication (i.e., gaze aversion, body posture, gestures and cues, and facial expression). In part (as discussed above), there is a body of research to suggest that children with Asperger syndrome show no dysfunction in content of speech, but none to suggest that they do not display deficits in the areas of dysprosody and nonverbal communication. Although the WHO and the APA differentiate Asperger syndrome and childhood autism on the basis of language, others would argue that it is premature to suggest that verbal and nonverbal language dysfunction (especially when viewed from the context of communication) are not a diagnostic part of Asperger syndrome (Bishop 1989; Gillberg, & Coleman, 1992).

Clumsiness and Neuromotor Development

Lorna Wing (1981) resurrected the 1944 case study of Hans Asperger because of her conviction that there was a group of children with PDD who had a significantly different neuropsychological profile than that of infantile autism yet still had the same characteristic core findings of social impairment, communication deficit, and restrictive behavior, interests, and activities, all of which present with the developmental constructs of *deviancy* (the "qualitative" aspect in the ICD-10 and DSM-IV), *delay*, and *dissociation* (i.e., language and cognition). Wing described her subjects with Asperger syndrome as actually having better verbal abilities on the Wechsler Intelligence Scale for Children–Revised (1974) than performance abilities. She vigorously contended that motor clumsiness represented an aspect of Asperger syndrome.

In a study of a population of children diagnosed by Kanner's criteria as having autism, Gillberg (1989) used Wing's classification system and separated those with Asperger syndrome from those with classic autism. However, he did not include motor clumsiness as a feature. He then compared the two groups to determine if any other variables separated them. He found significant differences between the Asperger syndrome and Childhood Autism groups in the areas of echolalia, bilingual development, motor clumsiness, and circumscribed interests. The two areas that were most significant were motor clumsiness and circumscribed interests. The Asperger syndrome group had more circumscribed interests than the Childhood Autism group.

Ghaziuddin, Tsai, and Ghaziuddin (1992) reviewed 42 papers on Asperger syndrome, of which 20 were case reports, 10 were case-control studies, and the rest were case series or comments. Only four of these were prospective studies using standardized measures. A problem with all of these studies was that they did not define clumsiness. Ghaziuddin et al. found a problem with the four studies that utilized standardized tests in that they did not use standardized tests that were specifically intended for determining motor performance, and they did not differentiate between upper extremity and lower extremity motor performance. Nevertheless, the studies utilizing standardized measures (Gillberg, 1989; Szatmari, Bartolucci, & Bremmer, 1989; Szatmari, Tuff, Finlayson, & Bartolucci, 1990; Tantam, 1988) all concluded that children with Asperger syndrome were clumsy in some way. At this point, there seems to be consensus that clumsiness is associated with Asperger syndrome to some degree, but little evidence of its specificity or specific information concerning what "clumsiness" means with regard to Asperger syndrome has been gathered.

Deficits of Right-Hemisphere Function

Voeller (1986) described 15 children diagnosed as having a right hemisphere deficit. These children lacked the ability to interpret social cues, some appeared to be unable to express their feelings, 87% had poor peer relationships, 60% had atypical prosody, 40% had gesturing deficits, and 93% had attention-deficit disorders. In addition, eye contact was deficient in the majority of these children; 53% were said to be withdrawn and isolated. Based on these findings, as well as the findings of other neuropsychological studies, one might conclude that it is difficult to differentiate the high-functioning child with Asperger syndrome from a child with a severe nonverbal learning disability (Rumsey, 1992; Semrud-Clikeman, & Hynd, 1990). However, children with right hemisphere deficits have not been reported to have the severely restricted range of interests, nor the motor stereotypies, that are core elements typically associated with Asperger syndrome. No study has investigated whether children with Asperger syndrome without mental retardation display dyscalculia, dysgraphia, significant problems with directionality, and finger agnosia.

Neurodevelopmental and Behavioral Differences

Currently, many questions remain with regard to high-functioning children and adolescents with PDD. Tables 2 and 3 compare current thought with regard to various functional abilities (Table 2) and behavioral findings (Table 3) as they relate to three disorders: childhood autism without mental retardation, Asperger syndrome, and nonverbal learning disabilities. From a neurodevelopmental perspective, very little can be concluded at this point with regard to Asperger syndrome. Some neurodevelopmental functions show delay disproportionate to mental age but do so only on the basis of very limited clinical research. These areas include nonverbal communication, attention, visual-motor processing, gross motor skills, math reasoning, written language, praxis, directionality, and finger gnosia.

From a neurodevelopmental perspective, it is not clear exactly how one would differentiate

Table 2.   Developmental differences in functional abilities between PDD and nonverbal learning disability (LD)

Functional area	Autism	Asperger	Nonverbal LD
Verbal language	DD	DP	DP
Nonverbal language	DD	DD?	DD?
Peer relations	DD	DD	DD
Attention	DP	DD?	DD
Visual-motor skills	ND	U	DD
Gross motor skills	ND	DD?	DD?
Math reasoning	U	U	DD
Writing	DD	U	DD
Social skills	DD	DD	DD
Praxis	U	DD?	DD?
Directionality	DP	U	DD
Finger gnosia	DP	U	DD
Cohesive links			
Endophoric references	DD	DP	U
Exophoric references	DD	DP	U
Unclear conversation	DP	DD	U

Key: DD, delay disproportionate to mental age; DP, delay proportionate to mental age; ND, no delay or function may exceed mental age; U, unknown on the basis of clinical research; ?, research is in no way conclusive.

Asperger syndrome from a nonverbal learning disability. In contrast, if one compares the behavioral manifestations of Asperger syndrome to those of nonverbal learning disabilities, it becomes much less difficult to differentiate these two conditions based on current nosology. In fact, with the exception of language behaviors, the inverse holds true when one compares children with Asperger syndrome to children with childhood autism without mental retardation. In the case of Asperger syndrome and high-functioning childhood autism, the differentiation is more difficult when comparing behavior, and less difficult when comparing neurodevelopmental functions. In addition to differentiating both of these conditions from nonverbal learning disabilities, it is very important for the developmental physician to differentiate Asperger

syndrome from the early onset of schizophrenia (APA, 1994). This has been a particular concern recently. From a developmental perspective, the history will play a major role in making this determination. Other major distinctions would include the relationship to behavioral experiences and language dysfunction (Baltaxe & D'Angiola, 1992).

MANAGEMENT AND INTERVENTIONS FOR HIGH-FUNCTIONING CHILDREN WITH PDD

Education

Lord and Venter (1992) reported a strong positive relationship between early intelligence and aggregate measures of academic achievement.

Table 3.   Developmental differences in behaviors between PDD and nonverbal learning disability (LD)

Behavior	Autism	Asperger	Nonverbal LD
Language repetition	+ + +	+	−
Echolalia	+ + +	+/−	−
Motor stereotypies	+ + +	+ + +	−
Object perseveration	+ + +	+ + +	−
Rigidity	+ + +	+ + +	+
Unimaginative play	+ + +	+ +	−
Hyperacusia	+ + +	+ + +	−
Tactile defensiveness	+ + +	+ + +	−
Isolation	+ + +	+ + +	+ + +

Key: + + +, striking; + +, noticeable; +, present; −, absent.

Visual problem solving and intelligence were related to achievement in all subjects with the exception of reading comprehension and oral comprehension, which correlated with verbal intelligence. High-functioning children with PDD are able to achieve in academic settings; typically the school will need to provide special education supports and make general education modifications. Although some high-functioning school-age children with PDD may be hyperlexic, even hyperlexic children with semantic pragmatic presentations may have difficulties with reading comprehension.

If the parents of a high-functioning child with PDD hope to get a general education teacher to make classroom modifications for their child with Asperger syndrome or with childhood autism without mental retardation, it is imperative that the teacher communicate with the special education teacher and have a general understanding of autism and the problems of children with PDD, including behavioral and processing impediments. In addition, an elementary teacher who is considered to have a goal-directed approach to education and classroom creativity will be more comfortable working with high-functioning children with autism or Asperger syndrome. Teachers whose style and methods lack flexibility may be unable to make the changes that are necessary to include the child with PDD, who has significant odd and stilted behaviors and a range of processing disabilities. No matter how creative the teacher might be, some background knowledge about PDD and the difficulties he or she may encounter because of the condition is nearly essential.

General education *modifications* will include strategic seating and frequent feedback aimed at maximizing work output by interrupting perseverative behavior and inattention. Modifications that general teachers must be ready to incorporate might include 1) avoiding the use of abstract terms when directing or questioning students with PDD, 2) using visual aids when teaching abstract concepts, 3) preparing students for changes in routine, 4) breaking down tasks into several steps, 5) avoiding the use of language that demands interpretation (metaphors, idioms, etc.), 6) privately communicating

to the child with PDD when he or she should no longer share a topic or idea in class that has become on occasion an object of ridicule within the class, and 7) redirecting the child with PDD's narrow interest into a learning action, such as researching and writing about it rather than dwelling on it in group settings. Once the teacher understands responses necessitated by the condition of the child with PDD without mental retardation, other more individualized modifications can be generated.

In some school settings, it may not be possible to consider general education, no matter how high functioning and well behaved a child with PDD may be. Likewise, some children with PDD without mental retardation make less progress in a general classroom than in a more specialized setting. The educational needs of these children must be determined on a case-by-case basis, especially whenever mainstreaming is recommended. When a school district is intransigent and its program is unable to provide the programming to accommodate the educational needs of a child with PDD without mental retardation, the developmental pediatrician should discuss with the family the possibility of private schools that support children with complex learning problems. The developmental pediatrician must be available to support the family's decision and provide advocacy information with respect to legal rights, protection, and advocacy, as well as support groups.

Counseling

High-functioning children with PDD benefit from ongoing counseling throughout middle childhood and adolescence and into adulthood. Counseling allows the child to develop a trusting relationship with an adult. Because this person is not a parent, he or she is able to make suggestions to the high-functioning child with PDD that may be met with less resistance than had the suggestion come from the parent. Successful counseling is able to help the child to better understand how emotions work. The counselor will try to demonstrate how events that occur to the child are interrelated (Mesibov, 1992). The counselor also works with the child on the need to control motor stereotypies and to set limits on obsessive interests and activities. Most importantly, counseling should help the child with PDD to better understand the nature of his or her problem and to express his or her emotions.

Parent counseling is equally important to allow parents to express their concerns, to understand the nature of the child's problems, and to let the parents know how their child perceives his or her relationship with them and any siblings. Parents need to find help with concerns beyond advocacy and legal rights. In the case of a family that is dysfunctional, family counselors must have some understanding of autism and how it affects a family to be helpful. The developmental pediatrician must take time to identify psychologists, social workers, and psychiatrists who are trained to support families to nurture, shape, and care for children without mental retardation within the autistic spectrum of disability. Professionals must be able to offer the family the support they need. Here is where the developmental pediatrician must be knowledgeable. There are few more heartbreaking diagnoses that a physician can deliver to a parent than PDD. The developmental pediatrician must make this diagnosis, should if at all possible have a social worker sensitive to the issues present to support the family during diagnostic counseling, and should be ready to offer to help the family arrange for a second opinion. Because of the high-functioning capacity and presentation of the child, the parents doubt the diagnosis in many cases. The typical conceptualization of autism is far different from parents' perception of their bright although unusual child.

Adaptation to and acceptance of this diagnosis is only the beginning. If the child has the capability of inclusion within a general school setting, he or she will most likely endure difficulty in completing work within time constraints, in facing ongoing peer ridicule, and in failing to find a friend. It is difficult for children with PDD to control the drive to engage in perseverative sterotypies and other socially unacceptable behaviors. The child will require enormous effort by the parents to succeed and progress to his or her maximum potential. This is a child who may eventually achieve partial or complete independence but whose potential for developing an intimate relationship is at best poor. Temple Grandin is such a person, and her story has been put in perspective in an article by Oliver Sacks (1994). In addition, the family counselor must include the sibling(s) of the child with PDD. In a functional family, siblings will receive less attention at times, especially if they are fortunate enough to have average or above-average competency. The sibling of a child with PDD not only may experience less attention but, if he or she is close enough in age and attends the same school, may also be teased about his or her sib. At some point, a situation may arise in which he or she experiences the harrassment of the sib with PDD. In short, even the family counselor who is working with a stable, functional family has a large number of issues to address. In the case of a dysfunctional family, the impairments may overwhelm the situation, making family therapy painful and discouraging.

The developmental pediatrician should follow the child with Asperger syndrome or childhood autism and should monitor the child's adaptive and functional development. Because he or she is charged with possessing developmental information and knowledge relating to the life cycle, the pediatrician can be of great importance in helping the family meet year-to-year needs and can act as an ombudsman. Information about school placement, adaptive development, social stimulation, summer camps that integrate children with learning disabilities without mental retardation, controversial treatments, pharmacotherapy, and vocational and college opportunities will be meaningful throughout the child and adolescent phases of development (see Chapters 25, 26, 31, and 33, Volume I).

Language Intervention

Both the WHO and the APA stipulate that children with Asperger syndrome should not have a language deficit. The study reviewed earlier by Fine et al. (1994) demonstrated that high-functioning children with childhood autism have significantly greater difficulty with language than children with Asperger syndrome. It remains controversial whether the communication deficit of the child with Asperger syndrome is due to language, but until the efficacy of pragmatic language therapy is seriously questioned, the pediatrician should be willing to prescribe this or social skills training. Because of problems with comprehension, and very often ability to learn the nuances of grammer, frequently high-functioning children in *both* the childhood autism and Asperger syndrome groups can benefit from both speech and language pathologist and learning disability teacher interventions to help them with speaking and listening, comprehension, and writing.

As high-functioning children with PDD enter adolescence, they experience shifts in interests. The range of communication abilities at this level becomes much broader. Even the verbal high-functioning child with PDD experiences great difficulty coping with the increasingly complex issues with which all teenagers are faced. Communication at this level is a major challenge for the high-functioning child with PDD; goals should include 1) participation in age-appropriate social relationships outside of the family, and 2) to learn language that will maximize the opportunity to develop individualized interests. Strategies to help adolescents with PDD to develop these skills include word-oriented games, computer games, journals, writing stories, volunteer work in libraries, and supervised teenage group discussions (Lord, 1988).

Social Skills Training

The TEACCH program developed in Chapel Hill, North Carolina, has had success in including social skills group training as part of the habilitation of the high-functioning child with PDD (Mesibov, 1992). At the center of this approach is a cognitive social learning scheme that includes role playing, rehearsal, participating in social activities in a natural social setting, and coming to an understanding of social expectations through social encounters. TEACCH sought to include adolescents and adults without PDD in these groups and had success recruiting college students who had an interest in learning about developmental dis-

abilities. The goals of this intervention have been skill development and environmental adaptation.

Management of the Autistic Savant

High-functioning children with PDD sometimes demonstrate abilities that significantly exceed measured intelligence. People with such abilities are often referred to as "savants." Savant abilities among children with PDD have been noted in many different areas, including music, art, calender calculations, and general calculations. Rimland and Fein (1988) reported that 1 of 10 children with autism demonstrates savant capacities. Certainly, high-functioning children with PDD would demonstrate these capacities at a rate exceeding that of the general population with PDD.

Very little has been proven with regard to the evolution of autistic savant capacities. Some anecdotal observations have been reported. Some researchers contend that the savant ability plateaus and may regress by adolescence. Another unscientific observation is that, as the autistic child progresses toward more independence and social control, the savant ability regresses (Rimland & Fein, 1988). These abilities have been related to isolated areas of superior processing, notably Wechsler subtests that include digit span, arithmetic, and information. If an autistic child tends to obsess on a particular subject, some contend that he or she should be encouraged to expand involvement in the area. For example, if an autistic child has a keen interest in animal life, learning about various aspects of animal life ultimately may be useful to him or her. Temple Grandin contends that such encouragement led to her success and vocation (Grandin & Scariano, 1986). However, it is difficult to see how this approach could be useful in someone whose area of interest is calendrical calculations.

Psychopharmacological Intervention

There is recent evidence that fluoxetine hydrochloride (Prozac) and clomipramine hydrochloride (Anaphranil) may be effective for at least some patients with autism (Cook, Rowlett, Jaselskis, & Leventhal, 1992; Garber,

McGonigle, Slomka & MonteVerde, 1992; McDougle et al., 1992). These drugs have established efficacy in the child with obsessive-compulsive disorder (Green, 1991). In a number of these children, the stereotypies and obsessive behaviors have been significantly reduced. Both of these drugs are serotonin inhibitors, and the primary metabolite of clomipramine (desmethylclomipramine) inhibits norepinephrine uptake as well. Because of the side effects of both of these drugs, usage is recommended for children who have reached 11 years of age (Green, 1991).

Fluoxetine reaches peak plasma levels in 6–8 hours, and its elimination half-life is 24–36 hours. It takes several weeks for steady-state plasma levels to be achieved. Untoward effects of fluoxetine include nausea, weight loss, anxiety, nervousness, insomnia, and excessive sweating. Dosage is usually initiated at 20 mg orally every morning, and in many cases this is an optimal dosage.

Clomipramine belongs to the tricyclic antidepressant class of psychopharmacologic agents. The mean half-life is 32 hours, and that of its major metabolite is 70 hours. Peak plasma levels generally are reached 3–4 hours after ingestion. As with all tricyclic antidepressants, it is imperative to examine the child's electrocardiogram prior to initiating the drug. Any abnormality of the P-R interval or QRS complex is a contraindication to use. Electrocardiograms also should be checked once medication is initiated, because the drug will increase these intervals. Apart from cardiac arrhythmias, other possible side effects include seizures (risk is approximately 1.5% after 1 year of usage), somnolence, tremor, dizziness, headache, sleep disorders, increased diaphoresis, postural hypotension, tachycardia, and syncope; gastrointestinal problems, dysmenorrhea, and ejaculation failure are also untoward effects of the drug. Serum levels should be monitored and should be maintained below 60 ng/ml. Abrupt withdrawal can result in significant side effects as well. The initial dosage is generally 25 mg/day, and it is titrated to a maximum dosage of 100 mg/day or 3 mg/kg (whichever is less). Over time, the dosage can be increased gradually. This drug carries significant risks, and this class of drugs has been responsible for childhood deaths resulting from cardiac arrhythmias. The developmental pediatrician who is inexperienced in the use of clomipramine should seek guidance from a child psychiatrist who has experience or should refer the child to an experienced psychiatrist to evaluate him or her as a potential candidate for pharmacotherapy.

If a child has a significant problem with attention that appears to be interfering with learning and behavior, a trial of stimulants should be considered. This should be monitored with the help of the classroom teacher. In addition to the side effects usually associated with stimulants, in the child with PDD there exists the risk that the drug may increase the frequency of stereotypies and perseverations. The parents should monitor the frequency of these behaviors before the drug trial is initiated.

OUTCOME STUDIES

Recent outcome investigations of high-functioning adolescents and adults with PDD are much more encouraging than those completed in the 1970s. With the exception of the area of reading comprehension, most recent studies demonstrate that adolescents with PDD with full-scale IQs above 80 can develop functional academic skills (Lord & Venter, 1992). More children with PDD appear to be achieving some measure of independent living. However with the exception of one study (Szatmari, Bartolucci, Bremner, Bond, & Rich, 1989), studies have been less encouraging with regard to the development of adaptive skills and vocational independence. Outcome still appears dependent on the expansion of community vocational and residential support services for high-functioning individuals with PDD. Recent outcome studies suggest that the high-functioning subgroup of children with PDD have the potential to achieve a better outcome (Tantam, 1991). Mental health support as an adult would seem to be of great importance to the child with PDD who achieves independence.

REFERENCES

American Psychiatric Association. (1994). *Diagnostic and statistical manual of mental disorders* (4th ed.). Washington, DC: American Psychiatric Press.

Asperger, H. (1991). "Autistic psychopathy" in childhood (U. Frith, Trans. and Annotator). In U. Frith (Ed.), *Autism and Asperger syndrome* (pp. 37–92). Cambridge, England: Cambridge University Press.

Baltaxe & D'Angiola (1992). Cohesion in the discourse-interaction of the autistic, specifically language impaired and normal children. *Journal of Autism and Developmental Disorders, 22*, 1–21.

Baron-Cohen, S. (1988). Social and pragmatic deficits in autism: Cognitive or affective? *Journal of Autism and Developmental Disorders, 18*, 379–402.

Bartolucci, G., & Fine, J. (1987). The frequency of cohesive weakness in psychiatric syndromes. *Applied Psychologist, 8*, 67–74.

Cook, E.H., Rowlett, R., Jaselskis, C., & Leventhal, B.L. (1992). Fluoxetine treatment of children and adults with autistic disorder and mental retardation. *Journal of Child and Adolescent Psychiatry, 31*, 739–745.

Farber, J. (1991). Autism and other communication disorders. In A.J. Capute & P.J. Accardo (Eds.), *Developmental disabilities in infancy and childhood* (pp. 305–323). Baltimore: Paul H. Brookes Publishing Co.

Farber, J., & Capute, A. (1984). Understanding autism. *Clinical Pediatrics, 23*, 199–202.

Fine, J., Bartolucci, G., Szatmari, P., & Ginsberg, G. (1994). Cohesive discourse in pervasive developmental disorders. *Journal of Autism and Developmental Disabilities, 24*, 315–329.

Frith, U. (1991). Asperger and his syndrome. In U. Frith (Ed.), *Autism and Asperger syndrome* (pp. 1–36). Cambridge, England: Cambridge University Press.

Garber, H.J., McGonigle, J.J., Slomka, G.T., & Monteverde, E. (1992). Clomipramine treatment of stereotypic behaviors and self-injury in patients with developmental disabilities. *Journal of the American Academy of Child and Adolescent Psychiatry, 31*, 1157–1160.

Ghaziuddin, M., Tsai, L.Y., & Ghaziuddin, N. (1992). Brief report: A reappraisal of clumsiness as a diagnostic feature of Asperger syndrome. *Journal of Autism and Developmental Disorders, 22*, 651–656.

Gillberg, C. (1989). Asperger syndrome in 23 Swedish children. *Developmental Medicine and Child Neurology, 31*, 520–531.

Gillberg, C., & Coleman, M. (1992). *The biology of the autistic syndromes* (pp. 85–95). Oxford, England: Blackwell Scientific Publications Ltd.

Grandin, T., & Scariano, M.N. (1986). *Emergence: Labeled autistic*. Novato, CA: Arena Press.

Green, W.H. (1991). Principles of psychopharmacotherapy and specific drug treatments. In M. Lewis (Ed.), *Child and adolescent psychiatry* (pp. 770–795). Baltimore: Williams & Wilkins.

Kanner, L. (1943). Autistic disturbances of affective contact. *Nervous Child, 2*, 217–250.

Kanner, L. (1971). Follow-up study of eleven autistic children originally reported in 1943. *Journal of Autism and Childhood Schizophrenia, 1*, 119–145.

Klin, A. (1994). Asperger syndrome. *Child and Adolescent Psychiatric Clinics of North America, 3*, 131–148.

LeCouteur, A., Rutter, M., Lord, C., Rios, P., Robertson, S., Holdgrafer, M., & McLennan, J.D. (1989). Autism diagnostic interview: A standardized investigator-based instrument. *Journal of Autism and Developmental Disorders, 19*, 363–387.

Lord, C. (1988). Enhancing communication in adolescents with autism. *Topics in Language Disorders, 9*, 72–81.

Lord, C., Mulloy, C., Wendelboe, M., & Schopler, E. (1991). Pre- and perinatal factors in high-functioning females and males with autism. *Journal of Autism and Developmental Disorders, 21*, 197–209.

Lord, C., & Venter, A. (1992). Outcome and follow-up studies of high-functioning autistic individuals. In E. Schopler & G.B. Mesibov (Eds.), *High-functioning individuals with autism* (pp. 197–200). New York: Plenum Press.

McDougall, C.J., Price, L.H., Volkmar, F.R., Goodman, W.K., Ward-Obrien, D., Nielsen, J., Bregman, J., & Cohen, D.J. (1992). Clomipramine in autism: preliminary evidence of efficacy. *Journal of the American Academy of Child & Adolescent Psychiatry, 31*, 746–750.

Mesibov, G.B. (1992). Treatment issues with high-functioning adolescents and adults with autism. In E. Schopler & G.B. Mesibov (Eds.), *High-functioning individuals with autism* (pp. 143–156). New York: Plenum Press.

Mesibov, G.B., & Schopler, E. (1992). Introduction to high-functioning individuals with autism. In E. Schopler & G.B. Mesibov (Eds.), *High-functioning individuals with autism* (pp. 3–9). New York: Plenum Press.

Rimland, B., & Fein, D. (1988). Special talents of autistic savants. In L.K. Obler & D. Fein (Eds.), *The exceptional brain* (pp. 474–492). New York: Guilford Press.

Rumsey, J.M. (1992). Neuropsychological studies of high-level autism. In E. Schopler & G.B. Mesibov (Eds.), *High-functioning individuals with autism* (pp. 41–59). New York: Plenum Press.

Rutter, M. (1983). Cognitive deficits in the pathogenesis of autism. *Journal of Child Psychology and Psychiatry, 24*, 513–531.

Rutter, M., & Schopler, E. (1987). Autism and pervasive developmental disorders: Concept and diagnostic issues. *Journal of Autism and Developmental Disorders, 17*, 159–186.

Sacks, O. (1993, December 27–January 3). A neurologist's notebook: An anthropologist on Mars. *The New Yorker*, pp. 106–125.

Semrud-Clikeman, M., & Hynd, G.W. (1990). Right hemispheric dysfunction in nonverbal learning disabilities: Social, academic, and adaptive functioning in adults and children. *Psychological Bulletin, 107*, 196–209.

Simon, C. (1986). *Evaluating communicative competence*. Tucson, AZ: Communication Skill Builders.

Szatmari, P., Bartolucci, G., & Bremner, R. (1989). Asperger's syndrome and autism: Comparison of early history and outcome. *Developmental Medicine and Child Neurology, 31*, 709–720.

Szatmari, P., Bartolucci, G., Bremner, R.S., Bond, S., & Rich, S. (1989). A follow-up study of high functioning autistic children. *Journal of Autism and Developmental Disorders, 19*, 213–226.

Szatmari, P., Tuff, L., Finlayson, M.A., & Bartolucci, G. (1990). Asperger's syndrome and autism: Neurocognitive aspects. *Journal of the American Academy of Child and Adolescent Psychiatry, 29*, 130–136.

Tantam, D. (1988). Lifelong eccentricity and social isolation. II. Asperger's syndrome or schizoid personality disorder. *British Journal of Psychiatry, 153*, 783–791.

Tantam, D. (1991). Asperger syndrome in adulthood. In U. Frith (Ed.), *Autism and Asperger syndrome* (pp. 147–183). Cambridge, England: Cambridge University Press.

Voeller, K.K.S. (1986). Right-hemisphere deficit syndrome in children. *American Journal of Psychiatry, 143*, 1004–1009.

Volden, J., & Lord, C. (1991). Neologisms and idiosyncratic language in autistic speakers. *Journal of Autism and Developmental Disorders, 21*, 109–130.

Wechsler, D. *Wechsler Intelligence Scale for Children–Revised*. New York: Psychological Corporation.

Wiig, E., & Secord, W. (1989). *Test of language competence*. San Antonio, TX: Psychological Corporation.

Wing, L. (1981). Asperger's syndrome: A clinical account. *Psychological Medicine, 11*, 115–129.

Wing, L., & Atwood, A. (1987). Syndromes of autism and atypical development. In D.J. Cohen, A.M. Donnellan, & R. Paul (Eds.), *Handbook of autism and pervasive developmental disorders* (pp. 3–19). New York: John Wiley & Sons.

Wolff, S., & Barlow, A. (1979). Schizoid personality in childhood: A comparison study of schizoid, autistic, and normal children. *Journal of Child Psychology and Psychiatry, 20*, 19–46.

World Health Organization. (1992). *International classification of diseases: Tenth revision* (pp. 253–258). Geneva: Author.

World Health Organization. (1993). *1993 draft of Chapter 5 categories for-F99 (mental, behavioral, and developmental disorders)*. Geneva: Author.

Zachman, L., Jorgensen, C., Huisingh, R., & Barrett, M. (1984). *Test of Problem Solving*. Moline, IL: Linguisystems.

Chapter 25

The Discovery and Study of Rett Syndrome

Lessons for the Understanding of Developmental Disabilities

Hugo W. Moser, M.D., and Sakkubai Naidu, M.D.

In 1966, Professor Andreas Rett, working in his Vienna clinic, observed two thin girls sitting next to each other on their mother's laps, both rocking back and forth, and both constantly wringing their hands (Haas, 1988). He noticed that the behavior of the two girls was identical, and that it differed from the varied stereotypical movements that are often observed in people with severe or profound mental retardation. Most significantly, with the aid of his chief nurse, Rett remembered six other girls whose behavior matched that of these two patients. This moment represented the first step in the ongoing study of a disorder that causes mental retardation and developmental disability—a disorder that rivals in frequency the most common metabolic cause of severe or profound mental retardation, phenylketonuria.

EXISTENCE OF RETT SYNDROME

The combination of signs and symptoms that are now designated as constituting Rett syndrome has been described by Hagberg, Aicardi, Dias, and Ramos (1983). The diagnostic criteria, summarized by the Rett Syndrome Diagnostic Criteria Work Group (1988), are listed in Table 1. Table 2 lists the four clinical stages of the disorder delineated by Hagberg and Witt-Engerstrom (1986). By 1987, this complex pattern of behavioral and neurologic disturbances had been noted in over 2,500 girls in all parts of the world. The pattern of evolution and symptomatology in these patients has been remarkably consistent. Thus, at the phenomenological level, Rett syndrome clearly exists.

RETT SYNDROME AS A DISTINCT DISEASE ENTITY

Given the fact that many patients show the consistent pattern of symptoms and signs that are now referred to as Rett syndrome, the most important next question is whether all, or at least a significant proportion, of these cases represent a single disease entity. This question exemplifies the complex relationships between phenotype and genotype raised by McKusick in 1969. McKusick cited the concepts of *genetic heterogeneity*—that is, a similar phenotype may be associated with several genetic disorders—and *phenotypic variability*—that is, a single genetic disorder may be associated with varying phenotypic manifestations. Because of its occurrence only in girls, and the results of twin studies (Zoghbi, 1988), Rett syndrome is now considered likely to be genetically determined. The degree to which genetic heterogeneity exists cannot be determined until a biologic marker is identified. The search for such a marker is a research priority. Hyman and Batshaw (1986) described an 8-year-old girl with ornithine transcarbamylase deficiency whose phenotype corresponded to Rett syndrome except for the presence of the exclusion criterion of hyperammonemia and a history of episodes of severe vomiting and hyperammonemic coma. Because no biologic marker has been identified, the

Table 1.   Diagnostic criteria for Rett syndrome

Necessary criteria
1. Apparently normal prenatal and perinatal period
2. Apparently normal psychomotor development through the first 6 months
3. Normal head circumference at birth
4. Deceleration of head growth between ages 5 months and 4 years
5. Loss of acquired purposeful hand skills between 6 and 30 months temporally associated with communication dysfunction and social withdrawal
6. Development of severely impaired expressive and receptive language, and presence of apparent severe psychomotor retardation
7. Stereotypic hand movements, such as hand wringing/squeezing, clapping/tapping, mouthing, and "washing"/rubbing automatisms, appearing after purposeful hand skills are lost
8. Appearance of gait apraxia and truncal apraxia-ataxia between 1 and 4 years
9. Diagnosis tentative until 2–5 years of age

Supportive criteria
1. Breathing dysfunction
   Periodic apnea during wakefulness
   Intermittent hyperventilation
   Breath-holding spells
   Forced expulsion of air or saliva
2. EEG abnormalities
   Slow waking background and intermittent rhythmic slowing (3–5 Hz)
   Epileptiform discharges, with or without clinical seizures
3. Seizures
4. Spasticity often with associated development of muscle wasting and dystonia
5. Peripheral vasomotor disturbances
6. Scoliosis
7. Growth retardation
8. Hypotrophic small feet

Exclusionary criteria
1. Evidence of intrauterine growth retardation
2. Organomegaly or other signs of storage disease
3. Retinopathy or optic atrophy
4. Microcephaly at birth
5. Evidence of perinatally acquired brain damage
6. Existence of identifiable metabolic or other progressive neurologic disorder
7. Acquired neurologic disorders resulting from severe infections or head trauma

From Trevathan, E., & Naidu, S. (1988). The clinical recognition and differential diagnosis of Rett syndrome. *Journal of Child Neurology, 3*(Suppl.), 6–16; reprinted by permission.

degree of phenotypic variability is also unknown. By analogy with other disorders, Opitz has cautioned that

> since cause in the Rett syndrome is not known, it is impossible to determine the true degree and complete extent of its variability, and we may be in danger of severely truncating the phenotypes by drawing the diagnostic criteria too narrowly and exclusively. (Opitz, 1986, p. 29)

Hagberg and Gillberg (1993) have summarized the growing literature on atypical or "forme fruste" children with Rett syndrome. These include children in whom developmental regression is less severe than in the classic syndrome, a preserved speech variant, an infantile seizure onset variant, a congenital variant, and a late childhood regression variant. The relationship of these variants to classic Rett syndrome cannot be determined until the underlying defect of Rett syndrome or a diagnostic marker is identified.

DISCOVERY OF RETT SYNDROME

Discussions with many pediatricians and neurologists indicated that they had seen children with Rett syndrome prior to its description, but had viewed them as individual cases that defied

Table 2. Clinical characteristics of Rett syndrome and differential diagnosis by stage

Stage	Clinical characteristics	Differential diagnosis
I Onset: 6–18 mos. Duration: Months	Developmental stagnation Deceleration of head/brain growth Disinterest in play activity and environment Hypotonia EEG: normal or minimal slowing of posterior rhythm	Benign congenital hypotonia Prader-Willi syndrome Cerebral palsy
II Onset: 1–3 yrs. Duration: Weeks to months	Rapid developmental regression with irritability Loss of hand use Seizures Hand stereotypies: wringing, clapping, tapping, mouthing Autistic manifestations Loss of expressive language Insomnia Self-abusive behavior (e.g., chewing fingers, slapping face) EEG: slowing and gradual loss of normal sleep activity; focal or multifocal spike and wave	Autism Psychosis Hearing or visual disturbance Epileptic encephalopathy Neurocutaneous syndromes Neurodegenerative disorders Various disorders of organic acid and amino acid metabolism
III Onset: 2–10 yrs. Duration: Months to years	Severe mental retardation/apparent dementia Amelioration of autistic features Seizures Hand stereotypies; wringing, clapping, tapping, mouthing Prominent ataxia and apraxia Hyperreflexia and progressive rigidity Hyperventilation, breath-holding, aerophagia during waking Weight loss with excellent appetite Early scoliosis Bruxism EEG: gradual disappearance of posterior rhythm, generalized slow, absent vertex and spindle activity, epileptiform abnormalities activated during sleep	Spastic ataxic cerebral palsy Spinocerebellar degeneration Leukodystrophies or other storage disorders Neuroaxonal dystrophy Lennox-Gastaut syndrome Angelman syndrome
IV Onset: 10 + yrs. Duration: Years	Progressive scoliosis, muscle wasting and rigidity Decreasing mobility, wheelchair use Growth retardation Improved eye contact Virtual absence of expressive and receptive language Trophic disturbance of feet Reduced seizure frequency EEG: poor background organization with marked slowing and multifocal spikes and slow spike and wave pattern activated by sleep	Unknown degenerative disorder

From Trevathan, E., & Naidu, S. (1988). The clinical recognition and differential diagnosis of Rett syndrome. *Journal of Child Neurology, 3*(Suppl.), 6–16; reprinted by permission.

understanding, or as examples of autism. Rett's spark of recognition, although in part a matter of chance, reflected his remarkable powers of observation and his vast clinical experience. It may also reflect the organization of health ser-

vices in Austria at that time. As part of his responsibility for mental retardation services in Austria, Rett saw a considerable proportion of all patients with severe and profound mental retardation. Patients were first examined by more junior staff and then seen by Rett at the final stage of this evaluation process. This organizational pattern meant that one physician saw a large number of patients with mental retardation, thus increasing the likelihood of the "two-hit phenomenon" that led to the recognition of Rett syndrome. Such an organizational structure is not common in the United States.

RECOGNITION OF RETT SYNDROME

Three factors may have contributed to the 17-year interval between the initial description of Rett syndrome and its general recognition: 1) the first description of the syndrome was published in an Austrian journal, whose readership was largely limited to Austrians; 2) behavioral abnormalities and movement disorders were difficult to describe without photographs, videotapes, or motion pictures; and 3) the syndrome initially was associated erroneously with hyperammonemia. These factors are cited here because they may well apply to other disorders that are as yet unrecognized and unnamed. Efforts should be made to recognize and correct these impediments.

The 1983 publication on Rett syndrome by Hagberg et al. proved to be the main catalyst in making the world aware of the disorder. This publication appeared in English in a widely read and indexed journal and included photographs.

IMPLICATIONS FOR DEVELOPMENTAL DISABILITIES

The delineation of Rett syndrome facilitates targeted study of a significant number of people with severe developmental disabilities. In this way it is analogous to fragile X syndrome. The establishment of such groupings is important because it is difficult and probably impossible to understand developmental disabilities unless they are separated into meaningful subdivisions. The higher the proportion of people with developmental disabilities that can be assigned to specific etiologies or categories, the better our opportunity to prevent or treat these disorders.

Two major research challenges emerge with respect to Rett syndrome: the clarification of the genetics and the pathophysiology of behavioral and neurologic features. The genetics of Rett syndrome are unique and cannot be accounted for fully by known mechanisms. Along with the Lesch-Nyhan syndrome, Rett syndrome represents a striking behavior disorder that surely has a biologic basis. Anatomic, biochemical, and neurophysiologic studies may yield new information about how these characteristic behavior patterns come about and how they can be treated. To the extent to which this can be accomplished, the study of Rett syndrome may also throw light on autism, movement disorders, self-mutilation, and respiratory control mechanisms.

SEARCH FOR A DIAGNOSTIC MARKER

The major barrier to understanding Rett syndrome is the absence of a biologic marker. The situation may be likened to the status of Down syndrome during the 90 years between the identification of the disorder and the identification of the chromosomal abnormality. The consistency of the highly complex manifestations, combined with the data that support a genetic basis, suggest that at least a proportion of cases will be found to represent a single disease entity. This supposition underlies current research efforts to define the genetic basis and disease mechanisms.

The first step in identifying a diagnostic marker is to assemble and study a sufficiently large group of children who have the classic Rett syndrome phenotype and no other known etiology. The exclusion of phenocopies is an important and difficult challenge. Contamination of the study sample with only a few subjects with disorders other than Rett syndrome may lead to erroneous conclusions. It may be difficult, for example, to distinguish Rett syndrome from ceroid lipofuscinosis (Batten disease). The ocular abnormalities characteristic of Batten disease often do not manifest themselves until after age 4, the early clinical features resemble those of Rett syndrome, and demonstration of the most specific markers of Batten disease requires specialized and moderately invasive procedures that become appropriate only when there are significant reasons to suspect the diagnosis. Because of the risk of misdiagnosing Batten disease as Rett syndrome, the diagnosis of Rett syndrome should be considered as tentative in children less than 4 years old. Table 2 lists other conditions that must be excluded. At this time, the search for a diagnostic marker has been unsuccessful.

GENETICS

The Rett syndrome gene is believed to be X-linked dominant and lethal in boys, with reproductive lethality in girls. The great majority of cases are believed to represent new mutations (Comings, 1986). This hypothesis, although consistent with the observed patterns of inheritance, has not yet been proved, and other mechanisms have been cited (Ellison et al., 1992).

In the absence of a diagnostic marker, suppositions about the genetics of Rett syndrome are based on the analysis of the familial occurrence of cases with the classic phenotype. The fact that the classic phenotype has been observed only in girls raised the suspicion that the disorder was genetically determined. The most convincing support for a genetic basis is provided by the concordance in identical twins and the discordance in nonidentical twins (Table 3).

Approximately 0.5% of children with Rett syndrome have relatives other than twins with Rett syndrome. Although this relatively low recurrence risk permits genetic counselors to be optimistic, this familial incidence is in excess of the 1 in 15,000 expected from chance alone. The confinement of Rett syndrome to girls suggests that it is linked in some way to the X chromosome. McKusick's catalogue lists 139 disorders that are X linked (McKusick, 1994). Most of these disorders are recessive; that is, only boys are affected, whereas girls are phenotypically normal or only mildly involved. Only four disorders have been designated as X-linked dominant: the Aicardi syndrome (McKusick 30405), incontinentia pigmenti (McKusick 30830), the oral-facial-digital syndrome (McKusick 31120), and focal dermal hypoplasia (McKusick 30560).

The hypothesis that the great majority of Rett syndrome cases represent new mutations is based on the observation that people with the disorder have as many brothers as sisters, and that the rate of spontaneous miscarriages is not abnormally high. If a gene lethal to boys had been transmitted by a carrier mother, the ratio of male to female siblings would have been 1:2, and the rate of spontaneous miscarriages would have been above average. The rarity of familial cases is also consistent with the hypothesis that most cases represent new mutations. The few cases that are familial have been hypothesized to be examples of germinal mosaicism (Comings, 1986) (i.e., some but not all of the germline cells have the Rett mutation). Under these circumstances, some but not all the female offspring would have the disorder, with male fetuses failing to survive. If this hypothesis is correct, in these families the ratio of male to female siblings should be 1:2 and the rate of spontaneous miscarriages higher than normal. Although the number of such families is too small to permit statistically valid comparisons, in one of these families the number of spontaneous miscarriages was high (Hanefeld, 1985). Comings has used studies of families with Rett syndrome members to derive an estimate of the relative frequency of mutations that result in germinal mosaicism versus total germinal mutations, a ratio that at present cannot be estimated from other sources. With 2 in 600 families having affected sisters, the ratio would be 1:300. However, because affected brothers would be missed, the ratio is probably closer to 1:150 (Comings, 1986).

Detailed genealogic studies conducted in Sweden by Akesson, Hagberg, Wahlstrom, and Engerstrom (1992) provide additional evidence for a genetic basis of Rett syndrome. These

Table 3. Familial cases in Rett syndrome

Relationship	Number of pairs
Monozygotic twins, concordant	7
Dizygotic twin, discordant	
Female/female	2
Female/male	4
Full sisters	3
Half-sisters	2
Second half-cousins	1
Aunt–niece	1

From Zoghbi, H. (1988). Genetic aspects of Rett syndrome. *Journal of Child Neurology, 3*(Suppl.), 576–578; reprinted by permission.

authors were able to trace 77 families for 7–10 generations. Thirty-nine of the families were traced to nine small and separate rural areas. Common origins were traced with equal frequency to paternal and maternal ancestry, and there was a raised rate of consanguineous marriages in the paternal as well as in the maternal ancestry. These findings, although not conclusive, would be most compatible with an autosomal recessive mode of inheritance.

Although the preponderance of evidence strongly supports a genetic basis for Rett syndrome, the nature of the genetic defect remains undefined. Ellison et al. (1992) have excluded a substantial portion of the X chromosome as a candidate for the Rett syndrome gene. Searches for the presence of abnormal X inactivation patterns or uniparental disomy so far have not revealed definitive abnormalities.

NEUROPATHOLOGIC AND NEUROCHEMICAL CHANGES

Oldfors, Sourander, and Percy (1993) have reviewed the neuropathology and neurochemistry of Rett syndrome. The major and consistent macroscopic change is a reduction in brain size associated with a 12%–41% reduction in brain weight (Jellinger, Armstrong, Zoghbi, & Percy, 1988). These postmortem findings are consistent with recent in vivo volumetric magnetic resonance imaging (MRI) studies of 11 children with Rett syndrome and age-matched controls performed by Reiss et al. (1993). The children with Rett syndrome showed a 30% overall reduction in brain volume that affected gray matter somewhat more than white matter. The caudate nuclei were reduced disproportionally in size, even in comparison to the overall reduction in brain volume. The youngest (4-year-old) child showed the same degree of volume reduction as the teenage and 20-year-old patients.

Microscopic studies have shown no defects of neuronal migration or white matter degeneration. The most consistent finding has been hypopigmentation of the zona compacta of the substantia nigra, with reduced neuromelanin in many of the neurons. Belischenko, Oldfors, Magberg, and Dahlstrom (1994) demonstrated abnormalities in the dendritic architecture. Neu-

rochemical studies have revealed a reduction in the levels of dopamine in several cortical regions and the putamen and reduced levels of choline acetyltransferase activity, particularly in the thalamus (Wenk, Naidu, Casanova, Kitt, & Moser, 1991). The reduced dopamine content in the basal ganglia is consistent with the hypopigmentation of the substantia nigra and is indicative of an abnormality of the dopaminergic system. The reduced level of acetyltransferase activity suggests that there may also be an abnormality of the cholinergic system. Analysis of complex brain lipids revealed an apparently selective reduction of gangliosides GD1A and GT1b (Lekman, Hagberg, & Svennerholm, 1991a, 1991b). Because GD1A is prominent in synaptic terminals, its reduction may be related to the dendritic abnormalities noted in the morphologic studies.

PATHOGENESIS OF RETT SYNDROME

The coordinated analysis of clinical, pathologic, and radiologic findings has led to the hypothesis that Rett syndrome differs fundamentally from the classic neurodegenerative disorders. Studies in our clinic and elsewhere indicate that, subsequent to Stage III (see Table 2), Rett syndrome appears to be a static rather than a progressive disorder, and individuals in Stage IV of the illness may remain in a static condition for decades. The volumetric MRI studies of Reiss et al. (1993) also failed to show progressive alterations in older children, and the same conclusion was reached by Belischenko et al. (1994) in their neuropathologic studies. The rapidly progressive Stages I through III of Rett syndrome coincide temporarily with the period of synaptogenesis (Huttenlocher & deCourten, 1987). It is our hypothesis that Rett syndrome involves an as yet undefined abnormality in synaptogenesis and that this leads to the profound failure in early development, and a static course once this stage of development has passed. Retrospective developmental histories obtained in our clinic suggest that even the presymptomatic development of girls with Rett syndrome falls somewhat short of typical (S. Naidu, unpublished observation, 1995). Recent pathologic studies by Baumann and Kemper

(1992) have demonstrated changes in the inferior olivary nuclei that suggest abnormalities in the late prenatal period. The nature of the postulated early developmental abnormality is speculative. One possibility involves one of the brain growth factors that are currently under intensive study (Koliatsos et al., 1991; Ozcelik, Rosenthal, & Francke, 1991).

THERAPY OF RETT SYNDROME

Children with Rett syndrome require a carefully integrated program aimed to maintain general health, nutrition, physical therapy, and communication skills. Nutrition management includes a high caloric intake and the symptomatic treatment of constipation with high-fiber diets and mineral oil. A communication board can be of great value as an alternative means of communication. Special attention must be directed toward the prevention and therapy of scoliosis. This condition may advance more rapidly in children with Rett syndrome than in children with idiopathic scoliosis, and treatment includes bracing and at times primary fusion (Stokland, Lidstrom, & Hagberg, 1993). Seizures have been managed successfully in 75% of children with customary medications such as carbamazepine and sodium valproate. Care must be taken to distinguish between seizures and the intermittent periods of apnea and hyperventilation that are a frequent feature in children with Rett syndrome in the waking state. Therapies directed toward the postulated basic mechanisms of Rett syndrome have not been successful so far. Administration of L-dopa or dopamine agonists, such as bromcriptine, or the opiate antagonist naltrexone, have not been of benefit (Percy et al., 1994).

REFERENCES

Akesson, H.O., Hagberg, B., Wahlstrom, J., & Engerstrom, I.W. (1992). Rett syndrome: A search for gene sources. *American Journal of Medical Genetics, 42,* 104–108.

Bauman, M.L., & Kemper, T.L. (1992). Pervasive neuropathological abnormalities of the brain in Rett syndrome. *Journal of Neuropathology and Experimental Neurology, 51,* 340.

Belischenko, P.V., Oldfors, A., Hagberg, B., & Dahlstrom, A. (1994). Rett syndrome: 3-D confocal microscopy of cortical pyramidal dendrites and afferents. *NeuroReport, 5,* 1509–1513.

Comings, D.E. (1986). The genetics of Rett syndrome: The consequence of a disorder where every case is a new mutation. *American Journal of Medical Genetics, 24,* 383–388.

Ellison, K.A., Fill, C.P., Terwilliger, J., DeGennaro, L.J., Martin-Gallardo, A., Anvret, M., Percy, A.K., Ott, J., & Zoghbi, H. (1992). Examination of X chromosome markers in Rett syndrome: Exclusion mapping with a novel variation on multilocus linkage analysis. *American Journal of Human Genetics, 50,* 278–287.

Haas, R.H. (1988). The history and challenge of Rett syndrome. *Journal of Child Neurology, 3,* 53–55.

Hagberg, B., Aicardi, J., Dias, K., & Ramos, O. (1983). A progressive syndrome of autism, dementia, ataxia and loss of purposeful hand use in girls: Rett's syndrome. Reports of 35 cases. *Annals of Neurology, 14,* 471–479.

Hagberg, B., & Gillberg, C. (1993). Rett variants—rettoid phenotypes. In B. Hagberg (Ed.), *Rett syndrome—clinical and biological aspects* (pp. 40–60). London: McKeith Press.

Hagberg, B., & Witt-Engerstrom, I. (1986). Rett syndrome: A suggested staging system for describing the impairment profile with increasing age toward adolescence. *American Journal of Medical Genetics, 24*(Suppl. 1), 47–59.

Hanefeld, F. (1985). The clinical pattern of the Rett syndrome. *Brain Development, 7,* 320–325.

Huttenlocher, P.R., & deCourten, C. (1987). The development of synapses in striate cortex of man. *Human Neurobiology, 6,* 1–9.

Hyman, S.L., & Batshaw, M.L. (1986). A case of ornithine transcarbamylase deficiency with Rett syndrome manifestations. *American Journal of Medical Genetics, 24*(Suppl. 1), 339–343.

Jellinger, K., Armstrong, D., Zoghbi, H.Y., & Percy, A.K. (1988). Neuropathology of Rett syndrome. *Acta Neuropathologica, 76,* 142–158.

Koliatsos, V.E., Clatterbuck, R.E., Nauta, H.J.W., Knusel, B., Burton, L.E., Hefti, F.F., Mobley, W.C., & Price, D.L. (1991). Human nerve growth factor prevents degeneration of basal forebrain cholinergic neurons in primates. *Annals of Neurology, 30,* 831–840.

Lekman, A., Hagberg, B., & Svennerholm, L. (1991a). Altered cerebellar ganglioside pattern in Rett syndrome. *Neurochemistry International, 19,* 505–509.

Lekman, A.Y., Hagberg, B.A., & Svennerholm, L.T. (1991b). Membrane cerebral lipids in Rett syndrome. *Pediatric Neurology, 7,* 186–190.

McKusick, V.A. (1969). On lumpers and splitters, or the nosology of genetic disease. *Perspectives in Biology and Medicine, 12,* 298–318.

McKusick, V.A. (1994). *Mendelian inheritance in man: Catalog of autosomal dominant, autosomal recessive, and X-linked phenotypes* (11th ed.). Baltimore: Johns Hopkins University Press.

Oldfors, A., Sourander, P., & Percy, A.K. (1993). Neuropathology and neurochemistry. In B. Hagberg (Ed.), *Rett syndrome—clinical and biological aspects* (pp. 86–98). London: McKeith Press.

Opitz, J.M. (1986). Rett syndrome: Some comments on terminology and diagnosis. *American Journal of Medical Genetics, 24*(Suppl. 1), 27–37.

Ozcelik, T., Rosenthal, A., & Francke, U. (1991). Chromosomal mapping of brain-derived neurotrophic factor and neurotrophin-3 genes in man and mouse. *Genomics, 10,* 569–575.

Percy, A.K., Glaze, D.G., Schultz, R.J., Zoghbi, H.Y., Williamson, D., Frost, J.D., Jankovic, J.J., delJunco, D., Skender, M., Waring, S., & Myer,

E.C. (1994). Rett syndrome: Controlled study of an oral opiate agonist, naltrexone. *Annals of Neurology, 35,* 464–470.

Reiss, A.L., Faruque, F., Naidu, S., Abrams, M., Beaty, T., Bryan, R.N., & Moser, H.W. (1993). Neuroanatomy of Rett syndrome: A volumetric imaging study. *Annals of Neurology, 34,* 227–234.

Rett Syndrome Diagnostic Criteria Work Group. (1988). Diagnostic criteria for Rett syndrome. *Annals of Neurology, 23,* 425–428.

Stokland, E., Lidstrom, J., & Hagberg, B. (1993). *Scoliosis in Rett syndrome—Clinical and biological aspects* (pp. 61–71). London: McKeith Press.

Trevathan, E., & Naidu, S. (1988). The clinical recognition and differential diagnosis of Rett syndrome. *Journal of Child Neurology, 3* (Suppl.), 6–16.

Wenk, G.L., Naidu, S., Casanova, M.F., Kitt, C.A., & Moser, H. (1991). Altered neurochemical markers in Rett's syndrome. *Neurology, 41,* 1753–1756.

Zoghbi, H. (1988). Genetic aspects of Rett syndrome. *Journal of Child Neurology, 3*(Suppl.), 576–578.

PART VI

THE SPECTRUM OF DISORDERS OF LEARNING AND ATTENTION

Chapter 26

Neurologically Based Specific Learning Disabilities

Bruce K. Shapiro, M.D.

Neurologically based specific learning disabilities have been recognized for approximately 100 years. Over that time, the definition has evolved but has not been substantially altered. Currently, the definition of specific learning disability most commonly used is that written by the federal government:

> Those children who have a disorder in one or more of the basic psychological processes involved in understanding or in using language, spoken or written, which disorder may manifest itself in an imperfect ability to listen, think, speak, read, write, spell, or do mathematical calculations. Such disorders include such conditions as perceptual handicaps, brain injury, minimal brain dysfunction, dyslexia and developmental aphasia. Such term does not include children who have learning problems which are primarily the result of visual, hearing, or motor handicaps, of mental retardation, of emotional disturbance or environmental, cultural, or economic disadvantage. (Office of Education, 1977, p. 65,083)

This definition has three fundamental characteristics. The first characteristic establishes the boundaries of specific learning disability. Children with specific learning disabilities are distinguished operationally from those with more general mental retardation by the requirement for imperfection in academic abilities (reading, spelling, writing, or mathematical calculations) or the skills necessary for academic performance (thinking, listening, speaking) relative to their cognitive potential. The definition also attributes the mechanism of specific learning disabilities to dysfunction of the central nervous system (basic psychological processes) and focuses on processes that give rise to deficient language.

There are no pathognomonic criteria for the diagnosis of specific learning disability; the definition reflects a functional grouping. This has resulted in difficulty in implementing the definition. Because the criteria are subject to interpretation, there have been many attempts to operationalize the definition and facilitate a standard approach to diagnosis. Most attempts have sought to define and measure "an imperfect ability" or the requisite basic psychological processes. However, substantial variation remains in the techniques and measurements used to diagnose specific learning disability.

The second characteristic of the definition is incorporation. Specific learning disabilities are pervasive disorders and have many manifestations. As a result, many characterizations focus on single aspects of dysfunction. The definition groups children with multiple dysfunctions under a single diagnostic umbrella. Although such grouping has brought attention to children with academic underachievement and has made investigators more cognizant of the breadth of the disorder, consolidating the various neurologically based specific learning disabilities obscures the heterogeneity of the populations. Attention-deficit/hyperactivity disorder, for example, is not part of the definition because it did not enter the diagnostic lexicon until after specific learning disabilities were defined.

The third characteristic is the most misunderstood aspect of the definition. The exclusionary phrases were not meant to imply that specific learning disability could *not* occur with motor dysfunction, poverty, or social or cultural disadvantage. Clearly, social risk can be manifested as biologic dysfunction. The reasons for the exclusionary phrases were fiscal: Congress already had programs that addressed these problems and sought to prevent duplication of funding.

The National Joint Committee on Learning Disabilities has sought to clarify some of the aspects of this earlier definition. Their definition emphasizes the heterogeneity of learning disability, recognizes that it extends beyond childhood, and acknowledges that there is comorbidity with other developmental disabilities and cultural disadvantages:

> Learning disability is a generic term that refers to a heterogenous group of disorders manifested by significant difficulties in the acquisition and use of listening, speaking, reading, writing, reasoning, or mathematical abilities. These disorders are intrinsic to the individual and are presumed to be due to central nervous system dysfunction. Even though a learning disability may occur concomitantly with other disabling conditions (e.g., sensory impairment, mental retardation, social and emotional disturbance) or environmental influences (e.g., cultural differences or insufficient/inappropriate instruction), it is not the direct result of those conditions or influences. (Hammill, 1990, pp. 77–78)

ASSOCIATED DEFICITS

Children with specific learning disabilities are likely to have additional neurologic dysfunctions because developmental dysfunction is usually diffuse in children. The additional deficits are so closely associated with specific learning disabilities (e.g., hyperactivity) that some researchers have attempted to incorporate the associated deficits into the syndrome. Associated deficits may be more limiting than the primary diagnosis and therefore must be considered in developing a comprehensive management program. However, lumping all the associated dysfunctions into a single syndrome is likely to obscure different clinical patterns, prognostic factors, and treatment effects.

Strauss and Lehtinen (1947) brought attention to one of the most common accompaniments of learning dysfunction. Based on their work with children and young adults who contracted von Economo's encephalitis in the pandemic of 1918, they described a syndrome of behaviors that were seen in association with "brain damage." These components of the Strauss syndrome included hyperactivity, attentional peculiarities, impulsivity, emotional lability, and perceptual dysfunction. These behaviors later came to be associated with brain dysfunction,

even though no clear neural insult had been substantiated and no brain lesion could be demonstrated. The Strauss syndrome was the precursor of minimal brain dysfunction and hyperkinetic syndromes. Later it came to be called attention-deficit/hyperactivity disorder (ADHD). Controversy persists as to whether the Strauss syndrome is a unique condition and how specific it is for brain damage or dysfunction. The frequency of ADHD behaviors range from 25% to 80% in children with learning disability, while the frequency of learning disabilities in children with ADHD is much lower, ranging from 10% to 43% (Shaywitz & Shaywitz, 1988).

In addition to ADHD, other behavioral disturbances have been associated with learning disabilities. Affective disorders may be seen in conjunction with nonverbal learning disorders or disorders of written expression. Oppositional defiant disorders and conduct disorders are not rare. Whether the behavioral/emotional disturbances are part of the learning disability, the result of maladjustment to it, or some other interaction is unclear.

In addition to the behavioral disturbances described by Strauss, Lehtinen, and others, Paine (1962) recognized a continuum of minimal chronic brain syndromes in children. These were formes frustes of the major brain dysfunctions: cerebral palsy, seizure disorders, mental retardation, and sensory impairments. As a result, children with learning disabilities may have many different presentations. Table 1 lists a proposed classification of minimal brain dysfunctions. Each of these dysfunctions has a spectrum of severity. Not infrequently, the associated minimal brain dysfunction may predominate the clinical presentation and obscure the specific learning disability. Minimal brain dysfunctions are associated with disorders of higher cortical function but are not unique to specific learning disability. Thus, minimal brain dysfunctions may be associated with specific learning disability, but they can also be seen without significant academic underachievement or with mental retardation.

NOSOLOGY

If there is no "garden variety" of learning disability, can children with specific learning

Table 1. Proposed classification of disorders that usually have globally typical cognition but show specific deficits in brain function/processing

Peripheral disorders of processing
  Deafness
  Blindness
Central processing disorders—minimal brain dysfunction
  Motor
    Minimal cerebral palsy
    Central hypotonia
    Apraxia
    Clumsy child syndrome
    Complex tic disorder/Tourette syndrome
  Language
    Autism
    Preschool communication disorders
    Developmental dysphasias
      Expressive
      Receptive
      Mixed
    Articulation disorders
    Specific learning disability
      Reading
      Mathematics
      Written expression
  Minor perceptual dysfunction (visual–motor dysfunction)
  Behavior
    Strauss syndrome
    Hyperkinetic syndrome
    Attention-deficit/hyperactivity disorder
    Oppositional defiant disorder
    Conduct disorder
    Disorder in pragmatic language use

disabilities be distinguished from the population without learning disabilities? When compared to groups of typical children, children with specific learning disabilities are deficient on almost any measure. However, the ability to distinguish individual children on any single factor is poor. The overlap between typical ability and learning disability is too great to distinguish groups. This may be because the child with specific learning disability is not grossly abnormal but qualitatively different, and the parameters measured may not be fine enough to permit classification of individual children. Alternatively, it may be that neurologically based learning disabilities are not distinct entities but final pathways for many different types of dysfunction. In response to the lack of pathognomonic signs or tests, a "hydraulic parfait" (Arnold, 1976) critique of diagnosis has been proposed. This occurs when one repeats, "yes, but typical children also do this" several times. At present, the diagnosis of specific learning disability suffers from a lack of unique distinguishing characteristics, and clinicians are left with little more than hydraulic parfaits.

Temporal factors further complicate the understanding of learning disability. The manifestations of the condition are not stable throughout the person's life (Accardo, 1980). Although children who have not experienced formal schooling cannot be said to have learning disability, the abnormal neurologic substrate is present before academic learning takes place and may manifest itself in motor or language disorders. Whether children who present with early learning dysfunction are the same as those who present later is not known. At the other end of the age spectrum is the adult who has attained the requisite reading skills, albeit in an imperfect and labored fashion, and is functionally literate (reads for information) and therefore does not have a disability.

Current classification schemata focus on the dysfunction rather than the mechanism of dysfunction. The number of diagnoses used underscores the heterogeneity and pervasiveness of the dysfunction (see Table 2). As a result, multiple diagnostic labels are used to describe various aspects of a single dysfunction. Typically, diagnoses focus on neurologic, behavioral, psychological, or pedagogic areas. Thus a single child may be diagnosed as having minimal brain dysfunction, ADHD, specific reading disorder, and a developmental language disorder. Although the diagnoses do serve to describe the child, care must be taken lest the surfeit of diagnoses cause the child to be perceived as having multiple disabilities instead of having a single, multidimensional problem.

Learning disabilities commonly affect multiple areas of learning. In some cases they are global and affect all areas, whereas in others they may represent an isolated deficit. The age of identification of specific learning disability depends both on the type, severity, and number of deficits and on whether there are associated behavior and attention problems.

Table 2. Classification of academic disabilities secondary to neurologic dysfunction

Attention-deficit/hyperactivity disorder
Central communication disorder
Congenital word blindness
Developmental arithmetic disorder
Developmental language disorder
Developmental dyslexia
Developmental reading disorder
Disorders of auditory discrimination
Disorders of auditory memory
Disorders of visual memory
Disorders of visual–motor function
Disorders of visual perception
Disorders of visual sequencing
Dyscalculia
Dyslexia
Hyperkinetic syndrome
Memory disturbance
Minimal brain dysfunction
Specific reading disorder

Reading is the first skill learned, and usually reading disorders are detected before disorders of spelling and written expression. Among the specific subtypes of reading disability, children with decoding problems (learning to identify letters and sound out phonics) tend to present with difficulties by the end of first grade, whereas children whose reading disability primarily involves comprehension may escape early detection. Such a child may be able to decode and comprehend simple paragraphs but will be unable to understand the complexities of a book. He or she may not experience difficulty until the latter part of elementary school, when the curriculum moves from reading paragraphs to reading chapters in books. Because these children have performed adequately in the early grades, they may be mistakenly viewed as doing poorly because of a lack of motivation.

Specific learning disabilities in written expression may result from several causes: language disorder, spatial disorder, memory and attention deficits, and motor disorder (Sandler et al., 1992). Written expression disorders may be discovered because of poor handwriting, failure to complete written assignments, difficulty copying board work, and poor grades in math or spelling. They may also be detected incidentally as part of the evaluation of poor reading. The difficulty in their identification results from a failure to reconcile the fact that the child may be able to write (often neatly) if given sufficient time, but fails under pressures of time or volume.

Most often specific learning disability in mathematics is seen in conjunction with deficits in either reading or written expression. Dyscalculia is rarely an isolated finding. Children who have a fundamental conceptual problem in mathematics should be distinguished from children whose mathematics difficulties arise from a more general dysfunction (e.g., reading word problems or memorizing math facts) (see Chapter 27, this volume).

PREVALENCE

It is difficult to estimate how many children have neurologically based learning disorders. Overall, learning disability is diagnosed in approximately 6% of school-age children, with boys being affected about twice as frequently as girls. This prevalence is probably an *underestimate* because it does not account for those children who have not been identified, the way in which children with learning disability are identified, those who receive services under a different category, or those who drop out of school. In addition, not all children who show neurologic or behavioral dysfunction have learning problems and not all children with learning problems show neurologic signs. This is supported by the small number of children in the National Collaborative Perinatal Project (NCPP) who demonstrated learning, neurologic, and behavioral dysfunctions (prevalence of 0.18%). When individual factors are considered, the prevalence is higher. A total of 7.88% of the children in the NCPP demonstrated neurologic signs, 7.90% revealed hyperactivity/impulsivity, and 8.36% had learning disorders (Nichols & Chen, 1981).

ROLES OF THE PEDIATRICIAN

The role of the pediatrician in the care of the child with learning disabilities has been somewhat controversial. Some have maintained that this is an educational problem and not within the purview of pediatrics. Others have advocated more active participation in early identification, confirmation of the diagnosis, treatment, and monitoring. Clearly, the primary care roles are within the purview of pediatrics. However, if one accepts the premise that specific learning disabilities are problems that extend beyond the classroom and impact on the child's ability to develop, then at least four additional roles can be identified.

Pediatricians are the professionals whom parents most commonly encounter in relationship to their infants and toddlers. Thus the pediatrician is in a position *to identify preacademic learning disabilities*. Although specific learning disabilities cannot be diagnosed until the child is exposed to a school environment, the aberrant neurologic substrate may be identified well before formal education begins. This may be manifested as early developmental delays or nonsequential developmental patterns and may be identified more easily than later, more traditional learning disability patterns. Recognition of the neurologic basis for the child's unusual development permits appropriate counseling of the parents, increases surveillance of the child's development, allows for and promotes early interventions, and may facilitate entrance into school.

The pediatrician is often asked to *confirm the diagnosis of specific learning disability*. The child's academic underachievement, behavioral disturbance, or neurologic dysfunction may be first noted by the classroom teacher. Commonly this results in either the parent or teacher referring the child for evaluation of the abnormality and diagnosis. This requires the pediatrician to interact with the school to acquire needed information, diagnose syndromes and disorders that may mimic or be associated with specific learning disabilities, and secure the necessary evaluations to establish a diagnosis.

After the diagnosis is established, the pediatrician may be called on to participate in *management*. In this role, the pediatrician acts as an advocate for the child and the child's family. Pediatricians may have to assist in the setting of treatment priorities, coordinate the efforts of multiple disciplines, help the family make choices, and/or administer drug therapy.

After the initial management program has been devised, the pediatrician should *monitor* the results. Because there is no "garden variety" of specific learning disability, therapy programs must be individualized and modified as the conditions change. By ensuring communication between parents, school, child, and others, the pediatrician can assess the overall effectiveness of the management program and modify it as needed.

DIAGNOSIS

History

Although a general pediatric history is the foundation of clinical evaluation, the history must be neurodevelopmentally modified for children suspected of having learning disorders. The history in these children may be obtained from several sources: mother, father, school, and child. Not infrequently the perceptions of these sources differ. The differences must be reconciled by clarifying differing perceptions and weighing the various sources of information.

The purpose of the history is to describe the child. The nature of school problems must be delineated. What areas does the child find difficult? How long has he or she had problems? How severe are the learning problems? What is currently being done about the problem, and what has previously been tried?

The child's behavior should also be evaluated. Learning problems and behavior problems frequently, but not always, coexist. Learning and behavior must be evaluated independently of each other. Not only should children be assessed for Strauss syndrome, but other behavioral disturbances consistent with poor social interactions, school avoidance, conduct disorders, oppositional defiant disorders, and depression also should be investigated.

It is in the area of behavior that parents are most likely to disagree with the school. Frequently school and home behaviors are different. Usually it is not that the reporters are unreliable but that the conditions differ. The method used to measure behavior is of major importance because it influences the type of information obtained. Directly observing the child in various settings is most likely to yield an accurate view of behavior problems. This is suitable for research studies but is not practical in a clinical setting. Interviewing the teacher, parents, and child will usually give valid information, but this is also usually impracticable because of the difficulties with information gathering and the need to synthesize the various reports. Most practitioners use questionnaires to collect information about a child because it is a technique of obtaining information that requires only a modest investment of time and effort. However, all of the many different questionnaires available are flawed because they limit the scope of behavior to be assessed; they depend on the validity of the respondent; they provide information of uncertain value; and they fail to allow the evaluation or weighing of the various responses, thus making it difficult to resolve questions. Ultimately the practitioner must balance the expediency of questionnaires against the often superior information of interviews and develop a personal system of behavioral assessment.

The history will explore neurologic dysfunction only minimally. In addition to standard questions about neurologic dysfunction, the history for children with learning dysfunction should focus on clumsiness of fine and gross motor abilities. Despite attempts to objectify clumsiness, this is much better observed than reported. A history of delayed shoe tying, cutting, buttoning, or tricycle riding may be an indicator of clumsiness.

Describing the child's early development gives information about the time course of the child's dysfunction. Many children manifest deviant or mildly delayed early development and are called immature. These immaturities are commonly seen in fine motor, social, and language areas in preschool children. Some children exhibit a pattern of nondisabling motor delay in the first year or two, with modest language delays becoming evident later and subsequent learning disorders by school age. Still others show extremes of fetal activity, prolonged colic, difficulty establishing periodicity, and ongoing behavior problems.

The history should also attempt to determine the cause of the learning disability and exclude other conditions that may imitate or be associated with specific learning disabilities. Perinatal events, although statistically related, are not a frequent cause of learning disabilities (Balow, Rubin, & Rosen, 1975-1976). Traditional markers of perinatal risk are more closely related to cerebral palsy than to specific learning disabilities, although follow-up of very low birth weight infants suggest a high prevalence of specific learning disorders. Therefore, the possible contribution of perinatal events should be explored. Similarly, major neurologic events such as meningitis, seizures, or loss of consciousness should be ascertained and a thorough review of systems performed.

Specific learning disabilities cluster in families (Childs & Finuccci, 1983). The family history should ascertain the level of parental educational achievement. In addition, information should be obtained about parental reading status, parental receipt of special education services, and parental performance in early elementary school. Deviations in the parents' early development, such as late walking or talking, should also be ascertained. Similar information should be sought about siblings, uncles and aunts, and first cousins.

The same general principles apply to children who are being considered for a diagnosis of preacademic learning disabilities. In these children, nonspecific neurobehavioral signs of developmental dysfunction may be present before academics are attempted—hyperactivity, immaturity, gross and fine motor delays (clumsiness), and central processing dysfunction (e.g., deviant language development or visual–perceptual dysfunction). However, specific clinical signs may not be evidenced until the teaching of reading is attempted. Although the unusual development of these children may be recognized at an early age, the diagnosis of specific learning disability may be delayed by the inability of the child to meet diagnostic criteria for "significant" discrepancy, or by the presence of confounding circumstances (e.g., male sex, date of birth, familial discord).

Physical Examination

The physical examination does not yield specific diagnostic information. There are no pathognomonic signs of learning disability.

Neurologic dysfunction may exist in the absence of learning disorders and vice versa. Thus the purposes of the physical examination are to delineate neurologic dysfunction that may or may not be associated with learning problems, and to detect disorders that may be associated with specific learning disabilities.

A complete physical examination should be performed as part of the evaluation of learning disorders. Abnormal growth patterns, as would be seen in chronic conditions (such as inflammatory bowel disease), fetal alcohol syndrome, or cerebral gigantism, may be seen in children with academic underachievement. Defects in vision and hearing should be excluded. Visual disturbance to a degree that would cause academic underachievement is usually noted early in school. The ability of conductive hearing loss to cause learning disabilities remains controversial. However, sensorineural hearing loss may progress insidiously and cause communicatively disabling hearing losses. Physical anomalies have been associated with specific learning disabilities and hyperactive behavior, although the association has not been strong enough to permit diagnoses based on anomalies (Burg, Rapoport, Bartley, Quinn, & Timmins, 1980). Many medical conditions present with learning difficulties; most are excluded by a thorough history and physical examination.

The traditional neurologic evaluation is rarely helpful in the evaluation of the child with specific learning disabilities. As is true for vision, most significant neurologic abnormalities, save for forme frustes, are detected before school age. Soft neurologic signs are of particular interest when assessing children with learning disabilities (H.G. Taylor, 1987). These signs are developmental in nature and are more common in children with learning and behavior problems. However, soft neurologic signs are difficult to measure reliably, do not correlate directly with learning or behavior, do not have localizing value, and do not contribute to educational intervention. Soft signs are of most use in the groups that are at the extreme—gifted children with academic underachievement, intellectually limited children, and young children who may not be old enough to permit detection of a significant discrepancy. Soft signs may be found in motor, cortical sensory, or central processing modalities. Motor soft signs demonstrate asymmetry of function, abnormal tone, or difficulty with motor control as evidenced by synkinesias or poor modulation of volitional acts. Cortical sensory signs such as extinction, finger agnosia, dysgraphesthesia, or poor kinesthesia may also demonstrate asymmetry, but more often are used to define neural immaturity. Soft signs of processing dysfunction are usually assessed as part of the psychological evaluation. However, visual and auditory processing tasks may be evaluated by pediatricians as part of the neurodevelopmental examination.

Confirmatory Tests

The history and physical examination can lead the physician to suspect specific learning disabilities as the cause of a child's academic problems, but the confirmatory testing must be obtained from consultants. The presence of behavioral problems or neurologic findings does not make the diagnosis of specific learning disabilities. Table 3 lists the conditions to be considered in the differential diagnosis of academic underachievement. Children with specific learning disabilities are not intellectually limited, but they are achieving academically at a degree that is less than that predicted from their IQ. Although intellectual deficiency is a common cause of academic dysfunction, IQ is not directly related to academic performance in children (Siegel, 1989). Although there is an intellectual threshold for reading, gifted children may be nonreaders.

To make a diagnosis of specific learning disabilities, it is necessary to demonstrate a severe discrepancy between cognitive potential and

Table 3. Differential diagnoses of the school-age child with academic underachievement

Specific learning disability
Central communication disorder
Attention-deficit/hyperactivity disorder
Intellectual limitation (mental retardation or borderline retardation)
Progressive loss of hearing or vision
Chronic physical disorder
Deprivational home environment
Major psychiatric dysfunction
Motivation (in older children)

achievement. Usually this entails administration of standardized tests to measure both IQ and educational achievement. However, discrepancy approaches to specific learning disabilites do not have adequate concurrent or predictive validity. As a result, discrepancy approaches do not permit early diagnosis (Shapiro et al., 1990), nor do they facilitate the provision of educational assistance (Shaywitz, Escobar, Shaywitz, Fletcher, & Makuch, 1992).

Despite the lack of a direct relationship between IQ and academic achievement in specific learning disabilities, psychologists have sought to define patterns of test performance that would permit the diagnosis of specific learning disability to be made solely on the basis of the processing dysfunction observed on psychological tests. The Wechsler Intelligence Scale for Children (original, revised, and third editions; Wechsler, 1949, 1981, and 1991, respectively) has been studied most extensively in this regard. Attempts have been made to define specific learning disability by discrepancies between verbal and performance portions of this test, variability among subtests (scatter), and pattern analysis (e.g., ACID profiles: low Arithmetic, Coding, Information, and Digit Span scores). These profiles are associated with specific learning disabilities but do not possess sufficient classification abilities to permit diagnosis (Kaufman, 1981).

There are many more tests of academic achievement than of intellectual potential. Each of these tests have their proponents and their shortcomings (see Salvia & Ysseldyke, 1984; R. L. Taylor & Warren, 1984). Because reading is the academic focus in the early grades, it is measured in a much more standardized fashion than mathematics. As a result, there is greater agreement among reading tests than math tests. Despite this, reading tests may be criticized for their inability to assess young children, their lack of predictive validity, and their lack of relationship to classroom performance. (For example, in later elementary school, children are expected to comprehend and retain material based on several pages of reading, but most reading tests require the student to read a paragraph or less. These children may test well but perform poorly in the classroom.)

The routine use of academic tests to establish the diagnosis of specific learning disability is questionable. When the referral is made to confirm the diagnosis, it is already apparent that the child is underachieving in the classroom. If the child is of average intelligence and otherwise unimpaired, then specific learning disability is the diagnosis. Testing then is being done not to demonstrate a cognition–achievement discrepancy but to delineate a discrepancy that is severe enough to warrant intervention. In the ideal setting, academic assessment would not be used as a gate-keeping device to exclude children from services but rather as a means of defining the type of help a child required.

After the Initial Evaluation

The number of disciplines that claim expertise in the evaluation or treatment of disorders that are chronic, complex, and incurable is large. The number of professionals involved with children with learning disabilities is so large that the family's financial resources can be quickly exhausted. It is up to the primary care pediatrician to help the family decide which diagnostic and therapeutic services are needed to ensure the completion of the evaluation and to coordinate the setting of treatment priorities.

For many children the evaluation will be largely completed in the school setting. Some families will opt for evaluations outside of school. However, following completion of the evaluation, the family will be interacting with the school to develop the educational portion of the treatment plan. The school is required under the Education for All Handicapped Children Act of 1975 (PL 94-142) to provide a free, appropriate education in the least restrictive environment to children with disabling conditions. The time frame for implementation of an individualized education program is outlined in Table 4.

MECHANISMS OF DYSFUNCTION

Learning disabilities were distinguished from mental retardation and other neurologically based disorders in the late 19th century. Kussmaul (1877) described an adult with an acquired brain lesion whose ability to read was lost but whose intellect, speech, and vision were spared.

Table 4. PL 94-142: Legislated time frame for the implementation of the individualized education program (IEP)

	Maximum number of days permitted	Cumulative calendar days elapsed
Parents request screening	0	0
Screening completed	30	30
Assessment completed	45	75
Meeting of Admission, Review, and Dismissal Committee (ARD) held	30	105
IEP written and approved by ARD	30	135
IEP implemented	30 school days	177
IEP review	60 school days	261
Written report presented to parents	10 school days	275

He coined the term *word blind* to describe these symptoms. Morgan (1896) reported an otherwise normal 14-year-old who had difficulty in reading and spelling but seemingly typical arithmetic abilities. Hinshelwood (1900, 1917) comprehensively described the condition. He defined congenital word blindness as a congenital defect occurring in children with otherwise normal and undamaged brains that is characterized by a disability in learning to read so great, and so unamenable to traditional teaching, that it is manifestly due to a pathologic condition. Hinshelwood's 1917 monograph marks the end of the period of clinical description of learning disabilities. Subsequent researchers have sought to further define the nature of the dysfunctions, both in terms of mechanism and associated dysfunctions.

Whereas early work sought to define the cause of learning disorders, later studies have associated disordered learning with a variety of deficits: There is no one single cause for learning disorders. In addition, specificity to the processing dysfunction is lacking: Children may have the same processing deficit and show different types of learning disorders, or they may have the same type of learning disorder yet have different underlying deficits in processing. As is true of developmental milestones, learning abilities are a final pathway for the interaction of multiple different processes. Researchers who first encountered learning disorders thought that deficits in the visual or visual–motor systems were the most likely etiology for learning disorders. Morgan (1896) hypothesized a basic defect in storing visual impressions of words. Orton (1925) believed that learning disabilities

resulted from a delay in the normal maturation of hemispheric dominance. He emphasized the letter and word reversals in reading and writing and coined the term *strephosymbolia* to describe the "twisted symbol" system of children with learning disability. Bender (1956) proposed disordered visual organization as the etiology; this could be identified in how the child was able to copy figures. Hermann and Norrie (1958) also focused on children with directionality problems and diagnosed those with left–right disorientation, finger agnosia, acalculia, and agraphia as having "developmental" Gerstmann syndrome. Birch (1962) proposed an intersensory integration deficit: the inability of the child with learning disability to combine and compare information processed through different sensory modalities. Questions remain about the validity of these findings, whether these dysfunctions were demonstrable in real life outside of the testing situation, and whether the poor visual–motor abilities represented just another aspect of abnormal development and were therefore a covariant rather than a causal factor.

Some researchers hold sequential memory deficits in the form of temporal order recall deficits as responsible for learning dysfunction (Bakker, 1972). Memory deficits are frequently seen in children with ADHD. In some children these deficits improve with stimulant medications. Although stimulants may improve test performance, correction of the deficits in temporal order recall tasks yields more ambiguous results. Others have suggested that the temporal order recall tasks are verbally mediated.

Later research has centered on verbal processing as a cause of reading disorders (Vellutino, 1978). Children with reading disorders have shown weaknesses in almost all areas of verbal function. Deficiencies have been noted in syntax, semantics, and phonologic processing. However, the findings are confined to group differences and do not identify individual children with learning disorders. Studies have suggested that early language problems lead to reading disorders (Bashir & Scavuzzo, 1992), but another study has suggested a better prognosis if the gap is closed by age 5 1/2 (Bishop & Adams, 1990). Thus, blanket assertions that verbal processing dysfunction is the cause of learning disorders must be viewed with caution.

Trying to determine the underlying etiology for subtypes of learning dysfunction may prove to be impossible with current capabilities. Perhaps the factor that most limits attempts to define psychological mechanisms of learning disorders is the lack of an operational definition of specific learning disability. The current definition is a definition of exclusion and is limited by the patient's age, intellectual capacity, and socioeconomic status and the presence of other neurologic dysfunctions. In addition, psychological processes focus on the content and not the mechanism of brain function and therefore do not represent distinctive functions.

SUBCLASSIFICATION

Although it may not be possible to delineate the underlying mechanisms, subclassifying learning disorders may nevertheless be valuable for several reasons. Perhaps the most important is prognosis. If children with a universally good prognosis can be identified, then remediation may be withheld until the child closes the gap. Similarly, if the prognosis is good, then alternate strategies may be employed. Grouping similar children permits the study of possible etiologies and mechanisms of learning disorders and allows the effect of therapy to be fairly evaluated. Heterogeneity of groups may obscure mechanisms or etiologic factors, or may cause an effective therapy to be discarded or an ineffective therapy to be endorsed. Several approaches used to subclassify children with learning disorders are based on test performance, anatomy, physiology, and genetics.

Performance on different tests is an obvious way of dividing children who have learning disorders. Subclassifying by test performance assumes that the tests are measuring a factor that is meaningful, that the population on which the schema is based is representative of the total population, and that the factors measured are stable. Children who perform poorly on arithmetic may be separated from poor readers. Visual learners may be distinguished from auditory learners, analytic readers discriminated from gestalt readers, language disorders from articulatory disorders, and graphomotor disorders from visuospatial disorders. Clinical heterogeneity is also noted in presentation and ranges from word blindness to inefficient, but functional, reading. The gifted child with dyslexia may have high scores on intellectual testing but only average reading scores. Similar variation is noted in neuropsychological function and in studies of the type of errors made by children with learning disabilities. All children with dyslexia do not make the same type of reading errors. Consequently, attempts to subclassify dyslexia by neuropsychological profiles have been unsuccessful.

Since the early 1980s, it has become possible to define neuroanatomic structures in a more sophisticated fashion, and to image brain structures in living patients. These approaches have focused on children with dyslexia. Neuronal ectopias and architectonic dysplasias, predominantly in the perisylvian region, have been described. In addition, abnormal symmetry of the planum temporale was noted (Galaburda, Sherman, Rosen, Aboitz, & Geschwind, 1985). However, neuropathologic studies have been few. Using computerized tomography scans, some investigators have reported findings compatible with the pathologic studies and described a lack of normal brain asymmetry in patients with dyslexia (Rosenberger & Hier, 1980). However, others have failed to confirm this finding (Haslam, Delby, Johns, & Rademaker, 1981). Magnetic resonance imaging has not revealed consistent abnormalities, although one study alluded to unusual symmetrical temporal lobe volumes (Rumsey et al., 1986). Hynd and co-workers found that children with dyslexia had a lower rate of left versus right plana asymmetry than typical chidren or those with ADHD. However, the finding was not sufficient to allow classification of individual children (Hynd, Semrud-Clikeman, Lorys, Novey, & Eliopulos, 1990).

Physiologic approaches have also concentrated on reading disorders. These have included electroencephalograms, brain electrical activity mapping (BEAM), and positron emission tomography (PET). Electroencephalography has long been shown not to distinguish groups of children with learning disorders. More recent attempts to distinguish dyslexic from nondyslexic children using electroencephalographic techniques have also been unrewarding. BEAM is a method for summarizing and recording encephalographic spatiotemporal information contained in recordings from multiple scalp electrodes. Using BEAM technology, 10 different testing conditions or states were used to define diagnostic rules that properly classified subjects 80%–90% of the time as to presence or absence of dyslexia (Duffy, Denckla, Bartels, Sandini, & Kiessling, 1979a). Although most of the abnormalities were seen on the left hemisphere, the greatest between group difference was in the bilateral medial frontal region (Duffy, Bartels, Denckla, & Sandini, 1979b). Unfortunately, these findings could not be replicated in a younger population (Badian, McAnulty, Duffy, & Als, 1990). PET scanning is a research tool that assesses brain activity as evidenced by changes in regional glucose metabolism or regional blood flow. During a phonologic rhyme task, severely dyslexic men failed to activate those left temporoparietal regions near the angular gyrus activated by typically reading controls (Rumsey et al., 1992).

Genetic approaches to specific learning disability are based on studies that suggest substantial familial clustering. Further evidence is derived from twin studies that have found a 90% concordance for monozygotes and a 32% concordance for dizygotic twins (Lewitter, DeFries, & Elston, 1980). However, the imprecision of the diagnostic criteria and the lack of definition of the pathophysiology probably contributed to obscure a number of hereditary dyslexia syndromes. As a result, studies that rely on clinical criteria have not yielded consistent results, and several different modes of inheritance have been proposed. Attempts to discern a possible linkage between reading disability and chromosome 15 were met with enthusiasm because it raised the possibility of an objective marker for reading disorders that was free from the shortcomings of the usual methods of diagnosis. However, repeating the analysis with chromosome 15–specific DNA probes failed to confirm the initial findings (Bisgaard, Eiberg, Moller, Niebuhr, & Mohr, 1987). It is doubtful that a single major locus would account for all reading disability (Pennington et al., 1991).

Although the techniques proposed to subclassify learning disability are enticing because they are objective, endorsement of any approach must be withheld until validity, with respect to the reasons for subclassification, can be demonstrated. Primary mechanisms must be differentiated from secondary phenomena. Currently, the published studies are small and the generalizability of the findings has not been shown. Despite the current limitations, more objective ways of defining specific learning disabilities will facilitate understanding of the syndrome.

MANAGEMENT

There is no effective treatment for specific learning disability. Although certain techniques may modify the manifestations of the neural dysfunction, no method has been consistently shown to cure specific learning disability. The complex and pervasive nature of specific learning disabilities requires that a comprehensive, coordinated, multimodal approach address educational, parental, and child issues.

Educational Therapy

Educational achievement is the major developmental task of school-age children. If children are unsuccessful in school, it carries over into other aspects of their lives, and diminished self-esteem may result. Consequently, the major focus of habilitation of children with specific learning disorders is to ensure that the child is in a satisfactory school environment (see Chapter 29, this volume).

Educational therapy is not a unitary entity and must be tailored to the individual needs of the child. Educational therapy may be delivered in a variety of settings ranging from consultative services and resource rooms to self-contained classes or special schools. Although clinical impressions support the efficacy of special education in prevention of secondary emotional defects, data to prove the effectiveness of special education in ameliorating the educational deficits are lacking (Yule, 1976). Although each of the pedagogic approaches (Johnson, 1978) to the management of specific learning disabilities has its advocates, it has not been shown that any educational intervention alters the child's rate of learning, nor that the outcome is modified over what can be expected from maturation. Debate still rages as to the best remedial technique for reading disability: Is it better to use an analytic approach that focuses on smaller units (e.g., graphophonemes and words) or to use knowledge of higher order language to anticipate oncoming text (e.g., language experience) or a parallel interaction model that uses all parts simultaneously (e.g., basal reader) (Silver & Hagin, 1990)? This debate is due, in part, to the lack of knowledge of the long-term consequences of specific learning disability and to the inability to generalize across programs and students.

Tutoring may prove effective for those children who do not receive special education services or for treatment over the summer. Specific training in study strategies may enable students to utilize their existing academic skills better. Many children with milder forms of learning disability can be maintained in a general classroom with accommodations made for areas of weakness. Retention is rarely useful because it does not alter the natural history of learning disability, has a negative effect on self-esteem, and adversely affects socialization.

Circumvention of reading problems may enhance performance in written language and mathematics. Oral presentation of material, reading to the child, books on tape, and study "buddies" may prove helpful. Circumvention techniques seem more appropriate for disorders of written expression. Similarly, calcula-tors can be helpful for children with mathematics disorders.

Attempts to improve the child's academic ability may result in assigning too much homework because the child must make up classwork that was not completed or because the child is unable to do the same amount of homework that others find reasonable. Techniques to facilitate homework performance may include reading and reviewing difficult material with the child, minimizing need for peripheral activity (e.g., copying of math problems or writing only spelling words rather than full sentences), and provision of secretarial support. Homework should be limited to a preestablished time allotment. Homework also should be closely monitored because difficulty may indicate that readiness for the topic areas has not been achieved and adjustment is required.

Although most children with learning disabilities will attain the academic skills required for everyday function, some do not achieve functional literacy in reading and mathematics during traditional education but do so as young adults. Individual differences in skills readiness should be accommodated and traditional education should be supplemented (e.g., functional curricula, computers, vocational training, work study). Alternative approaches usually are not offered until secondary school to ensure that remediation attempts have not been successful. For children with severe learning disability, this may not be early enough to maintain self-esteem.

Parental Counseling

A comprehensive management program must also include parent counseling. Parents are frequently anxious and confused because they are unsure why their child is not developing as expected. If there are educational problems, there is commonly a feeling that the school is shirking its responsibility. When home behavior is affected, there may be considerable disagreement over how to manage it. In counseling parents, the physician should diminish anxiety by helping the parents recognize that the child's problem does not result from inappropriate parenting. Similarly, the blame for the child's learning disorder does not lie with the school. Finally, the parent must be restored to the position of parent. To this end, literature and parent organizations (such as the Learning Disabilities Association, 4156 Library Road, Pittsburgh, PA 15234) are helpful.

Child-Oriented Therapy

Recommendations regarding management of the child's behavior may be sought from teachers, clergy, or mental health professionals (see Chapter 30, this volume). The child may be incorrectly perceived by the parents or teachers as lazy, stubborn, willful, or incorrigible. It is important to interpret this from the child's perspective and to identify those behaviors that are thought to be abnormal but are not unusual for a child with specific learning disabilities. For example, social immaturity, difficulty following directions, and a smaller than normal number of friends are not uncommon. Techniques to reward good behavior are commonly of help to parents who have been saying "No" for too long. In this regard, contracts are helpful, but they must be simple, clearly defined, attainable, and not revoked when other unacceptable behavior manifests.

Child guidance is also necessary. The nature of the child's disability must be explained to him or her in terms that can be understood. As the child grows, the explanation must be adjusted to meet the child's level of understanding. Approaches that seek to preserve and enhance feelings of self-worth may be warranted. Children must feel that they are capable, effective people, at least outside of school. Extracurricular activities and nonschool learning should be encouraged.

Although attempts to improve the fit between the child and the environment may ameliorate the current situation, they have not been shown to improve the long-term outcome. Further study is needed to determine to what degree and under what circumstances approaches that alter the environment are effective in the short term and affect long-term prognosis. The relationship between innate characteristics of the child with specific learning disability and his or her behavioral dysfunction also merits investigation.

Psychiatric evaluation and counseling may be required to treat coexisting mental health disorders. Stimulant medications may be an important adjunct to children with specific learning disabilities (see Chapter 29, this volume). They can be effective in treating ADHD. They are not a quick fix, however, and do not substitute for a comprehensive management program. Whether they positively influence learning in a clinically meaningful fashion is still not completely established. Other agents such as tricyclic antidepressants, α-adrenergic blockers, and major tranquilizers have all been recommended for children with complex learning disorders and behavioral disturbance.

The only way to determine who will be helped by pharmacologic agents is to undertake a therapeutic trial. A therapeutic trial requires a clear understanding of the desired changes (target behaviors), cooperative parents, good communication, and a source to report on the effects of the drug trial (usually a teacher). Drug effects may be noted very quickly. Therefore, contact with the parents should be within the first week. This allows for questions to be answered and anxieties alleviated. However, the decision to continue drugs is best deferred until a full month has elapsed. This allows transient side effects to diminish and provides enough time for an adequate assessment of behavior changes.

OUTCOMES

Neurologically based specific learning disabilities may be of little functional import or may cause significant, lasting disability. The outcomes vary and may be confined to a single area such as academics, behavior, or neurologic function, or may involve several areas. Although the academic dysfunctions are responsible for defining the syndrome, the associated dysfunctions may be more limiting than the primary academic deficits.

Four academic outcomes can be defined. The first is the child who normalizes his academic performance and, after a slow start, performs at grade level. This child demonstrates a developmental lag and this pattern of unusual development has a good prognosis. School programs that in the past delayed intervention until third grade were based on the expectation that many children would catch up and have a normal academic performance. The second academic outcome is characterized by the student who does not require long-term remedial instruction but may need training in study skills. While in a regular classroom, he or she may be considered to be an underachiever. The third outcome is the child who continues to have major difficulty in mastering reading and requires continued remedial teaching. The last group is composed of the children who fail to master functional academic skills.

Lasting academic disabilities are rare in children with specific learning disability unless intellectual limitation is an associated dysfunction. The long-term follow-up of children with specific reading disabilities suggests that they have adequate academic outcomes (see Schonhaut & Satz, 1983; Weiss & Hechtman, 1986). Most children ultimately attain functional literacy, but persistent deficits in reading, spelling, and written language may be noted in testing situations. The outcome for other academic deficiencies (e.g., mathematics) is less well studied. Circumvention of these areas may lessen the impact of impairments in other areas.

Behavioral dysfunction commonly accompanies specific learning disabilities. The primary behavioral disturbances of hyperactivity, impulsivity, lability of mood, distractibility, and altered reactivity may affect outcomes. Motor hyperactivity usually diminishes near puberty, but the other manifestations of the Strauss syndrome may persist. Although not necessarily disabling, these dysfunctions may give rise to less job satisfaction and the more frequent moves that are seen in young adults who were hyperactive as children. It is not clear whether these adverse outcomes are related to the primary dysfunction or to secondary problems arising from poor self-esteem. Other disorders, such as depression, conduct and oppositional defiant disorders, and alcoholism, rarely occur in adolescents and adults who manifested specific learning disability as children (Weiss & Hechtman, 1986).

Most studies of the social outcomes of children with learning disability have addressed criminal offenses, antisocial behavior, occupational achievement, or job performance. For the most part, studies have not demonstrated clear disadvantages for children who had learning disabilities. By contrast, as a group, children with hyperactivity do worse on these measures than controls (Weiss & Hechtman, 1986). Although it is likely that most children who have learning disabilities make satisfactory life adaptations, the studies should be viewed with caution because of population selection biases, small numbers, indistinct outcomes, improper controls, confounding variables (e.g., associated dysfunctions, socioeconomic status, or hyperactivity) and insufficient time of follow-up. In view of the variable outcomes, the diagnosis of specific learning disability, even with associated hyperactivity, should not forecast adverse social consequences.

CONCLUSIONS

Specific learning disabilities are neurodevelopmental disorders. As such, they are commonly associated with additional dysfunctions such as hyperactivity or clumsiness. The areas of deficit may change over time. Although the neurologic basis of these disorders has been established, the causes of specific learning disabilities are not known but are likely to be multifactorial. The final common pathway of specific learning disability is the brain's inefficient processing of information.

Although the most obvious manifestations of this disorder are in academic areas, the dysfunctions observed are frequently pervasive and extend beyond the school setting. The pediatrician is in an ideal position to assist in the management of the child with specific learning disability by confirming the diagnosis, prioritizing management objectives, providing anticipatory guidance, assisting in efforts to make a better fit between the environment and the child, prescribing stimulant medications as needed, and advocating for the child. Monitoring is necessary to ensure that the program remains appropriate to the child.

Long-term studies of academic, behavioral, and social outcomes suggest that most children with specific learning disabilities usually make a satisfactory life adjustment, although in some studies they do less well than comparison groups. Associated deficits such as low self-esteem, hyperactivity, poor social interaction, and family dysfunction may be of greater import to the outcome than the primary impairments in learning.

Further advances in the understanding of spe-

cific learning disabilities will require improved definitions. Homogeneous groups should permit the delineation of the mechanism of dysfunction, allow prognostication, and facilitate the determination of therapeutic effects. Anatomic, physiologic, and genetic methods hold promise for the successful subclassification of specific learning disabilities.

REFERENCES

Accardo, P. (1980). *A neurodevelopmental perspective on specific learning disabilities*. Baltimore: University Park Press.

Arnold, L.E. (1976). Minimal brain dysfunction: A hydraulic parfait model. *Diseases of the Nervous System, 37*, 171–173.

Badian, N.A., McAnulty, G.B., Duffy, F.H., & Als, H. (1990). Prediction of dyslexia in kindergarten boys. *Annals of Dyslexia, 40*, 152–169.

Bakker, D.J. (1972). *Temporal order in disturbed reading*. Rotterdam: University Press.

Balow, B., Rubin, R., & Rosen, M.J. (1975–1976). Perinatal events as precursors of reading disability. *Reading Research Quarterly, 11*, 36–71.

Bashir, A.S., & Scavuzzo, A. (1992). Children with language disorders: Natural history and academic success. *Journal of Learning Disabilities, 25*, 53–65.

Bender, L.A. (1956). *Psychopathology of children with organic brain disorders*. Springfield, IL: Charles C Thomas.

Birch, H.G. (1962). Dyslexia and maturation of visual function. In J. Money (Ed.), *Reading disability: Progress and research needs in dyslexia*. (pp. 161–170). Baltimore: Johns Hopkins Press.

Bisgaard, M.L., Eiberg, H., Moller, N., Niebuhr, E., & Mohr, J. (1987). Dyslexia and chromosome 15 heteromorphism: Negative LOD score in a Danish material. *Clinical Genetics, 32*, 118–119.

Bishop, D.V.M., & Adams, C. (1990). A prospective study of the relationship between specific language impairment, phonological disorders and reading retardation. *Journal of Child Psychology and Psychiatry, 31*, 1027–1050.

Burg, C., Rapoport, J., Bartley, L., Quinn, P.O., & Timmins, P. (1980). Newborn minor physical anomalies and problem behavior at age 3. *American Journal of Psychiatry, 137*, 791–796.

Childs, B., & Finucci, J. (1983). Genetics, epidemiology, and specific learning disability. In M. Rutter (Ed.) *Developmental neuropsychiatry* (pp. 507–519). New York: Guilford Press.

Duffy, F., Denckla, M., Bartels, P., Sandini, G., & Kiessling, L.S. (1979a). Dyslexia: Automated diagnosis by computerized classification of brain electrical activity. *Annals of Neurology, 7*, 421–428.

Duffy, F., Denckla, M., Bartels, P., & Sandini, G. (1979b). Dyslexia: Regional differences in brain electrical activity by topographic mapping. *Annals of Neurology, 7*, 412–420.

Education for All Handicapped Children Act of 1975, PL 94-142. (August 23, 1975). Title 20, U.S.C. 1401 et seq: *U.S. Statutes at Large, 89*, 773–796.

Galaburda, A., Sherman, G.F., Rosen, G.D., Aboitz, F., & Geschwind, N. (1985). Developmental dyslexia: Four consecutive patients with cortical abnormalities. *Annals of Neurology, 18*, 222–233.

Hammill, D.D. (1990). On defining learning disabilities: An emerging consensus. *Journal of Learning Disabilities, 21*, 74–84.

Haslam, R.H.A., Dalby, J.T., Johns, R.D., & Rademaker, A.W. (1981). Cerebral asymmetry in developmental dyslexia. *Archives of Neurology, 38*, 679–682.

Hermann, K., & Norrie, E. (1958). Is congenital word blindness a hereditary type of Gerstmann's Syndrome? *Psychiatria et Neurologia, 136*, 59–73.

Hinshelwood, J. (1900). *Congenital word blindness. Lancet, 1*, 1506–1508.

Hinshelwood, J. (1917). *Congenital word blindness*. London: H.K. Lewis.

Hynd, G.W., Semrud-Clikeman, M., Lorys, A.R., Novey, E.S., & Eliopulos, D. (1990). Brain morphology in developmental dyslexia and attention deficit disorder/hyperactivity. *Archives of Neurology, 47*, 919–926.

Johnson, D. (1978). Remedial approaches to dyslexia. In A. Benton & D. Pearl (Eds.), *Dyslexia: An appraisal of current knowledge* (pp. 397–422). New York: Oxford University Press.

Kaufman, A. (1981). The WISC-R and learning disabilities: State of the art. *Journal of Learning Disabilities, 9*, 520–526.

Kussmaul, A. (1877). Disturbance of speech. In H. vonZiemssen (Ed.), *Cyclopedia of the practice of medicine* (Vol. 14). NewYork: William Wood.

Lewitter, F.I., DeFries, J.C., & Elston, R.C. (1980). Genetic models of reading disability. *Behavior Genetics, 10*, 9–30.

Morgan, W.P. (1896). A case of congenital word blindness. *British Medical Journal, 2*, 1378.

Nichols, P.L., & Chen, T.C. (1981). *Minimal brain dysfunction: A prospective study.* Hillsdale, NJ: Lawrence Erlbaum Associates.

Office of Education. (1977). Assistance to states for education of handicapped children: Procedures for evaluating specific learning disability. *Federal Register, 42,* 65,083.

Orton, S. (1925). "Word-blindness" in school children. *Archives of Neurology and Psychiatry, 14,* 581–615.

Paine, R.S. (1962). Minimal chronic brain syndromes in children. *Developmental Medicine and Child Neurology, 4,* 21–27.

Pennington, B.F., Gilger, J.W., Pauls, D., Smith, S.A., Smith, S.D., & DeFries, J.C. (1991). Evidence for major gene transmission of developmental dyslexia. *JAMA, 266,* 1527–1534.

Rosenberger, P.B., & Hier, D.B. (1980). Cerebral asymmetry and verbal intellectual deficits. *Annals of Neurology, 8,* 300–304.

Rumsey, J.M., Anderson, P., Zametkin, A.J., Aquino, T., King, A.C., Hamburger, S.D., Pikus, A., Rapoport, J.L., & Cohen, R.M. (1992). Failure to activate the left temporoparietal cortex in dyslexia. *Archives of Neurology, 49,* 527–534.

Rumsey, J., Dorwart, R., Vermess, M., Deckla, M.B., Kruesi, M.J., & Rapoport, J.L. (1986). Magnetic resonance imaging of brain anatomy in severe developmental dyslexia. *Archives of Neurology, 43,* 1045–1046.

Salvia, J., & Yssledyke, J.E. (1984). *Assessment in special and remedial education* (3rd ed.). Boston: Houghton Mifflin.

Sandler, A.D., Watson, T.E., Footo, M., Levine, M.D., Coleman, W.L., & Hooper, S.R. (1992). Neurodevelopmental study of writing disorders in middle childhood. *Journal of Developmental and Behavioral Pediatrics, 13,* 17–23.

Schonhaut, S., & Satz, P. (1983). Prognosis for children with learning disabilities: A review of follow-up studies. In M. Rutter (Ed.), *Developmental neuropsychiatry* (pp. 542–563). New York: Guilford Press.

Shapiro, B.K., Palmer, F.B., Antell, S.E., Bikler, S., Ross, A., & Capute, A.J. (1990). Detection of young children in need of reading help. *Clinical Pediatrics, 29,* 206–213.

Shaywitz, S.E., Escobar, M.D., Shaywitz, B.A., Fletcher, J., & Makuch, R. (1992). Evidence that dyslexia may represent the lower tail of a normal distribution of reading ability. *New England Journal of Medicine, 326,* 145–150.

Shaywitz, S.E., & Shaywitz, B.A. (1988). Attention deficit disorder: Current perspectives. In J. F. Kavanagh & T. J. Truss, Jr. (Eds.), *Learning disabilities: Proceedings of a national conference* (pp. 369–523). Parkton, MD: York Press.

Siegel, L.S. (1989). IQ is irrelevant to the diagnosis of learning disabilities. *Journal of Learning Disabilities, 22,* 469–479.

Silver, A.A., & Hagin, R.A. (1990). Principles of educational remediation. In A. A. Silver & R. A. Hagin (Eds.), *Disorders of learning in childhood* (pp. 172). New York: John Wiley & Sons.

Strauss, A.A., & Lehtinen, L.E. (1947). *Psychopathology and education of the brain-injured child* (Vol. 1). New York: Grune & Stratton.

Taylor, H.G. (1987). The meaning and value of soft signs in the behavioral sciences. In D. Tupper (Ed.), *Soft neurological signs* (pp. 297–334). New York: Grune & Stratton.

Taylor, R.L., & Warren, S.A. (1984). Educational and psychological assesment of children with learning disorders. *Pediatric clinics of North America, 31,* 281–296.

Vellutino, P. (1978). Toward an understanding of dyslexia: Psychological factors in specific learning disability. In A. Benton & D. Pearl (Eds.), *Dyslexia: An appraisal of current knowledge* (pp. 61–112). New York: Oxford University Press.

Wechsler, D. (1949). *Weschler Intelligence Scale for Children.* New York: Psychological Corporation.

Wechsler, D. (1981). *Wechsler Adult Intelligence Scale—Revised.* New York: Psychological Corporation.

Wechsler, D. (1991). *Wechsler Intelligence Scale for Children—Third Edition.* New York: Psychological Corporation.

Weiss, G., & Hechtman, L.T. (1986). *Hyperactive children grown up.* New York: Guilford Press.

Yule, W. (1976). Issues and problems in remedial education. *Developmental Medicine and Child Neurology, 18,* 675–682.

Chapter 27

Dyscalculia

Ronald L. Lindsay, M.D.

Dyscalculia, or developmental disorder of mathematics, has been recognized for only 70 years. Despite being more common than many other forms of neurologically based specific learning disability, dyscalculia was not described in the medical literature until 40 years after the first descriptions of congenital reading disability and has not been as well researched as disorders of reading, writing, and spelling. Indeed, it has not been considered to be as debilitating as other forms of learning problems. This disability is considered by some to be socially acceptable, and thus unworthy of referral for neurodevelopmental assessment. Yet, because mathematics is a cumulative subject, it is in fact far less amenable to remediation once a child falls behind as compared to other areas of learning difficulty.

Henschen (1919) used the term *acalculia* to describe an acquired disturbance in calculating produced by a focal lesion of the brain. Acalculia was one of the components of Gerstmann syndrome, first proposed in the 1920s. Other components included finger agnosia, right–left disorientation, and agraphia (Gerstmann, 1940). This syndrome was considered to be the result of a lesion in the left parietal-occipital area. A developmental form of this acquired adult syndrome was also proposed (developmental Gerstmann syndrome) in which children exhibited the above four components and showed a strong difference between verbal and performance IQ, with verbal being stronger. Gerstmann's observations are not without controversy, because other researchers believe that there is no justification for grouping these four components into a separate syndrome.

Guttman (1937) suggested that children could have a form of congenital arithmetic disability. Cohn (1961) coined the term *dyscalculia* to refer

to mathematical disability. In time, dyscalculia has come to be used in describing children with developmental disorders of mathematics.

Kosc (1974) performed one of the first systematic studies of dyscalculia. He found that 6.4% of fifth-grade students in Czechoslovakia displayed symptoms of dyscalculia. Badian (1983), in a study of 1,476 students in grades 1 through 8, also found that 6.4% of students showed some form of dyscalculia, compared to 4.9% of students who showed some form of reading disability. There was some overlap in delayed skills: 2.7% of students were poor in both reading and mathematics, 2.2% were low in reading alone, and 3.6% were low in mathematics alone.

In another study (McLeod & Armstrong, 1982), learning disability teachers reported that 26.2% of students in special education were served primarily for mathematics disorders and that, for an additional 40.3% of students with learning disabilities, mathematics was an area of secondary concern.

MECHANISMS OF DYSFUNCTION AND SUBCLASSIFICATION

Dyscalculia is a neurologically based problem. Since Henschen's time, neurologic, cognitive, and neuropsychological researchers have attempted to localize the area of the brain that is injured or impaired in those persons with mathematics disabilities. Mathematics researchers have approached the study of dyscalculia from a number of perspectives (Table 1). One approach involves the subtyping of mathematics disabilities and the relationship of these subtypes with other forms of learning disorders. Research into the cognitive components of mathematics disability focuses on experimental

Table 1. Comparisons of mathematics subtyping studies

Kosc (1974)	Badian (1983)	Rourke (1993)	Geary (1993)

Verbal
  Inability to designate
  verbally mathematical
  terms
	Alexia and agraphia
	  Inability to read or
	  write numbers
		Group R-S: Psycholin-
		  guistic
			Semantic memory
			  Low frequency of
			  arithmetic fact retrieval
			  with high error rate

Practognostic
  Disturbance of mathe-
  matical manipulation
  with real or pictured
  objects
	Spatial
	  Spatial confusion
	
	Attentional-sequential
	  Difficulties with atten-
	  tion (operational signs,
	  decimal points) and
	  ability to remember
	  number facts
		Group A: Visual–Spatial
		  Spatial organization
		  Visual detail
		  Procedural errors
		  Failure to shift psycho-
		  logical set
		  Graphomotor
		  Memory
		  Judgment and
		  reasoning
			Procedural
			  Frequent use of imma-
			  ture procedures with
			  frequent errors in
			  execution

Lexical
  Disability in reading
  mathematical symbols
			Visuospatial
			  Difficulties in spatially
			  representing numerical
			  information

Graphical
  Disability in writing
  mathematical symbols
	Anarithmetria
	  Difficulties with mathe-
	  matical procedures
	
	Mixed		

Ideognostical
  Disability in under-
  standing mathematical
  ideas and relations and
  in performing
  mental calculations			

Operational
  Inability to carry out
  mathematical operations/
  computations			

studies of mathematics rather than the perfor-mance of students on achievement tests. A phenomenological approach can examine the subcomponents of mathematics ability and disability and their neurodevelopmental under-pinnings.

Beginning in 1975, Rourke and his col-leagues used a neuropsychological approach to subtyping mathematics disabilities by investi-gating the patterns of performance by students on standardized achievement tests. Rourke (1993) theorized that there were at least two profiles of neuropsychological deficits, with different patterns of neuropsychological assets and deficits leading to impaired mathematics performance in children.

One group of children with mathematics im-pairment (Group A; i.e., Arithmetic) had rela-tively intact reading and spelling skills. They performed poorly on measures of visuospatial skills, which was suggestive of right hemi-spheric dysfunction. These children were thought to have a form of nonverbal learning disability. A separate group of children (Group R-S; i.e., Reading-Spelling) with poor mathe-matics performance also had significant reading problems. These students performed well on nonverbal problem-solving tasks but had defi-ciencies in verbal/auditory–perceptual tasks. The problems that these students encountered with mathematics appeared to be due to a read-ing disability and inexperience with the subject material. Rourke (1993) suggested that there was a common verbal deficit underlying prob-lems in both mathematics and reading in Group R-S children.

Rourke further subdivided children with vi-suospatially based mathematics disabilities (his Group A) into seven overlapping categories on the basis of mechanical arithmetic errors: spa-tial organization, visual detail, procedural er-rors, failure to shift psychological set, grapho-motor, memory, and judgment and reasoning.

Denckla (1991) considered mathematical un-derachievement to be a form of nonverbal learning disability. In her classification system, nonverbal learning disabilities included a tri-ad of deficits in mathematics, visuospatial-constructive, and social skills. Weak spatial cognition was considered to be a major cause of mathematics disability, with the nature of this failure lateralized to the right hemisphere. Denkla noted that there were differing relative contributions of spatial ability at each stage of mathematics (arithmetic, algebra, geometry, etc.). At each stage, verbal–sequential compensation may be able to overcome weak spatial ability and permit a child to perform adequately in mathematics.

The development of skills underlying simple basic mathematics skills such as addition was examined using a cognitive approach in a series of studies by Geary (1993). These studies examined strategy use by students, error patterns, and the developmental changes in computational and memory retrieval skills. Geary found that the strategies used by elementary children to solve addition problems evolved over time as they progressed from a reliance on counting strategies to a reliance on retrieval memory. First-grade children use a mix of strategies, including counting fingers, verbal counting, and memory. Their performance was marked by procedural and memory errors.

Counting strategies ranged from the developmentally immature method of counting up both numbers (the *sum* or counting-all procedure) to the relatively more mature method of starting with the value of the larger integer and counting the number of the smaller integer until a sum was obtained (the *min* or counting-on procedure) used by children at the end of first grade.

Typical children, as they progressed into the second grade, placed an increasing reliance on memory retrieval, with decreasing reliance on counting strategies, and demonstrated a decrease in procedural and factual errors. Children with mathematics disabilities relied more on counting strategies and became more skilled in counting (although less so than typical children). They made the same number of procedural errors and their ability to retrieve number facts did not improve.

Geary (1993) found two distinct functional deficits in children with mathematics disabilities: procedural and memory retrieval. *Procedural deficits* followed a *developmental delay* pattern, in which the pattern of performance was similar to younger, academically typical children and tended to disappear over time. This

was thought to be mediated by poor attentional and active working memory skills. *Memory retrieval deficits* followed a *developmental difference* pattern that was qualitatively distinct from the pattern seen in same-age peers and younger, academically typical children and persisted throughout the elementary school years. Memory retrieval deficits often covaried with reading disabilities, suggesting a more general deficit in representation or retrieval from semantic memory. This deficit may involve the posterior regions of the left hemisphere.

Thus, Geary expanded the subtyping of mathematics disabilities outlined by Rourke. One of his subtypes was associated with a dysfunction of visuospatial skills (Rourke's Group A). Two other subtypes were proposed: one involving difficulties in arithmetic fact retrieval, including problems in the memorization of arithmetic tables (mathematics facts), and the other involving difficulties in the use of arithmetical procedures such as counting strategies, carrying, and borrowing.

As a student progresses through school, the increasing demands of mathematics require a multitude of developmental skills and processes. These include memory, sequential processes, language competency, higher order cognition (problem-solving skills and strategy use), visuospatial skills, and attention. These skills and processes must be integrated in distinctive patterns that address the requirements of individual mathematical tasks. Depending on the task, some of these processes are salient and others less so.

Using a phenomenological approach, it is possible to delineate a series of 16 interactive subcomponents of mathematics during the school years (Levine, Lindsay, & Reed, 1992). Each subcomponent has a distinctive set of neurodevelopmental underpinnings (Table 2). A phenomenological approach permits the investigation of the underlying dysfunctions that undermine an individual child's mathematical performance, as well as intact or superior skills that facilitate mathematics performance. Understanding these strengths and weaknesses permits more effective remediation without overconcern for the subtype of mathematics deficit the child possesses.

Table 2. Developmental–behavioral functions and their relationships to mathematics subcomponents[a]

	Interactive subcomponents						
	Attention	Memory	Language	Visuospatial	Sequential	Higher cognitive	Affective
Facts		+++	+				+
Details	+++	++					
Procedures	+	++			++	+	
Manipulations	+	++				+	
Patterns		+	+	+		++	
Words			+++			+	
Sentences			+++				
Images		+		+++			
Logic					+	++	
Estimations	+			+		++	
Concepts			+		+	+	
Approaches	+					++	
Accumulations		++			+		
Applications		+		+		+	
Apprehensions		+					++
Affinities		+				++	+

[a] Key to importance of function to subcomponent: +, mildly important; ++, moderately important; +++, salient.

Integrating a phenomenological approach with the findings of Rourke and Geary, one can follow the progression of skills used in mathematics during the first 4 years of school. In the first grade, students rely on spatially mediated counting strategies in solving addition problems. These skills, aided by the development of working memory, permit the child to develop long-term representations of basic addition facts and incorporate these into memory. The child's developing working memory and recall memory ability permit a reliance on these more efficient memory skills in solving addition problems, with counting strategies being utilized as a backup procedure if a satisfactory answer cannot be retrieved from memory. As the child progresses into late third and fourth grades and encounters multiplication, working memory and retrieval memory are increasingly salient because of the absence of effective or efficient counting strategies. Over a 3-year period, an early reliance on spatially based strategies develops into a reliance on memory-based strategies.

A review of the research on the development of mathematical talent (Benbow, 1988) echoes the research on mathematical disabilities. Students with superior mathematical skills not only developed higher order cognitive abilities earlier (i.e., entering the Piagetian stage of for-

mal operations), they also had superior spatial ability, excellent memory, and high verbal and reasoning skills. Bilateral cognitive representation of language and spatial abilities is thought to be associated with mathematical reasoning ability.

PROGRESSION OF MATHEMATICAL SKILL DEVELOPMENT

The development of mathematical reasoning ability and skills progresses in an orderly manner despite wide variations in culture (Piaget, 1965). In describing the child's concept of number, Piaget was not interested in computational ability, which was considered to be a process that could be carried out by rote without understanding. He focused instead on the child's ability to master basic ideas such as classification, ordering, one-to-one correspondence, and conservation.

It is unusual for a child to be significantly delayed in the development of these concepts. As a result, by the time a child enters kindergarten, he or she possesses an array of skills among which is the ability to count aloud to 10 or 20 or count fingers on a person's hands with one-to-one correspondence. By the end of kindergarten, a child could be competent in the ability to count to 20; identify sets up to 20; write the numerals 0–10 in order; identify certain geometric forms, such as a circle, square, rectangle, and triangle; and identify the inside and outside of a circle (Kurtz, 1978).

Beyond kindergarten, development of additional skills and competencies is dependent on a number of factors, including experience, curriculum, and the mastery of the above skills. As a result, it becomes difficult to establish mathematical developmental milestones.

Counting strategies are salient in kindergarten and first-grade mathematics (Figure 1). In the middle elementary grades (2 through 4), students should have developed mastery of basic addition and subtraction facts, thus relying on memory (semantic and procedural) strategies

in mathematics (Figure 2). During these years, students are introduced to regrouping, which adds additional burdens on active working memory. Learning multiplication facts adds additional burdens on recall memory. Fractions and decimals are introduced in the later elementary grades (5 and 6).

By middle school, students should have developed facility with word problems. This necessitates the development of higher cognitive skills such as conceptualization and estimation, as well as language skills and the development of a mathematical vocabulary (Figure 3). Automaticity and integration of skills also become important, placing additional demands on active working and procedural memory.

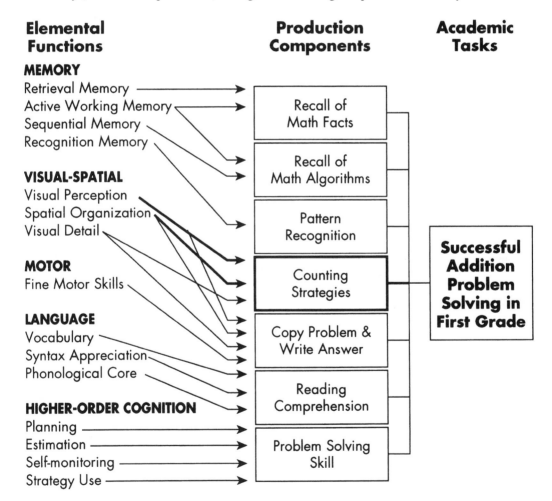

Figure 1. Solving addition problems in first grade. Strategy use in mathematics evolves depending on the nature of the task. Different strategies require that certain production components and elemental functions become salient. The thickness of lines and boxes reflects the degree of saliency.

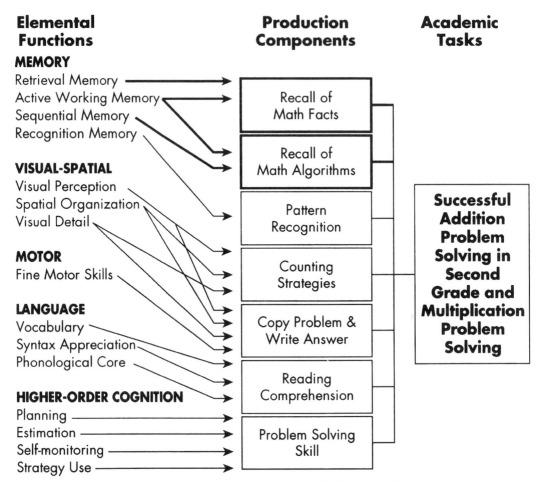

Figure 2. Solving addition problems in second grade and solving multiplication problems.

In high school, basic computational skills become less important as conceptualization and abstract symbolic reasoning become salient. Calculators become acceptable accessories in mathematics classes. Problem-solving skills such as estimation and the ability to be flexible in strategy use contribute to success in mathematics at this level. Acquisitions such as algebraic skills and geometric proofs require logical reasoning, the concepts of equivalence and proportion, and a high degree of language ability.

DIAGNOSIS OF DYSCALCULIA

History

As with all other developmental disabilities, a detailed history is an essential first step in the di-

agnostic process. Teachers, parents, and the child are all valuable sources of information. The child's teacher can provide observations of the child's performance in mathematics in the classroom setting. Similarly, a parent may be able to make observations of the child's performance when doing mathematics homework. Table 3 lists specific mathematics parameters that can be assessed by history and direct observation.

The child who is experiencing difficulty with mathematics may be able to provide details and possible causes for underachievement in this area. Some questions that may be helpful in this respect are listed in Table 4.

Physical Examination

A thorough physical examination, including a detailed neurologic assessment, should be performed as part of a neurodevelopmental evalua-

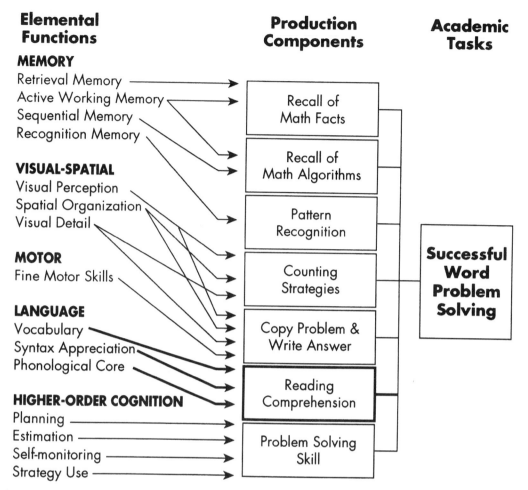

| Elemental Functions | Production Components | Academic Tasks |

Figure 3. Solving word problems.

tion of any learning disorder. The examination will not yield specific data leading to the diagnosis of a mathematics disability. However, certain neurologic diseases of childhood and forms of developmental disabilities with brain impairment are associated with an increased likelihood of mathematics disability (Table 5).

Geary (1993) reviewed studies on the potential heritability of mathematics disability and concluded that individual differences in basic numerical skills were at least partially heritable. He also pointed out that there was a need for specific behavioral genetic studies of mathematics disability.

Testing

Developmental and educational testing is necessary in order to confirm the diagnosis of mathe-

matics disability. Schools commonly use individually administered, standardized measures of cognitive ability and academic achievement in order to determine eligibility for special education services (Table 6). However, these tests contain inherent inadequacies involving content, scoring, and sensitivity (Reed, 1992).

An interdisciplinary approach to evaluation provides the child with a high level of expertise in the diagnosis and management of mathematics disability as well as any other form of learning disability. The role of the developmental pediatrician is often to serve as coordinator of the interdisciplinary team. In the diagnostic role, the developmental pediatrician conducts developmental and medical evaluations in order to define possible etiologies for the mathematics disability. These dysfunctions can include atten-

Table 3. Mathematics parameters meriting evaluation

Arithmetic fact retrieval—speed, accuracy, degree of automatization

Arithmetical procedural (algorithm) use—recall, use of developmentally immature strategies (e.g., counting strategies), degree of automatization

Strategy use and approaches to problem solving

Mastery of concepts underlying procedural use

Attention to detail

Work pace (reflective vs. impulsive)

Ability to interpret and solve word problems

Analysis of the child's affect in regard to mathematics

Table 4. Interview questions regarding mathematics performance

Do you understand when the teacher is explaining something in mathematics class?

Do you prefer to learn mathematics by having the teacher explain it to you, or would you prefer to see how a mathematics problem is solved correctly?

Do you have trouble remembering things in math? What kinds of things do you have trouble remembering?

Are word problems hard or easy for you to do?

Do you make a lot of careless mistakes in math?

Do you work too slow or too fast in math?

Does mathematics make you nervous?

Are there some parts of mathematics that are harder for you to do?

tion deficits, memory problems, poor conceptual ability, language disabilities, poor sequential organization, and visuospatial weaknesses.

Neurodevelopmental testing permits the developmental pediatrician to formulate a neurodevelopmental differential diagnosis and determine if further diagnostic assessments are needed. Constructive collaborations between pediatricians and educators can be very beneficial to children.

An educational diagnostician or psychoeducational specialist can perform an educational assessment that reflects the developmental demands of mathematical tasks, assess specific skill acquisition and application, and observe and analyze specific mathematical parameters (see Table 2). The evaluation should take into account the child's age and grade level.

Error analysis is one of the tools that can be utilized in the assessment of mathematics difficulties. There is more than one way that a student can make a mistake in mathematics, and many of these mistakes occur in recognizable patterns. By conducting error analysis, an educational diagnostician can collect sufficient information to be able to determine where the breakdowns in an individual student's performance occur, what neurodevelopmental subcomponents are involved, and how a plan for remediation can be developed.

A wider evaluation of learning strengths and weaknesses can provide additional insight into a child's difficulty with mathematics. Poor reading comprehension in addition to poor mathematics performance might suggest that a language disorder or poor semantic memory is the common impaired pathway. Problems with

spelling, writing, and mathematical procedures suggest impairment in sequential ability. Poor social skills, spatial deficits, and mathematical disabilities suggest nonverbal (right hemisphere) learning disabilities.

APPROACHES TO MANAGEMENT

Because of the cumulative nature of mathematics, remediation must be initiated early. It is far less likely that a child will catch up in mathematics than in any other type of learning disability. A child practices mathematics skills only in mathematics class, whereas reading and writing skills are utilized in all subjects.

It has been shown that children use mathematics performance as a basis for perceiving their own intellectual ability (Stipek & MacIver,

Table 5. Medical conditions associated with mathematics disability

Hydrocephalus

Myelomeningocele

Metachromatic leukodystrophy

Agenesis of the corpus callosum

Williams syndrome

Turner syndrome

Autism/Asperger syndrome

Female carriers of fragile X gene

Insulin-dependent diabetes mellitus

Congenital hypothyroidism

Velocardiofacial syndrome

Exposure to high-dose intracranial radiation

Table 6. Commonly used school assessments of mathematics achievement

Wide Range Achievement Test–Revised (1984)

For ages 5–75 years. Includes a timed subtest of arithmetic computation permitting assessment of rate of performance. Norms are recent and representative. Raw scores are converted to age standard scores, percentiles, and grade equivalents.

Wechsler Individual Achievement Test (1992)

For grades K–12. Norms and standardization are linked to the Wechsler Intelligence Scale for Children–III. Subtests include mathematical reasoning (including measurement, geometry, number concepts, and problem solving) and numerical operations (the ability to write dictated numerals and solve calculation problems). A mathematics composite score can be derived from the subtest scores. Mathematics reasoning subtest is included in the screening form of the test. The test provides standard scores, percentiles, and grade and age equivalents.

Woodcock-Johnson Psychoeducational Battery–Revised (1989)

For ages 2–90 years. On the Test of Achievement, there are two subtests assessing Calculation (basic operations as well as some geometric, trigonometric, logarithmic, and calculus operations), and Applied Problems (assessing skills in analyzing and solving practical problems in mathematics). The test is carefully standardized. Scoring manual includes standard scores, percentiles, and grade equivalents for individual subtests.

Kaufman Test of Educational Achievement (1985)

For ages 6–18 years. Has Brief and Comprehensive forms. The Brief form includes a global assessment of mathematic skills; the Comprehensive form has separate subtests for mathematics applications and computation. Standard scores and percentile ranks are provided based on age and grade, age and grade equivalents for each subtest, and a mathematics composite. Norms are recent and the test was carefully standardized.

Key Math–Revised (1988)

For grades K–9. An untimed, content-referenced test assessing mathematics. It is divided into three major areas and 13 subtests:

Basic concepts	Operations	Applications
Numeration	Addition	Measurement
Rational numbers	Subtraction	Time & money
Geometry	Multiplication	Estimation
	Division	Interpreting data
	Mental computation	Problem solving

Norms have improved from the original test and are representative. Behavioral objectives are included for each test item, permitting determination of the need for further assessment and remediation.

1989). Because this is a subject area that is taken so seriously by children, parents, and teachers, it is imperative that the nature of the individual child's mathematics disability be fully explained in terms that are developmentally appropriate. This must be accomplished in a manner that permits the child a measure of optimism. Clear explanations of individual neurodevelopmental strengths and weaknesses, and their relationships to mathematics performance, can be helpful.

Direct remediation may be necessary in order to strengthen weak neurodevelopmental subcomponents. This may require breaking down a complex mathematics problem into individual subcomponents and allowing the child to master each subcomponent as an end in itself. For example, a child who has difficulty recalling facts could be given practice drills to see how many problems can be solved in a limited period of time. A child who had problems recalling the

sequence of a procedure or algorithm can be allowed to explain the procedure, then attempt to solve it. If successful, the child could then try to teach it to another student. Students with stronger visuospatial skills could learn a procedure by watching a teacher solve a number of problems correctly.

Bypass techniques can be useful strategies in the classroom in order to circumvent weak mathematics subcomponents. This can allow a child to continue to progress in mathematics even as the weak subcomponent is being strengthened through remediation. Strategies can be as simple as allowing a child more time to finish a mathematics test, limiting the number of problems that are to be completed, or using a multiplication table or calculator if the child has difficulty recalling mathematics facts.

Identification and treatment of other neurodevelopmental disabilities that have an impact on mathematics is also an important component of management. If a child has an attentional problem, treatment with psychostimulant medication and cognitive management techniques is warranted. Language therapy for children with language disabilities may improve mathematics comprehension and the ability to understand and solve word problems.

Controlling the psychosocial sequelae of mathematics disability is also important. Parents and teachers must be made aware of the toll that mathematics disability has on a child's self-esteem. Anxiety over performance in mathematics negatively impacts memory function, affecting a wide array of mathematical procedures and leading to poorer performance and more anxiety. A measure of privacy in mathematics may be in order, whereby a child is not called to answer a problem in front of the class or have other students correct mathematics quizzes. Teachers and parents must be as supportive as possible when working with a child with mathematics disability.

CONCLUSIONS

Dyscalculia, or mathematics disability, is more common than disabilities in reading, writing, and spelling. Although the basis of dyscalculia appears to be multifactoral, on the basis of cognitive and neuropsychological research, there appear to be three main subtypes of dyscalculia based on weak neurodevelopmental skills: poor memory for mathematics facts, inability to perform mathematic procedures, and visuospatial deficits. Further research on the neurodevelopmental and genetic basis of mathematics disability is necessary.

Developmental pediatricians and special educators can collaborate in the evaluation and management of children with dyscalculia. The need for early intervention in children with mathematics disability is more acute than in other learning disabilities given the cumulative nature of mathematics. Intervention should include the use of remediation techniques, bypass strategies, and controlling the psychosocial sequelae of mathematics disability.

REFERENCES

Badian, N.A. (1983). Dyscalculia and nonverbal disorders of learning. In H.R. Myklebust (Ed.), *Progress in learning disabilities* (Vol. 5, pp. 235–264). New York: Stratton.

Benbow, C. P. (1988). Neuropsychological perspectives on mathematical talent. In L.K. Obler & D. Fein (Eds.), *The exceptional brain, neuropsychology of talent and special abilities* (pp. 48–69). New York: Guilford.

Cohn, R. (1961). Dyscalculia. *Archives of Neurology, 4*, 301–307.

Connolly, A. (1988). *Key Math—Revised: A Diagnostic Inventory of Essential Mathematics.* Circle Pines, MN: American Guidance Service.

Denckla, M.B. (1991). Academic and extracurricular aspects of nonverbal learning disabilities. *Psychiatric Annals, 21*, 717–724.

Geary, D.C. (1993). Mathematical disabilities: Cognitive, neuropsychological, and genetic components. *Psychological Bulletin, 114*, 345–362.

Gerstmann, J. (1940). Syndrome of finger agnosia, disorientation for right and left, agraphia and acalculia. *Archives of Neurology and Psychiatry, 44*, 398–408.

Guttman, E. (1937). Congenital arithmetic disability and acalculia (Henschen). *British Journal of Medical Psychology, 16*, 16–35.

Henschen, S. (1919). Uber Sprach-, Musik- und Rechenmechanismen und ihre Lokalisationen in Gehirn. *Zietschrift fur die gesamte Neurologie und Psychiatrie, 52*, 273–298.

Jastak, S., & Wilkinson, G.S. (1984). *Wide Range Achievement Test—Revised.* Wilmington, DE: Jastak Associates.

Kaufman, A.S., & Kaufman, N.L. (1985). *Kaufman Test of Educational Achievement.* Circles Pines, MN: American Guidance Service.

Kosc, L. (1974). Developmental dyscalculia. *Journal of Learning Disabilities, 7*, 164–177.

Kurtz, V.R. (1978). Kindergarten mathematics—A survey. *Arithmetic Teacher, 25*, 51–53.

Levine, M.D., Lindsay, R.L., & Reed, M.S. (1992). The wrath of math: Deficiencies of mathematical mastery in the school child. *Pediatric Clinics of North America, 39*, 525–536.

McLeod, T.M., & Armstrong, S.W. (1982). Learning disabilities in mathematics—skill deficits and remedial approaches at the intermediate and secondary level. *Learning Disability Quarterly, 5*, 305–311.

Piaget, J. (1965). *The child's concept of number.* New York: W.W. Norton.

Reed, M. (1992). Educational testing. In M.D. Levine, A. Crocker, & W. Carey. (Eds.), *Developmental behavioral pediatrics* (pp. 638–645). Philadelphia: W.B. Saunders.

Rourke, B.P. (1993). Arithmetic disabilities, specific and otherwise: A neuropsychological perspective. *Journal of Learning Disabilities, 26*, 214–226.

Stipek, D., & MacIver, D. (1989). Developmental changes in children's assessment of intellectual competence. *Child Development, 60*, 521–538.

Wechsler, D. (1992). *Wechsler Individual Achievement Test.* San Antonio, TX: Psychological Corporation.

Woodcock, R.W., & Johnson, M.B. (1989). *Woodcock-Johnson Psychoeducational Test Battery—Revised.* Allen, TX: DLM.

Chapter 28

Attention-Deficit Disorders and Hyperactivity

Thomas A. Blondis, M.D.

The delay thus gained might not be more than a second in duration—but that second might be critical; for in the constant rising and falling of considerations in the mind, where two associated systems of them are nearly in equilibrium it is often a matter of but a second more or less of attention at the outset, whether one system shall gain force to occupy the field and develop itself, and exclude the other, or be excluded itself by the other. (James, 1890/1952)

Although attention is a psychological process that is as old as the human being, William James was the first of the great Western thinkers to consider the varieties and components of attentional processing. Consideration of a specific neurodevelopmental condition that disrupts an executive system that controls impulses, attention, and activity, is in its infancy. It was not until Strauss's work that a central nervous system disorder of impulse and attentional control was proposed (Strauss & Lehtinen, 1947).

Although cases of almost complete disinhibition of control exist in childhood, these are the exception. The medical and psychiatric communities have yet to develop a system of recognition that includes boundaries that clearly distinguish a neurobehavioral condition of disordered activity and impulse control.

Various clinical scientists throughout the world have developed standards for the diagnosis of disorders that have different names in different countries (Conners & Kinsbourne, 1990). These disorders constitute a spectrum of central processing dysfunctions, but the trend has been toward splitting this spectrum in order to more clearly delineate the individual child's deficit(s). The so-called attention-deficit/hyperactivity disorder (ADHD) is one example

of this. It is possible for the thoughtful clinician to diagnose this dimensional disorder if a "goodness of fit" can be demonstrated between the symptom complex and the child's psychological and neurodevelopmental profile.

Clinical research to date corroborates that the(se) neurologic disease(s) underlying disordered attention, impulse control, and organization are linked to a genetic etiology (Whitman, 1991). At the present time, this symptom complex is one of the two most frequently diagnosed disabling conditions in North America. Although there exists greater consensus regarding the behavioral symptom complex of this disorder, most scientists do not view ADHD as a behavioral disorder, but rather as possibly several chronic neurologic disorders. The nature of each of these disorders is clearly not as well defined as the symptom complex definitions, and the scientific effort to determine specific categorical syndromes remains outside of the clinical arena. Because the behavioral symptom complexes are more widely accepted and are supported by recent multi-centered field trials, we have chosen to refer to attention deficits and hyperactivity disorders as AD/HD throughout this chapter and Chapter 29.

These two chapters describe the clinical problems inherent in the current behavioral nosology, outline a clinical approach for the developmental pediatrician that describes some of the pitfalls of misdiagnosis, and outline an approach toward habilitating children with a neurodevelopmental condition affecting the executive processes (Accardo & Whitman, 1991; Blondis, Accardo, & Snow, 1989a, 1989b; Roizen, Blondis, Irwin, & Stein, 1994).

FROM SPLITTING TO
LUMPING AND BACK TO SPLITTING

Historical Background

The first description of what today is called
AD/HD is generally traced back to the description of minimal brain damage by Alfred Tredgold (1908). Many of the children described in
Tredgold's book were like children with
AD/HD: They were described as being "mentally deficient" but not as functionally retarded.
They progressed if they received individualized
instruction.

Charles Bradley (1937) described the improved school performance and more reflective
behavior in 30 children with headaches he
treated with benzedrine to raise their blood
pressure. He later reported a wide range of children whose behavior immediately improved on
amphetamine.

Strauss and Lehtinen published literature in
the 1940s and 1950s that described the behavior
of children with brain injury. These researchers
excluded children who had behavioral problems
resulting from limited emotional relationships.
Children who had definite organic brain pathology also demonstrated short attention span, hyperactivity or motor disinhibition, perseveration
or exaggerated attentional fixation, emotional
lability, and conceptual rigidity (Strauss &
Lehtinen, 1947). The "Strauss syndrome" soon
was named *minimal brain dysfunction* (MBD).
A U.S. Public Health Service task force attempted to provide a standardized terminology
and definition for children with MBD. Children
were to be of at least "near average" intelligence, with certain learning or behavioral problems that ranged from mild to severe. These developmental and behavioral symptoms were to
be associated with neurologic signs (Clements
& Peters, 1966).

The World Health Organization (WHO) defined a hyperkinetic syndrome of childhood in
1978. Short attention span and distractibility
were the central features of this disorder. At that
time, features in early childhood included disinhibition and unregulated overactivity; under-
activity was thought to predominate during
adolescence. Other behavioral characteristics

included impulsivity, aggression, and marked
mood fluctuation.

In its *Diagnostic and Statistical Manual of
Mental Disorders*, third edition (DSM-III), the
American Psychiatric Association (APA) (1980)
separated this disorder into attention deficit disorder (ADD) and attention deficit disorder with
hyperactivity (ADD-H). Children could now
have ADD with "inattention" and "impulsivity,"
either with or without "hyperactivity." As a result of early field trials begun after the DSM-III
was published, the APA revised the nomenclature to highlight hyperactivity as part of the disorder by making the diagnosis attention-
deficit/hyperactivity disorder (ADHD). At the
same time they preserved an entity undifferenti-
ated attention deficit disorder (UADD), which
replaced attention deficit disorder without hyperactivity (APA, 1987). UADD became less
commonly used, especially among North American pediatricians and neurologists.

It must be remembered that AD/HD children
are only one segment of the original MBD
population. Although overlap exists between
children with ADHD(s) and those with hyperkinetic disorder(s), all of these children fit
within the construct of MBD. In Table 1, one
can see that AD/HD represented only one segment of the dysfunction represented within the
MBD framework.

Current Behavioral Diagnostic Nosologies

Two different groups reached independent
conclusions in trying to determine the core behaviors underlying ADHD. These studies were
notable in that they were among the first studies
that attempted to validate the APA ADHD
nomenclature. Table 2 depicts the core clinical
behavioral symptoms that these studies reported. Note that "can't concentrate," "day-
dreams," and "acts without thinking" were the
three behaviors both studies agreed were core
manifestations of ADHD (Achenbach, Conners,
Quay, Verhylst, & Howell, 1989; Lahey et al.,
1987).

In a U.S.-U.K. Cross-National Study of the
DSM-III and the *International Classification of
Diseases*, ninth edition (ICD-9) (Prendergast et
al., 1988), ICD-9 interrater agreement was high

Table 1. Differing diagnostic criteria for low severity developmental disorders

Disorder	Symptoms	Origin
Hyperkinetic reaction of childhood	Overactivity Restlessness Distractibility Short attention span	DSM-II (American Psychiatric Association, 1968)

Attention-deficit/hyperactivity disorder	8 of 14 behaviors:
	  impulsivity
	  hyperactivity
	  inattentiveness
	Onset before age 7
	Excludes:
	  pervasive developmental
	  disorder
		DSM-III-R (American Psychiatric Association, 1987)

Minimal brain dysfunction	Delayed behavioral controls
	  attention
	  impulse
	  motor
	Motor and sensory
	  impairments
	Intellectual impairment
	Specific learning disability
		Clements & Peters (1966) (NIH Task Force)

Hyperkinetic syndrome of childhood	Essential features:
	  distractibility
	  short attention span
	Early childhood:
	  extreme overactivity
	  disinhibition
	  poor organization
	Adolescence:
	  occasional underactivity
	Other symptoms:
	  impulsivity
	  marked mood fluctuation
	  aggression
	Exclusions:
	  symptomatic of another
	  disorder
		ICD-9
		(World Health Organization, 1980)

only for trained research teams, and DSM-III criteria led to more diagnoses of ADHD than ICD-9 criteria led to diagnoses of hyperkinetic syndrome of childhood. This difference reached significance for U.K.-trained clinicians but not for U.S.-trained physicians. The authors concluded that both the diagnostic criteria and physician training contributed to this difference.

In a controlled prospective study that included an interdiagnoser reliability check, complete environmental and social background analysis, behavioral analysis, and neurodevelopmental testing of 180 cases, only 4 children met DSM-III classification for conduct disorder alone, whereas 83 were diagnosed to have ADD. However, 35 children met diagnostic criteria for both conduct disorder and ADD. Among these children, one third had severely dysfunctional family backgrounds (Reeves, Werry, Elkind, & Zametkin, 1987). This group generated two lists of behavioral symptoms related to ADHD: a list of inattentive behaviors and a list of hyperactive-impulsive behaviors. These behavior lists were published in *DSM-IV Options Book: Work in Progress* (Task Force on DSM-IV, 1993). Next these symptom lists un-

Table 2. Core clinical behavioral symptoms of ADHD[a]

Core behavioral symptom	Achenbach et al. (1989)	Lahey et al. (1987)
Can't concentrate	+	+
Daydreams	+	+
Impulsive, acts without thinking	+	+
Acts too young	+	−
Can't sit still	+	−
Confused	+	−
Poor schoolwork	+	−
Stares into space	+	−
Poor coordination, clumsy	+	−
Difficulty finishing tasks	−	+
Motor restlessness	−	+
Always on the go	−	+
Difficulty waiting turns	−	+
Difficulty organizing work	−	+
Sluggish	−	+
Drowsy	−	+

[a]Most common ADHD behavioral symptoms according to factor analysis loadings in two different studies.

Key: +, present in study population; −, absent in study population.

derwent field trials to determine the associated level of impairment. These field tests (Frick et al., 1994; Lahey et al., 1994) utilized a structured interview instrument, the Diagnostic Interview Schedule for Children (DISC) questionnaire, and the Child Global Assessment Scale (C-GAS). The study found that only inattentive symptoms were associated with academic failure, whereas hyperactive-impulsive symptoms were associated with global impairment. By utilizing quantitative measures versus the symptom lists, the investigators determined the number of symptoms necessary for a child to be considered atypical in the neurodevelopmental areas of attention and activity-impulsivity. The field tests included the investigation of interrater reliability and validity.

In 1992, the World Health Organization published the 10th edition of the ICD (ICD-10), revised its nomenclature, and split "hyperkinetic disorders" into 1) disturbance of activity and attention, 2) hyperkinetic conduct disorder, 3) other hyperkinetic disorders, and 4) hyperkinetic disorder, unspecified. In 1994, the APA

published the fourth edition of the DSM (DSM-IV). This revision is based on the field trials carried out since the inception of the ADHD nomenclature. It provides a list of inattentive behaviors and a list of hyperactive and impulsive behaviors. Children who exhibit a majority of the symptoms on both lists will meet criteria for ADHD, combined type. Children who often engage in a minority of the behavioral symptoms (fewer than six) will be considered either predominantly inattentive or predominantly hyperactive-impulsive. Table 3 compares the ICD-10 criteria to the DSM-IV diagnostic criteria.

The Current Dilemma: Weak Boundaries

All previous studies of ADD-related diagnostic criteria conclude that a useful and universally accepted nosology remains problematic. Three stances are possible: 1) question whether such a diagnostic entity even exists, 2) contend that there exists a "syndromal/categorical" model, or 3) adhere to a "dimensional" model (Zametkin & Rapoport, 1987). Although these authors support the "syndromal" model, everyone would agree that a comprehensive pathophysiologically understood disease is not yet within reach. Furthermore, it appears that a sizable percentage of children presenting with behaviors consistent with the AD/HD diagnosis during the early elementary school years outgrow the "syndrome" by adolescence. Clearly, the current disorder represents a clinical spectrum both from the point of view of presentation of behaviors and from that of severity and duration of dysfunction.

From the clinical perspective, an umbrella definition with a set of minimal criteria ("dimensional model") is useful as long as the criteria are narrow enough that differentiation can be made from other disorders (Barkley, 1990). Problems with the DSM-III-R definition included "lumping" or overgeneralization; a "behavioral" orientation; recognition that the disorder can be a secondary phenomenon but absence of sufficient criteria within DSM-III-R to ensure that this error is not made commonly; lack of inclusion of dysfunctional parameters of attention (i.e., age norms for sustained attention span, reliability- and validity-tested measures

Table 3. Diagnostic criteria for attention-deficit hyperactivity disorder (ADHD) and hyperkinetic disorder (HD)

ADHD criteria in DSM-IV[a]	HD criteria in ICD-10[b]

A1. Inattentive behaviors (six or more)
  a. Often fails to give close attention to details or makes careless mistakes
  b. Often has difficulty sustaining attention in tasks or play
  c. Often doesn't seem to listen to directed conversation
  d. Often doesn't follow through on instructions and complete assignments
  e. Often has difficulties organizing tasks and activities
  f. Often avoids, dislikes, etc., tasks requiring sustained mental effort
  g. Often loses things necessary for tasks or activities
  h. Is often easily distracted by extraneous stimuli
  i. Is often forgetful in daily activities
A2. Hyperactive–impulsive behaviors (six or more)
Hyperactivity
  a. Often fidgets with hands or feet or squirms in seat
  b. Often leaves seat in classroom in which seating is expected
  c. Often runs about or climbs excessively at inappropriate times
  d. Often has difficulty playing quietly
  e. Is often "on the go" or often acts as if "driven by a motor"
  f. Often talks excessively
Impulsivity
  g. Often blurts out answers to incomplete questions
  h. Often has difficulty waiting in lines or awaiting turn
  i. Often interrupts or intrudes on others
B. Some hyperactive–impulsive or inattentive symptoms before 7 years
C. Some impairment from the symptoms is present in two or more settings
D. Disturbance causes significant distress in learning or adaptive function
E. Symptoms do not occur with pervasive developmental disorders, schizophrenia, or other psychoses and are not caused by mood disorder, anxiety disorder, dissociative disorder, or personality disorder
	A. The two cardinal features—1) Inattention and 2) overactivity must be evident in more than one situation
	1. Impaired attention
	  a. leave tasks unfinished
	  b. frequently shift activities
	  c. lose interest in one task because diverted by another
	  d. excessive for child's mental age
	2. Impaired activity (overactivity)
	  a. excessive restlessness even in situations of calm
	  b. various manifestations dependent on situation:
	    • running and jumping
	    • getting up from seat
	    • fidgeting and wriggling
	    • excessive talk/noise
	B. Associated features
	1. Social disinhibition
	2. Recklessness in situations involving some danger
	3. Impulsive flouting of social rules
	4. Cardinal features <6 years

Adapted from the criteria of the American Psychiatric Association (1994) and the World Health Organization (1992).

[a]Three types of ADHD are listed in the DSM-IV:

(314.00) ADHD, Predominantly Inattentive Type (if more than six behaviors under A1 present for last 6 months).

(314.01) ADHD, Predominantly Hyperactive–Impulsive Type (if more than six behaviors under A2 present for last 6 months).

(314.01) ADHD, Combined Type (if more than six behaviors under A1 and A2 present for last 6 months).

[b]Other key related factors for HD:

• Conduct disorder versus hyperkinetic disorder: symptoms of conduct disorder are neither exclusion nor inclusion criteria for the diagnosis of HD. When diagnosed, HD takes precedence over conduct disorder. When features of both conduct disorder and hyperactivity are present and the hyperactivity is pervasive and severe, "hyperkinetic conduct disorder" is the diagnosis.

• Pervasive developmental disorders take precedence over HD when they are present.

of selective attention); and other secondary disabilities that may occur as a result of either hyperactivity or inattention. Although the DSM-IV classification does not solve these problems, it has corrected several misconceptions. In the original diagnostic category of attention deficit disorder without hyperactivity, impulsivity was an essential component for making this diagnosis. Clinical studies since then have linked truly impulsive behavior to hyperactive behavior. The new consensus among the professionals participating on the APA Task Force (Lahey et al., 1994) was that the predominantly inattentive type of ADHD does not include a dysfunction of impulse control. Studies of the thought processes of hyperkinetic children clearly demonstrate the developmental nature of this disorder (Douglas, 1972; Kahneman & Treisman, 1984; Wright & Vlietstra, 1975). The child who struggles to focus attention has difficulty developing the higher order attentional processes that are essential to competence in a technological society. Table 4 highlights the differences between typical childhood attentional processes and AD/HD processes.

Other investigators contend that the disorder should be "split" into multiple subtypes (Conners & Wells, 1986; Denckla, 1992; Sunder, DeMarco, Frutiger, & Levey, 1988; Weinberg & Brumback, 1992). Table 5 illustrates the six different types of neuropsychological profiles that the Conners and Wells (1986) factor and cluster analysis yielded. The table shows which two subtype profiles proved to be nonresponders to stimulant medication as well as the four subtypes that were definite responders. These subtypes did not match Conners and Wells symptomatically defined subtypes exactly, and they viewed the profiles as hypotheses.

The focus in the United States has centered around the behavioral expressions of this disorder mainly because of the influences of the APA. Because child psychiatry has played the lead role in creating the current diagnostic standard, a more developmental focus that differentiates the severity of attentional delay and delineates the child's processing dysfunctions, problem-solving difficulties, and learning often is overlooked. Developmental pediatricians,

neuropsychologists, and child neurologists seek to link the behavioral symptom complexes that now define AD/HD to psychological processes that underlie these symptom complexes. Several lifetime clinical investigators believe that within the AD/HD construct exist a number of neurodevelopmental diseases and that a different central nervous system pathology may be responsible for each disease (Denckla, 1992).

ATTENTION AND CONTROL

Development of Attention and Control

Attention is an evolving cognitive process (Table 6). During infancy attention is stimulus bound. Although infants initially favor a familiar stimulus, by 3 months they prefer novel stimuli. Habituation reflects this waning of a response to a stimulus with repeated presentation (Thompson & Spencer, 1966).

Between 3 and 6 months, memory expands, visual attention becomes less stimulus bound, and decision rules develop (Sophian & Hagan, 1978). The infant begins to orient to the direction of a stimulus, and this central nervous system processing-dependent reflex further tunes the organism to refine its perception (Sokolov, 1963). By 8 months, the infant develops accommodative imitation (the ability to replicate an external event). By 9 months, object permanence is sufficient to allow the infant to search for an object that disappears from view.

This development of attention is closely linked to the development of memory. The memory of the preschool child is nonstrategic and involuntary; the attention of the young child is exploratory. In experiments on visual fixation, the attention of the young preschool child is more passive, whereas the older child more actively searches and explores. In color–form

Table 4. Comparison of AD/HD and normal attentional processes

Cognitive domain	AD/HD	Normal
Stimulus approach	Open ended	Goal directed
System	Divergent	Convergent
Tempo	Too slow/too fast	Modulation to task demand
Sustained attention	Short data sequence	Long data sequence
Storage	Random information	Essential features

Table 5. AD/HD Subtypes derived from cluster analysis of children

Profile description	Negative areas demonstrating response to stimulant according to teacher rating scale
Disinhibition, hyperactivity (frontal lobe dysfunction)	Defiance
	Hyperactivity
	Psychopathology
Learning disability, inattentiveness	None
Motor impulsivity (can't follow directions)	None
Anxious, intermittently inattentive, high achiever (very intelligent)	Inattention spectrum (daydreaming, social passivity, short span)
	Anxiety
Behavior problems at home, no learning problems (no cognitive dysfunction)	Inattention spectrum
	Improved inattention may reflect decreased anxiety
Poor visual–spatial abilities ("right hemisphere" impairment)	Inattention
	Anxiety
	Sociability (worse during placebo)

Adapted from Conners and Wells (1986).

experiments, young preschool children remembered a stimulus more on the basis of what color it was, whereas school-age children increasingly employed form (Corah & Gospodinoff, 1966; Sophian & Hagen, 1978; Wright & Vlietstra, 1975). If memory for color is essentially memory for salient stimulus and memory for form emphasizes information, then one could conclude that school-age children attend with more organization than young preschool children.

Selective exploration develops in the preschool years. The average 5- to 6-year old then uses a systematic approach to perceive novel stimuli. Most children by school age are to some extent able to inhibit movement and free flight of ideas, modulate arousal to meet cognitive demands, and sustain attention through mental effort. The elementary school–age child's attention includes not only perceptual search but also goal directedness. This process continues to expand and is quite developed in the average middle school–age child. The ability of children to attend to the critical feature(s) of a novel or other experience while simultaneously reducing incidental learning is called *selective attention*. This ability to focus primarily on central features generally begins during middle school and continues to expand throughout adolescence. Selective attention in the adolescent and the adult is further expedited by logical search (Hagen, 1967; Hale & Alderman, 1978).

Theories of Attention

Most theories of attention ignore the ontogenic aspects of attentional processing and thereby fail adequately to allow for important psychological differences between adults and children (Fletcher & Taylor, 1984). Like any psychological process, attention must be viewed within the construct of the child's developmental level in order to be understood.

The *filter theory* (Broadbent, 1982; Kahneman & Treisman, 1984) interpreted attention as consisting of three components: a selective fil-

Table 6. Development of attentional processes

Appearance	Attentional process
Early infancy	Dominated by salient features of stimuli
3–4 months	Decision rules, orienting reflex
Late infancy	Accommodative imitation, object permanence
Preschool years	Selective orientation
Early elementary school	Expansion of attention span, attend to form, retain information
Middle childhood	Selective attention (progress toward central features), modulate attention to meet task demands

ter, a limited-capacity channel, and a detection device. Ensuing research documented the ability to perceive several different stimuli at a time, and produced a modified paradigm, the *filter attenuation theory*. This theory takes into account the subjects's ability simultaneously to give deep processing to one stimulus and superficial processing to other stimuli. Shiffrin and Schneider (1977) differentiated information processing into two forms: automatic and controlled. *Automatic processing* is used if skill performance has already been achieved (e.g., driving a car); *controlled processing* is needed if one is attending to a task that is new or has not been fully learned. This approach modifies the filter attenuation theory in that the subject need not switch processes between stimuli.

Research on the spatial attention of normal adult humans and animals suggests that control of eye movements underlies attentional processing. Infants develop this control during the first years of life. Cognitive psychology has recently begun to combine information-processing data with the study of biologic mechanisms underlying attention (Posner & Rothbart, 1981). Posner and colleagues' research points to the parietal lobe as playing a role in the *disengagement* facet of the attentional process. Parietal lobe lesions do not cause problems of alerting and localizing, but, if another cue is given, the individual has a difficult time disengaging from the initial stimulus (Posner & Peterson, 1990).

Development of Hyperactivity

Ross and Ross (1982) defined hyperactivity as a class of heterogeneous behavior disorders in which the major presenting complaint is a high level of activity that is exhibited at inappropriate times and cannot be inhibited on command. The child's mother may recall an excessive amount of activity during fetal life, and often reports restlessness, excessive crying, or colic during infancy. This is the child who ran at almost the same time that he or she began to walk, the toddler who got into everything and worried the parents early about the child's safety. By preschool age, the child was constantly moving and would not stay occupied with an activity for any length of time. He or she may have resisted sitting through meals

with the family. The parents may have continued to worry that, if they were not near, the child would get into prohibited activities, some of which are dangerous (e.g., playing with matches). Such children can be distinguished from the average preschooler, who is able to stop and adjust with only slight protest when directed to. The hyperactive child has been noted to seek attention, which may be linked to a hyperactive need for frequent feedback. In a structured one-to-one situation with a minimum of distractors, the preschool hyperactive child can usually successfully relate to adults and professionals. Clearly, not all children with AD/HD exhibit this developmental profile during infancy and preschool years.

PREVALENCE

The prevalence of AD/HD remains unknown. It will vary significantly with physician training and the classification system used. The Isle of Wight survey of 2,199 children attempted to determine the prevalence of the hyperkinetic syndrome of childhood (Rutter, Graham, & Yule, 1970). Schachar, Rutter, and Smith (1981) reported that about 2% of the 10- to 11-year-old children in this study were experiencing hyperkinesis. Lambert and Sandoval (1980) found only 1.2% of children to have pervasive hyperkinetic syndrome (behavioral symptom complex clearly present at home, school, and the clinic). Teacher questionnaire studies have identified up to 13% of children as hyperactive. A Swedish study sampled 3,500 6- to 7-year-old children in a two-step epidemiologic study to determine if a relationship existed between behavioral problems and perceptual and motor problems (Hellgren, Gillberg, Gillberg, & Enerskog, 1993). The combined prevalence of the three neurodevelopmental diagnoses of ADD, motor output, and perceptual disorder reached 18%.

These wide variations demonstrate the problem underlying a behavioral symptom complex that may contain elements of other neurodevelopmental dysfunctions and can be confused with other psychiatric constructs that include many of these behavioral symptoms (e.g., pervasive development disorder, anxiety disorders, childhood depression). The truth is that the prevalence of AD/HD remains unknown, but a conservative estimate would be that 3%–5% of children have a primary attentional and/or hyperkinetic disorder, and that boys outnumber girls by approximately a 3:1 ratio (Lambert & Sandoval, 1980).

ETIOLOGY

Many etiologies have been documented to cause the AD/HD behavioral symptom complex. Teratogens, extremely low birth weight, prematurity, birth hypoxia, and head trauma, as well as many diseases, are just a few conditions that are associated with the AD/HD symptom complex. However, the vast majority of children presenting with this symptom complex do not present with a condition associated with AD/HD.

McMahon (1980) found significant methodologic problems with all genetics studies. Most investigators failed to include a heterogeneous subject sampling, interviewers blinded to the diagnostic status of the children whose parents were being interviewed, a concurrent validation of diagnostic subgroups of children with AD/HD on the basis of severity, and thorough diagnostic procedures.

A study of hyperactivity in 93 pairs of same-sex twins from a population without developmental disabilities showed a significant correlation for AD/HD between monozygotic twins. This study used an activity level questionnaire score, and the conclusion reached was that genetic transmission is responsible for temperament (Willerman, 1973).

In a 1986 adoption study, the index children had to have been diagnosed by a registered psychologist as meeting the criteria for ADHD (Alberts-Corush, Firestone, & Goodman, 1986). Biologic and adoptive parents of children with ADHD (adopted prior to 6 months of age) were evaluated and compared. Biologically hyperactive parents had more attentional difficulties, slower mean reaction times, and fewer correct recognitions on a span of apprehension task than did adoptive parents. The biologic parents did not evidence more impulsivity than the adoptive parents did, however. The authors concluded that there exists an association between childhood hyperactivity and attentional deficits among the biologic parents of hyperactive children.

Given the high concurrence of hyperactivity among monozygotic twin and adoptive versus biologic parents, a genetic etiology is accepted as the leading cause of AD/HD. It may also be that a genetic susceptibility to the disorder combines with other factors, such as asphyxia, to produce the symptom complex. Genetic linkage methods have yet to produce a major association for AD/HD, although linkages of chromosomes have been made for Tourette syndrome and dyslexia (Whitman, 1991).

PATHOPHYSIOLOGY

Physiologic studies have demonstrated a relationship between improved performance on attentional tasks and deceleration of heart rate. A decrease of heart rate variability also has been related to children's performance on attentional tasks: Children with normal attentional processes exhibit a decrease in respiratory activity (Porges, 1984).

It has been recognized for some time that a stroke occurring in the prefrontal regions of the frontal lobe causes disinhibition, impulsivity, and lack of organization (Chelune, Ferguson, Koon, & Dickey, 1986; Goldman-Rakic, 1984). Since 1990, imaging studies have supported this possibility. Positron emission tomography (PET) studies on adults with AD/HD demonstrate reduced glucose utilization in particularly the right posterior–medial orbital area of the frontal lobe (Zametkin et al., 1990). Lou, Henriksen, Bruhn, Borner, and Nielsen (1989) spent a decade researching the regional cerebral blood flow of children with attentional disorders and controls. Their results localized the regulation of activity control and attentional processing, based on decreased metabolic activity, to the striatum (thalamus and basal ganglia) as well as the frontal cortex to a less significant extent. The studies of Lou et al. also demonstrated an increase of metabolism in the left striatal area among subjects with AD/HD when medicated with methylphenidate. No scientist involved with imaging studies would deny that the prefrontal cortex and the thalamus appear to be key areas of the brain related to executive function; however, other studies have shown that other areas are linked to attention. Posner and Raichle (1994) described how various anatomic networks may carry out executive processes. Magnetic resonance imaging studies have demonstrated that the size of the right caudate nucleus is reduced among subjects with AD/HD when compared to control subjects (Hynd et al., 1993).

Peloquin and Klorman (1986) demonstrated a decreased amplitude among subjects with AD/HD of the late positive component (LPC) in an event-related potential study. The LPC amplitude increased in these subjects when they performed a continuous performance task after taking methylphenidate. Slow-wave activity in frontal regions and decreased beta activity in temporal regions of the brain have been noted in male children with AD/HD compared to matched controls in a quantitative analysis of electroencephalograms (Mann, Lubar, Zimmerman, Miller, & Muenchen, 1992).

Neurotransmitter research has been able to establish the role of catecholamines (Zametkin & Rapoport, 1987). Beyond this fact, much of current thinking is conjecture. When clonidine, a drug that inhibits noradrenaline activity, proved to be an effective treatment for some subjects with AD/HD, support for a single neurotransmitter system theory decreased. Research using a hyperactive animal model suggests that AD/HD may be the result of too much norepinephrine in the locus ceruleus combined with a dopamine deficiency in the frontal–mesolimbic system (Huessy, 1984). This has become the working hypothesis of a number of basic science investigators (Malone, Kershner, & Swanson, 1994).

DIAGNOSIS

The process for evaluating and diagnosing AD/HD remains tedious and data laden in many cases. Many children present with elements of the AD/HD symptom complex, but the developmental pediatrician must verify that this symptom complex is a longstanding condition occurring in various environments that cannot be attributed to another medical or psychiatric cause. Direct observation, questionnaires, child and family interviews, psychological testing, and physical and neurodevelopmental examinations are required to make the precise primary diagnosis and to elucidate what secondary conditions exist. It is not uncommon for the AD/HD symptom complex to represent a secondary problem rather than a primary diagnosis. An interdisciplinary problem-solving conference that includes the school professionals who work with the child on a day-to-day basis remains the gold standard for developmental pediatricians. Figure 1 depicts the components involved in this diagnostic process.

Medical History

AD/HD remains a diagnosis that must depend more on history than either medical or psychological evaluation. The *behavioral questionnaire* is the accepted instrument for documenting symptoms that are encountered outside of the range of the medical/developmental center (Blondis, Accardo, & Snow, 1989a, 1989b). Past records and behavioral questionnaires will help to determine which professionals are needed to formulate a successful habilitative program. It is important that the questionnaires used be dependable. Currently, the two most reliable and useful behavioral questionnaire systems that deal with the continuum of AD/HD are the Child Behavior Profile (CBP) and the revised Conners Parent and Teacher Scales. There are many other questionnaires that can help pinpoint other concerns, including parent AD/HD or other childhood difficulties the parents encountered, or both; parent depression; and the child's learning problems and self-esteem.

Reliability and validity for both the CBP and the revised Conners scales are considered to be very good for questionnaires (Achenbach & Edelbrock, 1979; Edelbrock & Achenbach, 1984; Goyette, Conners, & Ulrich, 1978). The CBP is normed to measure more behavioral areas than the Conners scales. The CBP scales are a bit longer than the Conners scales but are shorter than other scales that measure a wide spectrum of behavior. The reading age for adults responding to the questions on these

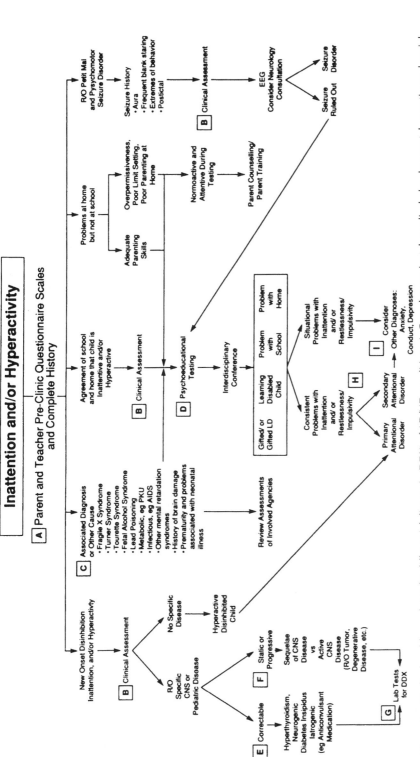

Figure 1. Medical problem solving for differential diagnosis (DDX) of AD/HD condition. *A,* Complete perinatal, medical, developmental, genetic, and social history must be obtained. *B,* The clinician must carry out a thorough examination that includes general, dysmorphology, and neurodevelopmental segments. *C,* Other diagnoses that include AD/HD behavioral symptoms should be determined or ruled out. *D,* Psychoeducational testing should include the clinical observation of behavior during testing or interview, as well as measures of verbal intelligence, visual intelligence, and achievement. *E,* Any correctable or partially correctable diseases, as well as diseases that might cause some AD/HD symptoms (e.g., seasonal allergies), must be determined. *F,* The clinician should rule out (R/O) active central nervous system (CNS) diseases. *G,* Laboratory test selection will vary depending on the clinical presentation of the patient. Any drug the child is taking that has known central nervous system side effects should be considered as the cause of the child's behavioral symptoms. *H,* Most likely, the child who manifests persistent problems with inattention and hyperactivity has either AD/HD, a specific learning disability, or a pervasive developmental disorder. *I,* Situational inattention or restlessness may be due to changes that are occurring at home, loss of self-esteem, and the like. Rarely would a depressed child be viewed by parents or professionals as having AD/HD, but either group may mistake AD/HD for a bipolar disorder. (AIDS, acquired immunodeficiency disorder; EEG, electroencephalogram; PKU, phenylketonuria.)

scales is approximately fourth grade for parents and fifth grade for teachers.

The drawbacks of questionnaires are well known. The halo effect leads the respondent to decide that the child has numerous behavioral problems on the basis of only a few severe symptoms. These questionnaires are well established and they do not account for the better validated behaviors that appear in the DSM-IV. The questionnaires underemphasize development and cognition. To minimize the distortion, the clinician must get several outside observers to complete the teacher report questionnaires, utilize current behavioral symptoms within the parent interview, and include several other questionnaires that can be tailored to meet the individual child.

Child and Parent Interviews

As in the case of any problem in the area of developmental medicine, it is essential that the clinician develop a thorough history. In addition, the developmental pediatrician should conduct an interview with the child who is being evaluated for the possible AD/HD.

The birth history should address the pregnancy (alcohol and drug consumption, fetal activity, infections, etc.), the labor and delivery (fetal bradycardia, fetal distress, breech presentation, traumatic delivery, etc.), and the neonatal course (resuscitation, prematurity, oxygen and ventilatory support, seizures or evidence of cerebral changes due to hypoxia, etc.). Perinatal insults have been shown to cause minor neurodevelopmental disabilities, as well as major disabilities (Drillien, Thompson, & Burgoyne, 1980; Nichols & Chen, 1981; Taylor, Klein, & Hack, 1994). The infant's behavior during the first few months of life may also support an early onset of this disorder.

The developmental history should focus on school-age milestones such as the age the child was able to tie his or her shoes, ride a bicycle without training wheels, identify letters of the alphabet, and sound out phonemes. It is important to inquire as to when the parents first perceived the child as having a problem with his or her development in behavioral control. The parents can be asked to rate their child's age level in various areas such as behavioral control and reading development.

A thorough medical history will review chronic diseases, major illnesses requiring hospitalization, major accidents that may have included a concussion, medications, allergies, surgical procedures, and special laboratory studies. The review of systems should cover enuresis, encopresis, constipation, appetite, sleep regulation, headaches, and stomachaches. If a medication trial is going to be entertained, it is worthwhile to have the parents grade the degree of severity of symptoms that would be considered side effects of a stimulant drug. This will be beneficial in determining whether concerns during the medication trial were present before the medication was initiated. Finally, the clinician must establish what care the parents have provided for in the areas of vision and dentistry and what holistic therapies the parents may be obtaining for the child.

The educational history will determine how the results of previous evaluations and interventions have been implemented by the school. In addition to evaluations by nonmedical disciplines, a profile of best and worst subjects, school attendance pattern, and other details about class size, individual teachers, and variations in methods of instruction (i.e., types of modifications within the regular education classroom) should be constructed.

The social history is often crucial. AD/HD is often a familial disorder, and primary caregivers may have this condition. In addition, primary caregivers often experience other neurobehavioral conditions (Roizen et al., 1994). Thus family function and family dynamics can be crucial in determining how possible it is to implement various recommendations. The family history is one way to lead into questions that deal with family function. It is important to know who in the family has/had chronic medical and psychological problems. The utilization of the Vineland Adaptive Scales can help the physician determine how this family operates. Ultimately, the physician must ask some questions that may require that the parents reveal more about the family than they initially anticipated. The physician needs this information, but he or she must use tact in obtaining it.

The clinician should determine what the child understands about the evaluation. He or she must also pursue how the child feels about him or herself. The use of a self-esteem inventory can help the clinician to obtain this information.

The Clinical Evaluation

The general physical examination should include careful attention to growth parameters (anthropometrics). Several causes of AD/HD are associated with short stature, and a number of others are also associated with macrocephaly and microcephaly. The presence of minor dysmorphic features has been associated with developmental problems, including disinhibition of behavioral control. If the number of minor dysmorphic features reaches four, the clinician may want to measure ear length, palpebral fissures, interpupillary distance, and finger length if any of these features are suspect for being outside the typical range. In the majority of cases in which development and minor dysmorphic features are detected, the finding is nonspecific for a genetic diagnosis (Accardo, Blondis, Roizen, & Whitman, 1991; Waldrop, Bell, McLaughlin, & Halverson, 1978). The list of associated minor dysmorphic findings is quite long, but the clinician should note the following:

Microcephaly or macrocephaly
Epicanthal folds
Hypertelorism
Low-set ears
Adherent ear lobules
High-arched palate
Single palmar crease
Short or incurved fifth fingers
Sandal gap deformity
Third toe longer than second toe

Pulse and blood pressure should be measured. This is not only of importance should a medication trial be indicated, but also may relate to several disorders that can cause the AD/HD symptom complex. Skin and hair should be inspected, and any unusual pigmentary deviancy is an indication for a Wood's lamp examination. The general examination should be complete and include genital observation.

The neurodevelopmental examination should include the classic neurologic examination. It is best to begin the exam by establishing handedness and preferred eye and foot. The clinician should incorporate a basic visual and hearing screen, and all cranial nerves should be evaluated. Both axial and extremity tone should be noted. Axial tone can be evaluated by the use of the posterior and anterior scarf signs. Soft neurologic signs should be examined, but, in the patient who is less than 12 years of age, soft sign norms for age and gender are an essential component of any useful examination. In particular, neurologic overflow in the form of exaggerated synkinesias and associated movements has been found among children with AD/HD (Blondis, Snow, & Accardo, 1990; Fog & Fog, 1963).

Behavior observation by the clinician is of utmost importance, although the absence of AD/HD behaviors is in no way conclusive with regard to diagnosis (Sleator & Ullman, 1981). The examiner observes the amount of intratask variability, ease of focus on academic tasks, reflective capacity, attention to detail, self-monitoring, and organization. It is important to differentiate attentiveness in visual and auditory domains. The developmental pediatrician may wish to utilize a direct observation measure for use during the examination. These measures are valid only in the context of a classroom or in other cases when the child is left alone and observed through a one-way mirror. Children with AD/HD in general perform much better if they are receiving one-to-one feedback.

Developmental screening measures such as a mini-intelligence test and a brief achievement test can give the developmental pediatrician insight into whether or not the child has a significant discrepancy between intelligence and achievement, and also more specific insight into how the child processes information. The use of a measure of visual-motor function can give the clinician valuable information with regard to the child's visual-motor development. Children who have a great deal of difficulty with pencil control or visual-motor skills are penalized in an educational system that requires that assignments be written (Blondis, Accardo, & Snow, 1989b; Levine, Oberklaid, & Meltzer, 1981).

Computerized continuous performance tasks can be a helpful adjunct to the developmental clinician in the diagnosis and treatment of AD/HD. The Test of Variable Attention (TOVA) and the Conners Continuous Performance Task are two such tests that have been marketed and undergo periodic change (Conners, 1992; Dupuy & Greenberg, 1993). The standardization of these tests has improved (Dupuy & Greenberg, 1993). These tests measure errors of commission and omission, reaction time, and the variability of attention over a period of approximately 20 minutes. Although the TOVA is the better normed test at this time, it is far more expensive because of the fee for scoring each test. Test results can be obtained in minutes by transmitting data via modem to a central computer. The cost of the Conners is reasonable, and it provides almost identical information. The clinician should not put a great deal of emphasis on the results of these tests. Other tests, like the *matching familiar figures* test originally developed by Kagan (1966), have been useful but are less well normed than the CPTs.

Differential Diagnoses

Various conditions, ranging from teratogens to neurodegenerative disorders, can cause an AD/HD symptom complex. Associated medical diseases are listed in Figure 1. Although medical causes represent the minority of case presentations, no one would dispute the importance of ruling out associated medical disorders. Recent research has demonstrated the influence of visual and hearing impairment on sustained attention (Ultmann & Kelly, 1991). The association of central perceptual deficits and motor output deficits with attentional deficits led to the Swedish diagnostic term *deficits in attention, motor control, and perception* (Hellgren et al., 1993). Certainly many children with AD/HD also have associated deficits in this area, but it is also possible that specific learning disability is the cause of the AD/HD symptom complex (Accardo, Blondis, & Whitman, 1990).

Fetal alcohol syndrome and fetal hydantoin syndrome (Hanson & Smith, 1975; Streissguth, Herman, & Smith, 1978) definitely have been associated with organic impulsivity and hyperactivity. The clinical research is less clear cut in

the case of cocaine. It is common for drug abusers to consistently drink alcohol. Recent studies have appeared that claim that nicotine is a teratogen, but these have not been well-controlled studies. Infections and postinfectious illnesses, such as acquired immunodeficiency syndrome and β-hemolytic streptococcal infections (Kiessling, Marcotte, & Culpepper, 1993), may cause attentional deficits. Toxic effects of chemicals such as lead and phenobarbital may cause inattentive and disinhibited behavior (Mitchell, Zhou, Chavez, & Guzman, 1993; Needleman et al., 1979; Vining et al., 1983). Claims have been made that iron deficiency can cause various neurodevelopmental deficits, including inattentive behavior (Lozoff, Jimenez, & Wolf, 1991). Brain injury is a well-known cause of hyperactivity and impulsive behavior (Mahoney et al., 1983). Metabolic causes include hyperthyroidism, hypothyroidism, and phenylketonuria (Johnson, 1969). Sex chromosome disorders, including XO, XXY, and XYY, are associated with various learning disabilities and behavioral disturbances (Eme, 1979). In addition, girls who are identified to have fragile X syndrome have been noted to have problems with selective attention (Hagerman, Kemper, & Hudson, 1985). Other genetic syndromes associated with AD/HD include neurofibromatosis, myotonic dystrophy (underarousal), Tourette syndrome, and Williams syndrome.

It is equally important to address childhood psychiatric diagnoses that may manifest many of the AD/HD behavioral symptoms. One must consider dysthymia, childhood depression, manic depression, high-functioning autism, anxiety disorder, conduct disorder, and schizophrenia. It may be quite difficult to discriminate between AD/HD and manic depression. In order to do so, the clinician must look for a pattern of dysphoria coupled with intermittent psychotic episodes. Aggressive symptoms frequently are observed among manic children (Nieman & De-Long, 1987; Weinberg & Brumback, 1992).

Laboratory Tests

The medical laboratory is generally of little use in the diagnosis of AD/HD. However, if other diseases that produce a similar symptom complex are considered in the differential diagnosis, then laboratory testing may be of great importance. The AD/HD symptom complex has been associated with a disease caused by mutations in the thyroid receptor–B gene. Generalized resistance to thyroid hormone (GRTH) is characterized by elevated serum thryroxine, elevated triiodothyronine (T_3), and normal or elevated thyrotropin concentrations (Hauser et al., 1993). Hauser and co-workers do not comment on the central nervous system comorbidity that other groups have noted (Weiss, Stein, Trommer, & Refetoff, 1993), and the comment that anecdotal evidence suggests that the behavioral symptoms of children with GRTH-AD/HD improve during therapy with T_3 remains uncertain (Weiss et al., 1993). Another disease that has been associated with the AD/HD symptom complex is poststreptococcal meningitis (Kiessling et al., 1993).

Dysmorphic features suggestive of a chromosomal syndrome or any other genetic syndrome should prompt the appropriate laboratory studies and genetic consultations.

Both the fragile X syndrome in girls and childhood myotonic dystrophy now can be identified by amplification of extracted DNA with the polymerase chain reaction and by Southern blot analysis. Obviously, if children live in poor urban areas, it is important to check their blood lead level regardless of whether they present with an AD/HD symptom complex.

An electroencephalogram may be indicated if, after a careful seizure history, the clinician has not ruled out this possibility. At this time, imaging studies and event-related potentials should not be used outside of the research tract.

Psychological and Educational Evaluations

Psychological testing is critical for the purpose of ruling out learning and psychiatric disabilities. Behavioral observations of the child during testing are as important as the test scores. The clinical psychologist should always describe the child's behavior during testing, and, based on the child's behavior, a good psychologist may decide that the test scores are not valid. The Wechsler intelligence tests are the most widely used psychological measures and penalize the child with AD/HD the least (Blondis et al., 1989b). Even though no norms exist for the population with AD/HD, both the freedom from distractibility factor and the "ACID" subscore factor (the subtests of Arithmetic, Coding, Information, and Digit Span) may help to establish a diagnosis. This factor only is meaningful if a significant developmental dissociation exists between the overall standard score and this factor standard score. The fact that this factor score is consistent with the test score does not rule out AD/HD.

Other intelligence tests may be more biased against populations of children with AD/HD or a specific learning disability. The Kaufman Assessment Battery for Children may be useful if one is investigating a simultaneous or sequential processing deficit that underlies the child's behavioral and output dysfunction. Children with learning disabilities tend to score lower on the Woodcock-Johnson Psychoeducational Battery and on the Detroit Test of Learning Aptitude. Both tests load for memory and should be avoided when testing children with a potential diagnosis of AD/HD. Neuropsychological tests represent a helpful tool for AD/HD diagnosis. These tests are becoming much more developmental in nature, and can get at executive processing deficits (Fletcher & Taylor, 1984; Snow & Cunningham, 1991; Vygotsky, 1962).

Individual achievement testing is equally important in the assessment of children presenting with possible AD/HD. Optimally, more in-depth achievement testing than the Wechsler Individual Achievement Test or the Wide Range Achievement Test should be incorporated as part of the evaluation. These tests are limited from both a diagnostic and a therapeutic perspective. Formal as well as informal testing is important. For example, although it is necessary to time the child's writing speed to determine if this represents another impediment to timely output for the child with AD/HD, it would be necessary to evaluate the slow writer with a test such as the Test of Written Language to rule out a comorbid specific learning disability in written language.

The Interdisciplinary Conference

The gold standard for accurate diagnoses and sound intervention is an interactive conference with the members of the various disciplines who have evaluated the child. A successful interdisciplinary evaluation must be organized in advance of the child's actual evaluation, and should include professionals from the child's school. The inclusion of representatives from the school increases the likelihood that the school will be satisfied that the evaluation was complete and the teaching interventions recommended will be given consideration. In this forum, the school professionals have the opportunity to challenge the findings and review the recommendations with the developmental pediatric team of professionals.

PROGNOSIS

Prospective and controlled studies (Hechtman & Weiss, 1986; Satterfield, Satterfield, & Schell, 1987) begin to offer some understanding of outcome for the hyperactive child. Both of these longitudinal studies used referral populations, and, from this standpoint, the resulting psychopathology of the adolescent and adult with AD/HD may be exaggerated in that the more severe AD/HD cases generally are referred to psychiatrists.

Satterfield et al. (1987) have conducted different longitudinal studies over a 20+-year span. Hyperactive children treated with stimulant medication produced a substantial number of delinquents across socioeconomic classes. In later studies with a multimodality treatment approach, children with AD/HD did significantly better than a group in which the only intervention was stimulant medication. Those receiving multimodality treatment evidenced fewer arrests and less antisocial behavior than the pharmacotherapy group. The Hechtman and Weiss (1986) 15-year study evaluated adults who had had AD/HD as children with psychiatric rating scales and biographical data. Differences between the hyperactive group and the control group reached significance in the area of observed antisocial behavior. However, results did not agree with previous studies that contended that antisocial personality disorder was definitively more prevalent among adults with AD/HD. There were nonsignificant trends for the adults with AD/HD to use too much alcohol and other drugs and to have more court appearances when compared to the control group.

Several generalizations can be made from these long-term studies. Approximately half of these children demonstrated some resolution of their problem, but the other half still evidenced significant disability. Twenty percent to 40% developed antisocial personality disorder, possibly secondary to poor peer acceptance and low self-esteem during childhood. Children with AD/HD do not appear to be at significantly increased risk for developing schizophrenia or psychosis. However, boys with hyperkinesis are at a substantially greater risk for conduct disorder and criminal conduct later in life. Drug management alone does not appreciably alter the outcome of hyperactive children, but neither does it produce a significantly increased risk of alcoholism or drug abuse. Stimulant medication in combination with other therapeutic interventions (e.g., individual, group, or family therapy; special education; parent training; cognitive training) probably does improve outcome (see Chapter 29, this volume).

CONCLUSIONS

AD/HD represents a group of disorders that present with deficits of sustained attention, control of impulses, and control of motor activity. Currently these disorders should be determined with the use of the behavioral criteria outlined in either the *Diagnostic and Statistical Manual of Mental Disorders* of the American Psychiatric Association or the *International Classification of Diseases* of the World Health Organization. Besides reviewing behavioral ratings from several different sources, the clinician will need to use his or her clinical acumen and differential diagnostic skills in determining if the child presenting with chief concerns of inattention, hyperactivity, or both has this symptom complex as a result of a specific disease or AD/HD. Clinical research clearly has shown the association of AD/HD with a continuum of other conditions. In particular, specific learning disability, delayed motor and perceptual processing, adaptive delay, and low self-esteem are common secondary conditions. This continuum requires the clinician to evaluate the delays, deviances, and dissociations of the child across central processing, adaptive, and emotional areas.

The pitfalls of misdiagnosis include

1. Exclusive reliance on or failure to use accepted behavioral criteria
2. Omission of a quantitative behavioral questionnaire system (parent, school, self, and other) to evaluate the behavior of the child across his or her environments
3. Inadequate medical or psychosocial history
4. Incomplete medical assessment characterized by overlooked dysmorphology, and an inadequate neurodevelopmental evaluation
5. Ignoring the possibility of other specific processing deficits that may be responsible

for the behavioral symtoms and signs of AD/HD
6. Disregarding other psychiatric conditions that mimic AD/HD behaviors

The biobehavioral scientist recognizes the *it* (Denckla, 1992) of what has become commonly referred to in North America as attention-deficit/hyperactivity disorder. In the future, it is probable that neuroscientists will be able to define the underlying neuroanatomy and neurophysiology behind the AD/HD disability(ies). When neuroscience reaches this stage, diagnostic methods will become less observation laden and more accurate. At this juncture, developmental pediatricians must follow the lead of our psychology and psychiatry colleagues who have worked toward defining more accurate behavioral symptoms of AD/HD.

REFERENCES

Accardo, P.J., Blondis, T.A., Roizen, N.J., & Whitman, B.Y. (1991). The physical examination of the child with attention deficit hyperactivity disorder. In P.J. Accardo, T.A. Blondis, & B.Y. Whitman (Eds.), *Attention deficit disorders and hyperactivity in children* (pp. 121–139). New York: Marcel Dekker.

Accardo, P.J., Blondis, T.A., & Whitman, B.Y. (1990). Disorders of attention and activity level in a referral population. *Pediatrics, 85,* 426–431.

Accardo, P.J., & Whitman, B.Y. (1991). The misdiagnosis of the hyperactive child. In P.J. Accardo, T.A. Blondis, & B.Y. Whitman (Eds.), *Attention deficit disorders and hyperactivity in children* (pp. 1–26). New York: Marcel Dekker.

Achenbach, T.M., Conners, C.K., Quay, H.C., Verhylst, F.C., & Howell, C.T. (1989). Replication of empirically derived syndromes as a basis for taxonomy of child/adolescent psychopathology. *Journal of Abnormal Child Psychology, 17,* 299–324.

Achenbach, T.M., & Edelbrock, C. (1979). The Child Behavior Profile: II, boys aged 12–16, girls aged 6–11 and 12–16. *Journal of Consulting and Clinical Psychology, 47,* 223–233.

Alberts-Corush, J., Firestone, P., & Goodman, J.T. (1986). Attention and impulsivity characteristics of the biological and adoptive parents of hyperactive and normal control children. *American Journal of Orthopsychiatry, 56,* 413–423.

American Psychiatric Association. (1968). *Diagnostic and statistical manual* (2nd ed.). Washington, DC: American Psychiatric Press.

American Psychiatric Association. (1980). *Diagnostic and statistical manual of mental disorders* (3rd ed.). Washington, DC: American Psychiatric Press.

American Psychiatric Association. (1987). *Diagnostic and statistical manual of mental disorders* (3rd ed. rev.). Washington, DC: American Psychiatric Press.

American Psychiatric Association. (1994). *Diagnostic and statistical manual of mental disorders* (4th ed.). Washington, DC: American Psychiatric Press.

Barkley, R.A. (1990). A critique of current diagnostic criteria for attention deficit hyperactivity disorder: Clinical and research implications. *Developmental and Behavioral Pediatrics, 11,* 343–352.

Blondis, T.A., Accardo, P.J., & Snow, J.H. (1989a). Measures of attention deficit, Part I: Questionnaires. *Chemical Pediatrics, 28,* 222–228.

Blondis, T.A., Accardo, P.J., & Snow, J.H. (1989b). Measures of attention deficit, Part II: Clinical perspectives and test interpretation. *Chemical Pediatrics, 28,* 268–276.

Blondis, T.A., Snow, J.H., & Accardo, P.J. (1990). The integration of soft signs in normal and academically at-risk children. *Pediatrics, 85,* 421–425.

Bradley, C. (1937). The behavior of children receiving benzedrine. *American Journal of Psychiatry, 94,* 577–585.

Broadbent, D.E. (1982). Task combination and selective intake of information. *Acta Psychologica, 50,* 253–290.

Chelune, G.J., Ferguson, W., Koon, R., & Dickey, T.O. (1986). Frontal lobe disinhibition in attention deficit disorder. *Child Psychiatry and Human Development, 16,* 221–234.

Clements, S.D., & Peters, J.E. (1966). Minimal brain dysfunction in the school age child: Diagnosis and treatment. *Archives of General Psychiatry, 6,* 185–197.

Conners, C.K. (1992). *CPT: Conners' Continuous Performance Test computer program version 2.0.* North Tonawanda, NY: Multi-Health Systems.

Conners, C.K., & Kinsbourne, M. (Eds.). (1990). *ADHD: Attention deficit hyperactivity disorder.* Munich: Medizin Verlag Munchen.

Conners, C.K., & Wells, K.C. (1986). *Hyperkinetic children.* Beverly Hills: Sage Publications.

Corah, N.L., & Gospodinoff, E.J. (1966). Color-form and whole-part perception in children. *Child Development, 37,* 837–842.

Denckla, M.B. (1992). Commentary: The myth of ADHD. *Journal of Child Neurology, 7,* 458–461.

Douglas, V.I. (1972). Stop, look, and listen: The problem of sustained attention and impulse control in hyperactive and normal children. *Canadian Journal of Behavioral Sciences, 4,* 259–282.

Drillien, C.M., Thompson, A.J., & Burgoyne, K. (1980). Low-birthweight children at early school-age: A longitudinal study. *Developmental Medicine and Child Neurology, 22,* 26–47.

Dupuy, T.R., & Greenberg, L.M. (1993). *T.O.V.A. Manual, Test of Variables of Attention computer program version 6.X for IBM PC or IBM compatible.* Los Alamitos, CA: Universal Attention Disorders.

Edelbrock, C., & Achenbach, T.M. (1984). The teacher version of the Child Behavior Profile: I, boys aged 6–11. *Journal of Consulting and Clinical Psychology, 52,* 207–217.

Eme, R. (1979). Sex differences in child psychopathology: A review. *Psychological Bulletin, 86,* 574–595.

Fletcher, J.M., & Taylor, H.G. (1984). Neuropsychological approaches to children: Towards a developmental neuropsychology. *Journal of Clinical Neuropsychology, 6,* 39–56.

Fog, E., & Fog, M. (1963). Cerebral inhibition examined by associated movements. In M. Bax & R. MacKeith (Eds.), *Minimal cerebral dysfunction* (Clinics in Developmental Medicine, No. 10, pp. 52–57). London: Spastics International Medical Publications in association with William Heinemann.

Frick, P.J., Lahey, B.B., Applegater, B., Kerdyck, L., Ollendick, T., Hynd, G.W., Garfinkel, B., Greenhill, L., Biederman, J., Barkley, R.A., McBurnett, K., Newman, J., & Waldman, I. (1994). DSM-IV field trials for the disruptive and attention deficit disorders: Diagnostic utility of symptoms. *Journal of the American Academy of Child and Adolescent Psychiatry, 33,* 529–539.

Goldman-Rakic, P.S. (1984). The frontal lobes: Uncharted provinces of the brain. *Trends in Neuro-Sciences, 7,* 425–429.

Goyette, C.H., Conners, C.K., & Ulrich, R.F. (1978). Normative data on the revised Conners Parent and Teacher Rating Scales. *Journal of Abnormal Child Psychology, 6,* 221–236.

Hagen, J.W. (1967). The effect of distraction on selective attention. *Child Development, 38,* 685–694.

Hagerman, R., Kemper, M., & Hudson, M. (1985). Learning disabilities and attentional problems in boys with the fragile X syndrome. *American Journal of Diseases of Children, 139,* 674–678.

Hale, G.A., & Alderman, L.B. (1978). Children's selective attention with variation in amount of stimulus exposure. *Journal of Abnormal Child Psychology, 26,* 320–327.

Hanson, J.W., & Smith, D.W. (1975). The fetal hydantoin syndrome. *Journal of Pediatrics, 87,* 285–290.

Hauser, P., Zametkin, A.J., Martinez, P., Vitiello, B., Matochik, J.A., Mixson, A.J., & Weitraub, B.D. (1993). Attention-deficit-hyperactivity disorder in people with generalized resistance to thyroid hormone. *New England Journal of Medicine, 328,* 997–1001.

Hechtman, L., & Weiss, G. (1986). Controlled prospective fifteen year follow-up of hyperactives as adults: Non-medical drug and alcohol use and anti-social behavior. *Canadian Journal of Psychiatry, 31,* 557–567.

Hellgren, L., Gillberg, C., Gillberg, I.C., & Enerskog, I. (1993). Children with deficits in attention, motor control, and perception (DAMP) almost grown up: General health at 16 years. *Developmental Medicine and Child Neurology, 35,* 881–892.

Huessy, H. (1984). Remarks on the epidemiology of MBD/ADD. In L.M. Bloomingdale (Ed.), *Attention deficit disorder: Diagnostic, cognitive, and therapeutic understanding* (pp. 1–9). Jamaica, NY: Spectrum.

Hynd, G.W., Hern, K.L., Novey, E.S., Eliopulos, R.T., Marshall, R., Gonzales, J.J., & Voeller, K.K. (1993). Attention deficit-hyperactivity disorder and asymmetry of the caudate nucleus. *Journal of Child Neurology, 8,* 339–347.

James, W. (1952). *The principles of psychology* (Great Books Series, Vol. 53, pp. 294–295). Chicago: Encyclopedia Britannica. (Original work published 1890)

Johnson, R.R. (1969). Behavioral characteristics of phenylketonuria and matched controls. *American Journal of Mental Deficiency, 74,* 17–19.

Kagan, J., Pearson, L., & Welch, L. (1966). Modifiability of impulsive tempo. *Journal of Educational Psychology, 57,* 359–365.

Kahneman, D., & Treisman, A. (1984). Changing views of attention and automaticity. In R. Parasuraman & D.R. Davies (Eds.), *Varieties of attention* (pp. 29–61). Orlando, FL: Academic Press.

Kiessling, L.S., Marcotte, A.C., & Culpepper, L. (1993). Antineuronal antibodies in movement disorders. *Pediatrics, 92*, 39–43.

Lahey, B.B., Applegate, B., McBurnett, K., Biederman, J., Greenhill, L., Hynd, G.W., Barkley, R.A., Newcorn, J., Jensen, P., Richters, J., Garfinkel, B., Kerdyk, L., Frick, P.J., Ollendick, T., Perez, D., Hart, E.L., Waldman, I., & Schaffer, D. (1994). DSM-IV field trials for attention-deficit hyperactivity disorder in children and adolescents. *American Journal of Psychiatry.*

Lahey, B.B., Pelham, W.E., Schaughency, E.A., Atkins, M.S., Murphy, H.A., Hynd, G., Russo, M., Hartdagen, S., & Lorys-Vernon, A. (1987). Dimensions and types of attention deficit disorder. *Journal of the American Academy of Child and Adolescent Psychiatry, 27*, 330–335.

Lambert, N.M., & Sandoval, J. (1980). The prevalence of learning disabilities in a sample of children considered hyperactive. *Journal of Abnormal Child Psychology, 8*, 33–50.

Levine, M.D., Oberklaid, F., & Meltzer, L.J. (1981). Developmental output failure—a study of low productivity in school age children. *Pediatrics, 67*, 18–25.

Lou, H.C., Henriksen, L., Bruhn, P., Borner, H., & Nielsen, J.B. (1989). Striatal dysfunction in attention deficit and hyperkinetic disorder. *Archives of Neurology, 46*, 48–52.

Lozoff, B., Jiminez, E., & Wolf, A.W. (1991). Long-term developmental outcome of infants with iron deficiency. *New England Journal of Medicine, 325*, 687–694.

Mahoney, W.J., D'Souza, B.J., Haller, J.A., Rogers, M.C., Epstein, M.H., & Freeman, J.M. (1983). Long-term outcome of children with severe head trauma and prolonged coma. *Pediatrics, 71*, 756–762.

Malone, M.A., Kershner, J.R., & Swanson, J.M. (1994). Hemispheric processing and methylphenidate effects in attention-deficit hyperactivity disorder. *Journal of Child Neurology, 9*, 181–189.

Mann, C.A., Lubar, J.F., Zimmerman, A.W., Miller, C.A., & Muenchen, R.A. (1992). Quantitative analysis of EEG in boys with attention-deficit-hyperactivity disorder: Controlled study with clinical implications. *Pediatric Neurology, 8*, 30–36.

McMahon, R.C. (1980). Genetic etiology in the hyperactive child syndrome: A critical review. *American Journal of Orthopsychiatry, 50*, 145–150.

Mitchell, W.G., Zhou, Y., Chavez, J.M., & Guzman, B.L. (1993). Effects of antiepileptic drugs on reaction time, attention, and impulsivity in children. *Pediatrics, 91*, 101–105.

Needleman, H., Gunnor, C., Leviton, A., Reed, R., Peresie, H., Maner, C., & Barrett, P. (1979). Deficits in psychologic and classroom performances of children with elevated dentine lead levels. *New England Journal of Medicine, 300*, 689–695.

Nichols, P.L., & Chen, T.-C. (1981). *Minimal brain dysfunction: A prospective study.* Hillsdale, NJ: Lawrence Erlbaum Associates.

Nieman, G.W., & DeLong, R. (1987). Use of the Personality Inventory for Children as an aid in differentiating children with mania from children with attention deficit disorder with hyperactivity. *Journal of the American Academy of Child and Adolescent Psychiatry, 26*, 381–388.

Peloquin, L.J., & Klorman, R. (1986). Affects of methylphenidate on normal children's mood, event-related potentials, and performance in memory scanning and vigilance. *Journal of Abnormal Psychology, 95*, 88–98.

Porges, S.W. (1984). Physiologic correlates of attention: A core process underlying learning disorders. *Pediatric Clinics of North America, 31*, 371–385.

Posner, M.I., & Peterson, S.E. (1990). The attention system of the human brain. *Annual Review of Neuroscience, 13*, 25–42.

Posner, M.I., & Raichle, M.E. (1994). Networks of attention. In *Images of the mind* (pp. 153–179). New York: Scientific American Library.

Posner, M.I., & Rothbart, M.K. (1981). The development of attentional mechanisms. In H.E. Howe, Jr. (Ed.), *Nebraska Symposium on Motivation* (Vol. 28, pp. 1–52). Lincoln: University of Nebraska Press.

Prendergast, M., Taylor, E., Rapoport, J.L., Bartko, J., Donnelly, M., Zametkin, A., Ahearn, M.B., Dunn, G., & Wieselberg, H.M. (1988). The diagnosis of childhood hyperactivity: A U.S.-U.K. cross-national study of DSM-III and ICD-9. *Journal of Child Psychology and Psychiatry, 3*, 289–300.

Reeves, J.C., Werry, J.S., Elkind, G.S., & Zametkin, A. (1987). Attention deficit, conduct, oppositional, and anxiety disorders in children: II. Clinical characteristics. *Journal of American Academy of Child Psychiatry, 26*, 144–155.

Roizen, N.J., Blondis, T.A., Irwin, M., & Stein, M. (1994). Adaptive functioning in children with attention deficit hyperactivity disorder. *Archives of Pediatrics and Adolescent Medicine, 148*, 1137–1142.

Roizen, N.J., Blondis, T.A., Rubinoff, A., Keiffer, J., Irwin, M., & Stein, M. (in press). High frequency of neurobehavioral disorders of children with attention deficit hyperactivity disorder (ADHD) compared to children with Down syndrome. *Archives of Pediatrics and Adolescent Medicine.*

Ross, D.M., & Ross, S.A. (1982). *Hyperactivity: Current issues, research, and theory.* New York: John Wiley & Sons.

Rutter, M., Graham, P., & Yule, W. (1970). *A neuropsychiatric study in childhood* (Clinics in Developmental Medicine, Nos. 35/36). London: Spastics International Medical Publications in association with William Heinemann.

Satterfield, J.H., Satterfield, B.T., & Schell, A.M. (1987). Therapeutic interventions to prevent delinquency in hyperactive boys. *Journal of American Academy of Child and Adolescent Psychiatry, 26,* 56–64.

Schachar, R., Rutter, M., & Smith, A. (1981). The characteristics of situationally and pervasively hyperactive children: Implications for syndrome definition. *Journal of Child Psychology and Psychiatry, 22,* 375–392.

Shiffrin, R.M., & Schneider, W. (1977). Controlled and automatic processing. II. Perceptual learning, automatic attending, and a general theory. *Psychological Review, 84,* 127–190.

Sleator, E.K., & Ullmann, R.K. (1981). Can the physician diagnose hyperactivity in the office? *Pediatrics, 67,* 13–17.

Snow, J.H., & Cunningham, K.J. (1991). Psychoeducational data. In P.J. Accardo, T.A. Blondis, & B.Y. Whitman (Eds.), *Attention deficit disorders and hyperactivity in children* (pp. 141–170). New York: Marcel Dekker.

Sokolov, E.N. (1963). *Perception and the conditional reflex.* New York: Macmillan.

Sophian, C., & Hagen, J.W. (1978). Involuntary memory and the development of retrieval skills in young children. *Journal of Experimental Child Psychology, 26,* 458–471.

Strauss, A.A., & Lehtinen, L.E. (1947). *Psychopathology and education of the brain-injured child.* New York: Grune & Stratton.

Streissguth, A.P., Herman, C.S., & Smith, D.W. (1978). Intelligence, behavior, and dysmorphogenesis in the fetal alcohol syndrome: A report on 20 patients. *Journal of Pediatrics, 92,* 363–367.

Sunder, T.R., DeMarco, S., Frutiger, A.D., & Levey, B. (1988). A developmental right hemisphere deficit syndrome in childhood. *Annals of Neurology, 24,* 322.

Task Force on DSM-IV. (1993). *DSM-IV draft criteria, 3-1-93.* Washington, DC: American Psychiatric Press.

Taylor, G., Klein, N., & Hack, M. (1994). Academic functioning in <750 gm birthweight children who have normal cognitive abilities: Evidence for specific learning disabilities. *Pediatric Research, 35,* 288A.

Thompson, R.F., & Spencer, W.O. (1966). Habituation, a model phenomenon for the study of neuronal substrates of behavior. *Psychological Review, 73,* 1–15.

Tredgold, A. (1908). *Mental deficiency (amentia).* New York: W. Wood.

Ultmann, M.H., & Kelly, D.P. (1991). Attention deficit in children with hearing or visual impairments. In P.J. Accardo, T.A. Blondis, & B.Y. Whitman (Eds.), *Attention deficit disorders and hyperactivity in children* (pp. 171–186). New York: Marcell Dekker.

Vining, E.P.G., Mellits, E.D., Cataldo, M.F., Dorsen, M.M., Spielberg, S.P., & Freeman, J.M. (1983). Effects of phenobarbital and sodium valproate on neuropsychological function and behavior. *Annals of Neurology, 14,* 360.

Vygotsky, L.S. (1962). *Thought and language.* Boston: MIT Press.

Waldrop, M.F., Bell, R.Q., McLaughlin, B., & Halverson, C.F. (1978). Newborn minor physical anomalies predict short attention span, peer aggression, and impulsivity. *Science, 199,* 563–565.

Weinberg, W.A., & Brumback, R.A. (1992). The myth of attention deficit-hyperactivity disorder: Symptoms resulting from multiple causes. *Journal of Child Neurology, 7,* 43 1–446.

Weiss, R.E., Stein, M.A., Trommer, B., & Refetoff, S. (1993). Attention-deficit hyperactivity disorder and thyroid function. *Journal of Pediatrics, 123,* 539–545.

Whitman, B.Y. (1991). The roots of organicity: Genetics and genograms. In P.J. Accardo, T.A. Blondis, & B.Y. Whitman (Eds.), *Attention deficit disorders and hyperactivity in children* (pp. 37–56). New York: Marcel Dekker.

Willerman, L. (1973). Activity level and hyperactivity in twins. *Child Development, 44,* 288–293.

World Health Organization. (1980). *International classification of diseases* (9th ed.). Geneva: Author.

World Health Organization. (1992). F90: Hyperkinetic disorders. In *The ICD-10 classification of mental and behavioural disorders.* Geneva: Author.

Wright, J.C., & Vlietstra, A.G. (1975). The development of selective attention: From perceptual exploration to logical search. In H.W. Reese (Ed.), *Advances in child development and behavior* (pp. 196–235). New York: Academic.

Zametkin, A.J., Nordahl, T., Gross, M., King, A.C., Semple, W.E., Rumsey, J., Hamburger, S., & Cohen, R.M. (1990). Cerebral glucose metabolism in adults with hyperactivity of childhood onset. *New England Journal of Medicine, 323,* 1361–1366.

Zametkin, A.J., & Rapoport, J.L. (1987). Neurobiology of attention deficit disorder with hyperactivity: Where have we come in 50 years? *Journal of the American Academy of Child and Adolescent Psychiatry, 26,* 676–686.

Chapter 29

Management of Attention-Deficit Disorders and Hyperactivity

Thomas A. Blondis, M.D., and Nancy J. Roizen, M.D.

The habilitation for children with attention deficit and/or hyperactivity disorder (AD/HD) is multifaceted and developmental. Modifications for preschool and early elementary children with AD/HD will be geared more toward decreasing the numbers of distractors, physical organization of the home and classroom that will allow the parent and teacher to accommodate the needs of hyperactive students, and behavior modifications that will provide incentives for improved home and classroom deportment as well as work output. As the child moves toward secondary school, modifications and interventions should shift toward improving self-monitoring, vigilance, and organizational skills.

Consequently, treatment goals must be individualized according to the child's age, level of maturity, degree of the AD/HD disorder, and associated problems. The paramount goal must be to develop a collaboration between the child, the parents, and all other professionals. Unless the parents can accept that the disorder is a lifetime condition, the child's ability to overcome the problem will be limited. The goal of successful treatment can be achieved only inasmuch as the child believes the problem can be overcome, realizes that areas of strength can be developed to compensate for poorly controlled and scattered thought processes, and senses that he or she can trust parents and involved professionals. For this reason, we recommend an *individualized home program*, which complements an individualized education program. The basis for this approach can be found in recent clinical studies.

Bloomquist, August, and Ostrander (1991) compared experimental cognitive–behavioral interventions for children diagnosed as having AD/HD. A multicomponent coordinated training program for parents, teachers, and children was compared to a training program that included only classroom teachers. At the end of the study, the multicomponent training program produced significantly less off-task/disruptive behavior in comparison to the classroom teacher training program.

The child's individualized home program must take into consideration the significant developmental dissociation between intelligence and adaptive skills (Roizen, Blondis, Irwin, & Stein, 1994). It has been demonstrated that parents of children with AD/HD evaluated in multiple disability clinics have a high incidence of neurobehavioral disorders, which include AD/HD, specific learning disabilities, alcoholism, and depression (Roizen et al., in press). If family psychopathology, dysfunction, or both exist and are ignored, then efforts directed from the school and pediatrician most likely will fall short of improving adaptive skills.

The pediatrician must guide the parents in developing short- and long-term goals that encourage goal-directed, responsible, and organized behavior. If it is or becomes apparent to the pediatrician that the family cannot model and be supportive of such a program for their child with AD/HD, then the pediatrician will need to direct the family to a family therapist who has experience in dealing with such children and their families.

MULTIMODALITY INTERVENTIONS

The need for a multimodal approach first became acknowledged when several investigative groups demonstrated poor outcomes in adults whose habilitation had been based only on stimulant medication during childhood (Satterfield, Satterfield, & Schell, 1987; Weiss, Hechtman, Milroy, & Perlman, 1985). Figure 1 is an example of how multimodality decisions can be made. Obviously the number and intensity of the modalities required to significantly improve the self-esteem of children with AD/HD, as well as the condition itself, will depend on how much failure they experience. However, modalities must be determined on a priority basis, and

in severe cases it may be that the habilitation team will change the prescription frequently if the individual is showing either no response or very rapid response to the interventions.

In general, modalities that have proven to help a large number of children with AD/HD improve their control and executive function can be broken down into five areas: demystification/counseling therapy (individual, family, and group); general classroom modifications; learning disability intervention (this includes

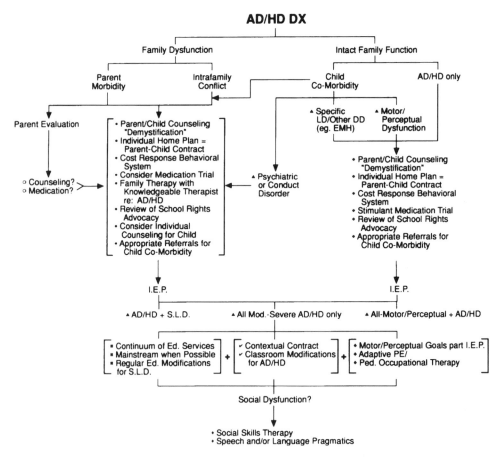

Figure 1. Important distinctions that the clinician must make in order to treat a child with AD/HD successfully. Once a diagnosis (DX) of AD/HD has been made, the clinician begins by asking two questions: Is the family dysfunctional, and is it possible that a parent in the home has a neurobehavioral disorder? If the family is having difficulty coping as a family despite the problems of the child who is undergoing evaluation, the inclusion of some form of counseling for the family becomes a necessary part of the child's treatment plan. If the child has engaged in criminal behavior or has a psychiatric diagnosis, then therapeutic interventions also will require either individual counseling, family therapy, or both. In any moderate to severe case of AD/HD, there will be adaptive dysfunction that will require contextual contracts with the child both at home and at school and the use of a behavioral modification *system*. If the child has a specific learning disability in addition to AD/HD, then a continuum of educational services is essential to successful treatment. Finally, the clinician must consider motor-perceptual and social deficits. (DD, developmental disability; EMH, educable mental handicap; IEP, individualized education program; LD, learning disability; PE, physical education; SLD, specific learning disability).

metacognitive and communication training); medication; and the development of organizational and study skills (this includes self-regulation and cognitive–behavioral therapy).

Counseling

Counseling, including parent, child, and family counseling, is the starting point of habilitation for the child with AD/HD and his or her family (Blondis, Clippard, Scroggs, & Peterson, 1991; Whitman & Smith, 1991). Even if the family was knowledgable about the disorder when they sought help, and even if there is no family dysfunction, important counseling with regard to "demystification," diagnosis, definition of problems, and prescription is undertaken by the pediatrician shortly after the evaluation is completed.

The pediatrician should discuss with the child the true nature of his or her problem. This demystification is very important because the child may fantasize that the disability is more severe than it actually is. The pediatrician can reassure children with AD/HD that, if they are able to develop their cognitive and personality strengths, then they have the opportunity to overcome weaknesses and to succeed in realizing goals that they set for themselves. Obviously, it is necessary for the pediatrician to define the strengths of the individual in order to make this counseling realistic. The pediatrician always must avoid any false reassurance; even children with severe AD/HD are able to intuit pseudo-support and pseudo-praise, which no doubt will affect negatively their relationship with the pediatrician. If a medication trial is to be undertaken, it is the pediatrician's role to discuss the prescription with the child. The nature of this dialogue will vary according to the age of the child.

The goal of parent counseling is to help the parents to accept and support their child. The pediatrician must adequately explain AD/HD to the parents, and explain that their child is not lazy, nor intentionally careless, and not purposefully trying to embarass the family. The parents' understanding of the disorder, coupled with a realistic assessment of the prognosis of AD/HD, will help direct the family toward acceptance and implementation of recommenda-

tions, such as the provision of more structure and organization within the home. The pediatrician must explain the importance of consistent expectations and modifications in order to create a proactive home life, which is crucial to the success of children with AD/HD. The pediatrician should provide a list of realistic behavioral, academic, social, and self-care goals for each child.

Once the parents have decided on a realistic set of short- and long-term goals for their child, they need to negotiate a contract with the child. The parents should first listen to goals that the child would set for him- or herself and try to incorporate these within their vision. In addition, the child should add to the contract in other ways, such as negotiating positive consequences for meeting the terms of the contract. The parents should base their behavior management on a response–cost system, so the atmosphere of the home in relation to the child with AD/HD is more positive than negative. A response–cost system is created when the child is given a number of tokens but has agreed to give up a certain number for specific inappropriate behaviors (see Chapter 30, this volume). Each token system must be shaped by the family based on the child's age, gender, culture, and the like.

Parents can benefit from some books and often parent training programs when it comes to promoting the development of the child with AD/HD. Books that are practical and readable for parents who read at a high school level include *The Difficult Child*, written by Stanley Turecki with Leslie Tonner (1985), *Attention Deficit Hyperactivity Disorder: What Every Parent Wants To Know*, written by David L. Wodrich (1994). In addition to these, there are many more good books available for parents and also some very helpful books at various levels for the child and adolescent with AD/HD. The parents may benefit from belonging to an organization such as Children and Adults with Attention Deficit Disorder (CH.ADD; 499 Northwest 70th Ave., Suite 308, Plantation, FL 33317; (305) 587-3700) or the Learning Disability Association (LDA; 4156 Library Rd., Pittsburgh, PA 15234; (412) 341-1515). Memberships to either of these organizations will give parents needed information through newsletters, professional speakers, and parent support groups.

In some cases, family therapy is indispensable to the entire family (Whitman & Smith, 1991). If the home environment is a "reactive" one, the process of habilitation of AD/HD will mean that the family must change this entirely to a "proactive" and flexible yet structured situation. If the pediatrician does not believe that the family is capable of making such a difficult transition, then mental health interventions must be considered. If the family is unwilling to consider family therapy, they should be made to understand the possible consequences of a poor outcome.

Individual counseling may improve the child's grasp of his or her problems and understanding about what must be done to change his or her course. Studies generally have not supported individual counseling as a primary intervention, but, if the goals of therapy are realistic, it may help the child avoid self-deprecation and reduce guilt. Group counseling in the form of role playing and working through common social conflicts that arise may be beneficial to the child with significant social delay and difficulty sustaining relationships with peers.

General Classroom Modifications

The general classroom teacher should develop realistic and sensitive expectations of the child (Blondis et al., 1991). The teacher can start by defining the period of time that the student with AD/HD can maintain attention to a task. Once this is defined, task demands can be very gradually increased. The teachers can develop contextual contracts or agreements with a student that couple various positive and negative consequences to specific behaviors. For example, a positive consequence can be contingent on time added to work completion.

The child with AD/HD has a great deal of underlying restlessness and often has a difficult time staying on task. Because of his or her inability to delay, the classic hyperactive child is an easy victim in the classroom for a revengeminded or manipulative fellow student. This child often engages in inappropriate behavior because he or she believes fellow classmates

enjoy these diversions. Children with both the predominantly hyperactive and predominantly inattentive types of AD/HD can be set up to look like the guilty party for classroom mischief, when in fact the child was not involved at all. In order to address these concerns, a number of strategies can be employed within the general classroom setting (Piontkowski & Calfee, 1979).

The child with AD/HD should be seated in the "teacher feedback zone." This is an area of the classroom that is continually within the teacher's visual field when he or she is teaching the class. This gives the teacher a clearer view of the child and also allows for frequent opportunities for teacher feedback. In addition, the organization of the classroom is important. Children with AD/HD should never be seated near a window or a door that is frequently open. This child will do better in a classroom where desks are arranged in rows so that the teacher can easily track what is going on and monitor children during work periods. Also, teachers should have several tables within the classroom where children can work on projects (or play educational games or use for other rewards if they finish their seat work). These tables should never have a partition separating them from the rest of the class because the teacher should be able to monitor activity (Haake, 1991; Paine, Radicchi, Rosellini, Deutchman, & Darch, 1983).

Lesson preparation and delivery are key components to successful teaching, and this is very important with regard to students with AD/HD. The teacher needs to use visual aids so that, if some material is missed, the child with AD/HD who has a slower processing speed can catch up. Because the child with AD/HD can incorporate small bits of information but gets lost if larger blocks of data are given, the teacher should make lessons brief without sacrificing significant content. It is always a good idea to use the student's name and to *quietly* redirect the child's attention. By simply using the child's name, the teacher may avoid sending a message of rejection. The general classroom teacher must make a conscious effort to give appropriate praise to students who have difficulty remaining on task. The teacher may decide to use self-reinforcement to aid in remembering to give appropriate praise.

The teacher needs to modify *worksheets and tests* for children with AD/HD who have learning difficulties. With younger children it is wise to use larger print. Students with AD/HD do better with a simple format and a few activities at one time. Worksheets and tests should include clear and simple directions. When a student with AD/HD must review for a test, the teacher should notify the parent that the child can cover a reasonable amount of review each night beginning several weeks before the test. Providing practice tests (e.g., the test from the year before) can help the child with the review. These are just a few of the modifications the teacher can make, but perhaps the most important is in some cases the limitation of written homework. Some motivated students with AD/HD spend their entire after-school time doing homework. If a teacher has the student do only every other problem, this child may have time to develop in areas that are related to life skills (communication, social, and motor). Learning is the goal of education, and, for the child with AD/HD, a burdensome assignment may cause further self-deprecation when the child is able to complete only part of the assignment, does not turn in the paper because he or she is ashamed that it is only half done, and receives a zero for the missing assignment.

Organizational modifications by general teachers become perhaps most important for the middle school and secondary school child. Children should learn to keep folders for each subject and to file old material on a weekly basis. The teacher should remind the class of due dates daily and can keep a list of important due dates on the board. The teacher can establish a daily routine and schedule and provide a list of daily activities on the chalkboard or an overhead. The teacher should have the student with AD/HD organize his or her desk weekly during elementary school and middle school years. There are many other organizational aids (e.g., semantic organizers) that the general teacher can provide or learn to provide.

Finally, *behavioral aids* are of utmost importance for the teacher's success. The teacher should implement a behavior program and stick to it (see Chapter 30, this volume). It should be a response–cost system, and every child with AD/HD should start off with a set number of tokens. In cases of serious intentional rule breaking, measures such as detentions and suspensions are indicated. In cases of rule breaking that are unintentional and caused because of the child's impulsivity and inattention, the infraction should constitute a loss of tokens. The teacher can let the class decide what they would like to include for positive reinforcers. Have class rules displayed and make them as simple as possible. The students should be reminded of the class rules more frequently during the initial phase of the year, and students who follow the rules should be praised and rewarded throughout the year.

The teacher should help focus teacher–student instruction on enhancement of the student's self-esteem. The teacher should be coached to make an effort to praise the child for appropriate behavior. The general teacher should also implement an individual behavior program for the child with AD/HD, and the student should earn points for sustained on-task behavior. The teacher should maintain vigilance in order to catch the child "being on-task," "being reflective," and "being in control." Both school rewards and nonschool rewards should be possible to earn for a set number of tokens. The teacher can let the child know when he or she is getting off task by a tactile cue, such as resting two fingers on the child's shoulder. The teacher also can encourage peer relationships. For example, the teacher may pair a child with AD/HD with another child when they have both completed their work and have a short period of time to play a school game together.

The teacher should introduce variety into the task. Novelty and humor will increase alertness in the classroom. What once were intriguing tasks can become boring if they are always presented in the same way to the child. Short periods of physical activity in between classes may relieve the child of some of his or her underlying restlessness. Children with AD/HD may enhance self-esteem and sense of responsibility by running an errand for the teacher.

It is important for the pediatrician to understand what possible modifications can work, in order to stimulate the parent and the child to see what may help. In this way, the pediatrician coaches and reinforces the parent's advocacy for the child, but also potentially the child's advocacy for him- or herself.

Learning Disability/ Behavior Disability Intervention

Because a substantial number of children with AD/HD also have other specific learning disabilities, and in some cases behavioral disabilities, this section of the habilitation program may include specific goals for academic areas such as writing or auditory comprehension and for behavioral goals such as decreasing aggressive outbursts. The emphasis is no longer on remediation of learning deficits, but rather on the utilization of strategies that tap into the child's cognitive and communication strengths. This applies also to the child's problems with inattention and lack of control.

Even in the absence of a definitive information-processing deficit, studies have demonstrated significant educational deficits that the child with AD/HD endures as a result of the inability to sustain attention (Zentall, 1993). Spelling is an example of a "selective attention" task. It has been demonstrated that children with AD/HD learn better when they are initially shown new words in black and white, and then color is added to highlight the irregular letters in the word (Zentall, 1989). Slower calculation speed has been demonstrated for learners with AD/HD, and these children have been shown to have poorer comprehension for *long passages* as opposed to short passages. These two areas of academic failure can be attributed to poor sustained attention. Visual-motor deficits appear to account for the problems that children with AD/HD have with handwriting (Zentall, 1993). Improvement in handwriting for children with AD/HD and visual-motor deficits requires significant increases in sustained attention.

The learning disability or behavior disability (LD/BD) teacher needs to establish trusting relationships with their students with AD/HD. The teacher should form a partnership and use contractual agreements to meet short- and long-term objectives that have been outlined for the child. The LD/BD teacher can orchestrate a continuity of care for this child with all of the other professionals that are involved with him or her.

The LD/BD teacher should utilize behavior modification and identify positive reinforcers just as the general classroom teacher does. The regular teacher has greater time constraints, and the LD/BD teacher can provide general classroom teachers with valuable information regarding successful reinforcers. If a particularly good reinforcer is identified, then this information should be shared between the school and the home. In fact, the more consistent the program, the better.

Medication

Approximately 70% and perhaps up to 95% of children with AD/HD respond dramatically to stimulant medication (Elia, Borcherding, Rapoport, & Keysor, 1991). Many parents and teachers of children with AD/HD have witnessed something close to Bradley's original depiction of this response:

> There appeared a definite "drive" to accomplish as much as possible during the school period, and often to spend extra time completing additional work. Speed of comprehension and accuracy of performance were increased in most cases. (Bradley, 1937, p. 578)

Although other drugs have proved beneficial to the child with AD/HD, only stimulants thus far have consistently demonstrated the potential to bring about an increased capacity to delay responses and an increased effort in the form of sustained attention in children with AD/HD asked to perform tests during both states (Elia et al., 1990, Rapport, DuPaul, & Kelly, 1989). Another advantage of stimulants is that fewer and less serious side effects accompany their use.

The pediatrician must consider the child with AD/HD within his or her social setting before deciding on medication. A decision to use stimulants if there is a high probability that the drug will be misused and that the family will not be supportive of the child while he or she is taking the drug may not be justifiable (Rapoport, 1980). Table 1 contains practical information for the pediatrician related to the drugs currently being used frequently for children with AD/HD. It does not contain some drugs that

Table 1. Psychopharmacological treatment for the child and adolescent with AD/HD

Agent: generic name (trade name)	Indications	Dosage	Common side effects
Methylphenidate (Ritalin)	AD/HD	0.3–0.7 mg/kg/dose (begin at low, short-acting dose with parents observing at home on weekends)	Hyporexia, failure to gain weight, insomnia, increased frequency of tics in a child with Tourette syndrome or complex tic disorder, nausea, dizziness, tachycardia, headaches, rigidity
Dextroamphetamine sulfate (Dexedrine)	AD/HD	0.15–0.6 mg/kg/dose (begin with small, short-acting dose as above, and titrate; on short-acting dosing, patient takes 8 A.M. and noon doses. Same is true for methylphenidate)	Anorexia, insomnia, failure to gain weight at normal rate, tachycardia, dizziness, headaches, rigidity
Pemoline (Cylert)	AD/HD	0.5–2.0 mg/kg/dose; child takes an A.M. dose (may consider adding a 2 P.M.–3 P.M. dose)	May not see effects for several weeks; hyporexia, failure to gain sufficient weight to keep pace with height, hypersensitivity, change in liver function and elevated liver enzymes
Clonidine hydrochloride (Catapres)	AD/HD, tic disorders, hypertension	Initial dosage 0.05 mg/day, (1/4 q.i.d.) and gradually titrate to a therapeutic dose (maximum 0.6 mg/day); divide into 3–4 doses during titration	Follow blood pressure closely; should discontinue slowly to avoid hypertension; initially drowsiness may occur even in slight doses
Imipramine (Tofranil)	Enuresis, depression, AD/HD with depressive mood or unresponsive to stimulants	For AD/HD: 0.5–3.0 mg/kg/day in one or two doses	Change in sensorium, anticholinergic effects: dry mouth, constipation, urinary retention
Desipramine (Norpramin)	Depression, AD/HD with depressed mood with stimulants	For AD/HD: to begin, 25-mg capsule/day; maintenance, 2.0–4.0 mg/kg/day	Fewer anticholinergic effects than imipramine; several cases of sudden death have been reported (baseline electrocardiogram should be evaluated before beginning treatment)
Thioridazine (Mellaril)	AD/HD unresponsive to stimulants; especially useful for disinhibited children with mental retardation	Begin with 0.5–1.0 mg/kg/day divided into 2–4 doses	Drowsiness, extrapyramidal symptoms, hyperactivity, tardive dyskinesia may result during discontinuation

show potential benefit but remain in the research stages.

Clearly, stimulant medication is not curative, and the collaboration of all parties, including the child, is imperative to successful management (Barkley, 1977; Rapoport, 1980). An alliance of doctor, family, teachers, and child will enhance the possibility of success. This alliance will help assure the family that has major questions about the use of medication, and may decrease future noncompliance. Problems that arise can be effectively supervised by the pediatrician, and decisions made by the family together with the AD/HD child should be communicated to the pediatrician. This alliance does not end after the pediatrician has spoken with the child about the benefits he or she may derive from taking the medication and the goals he or she should set for him or herself.

When initially counseling children with AD/HD that medication is recommended for them, the pediatrician should retrace his or her ideas about the causes of their current problems. Children with AD/HD should be told that the medication may help them to succeed in some aspects of school that they are having problems with and to control their impulses. These children should be informed that, if the medicine works, their success will depend on the resolve to improve concentration and on-task performance.

Basic Treatment Regimen

The pediatrician should recommend a medication trial for most children diagnosed as having AD/HD. The pediatrician first should discuss the issue of medication with the parents and, if the parent(s) are resistant to the idea of medication, they should be encouraged to read parent handouts before making a decision. If the parents are interested in a trial of medication, this can be a controlled study with both the child and teacher masked as to whether the placebo or medication is being used. The teacher completes a Conners abbreviated teacher questionnaire ("hyperactive index") daily, an ACTeRS questionnaire weekly (Blondis et al., 1991), or both. The Conners hyperactivity index covers behaviors that are measurable on a daily basis, whereas the ACTeRS questionnaire is longer and some of the questions pertaining to social skills and attention cannot be rated on a daily basis. The medication trial begins initially at home, with the parents administering the short-acting drug during a weekend day and observing their child to be sure that the child does not experience any untoward side effects. If the parent has a question regarding the child's response, the parent is encouraged to contact the pediatrician for clarification before continuing

or suspending the trial. Some children with AD/HD may not respond to methylphenidate until they reach a dose of 0.8 mg/kg. In general, most children will respond to a dosage of 0.3 mg/kg of methylphenidate and experience a minimum of side effects at this dosage.

Most recent studies show a great variability of response. Rapport et al. (1989) have demonstrated that factors such as gross body weight and age should play a limited role in determining the dosing of methylphenidate. This work disputed earlier studies (Sprague & Sleator, 1977) that had advocated dosages based solely on weight. Rapport et al. (1989) demonstrated that, in a group analysis, the relationship between dose and behavior response is primarily linear and unrelated to chronologic age, gross body weight, or body surface area. This study and two other studies carried out by Rapport all produced the same finding. The implication of these results is that the practitioner should titrate methylphenidate using various fixed dosages rather than according to body weight.

Although sustained-release methylphenidate has not demonstrated predictable drug absorption, Dexedrine spansules have demonstrated longer-acting treatment (Pelham et al., 1990). Anorexia as well as insomnia, headaches, and abdominal pains are side effects seen with a frequency above that of a placebo when administered to the childhood AD/HD population (Barkley, McMurray, Edelbrock, & Robbins, 1990). Tics are another side effect that deserve close attention even though they are reported as frequently by children with AD/HD who are taking a placebo. Clinical studies have clearly documented that children taking a stimulant developed tics and that the tics subsided when the stimulant was stopped. Claims that stimulant medication causes Tourette syndrome are unfounded. Tourette syndrome is associated with AD/HD and other learning disabilities. Actually, some children with Tourette syndrome have experienced a decrease in tics while on a stimulant. Nevertheless, if the child has experienced tics on Ritalin or Dexedrine, the pediatrician should give the child a trial of pemoline and, if the tics persist, then clonidine would be the drug of choice (Steingard, Biederman, Spencer, Wilens, & Gonzalez, 1993).

Several factors must be considered in regard to the number of doses prescribed for the child during the school week. Many children who are having no significant problems disrupting the home and who do not have a great deal of homework may be able to take two doses of short-acting stimulants. It is not clear exactly what the phenomenon of "rebound hyperactivity" actually represents, but parents of children with AD/HD definitely report this (Johnston, Pelham, Hoza, & Sturges, 1988). If significant rebound hyperactivity occurs on a regular basis, a third dose of stimulant medication generally is effective. There are other reasons for a regimen of either dextroamphetamine or methylphenidate that includes an after-school dose. Children beginning as early as third grade get homework and have a difficult time completing it, but may show significant benefit from an after-school dose of dextroamphetamine or methylphenidate.

Recent studies point to improvements in social development as well as improved performance in sports and reading output with stimulant medication use (Pelham, McBurnett, Harper, & Milich, 1990; Pelham et al., 1993). The results of other recent studies, although supportive of the ability of stimulants to suppress disinhibitory behavior, demonstrate the inability of stimulant medication to produce large effects on skills or higher cognitive processes (Swanson et al., 1993). If a child with AD/HD experiences no side effects and appears to benefit in multiple ways, dosing three times a day and on weekends makes the most sense. Some children with severe AD/HD with conduct disorder and other comorbidity cannot afford to take less than three doses per day if they truly respond to methylphenidate or dextroamphetamine. In our preliminary studies, the majority of children with AD/HD sleep better if they take two doses of medication, but some sleep better if they take a third dose. If the medication is causing insomnia, then a third dose may need to be administered earlier or discontinued. It is advisable to maintain the medication during the weekend unless one is unable to titrate the medication and avoid anorexia (Rapoport, Zametkin, Donnelly, & Ismond, 1985).

Long-Term Management

The long-term management of medication has been the most disappointing aspect of pediatric care of children with AD/HD (McBride, 1988). Very few pediatricians develop a system that encompasses regular monitoring of the child's progress at developing effective control over behavior, improved social relationships, and improved academic achievement. If the medicine is truly effective, the child is developing these competencies. If he or she is not, it may be that some other intervention ought to be considered as a part of the regimen. In a severe case the medication may help, but all modalities may be insufficient to substantially improve the outcome. The pediatrician must persist with this child and make sure that all modalities that are considered to be beneficial to some children with AD/HD are given an *optimal* trial. In some cases this may require a dialogue with members of the family who ordinarily do not accompany the child to clinic. In other cases it may require working with the family to advocate for a teacher who can competently integrate modifications in the school classroom, or the pediatrician may need to identify a mental health professional with expertise in the area of school problems to work with the child and his or her family.

If stimulants are being used, the pediatrician must monitor to see that weight and height maintain on the growth curve, and the first follow-up appointments should be spaced no more than every third month. Periodic withdrawal of the drug can be attempted at strategic times and with patient and family support, if the patient has made substantial improvements. Few long-term drug management studies have been conducted. Effective medication management requires the pediatrician to allow an adequate amount of time to truly address the issues of side effects; current behavioral and academic performance; changes in attentional processing; and social, emotional, and adaptive growth. The Test of Variable Attention (TOVA) is useful for evaluating the inattentive errors, impulsive errors, variability of attention, and reaction time of the child with AD/HD. This computerized test of attention and impulsivity is very expensive, however. The Conners Continuous Performance Task shows a great deal of promise at a much more reasonable price (see Chapter 29, this volume). Standardization has not progressed as rapidly as for the TOVA, but standardization is ongoing. Parents should be asked to complete questionnaires on side effects and behavior, and to have the schoolteacher(s) complete a short questionnaire just before the child's clinic visit.

Other Pharmacotherapeutic Agents

Pemoline is managed slightly differently than dextroamphetamine and methylphenidate even though the side effects are similar. A child with AD/HD may take up to a month to show a response to pemoline, whereas the response to the other stimulants is immediate. Pemoline need be administered only once a day in the morning, and herein lies its advantage—the stability of response. Pemoline is partially metabolized by the liver and carries the risk of liver dysfunction and a chemically induced hepatitis. For this reason, regular liver function tests should be performed every month initially until titration is achieved. Liver function should continue to be checked every 3–6 months. In some states, pemoline is not as strictly monitored by the drug enforcement agency, and the pediatrician is permitted to allow refills.

If the pediatrician has been successful with an adequate stimulant medication trial with methylphenidate, dextroamphetamine, and pemoline at dosages up to the maximum recommended amounts, then the pediatrician should consider clonidine hydrochloride. Although usually thought of as an antihypertensive agent, clonodine has proved to be a safe and effective medication for children with AD/HD symptoms (Hunt, Minderaa, & Cohen, 1985). For children who have problems with motor tics or Tourette syndrome, clonidine is one of the drugs of choice. The initial dose for children 8–13 years of age is 0.05 mg/day divided into three doses. Dosage is then titrated to meet target goals. Dry mouth and sleepiness are the two most common side effects. Sleepiness, if present initially, usually diminishes after several weeks. Baseline pulse and blood pressure determinations are essential because pulse and blood pressure must be monitored closely. Generally the blood pressure will decrease by approximately 10%.

Desipramine, a tricyclic antidepressant, has recently shown a good deal of promise for children with AD/HD who also meet criteria for other comorbid psychopathology. Desipramine consistently has decreased impulsive, hyperactive, and aggressive behaviors (Spencer, Biederman, Kerman, Steingard, & Wilens, 1993). It does not appear to improve performance on cognitive measures consistently, and, for this reason as well as for its more significant side effects, it cannot be recommended as a first-line drug for AD/HD (Biederman, 1991, Gualtieri, Keenan, & Chandler, 1991). Studies show decreased urinary methoxyhydroxyphenylglycol and vanillylmandelic acid, and to some extent a decreased norepinephrine excretion. In addition, pulse and blood pressure increase. Desipramine clearly involves norepinephrine mechanisms but may also involve dopaminergic mechanisms. This drug has caused significant arrhythmias in children with AD/HD, resulting in several fatalities. The child should have an electrocardiogram to rule out Wolff-Parkinson-White syndrome, a prolonged P-R interval, and any other conduction problems before initiating desipramine. Desipramine has been shown to cause a decline in motor performance. Because of the more severe side effects, desipramine should be reserved for children with AD/HD who have significant other psychopathologic comorbidity.

Cognitive–Behavioral Therapy and Language Pragmatics

The cognitive–behavioral methodology is based on the notion that if a child develops a process, he or she will be able to change a behavior (see Chapter 30, this volume). In the case of children with AD/HD, the process is one of self-regulation and organization for the purpose of overcoming unconscious daydreaming, impulsive reactions, and inability to sustain attention to complete a task. Cognitive–behavioral therapy is considered to be beneficial in selective cases, although group studies have not proved clearcut efficacy and several fail to show a trend. Some investigators believe that this intervention may benefit the child with AD/HD who is predominantly inattentive but will have little or no impact on hyperactive-impulsive children. No study has compared the effect of this treatment on these disparate subtypes.

It is important to identify the particular "thinking–behavior" that needs to be changed, and it is important before therapy begins to enlist the child's support. This can be done by counseling the child to try to change the "thinking–behavior" and by convincing the child that his or her control will determine consequences (Kendall & Braswell, 1993). Even in studies that have demonstrated a trend suggesting efficacy, some argue that the generalization of this methodology and the long-term maintenance have not yet been demonstrated.

Cognitive training includes teaching the child to regulate by self-verbalization. Initially the LD/BD teacher or the speech pathologist models this behavior for the child with AD/HD. In theory this behavior can be internalized (Meichenbaum & Goodman, 1971). Following the modeling sessions, the child is directed through the process by the instuctor. Next the child is asked to solve problems for the instructor while talking out loud. Later, the child demonstrates his or her competence to the instructor. As the child develops and perfects this skill, it becomes a silent and private technique for staying on task (see Table 2).

When language deficits exist, the speech and language teacher can integrate cognitive training by addressing language pragmatics, which is oftentimes a major problem for the child with AD/HD. Language pragmatics include establishing a referent, polite forms of requests, use of tactful deviousness, and keeping physical distance. These abilities are fundamental for developing good social skills, which is fundamental if this child is going to win social approval. If the child cannot qualify for speech and language services, possibly the LD/BD teacher can teach some basic pragmatics. Certainly the school and pediatrician should bring this to the parent's attention if it is a problem area.

UNCONVENTIONAL THERAPIES

Additive-free diets, sugar-free diets, and biofeedback are various controversial therapies touted sometimes as cures for children with vari-

Table 2. Steps to self-regulation training[a]

Teacher models self-talk
Teacher gives instructions, child performs task (overt, external)
Child performs task while guiding him- or herself out loud (overt, S-G)
Child guides him- or herself with whispered instructions (faded overt)
Child guides performance with private speech (covert, S-G)
Child processes without private speech
Child generalizes use of private self-regulation

Adapted from Meichenbaum & Goodman (1971).

[a]The professional first models self-guidance (S-G) through a task (e.g., math seat work). The child learns this process through the sequence outlined above under the supervision of the clinical professsional.

ous developmental disorders, including AD/HD. Despite lack of clear evidence, these therapies attract consumers who are frustrated with the progress that is occurring with standard treatment regimens.

Additive-free diets at one time were frequently dispensed therapies that parents of children with AD/HD utilized. To some parents, the diet consists of just using fruits instead of cakes for snacks. For other parents, the highly restrictive Feingold Kaiser-Permanente (K-P) diet is the choice (Feingold, 1975). Many studies of the K-P diet were conducted, but no controlled studies were supportive (Kinsbourne, 1994).

Refined sugar and aspartame have become food agents linked to possible change in personality and behavior. Studies and reviews (Accardo & Lindsay, 1994; Kinsbourne, 1994; Shaywitz et al., 1994; Wolraich et al., 1994) demonstrate the unscientifically founded conclusions drawn by investigators and proponents (Crook, 1975; Egger, Carter, Graham, Gumley, & Soothill, 1985) of this rigid, sacrificial, and stressful intervention.

The most recent controversial therapy to appear is biofeedback. Several studies of biofeedback have shown some promise for this intervention, but the majority of studies are uncontrolled group studies or case studies (Lee, 1991). Children with AD/HD most likely will have a difficult time generalizing this intervention, if studies are unable to show generalization for cognitive–behavioral interventions. At this time the pediatrician cannot encourage the use of this methodology.

AD/HD: A CONDITION
WORTH HABILITATING

The multimodality approach offers the most hope for the habilitation for the child with AD/HD. The medical management of this condition is demanding and requires frequent follow-up for the moderate to severely involved cases. The key to successful management, however, is not only in determining the child's neurodevelopmental continuum of disability, but also in reaching an understanding of the family dynamics and understanding the limits and capabilities of the family. The development and outcome of the child with AD/HD in a dysfunctional family is dependent on whether the interpersonal relationships and the mental health of the family can improve.

There is a great deal of proof that the AD/HD population is a population at risk for causing traffic accidents, abusing drugs, dropping out of school, becoming antisocial, and committing crimes against society. For this reason, competent management and follow-up will benefit not only a child who may be capable of a very creative and fulfilling life, but also society.

REFERENCES

Accardo, P.J., & Lindsay, R. (1994). Nutrition and behavior. *Pediatrics, 93,* 127–128.

Barkley, R.A. (1977). A review of stimulant drug research with hyperactive children. *Journal of Child Psychology and Psychiatry, 18,* 137–165.

Barkley, R.A., McMurray, M.B., Edelbrock, C.S., & Robbins, K. (1990). Side effects of methylphenidate in children with attention deficit hyperactivity disorder: A systemic, placebo-controlled evaluation. *Pediatrics, 86,* 184–192.

Biederman, J. (1991). Sudden death in children treated with a tricyclic antidepressant. *Journal of the American Academy of Child and Adolescent Psychiatry, 30,* 495–498.

Bloomquist, M.L., August, G.J., & Ostrander, R. (1991). Effects of a school-based cognitive-behavioral intervention for ADHD children. *Journal of Abnormal Child Psychology, 19,* 591–605.

Blondis, T.A., Clippard, D.C., Scroggs, D., & Peterson, L. (1991). Multidisciplinary habilitative prescriptions for the attention deficit hyperactivity disorder child. In P.J. Accardo, T.A. Blondis, & B.Y. Whitman (Eds.), *Attention deficit disorders and hyperactivity in children* (pp. 223–250). New York: Marcel Dekker.

Bradley, C. (1937). The behavior of children receiving benzedrine. *American Journal of Psychiatry, 94,* 577–585.

Crook, W.G. (1975). Food allergy—the great masquerader. *Pediatric Clinics of North America, 22,* 227–238.

Egger, J., Graham, P.J., Carter, C.M., Gumley, D., & Soothill, J.F. (1985). Controlled trial of oligoantigenic treatment in the hyperkinetic syndrome. *Lancet, 1,* 540–545.

Elia, J., Borcherding, B.G., Rapoport, J.L., & Keysor, C.S. (1990). Methylphenidate and dextroamphetamine treatments of hyperactivity: Are there true nonresponders? *Psychiatric Research, 36,* 141–155.

Feingold, B.F. (1975). *Why is your child hyperactive?* New York: Random House.

Gualtieri, C.T., Keenan, P.A., & Chandler, M. (1991). Clinical and neuropsychological effects of desipramine in children with attention deficit hyperactivity disorder. *Journal of Clinical Psychopharmacology, 11,* 155–159.

Haake, C.A. (1991). Behavioral markers and intervention strategies for regular and special education teachers. In P.J. Accardo, T.A. Blondis, & B.Y. Whitman (Eds.), *Attention deficit disorders and hyperactivity in children* (pp. 223–249). New York: Marcel Dekker.

Hunt, R.D., Minderaa, R.B., & Cohen, D.J. (1985). Condidine benefits children with attention deficit disorder and hyperactivity: Report of a double-blind placebo-crossover therapeutic trial. *Journal of the American Academy of Child Psychiatry, 24,* 617-629.

Johnston, C., Pelham, W.E., Hoza, J., & Sturges, J. (1988). Psychostimulant rebound in attention deficit disordered boys. *Journal of the American Academy of Child and Adolescent Psychiatry, 27,* 806–810.

Kendall, P.C., & Braswell, L. (1993). *Cognitive-behavioral therapy for impulsive children* (2nd ed.). New York: Guilford Press.

Kinsbourne, M. (1994). Sugar and the hyperactive child. *New England Journal of Medicine, 330,* 355–356.

Lee, S.W. (1991). Biofeedback as a treatment for childhood hyperactivity: A critical review of the literature. *Psychological Reports, 68,* 163–192.

McBride, M.C. (1988). An individual double-blind crossover trial for assessing methylphenidate response in children with attention deficit disorder. *Journal of Pediatrics, 113,* 137–145.

Meichenbaum, D.H., & Goodman, J. (1971). Training impulsive children to talk to themselves: A means of developing self-control. *Journal of Abnormal Psychology, 77,* 115–126.

Paine, S.C., Radicchi, J.A., Rosellini, L.C., Deutchman, L., & Darch, C.B. (1983). *Structuring your classroom for academic success.* Champaign, IL: Research Press.

Pelham, W.E., Carlson, C., Sams, S.E., Vallano, G., Dixon, M.J., & Hoza, B. (1993). Separate and combined effects of methylphenidate and behavior modification on boys with attention deficit-hyperactivity disorder in the classroom. *Journal of Consulting and Clinical Psychology, 61,* 506–515.

Pelham, W.E., Greenslade, K.E., Vodde-Hamilton, M., Greenstein, J.J., Gnagy, E.M., Guthrie, E.M., Hoover, M.D., & Dahl, R.E. (1990). Relative efficacy of long-acting stimulants on children with attention deficit-hyperactivity disorder—a comparison of standard methylphenidate, sustained-release methylphenidate, sustained-release dextroamphetamine, and pemoline. *Pediatrics, 86,* 226–237.

Pelham, W.E., McBurnett, K., Harper, G.W., & Milich, R. (1990). Methylphenidate and baseball playing in ADHD children: Who's on first? *Journal of Consulting Clinical Psychology, 58,* 130–133.

Piontkowski, D., & Calfee, R. (1979). Attention in the classroom. In G.A. Hale & M. Lewis (Eds.), *Attention and cognitive development* (pp. 297–329). New York: Plenum Press.

Rapoport, J.L. (1980). The "real" and "ideal" management of stimulant drug treatment for hyperactive children: Recent findings and a report from clinical practice. In C.K. Whalen & B. Henker (Eds.), *Hyperactive children: The social ecology of identification and treatment* (pp. 247–258). New York: Academic Press.

Rapoport, J.L., Zametkin, A., Donnelly, M., & Ismond, D. (1985). New drug trials in attention deficit disorder. *Psychopharmacology Bulletin, 21,* 232–236.

Rapport, M.D., DuPaul, G.J., & Kelly, K.L. (1989). Attention deficit hyperactivity disorder and methylphenidate: The relationship between gross body weight and drug response in children. *Psychopharmacology Bulletin, 25,* 285–290.

Roizen, N.J., Blondis, T.A., Irwin, M., Rubinoff, A., Keiffer, J., & Stein, M.A. (in press). Psychiatric and developmental disorders of children with ADHD: Utility of parent report. *Archives of Pediatrics and Adolescent Medicine.*

Roizen, N.J., Blondis, T.A., Irwin, M., & Stein, M. (1994). Adaptive functioning in children with Attention-Deficit Hyperactivity Disorder. *Archives of Pediatrics and Adolescent Medicine, 148,* 1137–1142.

Satterfield, J.H., Satterfield, B.T., & Schell, A.M. (1987). Therapeutic interventions to prevent delinquency in hyperactive boys. *Journal of American Academy of Child and Adolescent Psychiatry, 26,* 56–64.

Shaywitz, B.A., Sullivan, C.M., Anderson, G.M., Gillespie, S.M., Sullivan, B., & Shaywitz, S.E. (1994). Aspartame, behavior, and cognitive function in children with attention deficit disorder. *Pediatrics, 93,* 70–75.

Spencer, T., Biederman, J., Kerman, K., Steingard, R., & Wilens, T. (1993). Desipramine treatment of children with attention-deficit hyperactivity disorder and tic disorder or Tourette's syndrome. *Journal of the American Academy of Child and Adolescent Psychiatry, 32,* 354-360.

Sprague, R.L., & Sleator, E.K. (1977). Methylphenidate in hyperkinetic children: Differences in dose effects on learning and social behavior. *Science, 198,* 1274–1276.

Steingard, R., Biederman, J., Spencer, T., Wilens, T., & Gonzalez, A. (1993). Comparison of clonidine response in the treatment of attention deficit hyperactivity disorder with and without co-morbid tic disorders. *Journal of the American Academy of Child and Adolescent Psychiatry, 32,* 350–353.

Swanson, J.M., McBurnett, K., Wigal, T., Pfiffner, L.J., Lerner, M.A., Williams, L., Christian, D.L., Tamm, L., Willcutt, E., Crowley, K., Clevenger, W., Khouzam, N., Woo, C., Crinella, F.M., & Fisher, T.D. (1993). Effect of stimulant medication on children with attention deficit disorder: A "review of reviews." *Exceptional Children, 60,* 154–162.

Turecki, S., & Tonner, L. (1989). *The difficult child.* New York: Bantam Books.

Weiss, G., Hechtman, L., Milroy, T., & Perlman, T. (1985). Psychiatric status of hyperactives as adults: A controlled prospective 15-year follow-up of 63 hyperactive children. *Journal of the American Academy of Child Psychiatry, 24,* 211–220.

Whitman, B.Y., & Smith, C. (1991). Living with a hyperactive child: Principles of families, family therapy, and behavior management. In P.J. Accardo, T.A. Blondis, & B.Y. Whitman (Eds.), *Attention deficit disorders and hyperactivity in children* (pp. 187–222). New York: Marcel Dekker.

Wodrich, D.L. (1994). *Attention deficit hyperactivity disorder and your child: What every parent wants to know.* Baltimore: Paul H. Brookes Publishing Co.

Wolraich, M.L., Lindgren, S.D., Stumbo, P.J., Stegink, L.D., Appelbaum, M.I., & Kiritsy, M.C. (1994). Effects of diets high in sucrose or aspartame on the behavior and cognitive performance of children. *New England Journal of Medicine, 330,* 301–307.

Zentall, S.S. (1989). Attentional cueing in spelling tasks for hyperactive and comparison regular classroom children. *Journal of Special Education, 23,* 83-93.

Zentall, S.S. (1993). Research on the educational implications of attention deficit hyperactivity disorder. *Exceptional Children, 60,* 143–153.

Chapter 30

Nonpharmacologic Management of Disorders of Behavior and Attention

Susan E. Levy, M.D.

Learning and behavioral difficulties in children are very common complaints confronting a primary care physician. Prevalence estimates range from 5% to 30% of the pediatric population (Thompson, 1985). Attentional or behavior disorders may result in significant morbidity, suggesting that specific intervention be instituted as early as possible. Poor self-image, peer rejection, noncompliance, aggressive behavior, and family discord caused by behavioral dysfunction carry a poor prognosis for successful adult functioning (Patterson, Reid, & Dishion, 1992). Early identification and intervention is necessary to mitigate the secondary complications for children and families. Current treatment approaches include combinations of pharmacotherapy, educational intervention, behavior management, social skills training, and psychotherapy (see Chapter 29, this volume). Behavior management, in conjunction with pharmacotherapy, appears to be the most effective intervention for behavior and attentional disorders in children (Pelham et al., 1993).

Clinicians should be alert to the identification of common developmental and behavior disorders. They should be ready to intervene by referring to appropriate resources, by providing brief treatment and referring patients for whom brief interventions are not successful, or by providing long-term treatment (Silver, 1982). The primary care physician must be familiar with the range of diagnoses, types of available treatment, and availability of community resources for implementation of treatment and support of the family.

Behavioral symptoms may accompany developmental disorders, psychiatric illness, or poor social situations. The associated symptoms often overlap, making diagnosis of one specific behavioral syndrome difficult. In addition, children with chronic illness are at increased risk for superimposed behavioral and psychosocial problems (Thompson, 1985). Thus, children may meet diagnostic standards for more than one behavioral disorder under the criteria established by the *Diagnostic and Statistical Manual of Mental Disorders,* 4th edition (American Psychiatric Association, 1994). Diagnoses frequently associated with behavioral difficulties include attention-deficit/hyperactivity disorder (ADHD), conduct disorders, anxiety disorders of childhood or adolescence, oppositional defiant disorder, adjustment disorder with disturbance of conduct, and antisocial personality disorder. Specific behavioral symptoms include poor self-control, noncompliance, aggression, antisocial behavior, hyperactivity, oppositional behavior, poor peer relations, self-injurious behavior, and academic underachievement.

Programs using a combined, holistic approach to behavior disorders—taking into account the child, his or her underlying central nervous system dysfunction, and the family dynamics—appear to have the best outcome (Hansen & Cohen, 1984). As peer relationship skills, academic skills, and self-esteem improve, the rate of antisocial behavior generally will decline (Sleator & Pelham, 1986). One explanation is that the various treatments may interact synergistically, minimizing the shortcomings of each isolated treatment (Pelham & Murphy, 1986). For example, studies have shown that, when multimodal treatments are used, lower doses of stimulants at times may be sufficient (Carlson, Pelham, Milich, & Dixon, 1992). A disadvantage of combined treatment is that it is often more expensive and requires higher levels of compliance from children and their families. It may also be difficult to know which aspects of the treatment are most effective.

Noncompliance with intervention programs for behavior or emotional disorders may be as high as 50% (Firestone & Witt, 1982). The rate of compliance appears to be inversely correlated to the length and complexity of the intervention program (Brown, Borden, Wynne, Spunt, & Clingerman, 1987).

In children with ADHD, programs that combine pharmacologic, behavioral, and educational interventions are considered to be the most effective in ameliorating a wide range of symptoms (Barkley, 1990; see also Chapter 29, this volume). Given the chronic nature of ADHD, treatment programs that provide ongoing care to children with ADHD and their families appear to be more effective than brief treatment programs (Hinshaw, 1994). For instance, children who dropped out of a 3-year multimodal treatment program to be treated with stimulant medication alone did not do as well as those children who continued with the comprehensive program (Satterfield, Satterfield, & Cantwell, 1987). Intervention must be tailored to meet both the child's needs and the ability of the family to carry out the prescribed treatment. The most commonly used intervention for children with attentional or behavior disorders is medication. This includes stimulants, tranquilizers, antidepressants, and other neuromodulators. Too often, families and school personnel expect medication to cure the child's disability. The expectation cannot be fulfilled because of potential secondary symptoms. Drugs alone are rarely sufficient to bring children into an average range of academic and social functioning. Moreover, medication does not work for all children, and there is no clear evidence that children treated with medications show improvement in long-term prognosis (Jacobovitz, Sroufe, Stewart, & Leffert, 1990).

PRINCIPLES OF BEHAVIORAL INTERVENTION

The goal of behavioral intervention is to promote the acquisition of socially acceptable behaviors and decrease the frequency of problematic or unacceptable behaviors. Therapists and physicians often must teach the children, their families, and teachers to manage rather than eliminate many of the difficult behaviors. Interventions must be designed to facilitate coping, reinforce desired behaviors, and train the child and family to develop and implement alternative strategies. The interventions may need to be reintroduced periodically throughout the child's development.

Behavior management approaches use the observable responses or behaviors of children to guide assessment and intervention strategies. The techniques or treatments depend on understanding the function of a behavior and how it is influenced by antecedents and consequences. The appropriate behavioral intervention depends on understanding why a behavior occurs. For example, if a child is disruptive in the classroom in order to escape the demand of schoolwork beyond his or her capacity, timeout in the hall actually may reinforce the behavior by permitting escape from an undesirable situation.

The purpose of therapy is to either strengthen or weaken the bond between the antecedent stimulus and the child's response. The contingent relationships between observed behaviors and consequences are defined and then manipulated in a consistent manner, either by changing antecedent conditions or managing contingencies.

Management procedures are devised to increase behavior (e.g., positive reinforcement, negative reinforcement), decrease behavior (e.g., extinction, punishment), develop new behavior (shaping), or generalize behavior from one setting to another (Hirsch, 1992).

Positive reinforcement can be used to enhance the likelihood of occurrence of desired behaviors with concomitant decrease of undesired behaviors. Using this strategy, the contingencies are altered to provide attention and reward for the desired outcomes. Use of a token system is an example of a positive reinforcement technique. Chips or tokens are distributed for desirable behaviors and can be cashed in for prizes or privileges (for younger children) or converted to money (for older children) (Barkley, 1990).

Negative reinforcement occurs when an unpleasant stimulus is removed on the occurrence of an undesired or maladaptive behavior. It is not used often in behavior programs because it may involve aversive stimuli or result in undesirable emotional behavior (e.g., crying or aggression) (Hirsch, 1992). However, negative reinforcement is important for parents, teachers, and clinicians to understand because it may explain why children misbehave to avoid undesirable tasks (e.g., crying instead of going to bed).

In *extinction*, the frequency of a specific behavior is reduced by withdrawing reinforcing consequences that previously maintained the behavior. This is effective for attention-getting behaviors. Extinction is most effective when combined with positive reinforcement for a desirable alternative behavior.

Punishment is another means of decreasing undesirable behavior. This is when an aversive event occurs or a positive event is removed on the occurrence of the behavior problem. Although positive approaches should be emphasized, punishment has its place in behavior management, particularly when a problem behavior may be dangerous to the child or others. The mildest form of punishment is a time-out (from positive reinforcement) procedure. The child is removed from a rewarding context and placed in a nonstimulating environment, such as a time-out chair. Another example of a punishment is a response–cost procedure, in which a child forfeits tokens when undesired behaviors occur.

The behavioral approach of *shaping* involves the development of a new behavior pattern by reinforcing small steps or approximations toward the desired behavior. An important component of the management approach is the development of a plan to assure generalization of the changed behavior to other environments (e.g., home to school) and training of involved family and personnel to carry out the program consistently.

A combination of treatment strategies across settings may be indicated in certain situations. Behavior management techniques have been shown to be an effective approach used by both parents and teachers for changing many of the problematic behaviors associated with ADHD (Barkley, 1990). For instance, behavior therapy can improve child compliance with parent and teacher requests; help children pay attention for longer periods of time, enabling them to complete assignments; reduce the occurrence of impulsive, annoying behaviors; decrease the incidence of aggressive behavior; and increase the likelihood of cooperative social behavior. A number of formal training programs for parents of children who are aggressive or have ADHD, or both, have been developed.

APPLICATION OF BEHAVIORAL INTERVENTION

In this hypothetical example of behavioral intervention, a 3-year-old presented with a long history of frequent noncompliance with parental requests. The parents met with a behavior therapist and were instructed in the basic principles of behavior management. They were asked to record whether their child complied or not and whether an action was completed within 20 seconds of the parental request. At home, the parents completed a program in the context of a "parent's game" (Forehand & McMahon, 1981) that provides a semistructured situation in which one or both parents issue a series of one-step "do" requests, provide the child with a recommended response, and record the outcome (e.g., child complies or not). Ten "do" requests were selected by the parents (e.g., "Sit down," "Give me the _____ ," "Put the _____ in the _____ ."). The parents were instructed to issue "approvals" for child compliance, to implement chair time-out (not exceeding 3 minutes) for child noncompliance, and to return the child to the request situation subsequent to serving chair time-out and to reissue the request. Following reissuance and child compliance, no positive reinforcement was to be given.

During the 5 days of baseline observation, the child's compliance varied, averaging 24% (Figure 1). After parent training and during implementation of a program of positive reinforcement with chair time-out, the compliance steadily increased, averaging 84% over the last 5 days of recording.

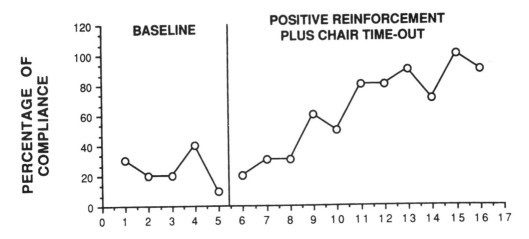

Figure 1. Rates of compliance with 10 "do" requests before parent training (baseline) and after parent training during implementation of a program of positive reinforcement with chair time-out.

LIMITATIONS TO BEHAVIORAL INTERVENTION

There are a number of limitations to behavioral intervention. Even though the children show improvement during treatment, problem behaviors often continue after treatment ends (Sleator & Pelham, 1986; Whalen & Henker, 1984). This is not unexpected because there is often an underlying central nervous system dysfunction that affects the child's understanding of order and may deter social understanding. There may be difficulties with generalization of treatment across settings. Another problem is parental compliance with the behavior regimen, which may be time consuming and costly. Clearly the effectiveness of behavior therapy is dependent on the motivation and capabilities of caregiving adults in the child's life (Firestone & Witt, 1982). Where parents are unable or unwilling to comply, stimulant medication may prove more effective.

TYPES OF BEHAVIORAL INTERVENTION PROGRAMS

Programs of behavioral intervention vary widely, ranging from informal suggestions of behavior management to parents or teachers to highly structured parent effectiveness training programs (Barkley, 1990). The individual re-

sponsible for implementation of a program also varies. Depending on the age, cognitive abilities, and motivation of the child and family, it may be the parent, the child, the teacher, or someone in the community who is responsible.

Parent-Mediated Intervention

Parent effectiveness training programs teach parents to implement behavior management techniques in their home (Barkley, 1990). Parent-mediated contingency management is most applicable to hyperactive, noncompliant, and oppositional children. It involves the manipulation of reinforcers and emphasizes the contingent relationship between behavior and consequences (Barkley, 1990; Kazdin, 1987).

The usual approach involves the following steps:

1. Identifying the target behavior to be changed. The problem must be defined in clear, precise terms so that the behavior can be observed reliably (e.g., Johnny has a tantrum when it's time to leave a store).
2. Determining what events usually precede the behavior (*antecedent stimuli*) (e.g., Mother saying, "It's time to go home now, Johnny," cues the behavior).
3. Determining the *consequences* that generally result when the child performs the behavior (e.g., increased parental attention).

4. Establishing a set of baseline measures (before intervention) demonstrating the frequency at which the problem behaviors occur.
5. Defining specific, realistic short- and long-term goal(s). (A short-term goal may be quiet verbal protest only; a long-term goal is full compliance without protest.)
6. Choosing an intervention. Reinforcement is the management of choice. It may need to be paired with extinction of behavior that is social attention mediated. In an older child this may be coupled with the imposition of a predetermined penalty or response–cost.
7. Monitoring the effectiveness of the intervention (recording the frequency of occurrence of the problematic behavior and comparing it against baseline levels).
8. Periodically evaluating the effectiveness of the intervention, with appropriate implementation of changes.

These steps also may be applied to management of behavioral difficulties in the classroom.

Behavior therapy makes common sense, but consistent, sustained implementation and ongoing professional supervision are necessary for a successful outcome. As part of this, parents often are asked to complete homework assignments. This may entail completing readings, collaborating with other caregivers and with teachers to implement a procedure, and implementing prescribed management strategies at home.

Child-Mediated Intervention

The child may be the mediator of change. Cognitive–behavioral therapy is an approach that teaches children self-instructional and self-reinforcement skills that they can use to guide their own behavior and systematically monitor their own progress (Kendall & Braswell, 1986). This intervention has demonstrated some success with aggressive children (Lochman, 1992), and somewhat less success with children with ADHD (Abikoff, 1985; Hinshaw, 1994).

The steps in self-instructional training include

1. Defining the problem
2. Approaching the problem—that is, helping the child initiate a strategy that will help move him or her toward a solution
3. Focusing attention
4. Choosing the answer
5. Self-praising and avoiding overly negative self-talk (e.g., a good response to a wrong answer would be "I made a mistake—Next time I'll try to go slower and concentrate more and maybe I'll get the right answer")

Cognitive–behavioral techniques are particularly attractive because they encourage children to become active participants of change in their own treatment programs. Children learn to set standards and goals, to evaluate their own actions, and to reward themselves on reaching specified criteria. This yields "portable coping strategies" (Kendall & Braswell, 1985).

Training programs in problem-solving skills focus on the child's underlying deficits in social perception, problem solving, attributions, and self-statement that result in maladaptive behavior (Kazdin, 1987). Behavior therapy programs emphasizing social skills training have resulted in significant short-term improvement in social skills and peer relationships in hyperactive children (Hinshaw, Henker, & Whalen, 1984).

School-Mediated Intervention

School-mediated intervention involves the collaboration of the family, the teacher, and the therapist. Teacher training for management of specific problematic behaviors and direct consultation by the therapist in the classroom are the most effective techniques. The principles are similar to those applied in parent management training and contingency management. General procedures include reinforcement contingencies (social or activity reinforcers or a token program for appropriate behavior; withdrawal of attention for minor inappropriate behavior), environmental restructuring (e.g., preferential seating in the front of the classroom, away from windows to decrease potential distractions), and punishment contingencies such as response–cost or time-out for more serious undesirable behavior (Abramowitz & O'Leary, 1991). The most important factor of management is close communication between family and school personnel and consistent carryover of the program.

Community-Based Intervention

Community-based activity programs promote carryover of acceptable behavior from treatment to community settings (Kazdin, 1987). Such programs work with community services to accomplish their goals through informal social activities, providing positive experiences in a structured setting. Approaches of other treatments (e.g., behavior therapy, social skills training, individual psychotherapy) may be part of such interventions.

SUMMARY

Behavior disorders are complex problems, affecting all aspects of the life of the child and his or her family. Intervention therefore must be comprehensive. A thorough evaluation must be completed to diagnose additional psychological, educational, and emotional problems that frequently accompany behavior disorders. Once the evaluation is complete, a multimodal approach to intervention may be designed. With the guidance of appropriate professionals, a comprehensive plan for behavioral intervention should be successful.

REFERENCES

Abikoff, H. (1985). Efficacy of cognitive intervention in hyperactive children: A critical review. *Clinical Psychology Review*, 5, 479–512.

Abramowitz, A.J., & O'Leary, S.G. (1991). Behavioral interventions for the classroom: Implications for students with ADHD. *School Psychology Review*, 20, 220–234.

American Psychiatric Association. (1994). *Diagnostic and statistical manual of mental disordes (4th ed.)*. Washington, DC: American Psychiatric Press.

Barkley, R.A. (1990). *Hyperactive children: A handbook for diagnosis and treatment*. New York: Guilford Press.

Brown, R.T., Borden, K.A., Wynne, M.E., Spunt, A.L., & Clingerman, S.A. (1987). Compliance with pharmacological and cognitive treatments for attention deficit disorder. *Journal of American Academy of Child and Adolescent Psychiatry*, 26, 521–526.

Carlson, C.L., Pelham, W.E., Milich, R., & Dixon, J. (1992). Single and combined effects of methylphenidate and behavior therapy on the classroom performance of children with attention-deficit hyperactivity disorder. *Journal of Abnormal Child Psychology*, 29, 677–688.

Firestone, P., & Witt, J.E. (1982). Characteristics of families completing and prematurely discontinuing a behavioral parent-training program. *Journal of Pediatric Psychology*, 52, 447–456.

Forehand, R., & McMahon, R.J. (1981). *Helping the noncompliant child: A clinician's guide to parent training*. New York: Guilford Press.

Hansen, C.R., & Cohen, D.J. (1984). Multimodality approaches in the treatment of attention deficit disorder. *Pediatric Clinics of North America*, 31, 499–513.

Hinshaw, S.P. (1994). *Attention deficits and hyperactivity in children*. Thousand Oaks, CA: Sage Press.

Hinshaw, S.P., Henker, B., & Whalen, C.K. (1984). Self control in hyperactive boys in anger inducing situations: Effects of cognitive-behavioral training and or methylphenidate. *Journal of Abnormal Child Psychiatry*, 12, 55–77.

Hirsch, D.L.O. (1992). Behavioral therapy. In M. Levine (Ed.), *Developmental-behavioral pediatrics* (2nd Ed., Chap. 80). Philadelphia: W.B. Saunders.

Jacobovitz, D., Sroufe, L.A., Stewart, M., & Leffert, N. (1990). Treatment of attentional and hyperactivity problems in children with sympathomimetic drugs: A comprehensive review. *Journal of Academy of Child and Adolescent Psychiatry*, 29, 677–688.

Kazdin, A.E. (1987). Current treatments. In *Clinical psychology and psychiatry: Vol. 8. Conduct disorders in childhood and adolescence* (pp. 29–53). Newberry, CA: Sage Press.

Kendall, P.C., & Braswell, L. (1985). *Cognitive-behavioral therapy for impulsive children*. New York: Guilford Press.

Kendall, P.C., & Braswell, L. (1986). Medical applications of cognitive-behavioral interventions with children. *Journal of Developmental and Behavioral Pediatrics*, 7, 257–264.

Lochman, J. (1992). Cognitive behavioral interventions with aggressive boy: Three year follow-up and preventative efforts. *Journal of Consulting and Clinical Psychology*, 60, 426–432.

Patterson, G.R., Reid, J.B., & Dishion, T.J. (1992). *Antisocial boys.* Eugene, OR: Castalia.

Pelham, W.E., Carlson, C., Sams, S.E., Vallano, G., Dixon, M., & Hoza, H. (1993). Separate and combined effects of methylphenidate and behavior modification on boys with attention deficit hyperactivity disorder in the classroom. *Journal of Consulting and Clinical Psychology, 61,* 506–515.

Pelham, W.E., & Murphy, H.A. (1986). Behavioral and pharmacological treatment of attention deficit and conduct disorders. In H. Hersen (Ed.), *Pharmacological and behavioral treatment: An integrative approach* (pp. 108–148). New York: John Wiley & Sons.

Satterfield, J.H., Satterfield, B.T., & Cantwell, D.P. (1987). Three-year multimodality treatment study of 100 hyperactive boys. *Journal of Pediatrics, 98,* 650–655.

Silver, L.B. (1982). The role of the pediatrician in the health-mental health delivery of care system in the United States. *Journal of Developmental and Behavioral Pediatrics, 3,* 217–224.

Sleator, E.K., & Pelham, W.E. (1986). Behavior therapy. In E.K. Sleator & W.E. Pelham (Eds.), *Attention deficit disorder* (Dialogues in Pediatric Management, Vol. 1, No. 3). East Norwalk, CT: Appleton-Century-Crofts.

Thompson, R.J. (1985). Delineation of children's behavior problems: A basis for assessment and intervention. *Journal of Developmental and Behavioral Pediatrics, 6,* 37–50.

Whalen, C.K., & Henker, B. (1984). Hyperactivity and the attention deficit disorders: Expanding frontiers. *Pediatric Clinics of North America, 31,* 397–427.

PART VII

ASSOCIATED DEFICITS

Chapter 31

Visual Impairments in Children

Alexander H. Hoon, Jr., M.D., M.P.H.

Vision plays an integral role in many aspects of childhood development. Given the importance of early intervention for children with visual impairment, those involved in assessment should be aware of the early signs and symptoms of visual loss to investigate etiology and initiate habilitation. Clinicians should develop the ability to integrate issues of diagnosis, prognosis, treatment, and possible recurrence risk to provide ongoing developmental surveillance and counseling as appropriate. Professionals providing services should have an understanding of prognosis in specific disorders and a knowledge of available community resources to plan appropriate habilitative programs for children with visual impairment. When issues of diagnosis and management are vigorously pursued and families are kept well informed, affected children have the best chance to reach their full potential.

This chapter is intended to address issues of diagnosis and management in children with visual impairments. Because an understanding of visual development is important to assessment, the normal sequence of visual milestones in premature and term infants is reviewed. Isolated visual impairments as well as those associated with systemic disorders and specific developmental disabilities including cerebral palsy and mental retardation are discussed. An approach to habilitation is included, emphasizing practical issues in management. For those interested in more specifics, selected sources of information and references have been included in the chapter appendix.

TERMINOLOGY

There are no universal definitions for visual impairment or blindness. The World Health Organization (1980) has published terminology for visual impairment including degree of impairment and visual acuity (Table 1). In the United States, legal blindness is defined as a visual acuity of 20/200 or less in the better eye with best correction, or a visual field of 20 degrees or less. This definition is frequently used to determine eligibility for services, including visual aids and schooling. For example, the American Printing House for the Blind, a federally funded

Table 1. World Health Organization terminology for visual impairment using metric nomenclature

	Degree of impairment	Best corrected visual acuity[a]	Alternative definition
Low vision	Moderate	6/18	Moderate low vision
	Severe	6/48	Severe low vision (counting fingers at 6 m or less)
Blindness	Profound	3/60	Profound low vision or moderate blindness (counting fingers at < 3 m)
	Near-total	1/60	Severe or near-total blindness (counting fingers at 1 m or less or hand movements at 5 m or less)
	Total	No light perception	Total blindness (including absence of the eye)

Adapted from the World Health Organization (1980).
[a]Acuity is measured in meters. For example: 3/60 (in meters) is equivalent to a visual acuity of 20/400 (6/6 = 20/20).

agency founded to provide educational materials for school-age children, uses this definition to establish eligibility.

Distinctions between visual disorder, impairment, disability, and handicap are important to understanding issues facing affected children and their families. For example, bilateral cataracts is a visual disorder that may cause an impairment in visual function and a disability by limiting expected abilities to perform visual tasks. The degree of handicap is subjective, and may be based on the child's perceptions, societal expectations, and social barriers. An appreciation of each will improve the care affected children receive.

Most legally blind children have functional vision. For example, visual acuity of 20/400 may permit mobility in unfamiliar surroundings. Useful vision less than 20/400 includes finger counting, the recognition of hand movement, light projection, and light perception (Table 2). Although light perception or projection represent minimal vision, it permits awareness of environment.

Visual impairment is a term used to describe children with visual acuities ranging from 20/70 to no light perception. The American Foundation for the Blind has suggested that the terms *visual impairment* and *low vision* be used for individuals with any degree of vision and that *blind* be employed only when there is no light perception. In this chapter, the terms *visual impairment*, *visual loss*, and *blindness* will all be used, recognizing that these terms may have differing meanings to various professionals.

Anatomical sites of visual loss may occur in anterior pathways (from the cornea to the lateral geniculate body) and/or in posterior pathways (Table 3). Posterior visual loss occurring from the optic radiations to the occipital lobe and cortical projections is termed *cortical visual impairment* or *cortical blindness,* depending on the degree of loss.

Visual impairment is not always a static process. In cortical visual impairment caused by hypoxic–ischemic encephalopathy, trauma, or meningitis, vision may improve over time. Vision will deteriorate gradually in disorders such as retinitis pigmentosa, or acutely worsen from a secondary retinal detachment in high myopia. A child who loses any degree of visual function, including light perception or projection, will feel the loss acutely.

Educators and habilitation specialists often divide blindness into congenital and adventitious groups. A child with *congenital blindness* either is born blind or develops blindness early in life, prior to memory of the visual world. *Adventitious blindness* is acquired later in life. Children with adventitious blindness have a visual concept of the world on which to build, which the congenitally blind child lacks. The approach to general education and to the development of unique skills such as braille reading or orientation and mobility instruction will differ in these two groups.

To obtain special education services under federal law, a child must have visual limitations interfering with the ability to learn (O'Brien, 1980). As stated in the Individuals with Disabilities Education Act (PL 101-476) visual impairment including blindness "means an impairment in vision that, even with correction, adversely affects a child's educational performance. The term includes both partial sight and blindness." Therefore, visual acuity does not directly determine eligibility for services.

PREVALENCE

It has been estimated that there are more than 1 million blind children worldwide, in addition to many others with less severe degrees of visual impairment (Foster, 1988). There is no national registry of blind individuals in the United States. Epidemiologic data have been collected by many public and private agencies, using different ascertainment criteria and definitions of visual loss. Surveys have been further compli-

Table 2. Terms used to describe abilities of children with visual impairments

Term	Definition
20/200 or 20/400	Largest letter on acuity charts
Finger counting	Calculated in feet from the child
Hand movements	To and fro movements also determined in feet
Light projection	Awareness of the direction of light
Light perception	Perception of light from dark

Table 3. Location of visual loss by anatomic site

Refractive error (requires glasses or contact lenses)
  Myopia
  Astigmatism
  Hyperopia
	Vitreous
	  Vitreous hemorrhage (due to trauma)

	Retina
	  Retinal detachment
	  Retinal degeneration—macular
	    degeneration
	  Macular dystrophy

Cornea
  Corneal opacity: trauma, metabolic, or dystrophy
  Corneal edema (glaucoma)	

Anterior chamber
  Iritis (inflammatory cells, protein)
  Hyphema (blood)
	Optic nerve
	  Optic atrophy or hypoplasia
	  Optic neuritis

Lens
  Cataract
	Cortical
	  Amblyopia
	  Cortical blindness

cated by changing etiologic factors in visual loss (Kirchner, 1988a). Incidence and prevalence figures represent estimates based on the best available data.

In the United States, the prevalence rates for legal blindness have been estimated at 1 in 1,000 children (Kirchner, 1988b). Between 30% and 70% of those with severe visual impairments have additional disabilities. In 1,067 children who were blind or had visual impairment, 62% had other educationally significant conditions (Kirchner, 1989). In a 39-year trend study in British Columbia, 64% of 576 children born with congenital ocular blindness excluding cortical visual loss had one or more associated disabilities, although in later years an increased percentage were without additional impairments (Robinson, Jan, & Kinnis, 1987).

ETIOLOGY

There are significant differences in etiology between developed and developing nations. Bilateral corneal scarring is responsible for over half the cases of childhood visual impairment in Africa but less than 1% in Europe and North America (Baird & Moore, 1993). By contrast, genetic causes are responsible for less than 10% of cases in Africa but approximately 50% in North America (Flowers, Tielsch, Enger, & Maumenee, 1993). In the developing world, preventable visual impairment often occurs in otherwise normal children from vitamin A deficiency and measles (Goldstein, 1980).

There have been temporal changes in the etiology of visual loss throughout the world. Since the rubella epidemic in 1964–1965, vaccination has markedly reduced the incidence of the congenital rubella syndrome (Cochi et al., 1989). Ophthalmia neonatorum and congenital syphilis are now rare causes of blindness. Reports in the 1980s document a resurgence of retinopathy of prematurity, primarily affecting infants with a birth weight of less than 1,000 grams (Gibson, Sheps, Schechter, Wiggins, & McCormick, 1989; Phelps, 1981). Cortical visual impairment is diagnosed more commonly now than in the past.

VISUAL PATHWAYS

The major characteristics of vision are color, binocularity (depth perception), and edge determination. Color vision is present at birth. Binocularity develops during the first weeks of life. Edge determination is the basis of visual acuity and develops to adult levels during childhood (Hoyt, Nickel, & Billson, 1982).

In the retina, rod and cone photoreceptors respond to photons of light. The macula, a small area of temporal retina containing predominantly cones, provides visual acuity. Ganglion cells in the retina integrate information from the photoreceptors and relay it through the axons of the optic nerve, transmitting a preliminary analysis of form, movement, and color of the visual image. Glutamate has been identified as an important neurotransmitter in photoreceptor, bipolar and ganglion cell function (Daw, Brienken, & Parkinson, 1989). The ganglion cell axons project to the lateral geniculate nucleus in the diencephalon and to mesencephalic nuclei, including the superior colliculus. The lateral geniculate nucleus also receives extensive input from the cortex, oculomotor centers, and reticular formation.

In the primary visual system known as the geniculo-striate system, fibers from the lateral geniculate nucleus are directed to the primary visual cortex (area 17 of Brodmann). One third to one half of these fibers provide the macular representation responsible for visual acuity. Fibers from the right side of each retina project to the right occipital cortex and those on the left to the left cortex. If there has been no disruption in this visual pathway, the brain is able to further process the visual information into a single, fused three-dimensional image. Disorders resulting in early amblyopia (e.g., congenital cataracts) can damage the fusional process irreversibly, although the acuity of the affected eye or eyes may improve with treatment.

The visual cortex has projections to many areas of the brain. Connections with the limbic system provide the emotional content to visually perceived information. Projections to the temporal cortex are involved in object recognition. Those to the parietal cortex provide spatial localization of objects and motion perception (Tusa, 1986).

There is evidence for a second visual system (extrageniculate), with ganglion fibers projecting to the superior colliculus and then through the pulvinar nucleus to parastriate cortex (areas 18–19). This system is believed to be involved with detection of movement, location of objects in space, and control of orienting responses. The site(s) of integration with the geniculostriate system are currently unknown (Jan, Wong, Groenveld, Flodmark, & Hoyt, 1986).

VISUAL DEVELOPMENT

The relative importance of genetic visual programming and environmental influences is a subject of continuing investigation. Understanding of the complexity of visual development stems from the research of Wiesel and Hubel, who demonstrated innate visual mechanisms modulated by early visual experience (Wiesel, 1982). For example, while early monocular deprivation in kittens leads to permanently altered visual function, later deprivation has little or no effect on vision.

This period of visual susceptibility has been called the critical period and is one of many ex-amples in central nervous system development where the effects of an insult depend on the timing. In children the critical period extends to 6–8 years of age, after which time visual deprivation does not lead to the visual loss associated with amblyopia.

Amblyopia has been defined as

a unilateral or bilateral decrease of visual acuity caused by form vision deprivation and/or abnormal binocular interaction for which no organic causes can be detected by the physical examination of the eye and which in appropriate cases is reversible by therapeutic measures. (von Noorden, 1977)

A difference of two lines on a visual acuity chart is the standard diagnostic criterion if the reduction is unilateral.

Amblyopia affects 1%–3% of school-age children. It may result from strabismus, anisometropia or early stimulus deprivation. Strabismic amblyopia is always unilateral and results from inhibition in retinocortical pathways from the fovea in the deviating eye. In anisometropic strabismus, where there is differing refractive power in each eye, the amblyopia may result from the anisometropia, the associated strabismus, or both. Amblyopia ex. anopsia is a unilateral or bilateral stimulus deprivation amblyopia, resulting from disuse or understimulation of the retina. It may result from congenital cataracts, severe ptosis, or corneal opacities (von Noorden, 1985). Children with developmental disabilities are at increased risk for strabismus, which if untreated may progress to amblyopia.

VISUAL FUNCTION AND ASSESSMENT

Preterm Infants

The development of vision begins prior to birth, with rapid maturation during infancy. The visual abilities of the human infant have been extensively studied in premature and term infants by tests of motor function and perception.

Optokinetic nystagmus emerges at 29–30 weeks' postconceptual age (Allen & Capute, 1986). It is commonly employed as a simple bedside tool to assess the integrity of the visual pathways. A drum with alternating black and white stripes is rotated in front of the baby with both eyes open or one eye covered. A positive response is horizontal jerk nystagmus, with the fast component opposite to the direction of rotation. There is both a subcortical and a cortical system involved in the generation of optokinetic nystagmus. Although the absence of optokinetic nystagmus is always of concern, a positive response does not guarantee that the cortical pathways are intact. An optokinetic response may be seen in infants with no calcarine cortex and those who are cortically blind, presumably generated from the subcortical system.

Other aspects of visual function in the premature infant have been well studied. Subcortical responses, including the blink response to light, develop at approximately 25 weeks' gestational age. Pupillary constriction to light begins between 29 and 31 weeks. Using the techniques of Fantz and Brazelton, Dubowitz and colleagues demonstrated the presence of discriminative visual function by 31–32 weeks' postconceptual age. However, there was little correlation between these two techniques in individual infants (Dubowitz, Dubowitz, Morante, & Vergote, 1980).

Research in the 1990s suggests that early visual experience in the low-risk preterm infant may not have a beneficial effect on visual development (Atkinson & Van Hof-van Duin, 1993). Morante and co-workers reported that visual function of maturing preterm infants and newborns of comparable postmenstrual age was comparable up to 36 weeks of age. However, by 40 weeks' postconceptual age, premature infants did not perform as well as term infants (Morante, Dubowitz, Levine, & Dubowitz, 1982). The issue of visual experience is confounded by risk factors, including intraventricular hemorrhage, hypoxia, and hypotension, that may affect the development and function of visual pathways.

Term Infants

At term, an infant's eyes are usually hypermetropic (farsighted), although as many as 25% may be myopic (nearsighted) (Cook & Glasscock, 1951). Although visual acuity is usually maximal near 18 cm, this may vary with accommodative ability as well as the testing paradigm used to assess acuity. Term newborns may

demonstrate pattern preference, fix and follow visual stimuli, and show optokinetic nystagmus.

Exodeviations are a normal finding in the newborn. In a study of 1,219 normal newborns, 33% were exotropic, 49% orthotropic, 3% esotropic, and 15% unclassified (Nixon, Helveston, Miller, Archer, & Ellis, 1985). The total incidence of constant and intermittent exotropia was 31% in a smaller comparison group of healthy premature infants examined near term. It was concluded that divergence may be normal at birth and that, over the first months of life, orthophoria develops as visual pathways mature.

The postnatal development of the anatomic structures and visual function progresses rapidly. Macular maturation begins in midgestation and continues until 4 months or later. Cone function is present at birth and well developed by 6 months. Accommodation reaches adult levels by 4 months. Binocular alignment develops within 3–4 weeks of life, corresponding to the development of the macula and increased power of accommodation. Depth perception is well developed by 4 months of age.

Optokinetic nystagmus, the ability to fix and follow, preferential looking paradigms, visual evoked potentials, pupillary responses, and eye movements have all been used to assess visual function in term infants. The responses may be influenced by attentional factors and vary according to state. Furthermore, the usefulness of visual evoked potentials is limited because the anatomic site of an abnormal response cannot be determined.

Using optokinetic nystagmus and preferential looking paradigms, neonatal visual acuities have been estimated to be between 20/400 and 20/800. In studies using visual evoked potentials, higher infant acuities have been reported (Hoyt, Nickel, & Billson, 1982). These differences may be due either to technique or to differing visual pathways being assessed.

The Teller cards utilize preferential looking to assess visual acuity between birth and 3 years in children with normal development and with developmental delay. The cards have black and white stripes of varying widths. Using a preferential looking paradigm involving patterned versus homogeneous stimuli, the finest stripe on which an infant preferentially fixates is a measure of visual acuity (Teller, McDonald, Preston, Sebris, & Dobson, 1986). Reported benefits of Teller cards include speed, accuracy, and a design that allows more objective judgment of individual subject responses (Mohn, van Hof-van Duin, Fetter, de Groot, & Gage, 1988).

In older studies, early visual abilities were reported to be predictive of later cortical function and neurologic integrity (Brazelton, Scholl, & Robey, 1966; Miranda, Hack, Fantz, Fanaroff, & Klaus, 1977). However, it is now believed that visual function as assessed by pattern preference and visual evoked potentials during the first months of life may be subcortically mediated and is not an index of cortical integrity (Dubowitz, Mushin, DeVries, & Arden, 1986). The predictive validity of novelty preference paradigms used in infancy has also been questioned.

Early Childhood

An accurate measure of visual function can often be obtained from parental report. In the toddler and preschooler, observing the child's response to visually interesting toys of various sizes is a valuable clinical assessment tool. This can provide useful information that may be otherwise difficult to obtain.

The formal assessment of visual function in the preschool child can be divided into objective tests requiring minimal cooperation (discussed above) and subjective tests in which active participation is needed. A key element is the time the examiner spends to obtain reliable results. If a unilateral visual loss is suspected, that eye should be tested first when cooperation is more likely to be optimal.

Subjective tests include the STYCAR Test, the Sonksen system, Allen cards, and Snellen letters. Mary Sheridan designed the STYCAR Tests to assess visual function in children older than 6 months who could not respond verbally and in those with impairments limiting responses (Sheridan, 1969). These tests utilize single-letter cards, charts, miniature toys, and graded white balls. More recently, Hyvarinen (the LH system) and Sonksen (the Sonksen Silver Acuity System) have utilized Sheridan's work to establish tests of visual function.

The Allen cards (Figure 1) are designed for children who can identify line pictures. They are used at 20 feet or less, giving a best acuity of 20/30. The Allen picture cards will usually give a higher acuity in the child between ages 4 and 6 than do the Snellen letters.

The Snellen chart is the most commonly utilized standard for children who can identify letters. The chart has 9 lines of letters, corresponding to visual acuities from 20/10 to 20/200. Snellen testing may underestimate visual acuity because some children may not read the letters if they lack confidence in their responses.

Vision screening tests identify children with refractive errors and amblyopia. Recognizing that many screening instruments have low specificity (Romano, 1990), clinicians should retest all children who fail an initial screening test prior to referral to an ophthalmologist. However, regardless of test results, an ophthalmological evaluation is warranted if the caregiver has persistent concerns about a child's visual function.

CLINICAL ASSESSMENT

The majority of blind children or children with significant visual impairment are identified in infancy on the basis of concerns by caregivers or clinicians (Hall & Hall, 1988). The presenting concern of visual loss should include an evaluation for ocular pathology, other central

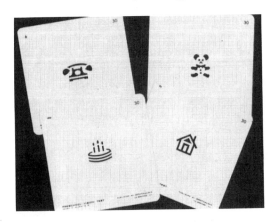

Figure 1. Allen cards are commonly used to test vision in young children. After the examiner determines that a child can correctly identify each picture, a distance determination is made for each eye individually using the cards sequentially (see text).

nervous system abnormalities, and findings suggestive of a systemic disorder. Children with a wide range of nonprogressive or progressive disorders with associated visual impairment may be seen by a primary care provider, developmental pediatrician, or pediatric neurologist for initial evaluation. Alternatively, an ophthalmologist may make the initial diagnosis of visual impairment, with referral to a clinician for comprehensive evaluation. In either case, it is important that the clinician be able to assess the degree of visual impairment and recommend appropriate diagnostic studies and habilitative evaluations.

A careful history from caregivers about visual function and ocular alignment should be obtained (Table 4). During the first 12–18 months of life, the most accurate assessment of visual abilities is usually obtained from caregivers, who have observed the child in many settings over time.

On examination, there are a number of signs, including visual inattentiveness, nystagmus, strabismus, and anatomic ocular asymmetry, that should alert the clinician to examine the eyes carefully. As part of the examination, the globes should be examined for microphthalmia, buphthalmos, or megalocornea. The iris may be absent (aniridia) or show a coloboma. A delayed or sluggish pupillary response suggests retinal or optic nerve disease. Extraocular mobility should be ascertained, as well as the presence or absence of nystagmus. The Hirshberg (pupillary light reflex) or cover–uncover test can be utilized to look for strabismus. By 3 months of age, infants should track in all directions and manifest a visual threat reponse.

In any child with strabismus, the evaluation should include the type of deviation, whether amblyopia is present, and whether there is associated ocular or systemic pathology (Fielder, 1989). The management of strabismus will vary by etiology, but treatment should include correction of any refractive error or amblyopia prior to surgical intervention. Any child presenting with esotropia in the first months of life should be promptly referred for ophthalmologic evaluation because the esotropia may be the presenting sign of a cataract or retinoblastoma.

Nystagmus occurring in the first months of life often heralds significant visual impairment. It has traditionally been divided into sensory and motor types, with sensory nystagmus being more common (Gelbart & Hoyt, 1988). Sensory nystagmus signifies an afferent defect in the neural control of ocular fixation and may be due to bilateral opacities of the cornea or lens, macular scars, macular hypoplasia as seen in albinism or aniridia, optic nerve hypoplasia, or retinal abnormalities such as achromatopsia or Leber congenital amaurosis. Motor nystagmus is thought to be due to a defect in the efferent control of eye movement. Ocular defects associated with motor nystagmus include mild refractive errors.

Children with sensory and motor nystagmus will frequently have a null point where the oscillations are minimized. They will often head turn to maintain the null point in the straight-ahead position to maximize distance acuity. Those with motor nystagmus will have better near vision than distance vision because convergence dampens the nystagmus (Burde, Savino, & Trobe, 1992). In any child with nystagmus, acuity should be assessed without blurring the fellow eye because further reductions in visual acuity will occur in the tested eye through occlusion of the fellow eye.

Minimal ophthalmoscopic evaluation should include the determination of a red reflex and an examination of the posterior pole, including optic nerve, retinal vessels, and macula. An absent red reflex (leukocoria) signifies corneal, lenticular, or vitreoretinal opacity. Common causes of leukocoria include cataracts, retinal detachment, coloboma, and retinoblastoma. The differential diagnosis of cataracts is extensive, and beyond the scope of this chapter (Table 5). Colobomas and optic nerve hypoplasia have been associated with midline central nervous system lesions, including those leading to endocrine dysfunction.

Table 4. Useful questions for assessing visual function

1. What can your child see? For example, can he or she see a brown M&M on a brown carpet? Reach for a cookie? Pick up a Cheerio?
2. Does your child have to turn his or her head to see best?
3. Are your child's eyes ever crossed? Do they ever jiggle or dance?
4. In what lighting situations does your child see best? Can he or she play after dark?

Table 5. Etiology of congenital and juvenile cataracts

Isolated hereditary cataracts (autosomal dominant, autosomal recessive, X linked)

Cataracts as part of a syndrome or systemic disease
1. Chromosomal disorders
   a. Down syndrome (trisomy 21)
   b. Edwards syndrome (trisomy 18)
   c. Patau syndrome (trisomy 13)
2. Metabolic disorders
   a. Albright pseudohypoparathyroidism
   b. Fabry disease
   c. Galactokinase deficiency
   d. Galactosemia
   e. Homocystinuria
   f. Lowe oculocerebrorenal syndrome
   g. Myotonic dystrophy
   h. Refsum disease
   i. Wilson disease
3. Skin diseases
   a. Congenital ectodermal dysplasia
   b. Incontinentia pigmenti
   c. Ito syndrome
   d. Rothmund-Thomson syndrome
   e. Werner syndrome
4. Mandibulofacial syndromes
   a. Hallermann-Streiff syndrome
   b. Pierre Robin syndrome (rarely)
   c. Rubinstein-Taybi syndrome (rarely)
5. Connective tissue and skeletal syndromes
   a. Conradi syndrome
   b. Marfan syndrome
   c. Syndromes with dislocated lenses
   d. Bone dysplasias
6. Renal disease
   a. Alport syndrome
   b. Lowe oculocerebrorenal syndrome
7. Central nervous system disease
   a. Marinesco-Sjogren syndrome
   b. Sjogren syndrome

Cataracts associated with ocular abnormalities
1. Aniridia
2. Microphthalmia
3. Norrie disease
4. Persistent hyperplastic primary vitreous (nongenetic)
5. Peters anomaly
6. Retinal degenerations
7. Sclerocornea

Postinflammatory congenital cataracts
1. Cytomegalovirus
2. Herpes simplex
3. Rubella
4. Other viral diseases during early pregnancy

Others
1. Hypoglycemia
2. Neonatal hypocalcemia
3. Retinoblastoma
4. Retinopathy of prematurity (retrolental fibroplasia)
5. Uveitis

Children with leukocoria should be promptly referred to an ophthalmologist.

Ophthalmologists have a number of instruments for diagnosis and management. In addition to an assessment of visual acuity, which may range from fix and follow function to Snellen testing, a standard examination includes a measure of intraocular pressure, retinoscopy, a slit lamp examination, and indirect ophthalmoscopy. If required, an examination may be done under anesthesia to get a more sustained view of relevant ocular structures or a measure of intraocular pressure.

Children with visual impairment should be referred to appropriate agencies responsible for providing early intervention services. In Maryland, the Maryland School for the Blind provides outreach services for children with suspected or confirmed visual impairment that can assist in the development of an individualized family service plan or an individualized education program, depending on the child's age. After a comprehensive assessment to best determine needs, an educational program is formulated to encourage sensorimotor development, orientation and mobility skills, language and communication, cognitive development, self-help skills, and social-emotional development.

Depending on age and visual function, referral to a low vision clinic may be beneficial. Ideally a low vision clinic should include ophthalmologists, optometrists, social workers, psychologists, orientation and mobility specialists, and others experienced with low vision services, working together to encourage the child to make the best use of residual vision. The assessment of functional vision should include distance and near acuity, visual fields, visual abilities and needs, and lighting. The clinic should provide a variety of habilitation and rehabilitation services, including optical aids.

ANATOMIC CLASSIFICATION

Visual impairment may be classified anatomically or by etiology. When an anatomic classification is used, the lateral geniculate body is often used to divide children with visual impairment into anterior and posterior pathway groups. There are important distinguishing features between the two groups.

Anterior pathway abnormalities include refractive errors as well as anterior segment, retinal and optic nerve findings. Pupillary reactions may be sluggish or nonreactive. Retinal disorders such as Leber congenital amaurosis may lead to digital manipulation of the eyes (eye pressing) (Jan et al., 1983). Lesions in the anterior visual pathways occurring during the first year of life with reduced visual acuity often lead to fixation (sensory) nystagmus.

By contrast, children with postgeniculate pathology may have either complete absence of visual function (cortical blindness) or, more commonly, a variable visual loss termed cortical visual impairment. The latter group are visually inattentive but may not act like "blind" children. When shown several items for identification, these children may correctly recognize each item presented individually but not when presented as a group (Jan, Groenveld, Sykanda, & Hoyt, 1987). Their visual function may fluctuate over time.

Ophthalmological examination may be normal or show an associated optic nerve atrophy. If the ocular examination is normal, pupillary reactions are normal. While fixation nystagmus is absent, there may be various other types of nystagmus, such as cerebellar nystagmus. If there is associated ocular pathology, the child may have a fixation nystagmus.

In some disorders where there is both anterior and posterior pathway involvement, these distinctions do not hold. For example, preterm infants may have both retinopathy of prematurity and injury to optic radiations or striate cortex (Hoon et al., 1988).

ETIOLOGIC CLASSIFICATION

Visual impairment may be classified into etiologic groups: 1) genetic disorders, 2) prenatal, 3) perinatal, and 4) postnatal causes. Environmental insults, including infections, hypoxia–ischemia, trauma, toxins, and increased intracranial pressure, can damage the visual pathways during various stages of development, with timing, location, and intensity affecting the severity of visual loss (Jan, 1993).

In North America, optic atrophy, microphthalmia, retinopathy of prematurity, cortical blindness, nystagmus, hereditary retinopathy, and congenital cataracts are common causes of visual impairment (Flowers et al., 1993). As was discussed previously, infectious and nutritional disorders are more common in developing nations.

Both the anatomic location and the onset of the visual loss can provide important etiologic clues. When a child presents with visual impairment of unknown cause, the initial steps in evaluation are to utilize history for insights into timing and to categorize the visual loss by location using physical examination. This will guide the etiologic workup and may provide information as to recurrence risk.

Because the majority of children with significant visual impairment present during the first year of life, it is important to know the differential diagnosis of "the blind infant." A useful division is into a group with primarily ocular/central nervous system involvement and a group with systemic disorders with ocular abnormalities. Important ocular causes (some of which may have associated central nervous system abnormalities) include Leber congenital amaurosis, optic atrophy, microphthalmia, nystagmus, congenital cataracts, retinopathy of prematurity, and optic nerve hypoplasia. Systemic causes include albinism, galactosemia, Marfan syndrome, storage diseases with corneal clouding, and mitochondrial and peroxisomal disorders. Cortical visual impairment may present without ocular or systemic abnormalities. Findings in many of these disorders are discussed later in this chapter.

Genetic Etiologies

Genetic causes of visual impairment include single-gene disorders; chromosomal deletions, rearrangements, and nondisjunctions; mitochondrial DNA abnormalities; and syndromes of unknown etiology. As many as 50% of legally blind children may have an underlying genetic cause (Bateman, 1983). Formal genetic consultation should be obtained in recognized hereditary ocular conditions such as aniridia, or if there are dysmorphic features or major malformations in addition to ocular pathology.

Advances in molecular biology have led to the gene localization for a number of ocular diseases to specific loci on nuclear and mitochondrial DNA. The chromosomal localization for retinoblastoma (13q14), aniridia (11p13), color blindness (Xq28), Norrie disease (Xp11.3), and some forms of autosomal dominant retinitis pigmentosa (3q) have been established. The mitochondrial 16-kB circular DNA has been sequenced. Mitochondrial disorders with point mutations (Leigh syndrome: nucleotide 8993) and deletions (Kearns-Sayre syndrome) have ocular abnormalities and significant visual impairment.

Aniridia is a complex ocular malformation with iris hypoplasia or absence, cataracts, foveal hypoplasia, and glaucoma. It may be inherited as an autosomal dominant trait with high penetrance or be found with an interstitial deletion on chromosome 11, mental retardation, and Wilms tumor. Visual acuity ranges from 20/30 to less than 20/200 (Helveston & Ellis, 1984).

Albinism includes a number of conditions affecting melanin metabolism, including oculocutaneous albinism; ocular albinism; and syndromes associated with albinism, some of which have abnormalities in the P gene (Lee et al., 1994). Ocular abnormalities include macular and optic nerve hypoplasia, nystagmus, reduced visual acuity, and translucent irides, as well as commonly associated refractive errors and strabismus for which close ophthalmologic follow-up is important (O'Donnell, 1984). The oculocutaneous forms are inherited as autosomal recessive traits. In ocular albinism, the pigmentary abnormalities are limited to the eye and may be inherited as an autosomal recessive or an X-linked trait. In all types, intelligence is normal.

There are several syndromes with albinism and associated developmental disorders. These include Waardenburg syndrome (autosomal dominant with partial albinism and deafness), Chediak-Higashi syndrome (autosomal recessive with mental retardation and immune defects), and Hermansky-Pudlak syndrome (autosomal recessive with bleeding disorder and pulmonary fibrosis).

The term *retinitis pigmentosa* includes a large number of retinal dystrophies with variable patterns of inheritance and dystrophy of the photoreceptors and pigment epithelium. A number

of mutations in the rhodopsin gene on the long arm of chromosome 3 have been identified in autosomal dominant retinitis pigmentosa (Dryja, 1992). There are numerous syndromes and systemic disorders with pigmentary retinal dystrophy and developmental disabilities. These include peroxisomal diseases (e.g., Zellweger syndrome and Refsum disease); mitochondrial diseases (e.g., Kearn-Sayre); Bardet-Biedl, and Laurence-Moon syndromes (Green et al., 1989; Schachat & Maumenee, 1982); neuronal ceroid lipofuscinosis; mucolipidoses; sphingolipidoses; Bassen-Kornzweig syndrome (abetalipoproteinemia); Hallervorden-Spatz syndrome; Usher syndrome; and Leber congenital amaurosis (Helveston & Ellis, 1984).

In the infant with signs of severe visual impairment, sluggish pupillary responses, and nystagmus, Leber congenital amaurosis should be considered. This designation covers a group of disorders with autosomal recessive inheritance, some of which may have associated mental retardation, deafness, seizures, and neurologic deterioration (Schroeder, Mets, & Maumenee, 1987). The retina may be normal or show a retinitis pigmentosa–like picture. The visual loss is severe but not progressive. The hallmark is a very abnormal or absent electroretinogram.

The neuronal ceroid lipofuscinoses represent a group of neurodegenerative conditions affecting the eye with progressive blindness and central nervous system deterioration. Depending on the age of onset, the disorder may be termed infantile, late infantile (Jansky-Bielschowsky), or juvenile (Batten disease). The diagnosis may be made by electron microscopic examination of a conjunctival biopsy (Francois, 1982).

Lowe syndrome is an autosomal recessive condition with congenital cataracts, glaucoma, hypotonia, mental retardation, rickets, and aminoaciduria (Tripathi, Cibis, Harris, & Tripathi, 1982). Alport syndrome has lenticonus, retinal dystrophy, sensorineural hearing loss and progressive interstitial nephritis (Govan, 1983). In Alport syndrome, the inheritance pattern is unclear, and either autosomal dominant with a sex influence or X-linked recessive is postulated.

The phakomatoses have associated ocular findings with both diagnostic and visual significance. In addition to the characteristic skin lesions, children with neurofibromatosis may have learning disabilities or mental retardation. The diagnosis is often confirmed by the presence of Lisch nodules, which are small iris hamartomas best seen by slit lamp examination. In tuberous sclerosis, as many as 50% of the patients will have fundus lesions, including retinal hamartomas. In ataxia–telelangectasia, which usually presents with progressive ataxia, cognitive impairment, and oculomotor apraxia, telangiectasias may subsequently appear on the bulbar conjunctiva. Sturge-Weber syndrome may have glaucoma and choroidal hemangiomas.

The cornea and retina are particularly vulnerable in metabolic (storage) diseases. Mucopolysaccharide, amino acid, and lipid disorders all may lead to corneal clouding and have associated central nervous system dysfunction, including mental retardation and seizures. Inheritance is varied and biopsy is often required to make the diagnosis. Storage diseases affecting the retina include the mucopoly/saccharidoses, mucolipidoses, and sphingolipidoses (Scriver, Beaudet, Sly, & Valle, 1989). The mucolipidoses and sphingolipidoses may have a cherry-red spot on ophthalmologic examination. This sign results from the storage of lipids in ganglion cells, obscuring the underlying red hue of the choroid except in the macular area, which has no ganglion cells. In these conditions, physical and mental deterioration are common.

Down syndrome is the most common of the chromosomal aberrations with associated ocular pathology. Common findings include strabismus, nystagmus, keratoconus, cataracts, severe myopia, astigmatism, glaucoma, and ptosis. Periodic ophthalmologic follow-up is recommended in this syndrome (Shapiro & France, 1985). Ocular findings do not correlate with the severity of the mental retardation (Ginsberg, Ballard, Buchino, & Kinkler, 1980).

Trisomy 13 is more often associated with microphthalmia and coloboma than trisomy 18. Ocular findings in Turner syndrome may include strabismus, cataract, and ptosis.

Mitochondrial disorders may have retinal dystrophy and optic atrophy. Recently, deletions in the 16-kB mitochondrial genome have been linked to the multisystem disorder Kearn-Sayre syndrome. This syndrome includes progressive external ophthalmoplegia, pigmentary retinopathy, heart block, sensorineural deafness, cerebellar ataxia, and mental impairment. It occurs sporadically with age of onset prior to 20 years. Relationships between the variably sized deletion, clinical presentation, and course remain to be determined (Moraes et al., 1989).

Finally, in syndromes of unknown etiology, Cornelia de Lange is often associated with significant visual impairment from optic atrophy, optic nerve colobomas, microcornea, and myopia. There are no characteristic ocular findings in Rett syndrome.

Prenatal Etiologies

Recognized nongenetic prenatal causes of visual impairment are commonly infectious (cytomegalovirus; toxoplasmosis; and, less commonly, rubella, herpes, and syphilis). Congenital cytomegalovirus infection—the most common congenital viral infection, occurring in 1% of newborns—may cause active chorioretinal inflammation with vitreous haze, retinal edema, and hemorrhage leading to chorioretinal atrophy. Toxoplasmosis may result in retinochoroiditis with focal atrophic and pigmented scars and destructive lesions in the macula. Rubella is associated with a "salt and pepper" retinopathy, cataracts, glaucoma, and microphthalmos. Later complications of congenital viral infections include mental retardation, autism, behavioral disturbances, sensorineural deafness, and cerebral palsy. Although herpes simplex usually presents as a perinatally acquired disease, it may also occur as an intrauterine infection with chorioretinitis, microphthalmia, and severe central nervous system malformations. Congenital syphilis is a rare cause of acute choroiditis in the infant.

As a teratogen, alcohol may have prenatal ocular effects in addition to effects on growth and cognition. In addition to small palpebral fissures and ptosis, corneal opacities, optic nerve hypoplasia, and retinal vascular tortuosity have been reported (Stromland, 1987).

Perinatal Etiologies

The most common etiologic risk factors of perinatally acquired visual impairment are related to two conditions: 1) hypoxia–ischemia in both the preterm and term infant and 2) hyperoxia in the premature infant. Hypoxia–ischemia may result in infarction of the optic radiations and/or visual cortex. Depending on the extent of injury, there may be cortical visual impairment or cortical blindness (Good et al., 1994).

Premature birth and the need for supplemental oxygen has been associated with retinopathy of prematurity (retrolental fibroplasia) since the 1950s. Acute complications include vitreal neovascularization and subtotal or total retinal detachment. Late complications include strabismus, myopia, dragging of the macula, retinal detachment, and acute glaucoma. The publication of an international classification of retinopathy of prematurity and the encouraging early results of cryotherapy represent attempts to control this often unpredictable disease of very immature infants (Cryotherapy Cooperative Group, 1988).

Postnatal Etiologies

Acquired visual impairment includes genetic and nongenetic visual loss in a child who previously had normal sight (Robinson & Jan, 1993). Nongenetic postnatal ocular disorders may result from a number of causes, the most common of which are accidents, infections, and tumors.

In the nongenetic group, the most common ocular finding is optic atrophy. In a review of 218 children seen at a tertiary neuro-ophthalmologic referral center with optic atrophy, the cause was tumors in 29% of cases, inflammation in 17%, trauma in 11%, unknown in 11%, hereditary in 9%, perinatal disease in 9%, hydrocephalus without tumor in 6%, neurodegenerative disease in 5%, and other in 4% (Repka & Miller, 1988). In other referral groups, the etiology of optic atrophy may be more likely to be genetically determined, including Leber optic atrophy or Kjer juvenile optic atrophy.

The human immunodeficiency virus (HIV) may have a wide spectrum of effects on the eye in the adult, some of which are treatable. Cotton wool spots are the most common ocular finding. A variety of viral, bacterial, fungal, and parasitic agents may infect the eye (Ai & Wong, 1988). As treatment modalities improve, children with HIV survive longer and may be afflicted with similar ophthalmologic problems.

VISUAL IMPAIRMENT IN SPECIFIC DISABILITIES

Delayed Visual Maturation

Delayed visual maturation is a term used to describe an infant presenting with visual impairment who subsequently demonstrates improved visual function. It is often considered in the infant more than 8 weeks of age who, despite normal pupillary reactions and eye movements, shows no signs of visual function. Although this condition often signifies broader central nervous system dysfunction, children with these signs have been described who subsequently developed without evidence of visual loss, mental retardation, or other disabilities (Mellor & Fielder, 1980). Delayed visual maturation has been subclassified into three groups with prognostic significance: 1) isolated; 2) with associated persistent neurodevelopmental abnormalities; and 3) with ocular abnormalities, including nystagmus (Tresidder, Fielder, & Nicholson, 1990).

In infants with a history of visual inattentiveness, a full developmental workup with ophthalmologic consultation should be obtained promptly. An anatomic or functional abnormality in the anterior visual pathway should be excluded. If there is no significant history (especially in the perinatal period) and no abnormalities on examination, then the delay may resolve without intervention, although close developmental surveillance is required. If significant findings are present, then appropriate interventions should be instituted.

Mental Retardation

The child with mental retardation has an increased incidence of anterior visual pathway pathology as well as cortical visual impairment. Many single-gene, chromosomal, multifactorial, and idiopathic genetic conditions leading to mental retardation have known ocular associations. If the cause is known, specific references should be sought for information on potential visual problems. In any child with unexplained cognitive delay or mental retardation, a thorough ophthalmologic assessment should be included in the initial workup, from both an etiologic and a habilitative perspective.

Children with mental retardation may have abnormalities in the anterior or posterior visual pathways or both. Recognized associations include an increased incidence of refractive errors, strabismus, and nystagmus as well as anatomic abnormalities such as cataracts, optic atrophy, microphthalmos, tapetoretinal degeneration, chorioretinitis, and ptosis (Bankes, 1974; Warburg, 1975). The prevalence of blindness or visual impairment in children with mental retardation ranges from 5% to 14%, with the most severe visual problems in those children with lowest intellectual function (Tuppurainen, 1983).

Cerebral Palsy

Many children with cerebral palsy will have associated ocular problems similar to those found in children with mental retardation (Black, 1980). These include a 15%–62% incidence of strabismus and a 50%–92% incidence of ocular abnormalities, with amblyopia, optic atrophy, nystagmus, and refractive errors being most common (Hiles, Wallar, & McFarlane, 1975).

There may be fluctuations between esotropia and exotropia in children with cerebral palsy (von Noorden, 1985). Although controversy remains over the optimal timing of strabismus surgery in these children, it does not appear that the timing of surgery affects either cosmetic appearance or functional outcome. The overall approach taken should be similar to that in unaffected children, with treatment of amblyopia and refractive errors prior to contemplation of surgical intervention (Fielder, 1989).

Cortical Visual Impairment

Cortical visual impairment may be congenital or acquired and either transient or permanent. Cortical visual loss may be total or vary in degree and setting as described previously. In the latter case, *cortical visual impairment* may be a more appropriate term (Whiting et al., 1985). Because of the varied visual deficits in individual children, there is no classification of the functional impairments.

Attempts at anatomic location have been mixed. Visual evoked responses have not been useful. Neuroimaging studies showing dilatation of the posterior horns as well as loss of brain tissue in the occipital cortex have been reported, but the ultimate visual outcome may not correlate with the observed pathology. Visual evoked potential mapping may be helpful in assessing cortical visual function in the future.

Transient cortical visual loss has been described following seizures, head injury, and meningitis. In cases of meningitis, immediate-onset visual loss has a better prognosis than visual loss acquired later in the course of the illness. Permanent cortical visual impairment may occur on a prenatal, perinatal, or acquired basis. When it is the result of malformation or intrauterine infection, mental retardation is usually present.

In one series of 50 children with cortical visual impairment, of whom 10 had prenatal causes (5 brain dysgenesis), 20 a perinatal etiology (15 asphyxia), and 20 acquired causes (7 shunt, 5 trauma), 34 had associated mental retardation, 6 had specific learning disabilities, and 10 had developmental delay. Thirty of these children had associated anterior visual abnormalities, the most common of which was optic nerve atrophy. Associated neurologic problems included cerebral palsy, mental retardation, and seizures (Whiting et al., 1985).

Children with hypoxic neurologic injury should be examined by an ophthalmologist. These children may have anterior pathway pathology as well as cortical visual loss.

FAMILY COUNSELING

Families often get their first information about visual impairment from a physician (Teplin, 1988). Taking an optimistic tone and focusing on factual content during the counseling is critical, because these will be remembered long after the visit. Ideally this information should be provided over more than one counseling session, because most families will remember little that is said after hearing the words "visual impairment" or "blindness." Although "visual impairment" is the preferred term, parents should also hear the word *blindness* because this remains a common public perception of these children.

In counseling, the clinician should answer questions involving etiology frankly and emphasize that development will continue, even with blindness and other disabilities that may be present. Myths about blindness, including the idea that to use residual vision is damaging, should be dispelled so that the child is encouraged to use vision to the best possible advantage. The importance of early intervention services and parent education should be discussed.

Answering questions about the acquisition of specific developmental milestones can be difficult. Although many of the milestones in the child with isolated visual impairment are known, in the child with multiple disabilities the clinician must be more circumspect in predicting cognitive, motor, and psychosocial outcome.

As with all developmental impairments, answers should include realistic expectations and hope. For example, it should be emphasized that the child with visual impairment is like any other child, requiring love, affection, understanding, and patience. The child with visual impairment will need to be shown how to do things. Depending on other impairments, the child may or may not be curious and may or may not be able to ask questions. The clinician should remember that the child will not develop an awareness of severe visual impairment either until informed of this disability or until he or she develops the realization of peer difference.

Timing is a key factor. The concept of anticipatory guidance must be carefully tailored to the individual family and child. At some point the child with glaucoma and his or her family must be made aware of the possibility of enucleation of the eye, especially if it becomes painful without relief. Likewise, the family of a child with retinopathy of prematurity should be informed of the risk and warning signs of retinal detachment and acute glaucoma.

EFFECTS ON THE CHILD

Visual impairment can produce barriers in the range and variety of childhood experiences in mobility and in interactions with others (Lowenfeld, 1975). A person with blindness must compensate by using other sensory modalities to learn form and function as well as to develop the concept formation necessary to permit generalization from the specific to the more general situation. (For example, will the child know that the shape of water is determined by its container?)

To move, a blind person must integrate position sense (orientation) with the ability to move (mobility). In the sighted population, orientation is effortless and automatic. Without sight, orientation and movement require the integration of many subtle auditory, olfactory, tactile, and kinesthetic cues. A congenitally blind child has only these senses with which to work. A person who has been adventitiously blinded relies on the same sensory cues within the context of visual memory of movement and locale.

Mobility may be facilitated with a sighted guide, a guide dog, or a prescription cane. Most blind people use a cane for mobility, although they may rely on a sighted guide in some situations, such as in a crowd. The cane has a white aluminum or Fiberglas shaft. It is fitted by a mobility specialist for height, stride, length, and comfort. The disadvantage of a cane is that it does not protect the person's upper body from overhanging objects such as branches or signs.

To qualify for a guide dog, a blind person must be 16 years of age or older and in good health, with at least average intelligence and good hearing. A dog is trained to protect the person's upper body and permits greater speed.

The child with visual and cognitive impairments faces additional obstacles. For example, with a relative lack of concept formation, the child may have learned a route map between two places but be unable to chose an alternative route in the presence of an obstacle.

Socialization represents a child's maturation from being self-centered to being socially conscious. It includes the acquisition of social skills such as eating and dressing as well as the development of interpersonal relationships. Environmental limitations on a blind child include the inability to recognize nonvisual cues in social situations as well as the reactions of others. These sensory restrictions may foster self-orientation and thereby inhibit normal socialization.

COGNITION AND EDUCATION

Cognitive development in a blind child differs from that in a sighted child. Mastering concepts such as huge, tiny, or fragile, which are primarily visually based, can be difficult. Cognition can be affected by the age of onset, the severity, and the cause of blindness.

The assessment of cognition in children with visual impairment and blindness is difficult because this is a heterogeneous population in terms of both etiology and associated impairments. Professionals who assess children with visual impairment should be cognizant of differences in cognitive development in these children and cautious in test interpretation.

Traditionally, children with visual impairment were educated in schools for blind persons. The trends in least restrictive environment have led to the increased inclusion of these children into general classrooms, with support services and instruction as required.

CONCLUSIONS

The assessment of a child with visual impairment requires rigorous attention to etiology and habilitative needs. Ongoing developmental surveillance is required to provide appropriate guidance for the many issues each child and family will face. Visual impairment requires adaptations by the child and caregivers to maximize the child's potential. As in other developmental disabilities an interdisciplinary approach with good communication between family and professionals will facilitate this result

REFERENCES

Ai, E., & Wong, K.L. (1988). Ophthalmic manifestations of AIDS. *Ophthalmology Clinics of North America, 1,* 53–61.

Allen, M.C., & Capute, A.J. (1986). Assessment of early auditory and visual abilities of extremely premature infants. *Developmental Medicine and Child Neurology, 28,* 458–466.

Atkinson, J., & Van Hof-van Duin, J. (1993). Visual assessment during the first years of life. In A.R. Fielder, A.B. Best, & M.C.O. Bax (Eds.), *The management of visual impairment in childhood* (Clinics in Developmental Medicine, No. 128, pp. 9–29). London: MacKeith Press.

Baird, G., & Moore, A.T. (1993). Epidemiology. In A.R. Fielder, A.B. Best, & M.C.O. Bax (Eds.), *The management of visual impairment in childhood* (Clinics in Developmental Medicine, No. 128, pp. 1–8). London: MacKeith Press.

Bankes, J.L.K. (1974). Eye defects of mentally handicapped children. *British Medical Journal, 2,* 533–535.

Bateman, J.B. (1983). Genetics in pediatric ophthalmology. *Pediatric Clinics of North America, 30,* 1015–1031.

Black, P.D. (1980). Ocular defects in children with cerebral palsy. *British Medical Journal, 281,* 487–488.

Brazelton, T.B., Scholl, M.L., & Robey, J.S. (1966). Visual responses in the newborn. *Pediatrics, 37,* 284–290.

Burde, R.M., Savino, P.J., & Trobe, J.D. (1992). *Clinical decisions in neuro-ophthalmology* (2nd ed., pp. 289–295). St. Louis: Mosby-Year Book.

Cochi, S.L., Edmonds, L.E., Dyer, K., Greaves, W.L., Marks, J.S., Rovira, E.Z., Preblud, S.R., & Orenstein, W.A. (1989). Congenital rubella syndrome in the United States, 1970–85. *American Journal of Epidemiology, 129,* 349–361.

Cook, R.C., & Glasscock, R.E. (1951). Refractive and ocular findings in the newborn. *American Journal of Ophthalmology, 34,* 1407.

Cryotherapy Cooperative Group. (1988). Multicenter trial of cryotherapy for retinopathy of prematurity: Preliminary results. *Pediatrics, 81,* 697–706.

Daw, N.W., Brienken, W.J., & Parkinson, D. (1989). The function of synoptic transmitters in the retina. *Annual Review of Neuroscience, 12,* 205–225.

Dryja, T.P. (1992). Doyne lecture: Rhodopsin and autosomal dominant retinitis pigmentosa. *Eye, 6,* 1–10.

Dubowitz, L.M.S., Dubowitz, V., Morante, A., & Verghote, M. (1980). Visual function in the preterm and fullterm newborn infant. *Developmental Medicine and Child Neurology, 22,* 465–475.

Dubowitz, L.M.S., Mushin, J., DeVries, L., & Arden, G.B. (1986). Visual function in the newborn infant: Is it cortically medicated? *Lancet, 1,* 1139–1141.

Fielder, A.R. (1989). The management of squint. *Archives of Disease in Childhood, 64,* 413–418.

Flowers, B., Tielsch, J., Enger, C., & Maumenee, I. (1994, May). Prevalence and causes of blindness among Canadian children [Abstract]. Presented at the annual meeting of the Association for Research in Vision and Ophthalmology, Sarasota, FL.

Foster, A. (1988). Childhood blindness. *Eye, 2*(Suppl.), 13–18.

Francois, J. (1982). Metabolic tapetoretinal degenerations. *Survey of Ophthalmology, 26,* 293–333.

Gelbart, S.S., & Hoyt, C.S. (1988). Congenital nystagmus: A clinical perspective in infancy. *Graefe's Archives of Clinical and Experimental Ophthalmology, 226,* 178–180.

Gibson, D.L., Sheps, S.B., Schechter, M.T., Wiggins, S., & McCormick, A.Q. (1989). Retinopathy of prematurity: A new epidemic? *Pediatrics, 83,* 486–492.

Ginsberg, J., Ballard, E.T., Buchino, J.J., & Kinkler, A.K. (1980). Further observations of ocular pathology in Down's syndrome. *Journal of Pediatric Ophthalmology and Strabismus, 17,* 166–171.

Goldstein, H. (1980). The reported demography and causes of blindness throughout the world. *Advances in Ophthalmology, 40,* 1–99.

Good, W.V., Jan, J.E., DeSa, L., Barkovich, A.J., Groenveld, M., & Hoyt, C.S. (1994). Cortical visual impairment in children. *Survey of Ophthalmology, 38,* 351–364.

Govan, J.A.A. (1983). Ocular manifestations of Alport's syndrome: A hereditary disorder of basement membranes? *British Journal of Ophthalmology, 67,* 493–503.

Green, J.S., Parfrey, P.S., Harnett, J.D., Farid, N.R., Cramer, B.C., Johnson, G., Heath, O., McManamon, P.J., O'Leary, E., & Pryse-Phillips, W. (1989). The cardinal manifestations of Bardet-Biedl syndrome, a form of Lawrence-Moon-Biedl syndrome. *New England Journal of Medicine, 321,* 1002–1009.

Hall, D.M.B., & Hall, S.M. (1988). Early detection of visual defects in infancy. *British Medical Journal, 296,* 823–824.

Helveston, E.M., & Ellis, F.P. (1984). *Pediatric ophthalmology practice* (2nd ed.). St. Louis: C.V. Mosby.

Hiles, D.A., Wallar, P.H., & McFarlane, F. (1975). Current concepts in the management of strabismus in children with cerebral palsy. *Annals of Ophthalmology, 7,* 789–797.

Hoon, A.H., Jan, J.E., Whitfield, M.F., McCormick, A.Q., Richards, D.P., & Robinson, G.C. (1988). Changing pattern of retinopathy of prematurity: A 37 year clinical experience. *Pediatrics, 82,* 344–349.

Hoyt, C.S., Nickel, B.L., & Billson, F.A. (1982). Ophthalmological examination of the infant: Developmental aspects. *Survey of Ophthalmology, 26,* 177–189.

Individuals with Disabilities Education Act of 1990 (IDEA), PL 101-476. (October 30, 1990). Title 20, U.S.C. 1400 et seq: *U.S. Statutes at Large, 105,* 587–608.

Jan, J.E. (1993). Neurological causes and investigations. In A.R. Fielder, A.B. Best, & M.C.O. Bax (Eds.), *The management of visual impairment in childhood* (Clinics in Developmental Medicine, No. 128, pp. 1–8). London: MacKeith Press.

Jan, J.E., Freeman, R.D., McCormick, A.Q., Scott, E.P., Robertson, W.D., & Newman, D.E. (1983). Eye-pressing by visually impaired children. *Developmental Medicine and Child Neurology, 25,* 755–762.

Jan, J.E., Groenveld, M., Sykanda, A.M., & Hoyt, C.S. (1987). Behavioral characteristics of children with permanent cortical visual impairment. *Developmental Medicine and Child Neurology, 29,* 571–576.

Jan, J.E., Wong, P.K.H., Groenveld, M., Flodmark, O., & Hoyt, C.S. (1986). Travel vision: "Collicular visual system?" *Pediatric Neurology, 2,* 359–362.

Kirchner, C. (1988a). *Data on blindness and visual impairment in the U.S.* (2nd ed.). New York: American Foundation for the Blind.

Kirchner, C. (1988b). National estimates of prevalence and demographics of children with visual impairments. In M.D. Wang, M.D. Reynolds, & H.J. Walberg (Eds.), *Handbook of special education: Research and practice* (Vol. 3, pp. 135–153). New York: Pergamon Press.

Kirchner, C. (1989). *Virginia database study on visually handicapped children* (Draft for NIDRR Report). New York: American Foundation for the Blind.

Lee, S-T., Nicholls, R.D., Bundey, S., Laxova, R., Musarella, M., & Spritz, R.A. (1994). Mutations of the P gene in oculocutaneous albinism, ocular albinism, and Prader-Willi plus albinism. *New England Journal of Medicine, 330,* 529–534.

Lowenfeld, B. (1975). *The changing status of the blind.* Springfield, IL: Charles C Thomas.

Mellor, D.H., & Fielder, A.R. (1980). Dissociated visual development: Electrodiagnostic studies in infants who are "slow to see." *Developmental Medicine and Child Neurology, 22,* 327–335.

Miranda, S.B., Hack, M., Fantz, R.L., Fanaroff, A.A., & Klaus, M.H. (1977). Neonatal pattern vision: A predictor of future performance? *Journal of Pediatrics, 91,* 642–647.

Mohn, G., van Hof-van Duin, J., Fetter, W.P.F., de Groot, L., & Gage, M. (1988). Acuity assessment of non-verbal infants and children: Clinical experience with the acuity card procedure. *Developmental Medicine and Child Neurology, 30,* 232–244.

Moraes, L.T., Dmauro, S., Zeviani, M., Lombes, A., Shanske, S., Miranda, A.F., Nakase, H., Bonilla, E., Werneck, L.C., Servidei, S., Nonaka, I., Koga, Y., Spiro, A.J., Brownell, K.W., Schmidt, B., Schotland, D.L., Zupanc, M., DiVivo, D.C., Schon, E.A., & Rowland, L.P. (1989). Mitochondrial DNA deletions in progressive external ophthalmoplegia and Kearn-Sayre syndrome. *New England Journal of Medicine, 320,* 1293–1299.

Morante, A., Dubowitz, L.M.S., Levene, M., & Dubowitz, V. (1982). The development of visual function in normal and neurologically abnormal preterm and fullterm infants. *Developmental Medicine and Child Neurology, 24,* 771–784.

Nixon, R.B., Helveston, E.M., Miller, K., Archer, S.M., & Ellis, F.D. (1985). Incidence of strabismus in neonates. *American Journal of Ophthalmology, 100,* 798–801.

O'Brien, R. (1980). Education of the child with impaired vision. *Pediatric Annals, 9,* 48–57.

O'Donnell, F.E. (1984). Congenital ocular hypopigmentation. *International Ophthalmology Clinics, 24,* 133–142.

Phelps, D.L. (1981). Retinopathy of prematurity: An estimate of visual loss in the United States-1979. *Pediatrics, 67,* 924–926.

Repka, M.X., & Miller, N.R. (1988). Optic atrophy in children. *American Journal of Ophthalmology, 106,* 191–193.

Robinson, G.C., & Jan, J.E. (1993). Acquired ocular visual impairment in children. *American Journal of Diseases of Children, 147,* 325–328.

Robinson, G.C., Jan, J.E., & Kinnis, C. (1987). Congenital ocular blindness in children. *American Journal of Diseases of Children, 141,* 1321–1324.

Romano, P.E. (1990). Vison/eye screening: Test twice and refer once. *Pediatric Annals, 19,* 359–367.

Schachat, A.P., & Maumenee, I.H. (1982). Burdet-Biedl syndrome and related disorders. *Archives of Ophthalmology, 100,* 285–289.

Schroeder, R., Mets, M.B., & Maumenee, I.H. (1987). Leber's congenital amaurosis. *Archives of Ophthalmology, 105,* 356–359.

Scriver, C.R., Beaudet, A.L., Sly, W.S., & Valle, D. (1989). *The metabolic basis of inherited disease* (6th ed.). New York: McGraw-Hill.

Shapiro, M.B., & France, T.D. (1985). The ocular features of Down's syndrome. *American Journal of Ophthalmology, 99,* 659–663.

Sheridan, M. (1969). Vision screening procedures for very young or handicapped children. In P. Gardiner, R. MacKeith, & V. Smith (Eds.), *Aspects of developmental and pediatric ophthalmology* (Clinics in Developmental Medicine, No. 32, pp. 39–47). London: Spastics International Medical Publications.

Stromland, K. (1987). Ocular involvement in the fetal alcohol syndrome. *Survey of Ophthalmology, 31,* 277–283.

Teller, D.Y., McDonald, M., Preston, K., Sebris, S.L., & Dobson, V. (1986). Assessment of visual acuity in infants and children: The acuity card procedure. *Developmental Medicine and Child Neurology, 28,* 779–789.

Teplin, S.W. (1988). Development of the blind infant and child with retinopathy of prematurity. The physician's role in intervention. *Birth Defects: Original Article Series, 24,* 301–323.

Tresidder, J., Fielder, A.R., & Nicholson, J. (1990). Delayed visual maturation: Ophthalmic and neurodevelopmental aspects. *Developmental Medicine and Child Neurology, 32,* 872–881.

Tripathi, R.C., Cibis, G.W., Harris, O.J., & Tripathi, B. (1982). Lowes syndrome. *Birth Defects: Original Article Series, 18,* 629–644.

Tuppurainen, K. (1983). Ocular findings among mentally retarded children in Finland. *Acta Ophthalmologica, 61,* 634–644.

Tusa, R. (1986). The visual cortex. *American Journal of EEG Technology, 26,* 135–143.

von Noorden, G.K. (1977). Mechanisms of amblyopia. *Documenta Ophthalmologica, 34,* 93.

von Noorden, G.K. (1985). *Binocular vision and ocular mobility* (3rd ed.). St. Louis: C.V. Mosby.

Warburg, M. (1975). Blindness in mentally retarded children. *Documenta Ophthalmologica, 39,* 343–349.

Whiting, S., Jan, J.E., Wong, P.K.H., Flodmark, O., Farrell, K., & McCormick, A.Q. (1985). Permanent cortical visual impairment in children. *Developmental Medicine and Child Neurology, 27,* 730–739.

Wiesel, T.N. (1982). The postnatal development of the visual cortex and the influence of environment (Nobel Lecture 1981). *Bioscience Reports, 2,* 351–377.

World Health Organization. (1980). *International classification of impairments, disabilities, and handicaps.* Geneva: WHO.

Sources of Additional Information

**American Academy of Ophthalmology
Public Education Program**
655 Beach Street
P.O. Box 7424
San Francisco, California 94109

American Foundation for the Blind
151 West 16th Street
New York, New York 10011

American Optometric Association
243 North Lindburgh Boulevard
St. Louis, Missouri 63141

American Printing House for the Blind
1839 Frankfort Avenue
Louisville, Kentucky 40206
(large print textbooks, tapes, Braille books,
and tangible aids)

Library of Congress Division of the Blind
Washington, DC 20225
(recorded poetry and literature, talking books)

**National Association for the Visually
Handicapped, Inc.**
3201 Balboa Street
San Francisco, California 94121

(large print textbooks, library material on request;
sources of information and guidance on resources for persons with visual impairments)

National Federation of the Blind
1800 Johnson Street
Baltimore, Maryland 21230

**National Society for the Prevention of
Blindness**
16 East 40th Street
New York, New York 10016

Recording for the Blind, Inc.
215 East 58th Street
New York, New York 10022
(recorded textbooks and reading materials from
elementary through college level)

Social Rehabilitation Service
Rehabilitation Services Administration
Washington, DC 20201
(information on state level relative to special
education and rehabilitation)

**U.S. Department of Health and Human
Services**
Division of Handicapped Children and Youth
Washington, DC 20225

Chapter 32

Hearing Loss

Nancy J. Roizen, M.D.

Professionals have long agreed that, in children, the earlier that a hearing loss is identified, the better the chances for remediation. In the 1982 and 1990 position statements by the Joint Committee on Infant Hearing, the committee endorsed testing the hearing of all children at risk for hearing loss in light of their asphyxia, congenital infections, family history, hyperbilirubinemia, malformations of the head and neck, meningitis, and prematurity. Even when physicians carefully followed these recommendations, they identified at most 50% of the children with hearing loss, making the average age at which professionals have identified hearing losses in children 25–30 months in the United States.

In 1990, the U.S. Department of Health and Human Services issued a report entitled *Healthy People 2000*, in which the federal government established goals to improve substantially the health of this country's citizens by the end of the decade. One of those goals was to "reduce the average age at which children with significant hearing impairment are identified to less than 12 months." Several other things have added momentum to the achievement of this goal. In 1988, Kemp described a new screening tool for evaluating hearing in infants and children, the otoacoustic emmission (OAE) (Kemp, 1988). Many of the early studies on OAE have had the drawbacks of studying small populations of high-risk children. In 1993, the Rhode Island Hearing Assessment Project (White & Behrens, 1993; White, Vohr, & Behrens, 1993) published promising preliminary studies on the use of OAE in 1,850 mainly low-risk infants from the well-baby nursery. In addition, the Rhode Island study (White et al., 1993) and other recent studies documented that the prevalence of significant hearing loss in newborns is

5–6 per 1,000, which is much higher than previous estimates of 1 per 1,000. In 1993, a National Institutes of Health Consensus Development Conference endorsed universal hearing screening prior to 3 months of age. In 1994, the Joint Committee on Infant Hearing endorsed the concept of universal hearing screening prior to 3 months of age.

Professionals have always recognized the significant effect of a severe to profound sensorineural hearing loss on the development of language and social skills. Only in the last few years, however, has research documented the significant effect of permanent unilateral hearing losses and mild to moderate hearing losses. These discoveries have supported the policy change to identify all children with unilateral and bilateral hearing losses. The effect of fluctuating hearing losses, particularly from otitis media, is controversial.

As of 1992, many states had partial or universal hearing loss identification programs, including 16 states with legislatively mandated programs, 5 with statewide programs, and 21 with individually operated birthing site programs. Most programs consisted of an initial screen with auditory brain stem response (ABR), behavioral testing, crib-o-gram, or OAE with follow-up with an ABR. Universal screening in the newborn period for hearing loss will take many years to be a reality. Until there is universal screening, early identification of such an impairment will depend largely on the physician's suspicions, a careful speech and language history, a search for risk factors, and subsequent referral for appropriate tests. With more infants being identified in the newborn period and the increased availability of early intervention, physicians should be knowledgeable about the causes and management of hearing loss. Physicians are responsible for the identification of hearing loss and its etiology and for guiding and supporting the parents through the evaluation and management of the hearing loss.

DEAFNESS

Experts do not agree as to when a hearing impairment should be classified as deafness. However, most experts would agree that a child can be considered deaf if his or her threshold for hearing across the speech frequencies (i.e., 500–2,000 cycles per second) is depressed to 80 dB in the better ear. Another criterion by which to define those children classified as deaf is to include those children who are being educated in a school or educational program for the deaf. The burden of the impairment and the need for special education for deaf children depends on several factors, including age at the onset of hearing loss, the audiologic characteristics of the hearing loss, the level of intelligence, the level of emotional stability, the presence of associated disabilities, and the ability to read lips (Table 1).

EPIDEMIOLOGY

Approximately one person in eight is a carrier of one of the many types of recessive hearing loss. The incidence of significant congenital sensorineural hearing loss (SNHL) is 1 per 1,000 births, with 4–5 more children having a hearing loss at birth. In 40%–60% of these children the SNHL is genetically based. Many more children acquire SNHL after birth, with 3% exhibiting some degree of hearing impairment by age 3. At 5 years of age, 10%–15% of children fail their hearing screen.

IDENTIFICATION OF HEARING LOSS

In the neonatal period, the indicators for an evaluation for sensorineural or conductive hearing loss or both, as described by the Joint Committee on Infant Hearing, have been refined in their 1994 position statement and include the following:

1. A family history of hereditary childhood sensorineural hearing loss

2. Congenital infections known to be associated with hearing loss
3. Craniofacial anomalies
4. Birth weight less than 1,500 g
5. Hyperbilirubinemia at a serum level requiring exchange transfusion
6. Ototoxic medications
7. Bacterial meningitis
8. Apgar score of 0–4 at 1 minute or 0–6 at 5 minutes
9. Mechanical ventilation for 5 days or longer
10. Stigmata of a syndrome known to include hearing loss

If all children with these risk factors are tested in the neonatal period, 20% of the newborn population would be tested. Of the children with hearing loss with risk factors, 40% have a family history of childhood hearing impairment and 25% have risks related to their neonatal intensive care unit experience, such as hyperbilirubinemia, with the remainder in other categories. When all children are screened for a hearing loss at birth, 68% of those identified with a hearing loss have risk factors and 32% are without risk factors.

Identification of a moderate to profound SNHL usually is made at an average age of 23 months; suspicions and concerns of parents usually are voiced an average of 12 months prior to this. Identification of milder losses frequently is made by age 3 or 4, and of unilateral or high-frequency losses by age 5 or 6. Early identification of hearing loss has important implications for speech therapy, amplification, educational placement, and behavior problems. The time-table for identification has changed little since the early 1970s despite advances in technology that enable accurate identification of children with hearing loss, the general thrust toward early identification of developmental disabilities, and the legal access to appropriate education brought by PL 94-142, the Education for All Handicapped Children Act, later reauthorized as the Individuals with Disabilities Education Act (IDEA, PL 101-476).

The importance of early identification of hearing loss cannot be overemphasized. The language experience of the early years is critical to the child's future learning capabilities. Once

Table 1. Degrees of hearing impairment

Level of hearing loss (Hz)	Description	Etiology	Sounds heard	Degree of disability	Possible needs
15–25 dB	Slight hearing loss	Serous otitis perforation, monmeric membrane sensorineural loss, tympanosclerosis	Hears vowel sounds clearly; may miss unvoiced consonant sounds	Mild auditory dysfunction in language learning	Hearing aid, lip reading, auditory training, speech therapy, preferential seating
25–40 dB	Mild hearing loss	Serous otitis perforation, tymphanosclerosis, monmeric membrane sensorineural loss	Hears only some louder-voiced speech sounds	Auditory learning dysfunction, mild language retardation, mild speech problems, inattention	Hearing aid, lip reading, auditory training, speech therapy
40–65 dB	Moderate hearing loss	Chronic otitis, middle ear anomaly, sensorineural loss	Misses most speech sounds at normal conversational level	Speech problems, language retardation, dysfunction, inattention	All of the above plus consideration of special classroom situation
65–95 dB	Severe hearing loss	Sensorineural or mixed loss from a sensorineural loss plus middle ear disease	Hears no speech sounds of normal conversation	Severe speech problems, language retardation, learning dysfunction, inattention	All of the above plus probable assignment to special classes
More than 95 dB	Profound hearing loss	Sensorineural or mixed loss	Hears no speech or other sounds	Severe speech problems, language retardation, learning dysfunction, inattention	All of the above plus probable assignment to special classes

Adapted from Northern and Downs (1974).

a hearing loss has been identified, much work must be done educationally, communicatively, audiologically, and medically. Research on early intervention programs for children with hearing loss confirms significantly higher levels of expressive language skills in children who receive early intervention relative to children for whom intervention was begun after age 3.

Prior to a diagnosis of hearing loss, parents most frequently complain of hearing-related problems such as a lack of response to speech and noise, followed by poor speech development. Less frequent complaints include behavior problems, such as inattention and hyperactivity, and problems related to the ears, such as infection, balance problems, and some ear fingering. Identification of the hearing loss is often delayed because of several factors. Sometimes the physician reassures the parents that the problem is mild and will go away. In up to 30%

of some series, the diagnosis of another developmental problem such as aphasia, mental retardation, learning disability, or emotional disturbance was made, thus delaying the identification of hearing loss. Children with developmental disabilities have an increased incidence of hearing loss (Table 2). The diagnosis can also be delayed because the physician lacks the knowledge that newer techniques can identify hearing loss at birth.

Critical to the early identification of children with hearing loss is obtaining a good language developmental history. Standardized historical scales, such as the Receptive-Expressive Emergent Language (REEL) Scale and the Clinical and Linguistic Auditory Milestone Scale (CLAMS), provide a quick, easy method of identifying language delays early. Because little expressive and receptive language competence is observed in the physician's office, a standardized historical scale is the preferred method of evaluation. The differential diagnosis for language delay includes autism, elective mutism, hearing loss, mental retardation, and primary language disorder (see Chapters 15, 22, and 23, this volume). Any child with a language delay or a lack of age-appropriate speech clarity should have a formal audiologic evaluation to rule out hearing loss. The infant vocalizations of the child with a significant SNHL include early babbling and are normal expressively until about 6–8 months of age. However, the expected 9-month milestones of imitation of sounds and response to his or her own name are not achieved.

Even if universal screening of infants becomes a reality, not all hearing loss will be present in the newborn period. The Joint Committee on Infant Hearing (1994) recommends hearing

evaluation when the following indicators are present:

1. Parent concern regarding hearing, speech, language, and/or developmental delay
2. Bacterial meningitis and other infections associated with sensorineural hearing loss
3. Head trauma associated with loss of consciousness or skull fracture
4. Stigmata or other findings associated with a syndrome known to include a sensorineural or conductive hearing loss or both
5. Ototoxic medication use
6. Recurrent or persistent otitis media with effusion for at least 3 months

The Joint Committee on Infant Hearing (1994) recommends a hearing evaluation every 6 months until age 3 years and at appropriate intervals thereafter in the following groups:

1. Groups with delayed onset sensorineural hearing loss
   a. family history of hereditary childhood hearing loss
   b. history of in utero infection (e.g., cytomegalovirus, rubella, syphilis, herpes, or toxoplasmosis)
   c. neurofibromatosis type II and neurodegenerative disorders
2. Groups associated with conductive hearing loss
   a. recurrent or persistent otitis media with effusion
   b. anatomic deformities and other disorders that affect eustachian tube function
   c. neurodegenerative disorders

HEARING EVALUATION

The peripheral auditory system includes the external auditory canal and tympanic membrane, the middle ear space and mechanical conduction system (ossicles and middle ear muscles), and the inner ear (cochlea and organ of Corti). Acoustic impedance (tympanometry) provides objective information on the status of the tympanic membrane and middle ear conductive mechanism. Behavioral pure-tone threshold audiometry reflects hearing sensitivity and, to a degree, the status of the middle ear and the

Table 2. Prevalence of hearing impairments in children with developmental disabilities

Disability	Percent with hearing impairment
Cerebral palsy	15.0
Developmental delay	4.6
Down syndrome	78.0
Mental retardation	3.0
Speech delay	1.0
Unclear speech	9.0

cochlea. Evoked OAEs also reflect hearing sensitivity but, more specifically, the status of the cochlea. The central auditory system includes the VIIth cranial nerve, the central auditory pathways through the brain stem to the radiations to the cortex, and the auditory areas of the temporal lobe. ABR provides objective information on hearing sensitivity, especially in infants, young children, and otherwise untestable patients. In addition to being a test of auditory function, ABR is at the same time a test of the neurologic integrity of the central auditory pathways at the level of the brain stem. An absent or reduced ABR can reflect loss of hearing sensitivity caused by middle ear, cochlear, or retrocochlear pathology; however, an abnormal ABR in the presence of normal hearing thresholds suggests possible central auditory nervous system dysfunction.

Evaluation Methods

There are several methods available to evaluate a child for hearing loss. These methods include ABR, behavioral play audiometry, OAE, and typanometry.

Auditory Brain Stem Response The ABR noninvasively measures the electrophysiologic responses of the brain stem auditory pathways to an acoustic stimulus. The response is obtained from a scale-derived electroencephalogram. Auditory stimuli are collected, averaged, and evaluated by a self-contained computer. The limitations of the ABR are as follows: 1) it tests primarily high-frequency sound ranges; 2) it is more expensive than other methods, in part because it requires professionally trained personnel and expensive equipment; 3) it usually requires sedation to place the child in the proper state; 4) it does not test behavioral responses to sound; and 5) in a child who has a neurologic impairment, it may not determine the child's hearing status. The positive aspects of the ABR include that it can determine the presence of a hearing loss (unilateral or bilateral); the degree of the loss; the frequencies of the loss; and usually whether the loss is sensorineural, conductive, or mixed. The ABR can test near-threshold stimuli, detecting mild losses. Because the response is physiologic, it is not affected by behavior or most commonly

used drugs. This is important for therapeutic interventions, prognosis, and directing an evaluation of the etiology.

Behavioral Play Audiometry Behavioral play audiometry uses visual reinforcement audiometry (VRA) and play conditioning techniques to quantify the child's response to different types of sound. VRA can yield relatively precise information about auditory sensitivity in typically developing infants as young as 6 months of age and in children up to 3 or 4 years. On the positive side, VRA gives the examiner an indication of the child's functional hearing. On the negative side, however, VRA may not represent the child's true hearing abilities and does not distinguish a conductive from a sensorineural hearing loss. Another limitation of VRA is that it tests the hearing in the better ear, and thus can miss a significant unilateral hearing impairment.

Otoacoustic Emission Otoacoustic emissions, or Kemp's echoes, are sounds that originate from the cochlea and can be detected in the external ear canal. Emissions of acoustic energy from the cochlea, whether spontaneous or evoked, are known collectively as OAEs. Spontaneous OAEs have little clinical utility, but evoked OAEs have considerable clinical potential as an infant screening test or method to differentiate cochlear from retrocochlear pathology. The presence of OAEs is indicative of a normally functioning cochlea. Obstruction of the outer ear canal with cerumen or a middle ear condition can interfere with or prevent detection of OAEs. OAE results in the first 24 hours of life are not always reliable.

Tympanometry A tympanogram does not test hearing but is used in conjunction with the tests described above to determine the mobility of the tympanic membrane and the possible contribution of fluid in the middle ear to a conductive hearing loss. The results in the first 6 months of life must be viewed with caution, however, in light of incorrect readings caused by the mobility of the ear canal.

Selection of Evaluation Method

The method chosen to evaluate the hearing of a child depends on several factors. An audiologist would use the OAE as a screening tool in the newborn period followed by the ABR for children failing the OAE. In children older than newborns, the initial method of evaluation of hearing status depends on the child's age, the possible etiology, and the degree of cooperation. Children who should undergo an ABR include those who are younger than 5 months of age, recovering from meningitis, uncooperative, or giving inconsistent responses to sound field and earphone evaluations. For children between 5 months and 3 years old who cannot cooperate with earphone testing, and in whom there are no indications for ABR, behavioral play audiometry is indicated. Earphone testing for children who can cooperate can identify unilateral responses and give specific information as to the degree and character of a hearing loss in all frequencies. Its limitations are that it depends on cooperative behavior with consistent responses and cannot distinguish a sensorineural from a conductive loss.

ETIOLOGY

The identification of a specific etiology for a hearing loss facilitates optimal management (Table 3) (Nadol, 1993). When a cause for the hearing loss is identified, parents seem relieved. In different types of SNHL, the high incidence of other organ involvement and the hereditary factors make identification of an etiology important (Paparella, Fox, & Schachern, 1989). A specific diagnosis—such as Usher syndrome, with its progressive visual loss, or Pendred syndrome, with its thyroid dysfunction—can facilitate the anticipation of associated deficits and their appropriate management. Facilitating the anticipation of the progression of hearing loss is important for amplification adjustment and for parent counseling. Occasionally, medical or surgical intervention may be helpful, as with syphilis or Alport syndrome (renal transplant). Knowledge of a specific etiology contributes to selecting the most appropriate habilitation alternatives.

The establishment of an etiology is especially important for genetic counseling in light of the high percentage of children whose hearing loss is hereditary (Arnos, Israel, Devlin, & Wilson, 1992). A careful history and physical examination will lead to the diagnosis of 60% of cases. The evaluation then becomes a process of excluding causes of SNHL with indicated laboratory tests and an ophthalmologic evaluation.

Bacterial Meningitis

Bacterial meningitis is the leading cause of acquired SNHL in infancy and childhood, accounting for 9% (Hotchkiss, 1989) of all cases of severe sensorineural hearing deficits. The SNHL with meningitis tends to be an isolated defect and is the most common persisting neurologic sequela of meningitis, occurring as a complication in about 10% (Fortnum, 1992) of cases. The incidence of hearing loss caused by bacterial meningitis has decreased as a result of several preventive measures. The use of *H. influenzae* B vaccine has decreased the incidence of meningitis by an estimated 50%–85%. The introduction of cephalosporins for the treatment of meningitis has decreased the incidence of hearing loss. Whether the treatment of meningitis with dexamethasone has decreased the incidence of hearing loss is controversial.

The literature on tuberculous meningitis comes from the early 1960s, when treatment included intramuscular and intrathecal streptomycin. The reported prevalence of SNHL in children who had tuberculous meningitis varied between 5% (Lorber, 1961) and 37% (Lincoln, Sordillo, & Davies, 1960) with some researchers reporting an additional 15% incidence of high-frequency loss. Ototoxic treatment may have contributed to the high incidence of SNHL. Studies indicate that the SNHL in meningitis develops within the first 48 hours of admission (Kaplan, Catlin, Weaver, & Feigin, 1984; Vienny et al., 1984). Studies of children with bacterial meningitis indicate that the number of days of symptoms before hospitalization and institution of antibiotic therapy does not correlate with the development of SNHL (Dodge et al., 1984).

Congenital Infections
and Other Viral Infections

Congenital infections account for about 10% of SNHL. Neonatal hearing loss is caused by a virus in 1 out of every 1,700 births. About 1%–2% of newborns are infected with cytomega-

Table 3. Etiologies of deafness

Cardiac

CHARGE (C and/or SN)

Jervell and Lange-Nielsen syndrome (AR) (SN)

Kartagener syndrome (C) (AR)

Kawasaki disease (SN)

Klipple-Feil sequence (C and/or SN)

Mitral insufficiency, joint fusion, and hearing loss (AD)

Noonan syndrome (SN)

Trisomy 13 syndrome (SN)

Turner syndrome (SN)

Degenerative

Friedreich ataxis

Huntington disease

Myoclonic epilepsy

External ear malformations

Ear malformation and conductive hearing loss (AD)

Malformed low-set ears and conductive hearing loss (AR)

Otofaciocervical abnormalities (AD)

Preauricular pits and neural hearing loss (AD)

Thickened ears and incudostapedial abnormality (AD)

Hereditary with no associated anomalies

Congenital moderate hearing loss (AR)

Congenital neural deafness (SL)

Congenital severe deafness (AD)

Congenital severe deafness (AR)

Early-onset neural deafness (AR)

Early-onset neural deafness (SL)

Low-frequency hearing loss (AD)

Midfrequency hearing loss (AD)

Moderate hearing loss (SL)

Otosclerosis (AD)

Progressive nerve deafness (AD)

Unilateral nerve deafness (AD)

Infectious

Bacterial

Acute meningitis (SN)

Otitis media (SN and/or C)

Pertussis (SN)

Streptococcal (scarlet fever) (SN)

Tuberculosis (SN)

Typhoid (SN)

Prenatal

Cytomegalovirus (SN)

Herpes simplex (SN)

Rubella (SN and/or C)

Syphilis (SN)

Toxoplasmosis (SN)

Viral

Adenovirus 3 (SN)

Infectious   *(continued)*

Herpes zoster (SN)

Infectious mononucleosis (SN)

Mumps (SN)

Rubella (SN)

Rubeola (SN)

Varicella (SN)

Viral encephalitis (SN)

Integumentary system disease

Albinism and congenital deafness (AD)

Anhidrosis and progressive hearing loss (AD)

Atopic dermatitis and neural hearing loss (AR)

Hereditary piebaldness and congenital deafness (AR?)

Keratopachydermia, digital constrictions, and deafness (AD)

Knuckle pads, leukonychia, and hearing loss (AD)

Leopard syndrome (lentigines and congenital deafness) (SN) (AD)

Onchodystrophy and congenital deafness (AD)

Onychodystrophy and deafness (AR)

Onychodystrophy, coniform teeth, and hearing loss (AD)

Onchodystrophy, digital abnormalities, and deafness (AR)

Pigmentary abnormalities and congenital deafness (SL)

Pilitorti and hearing loss (AR)

Pilitorti and hearing loss (AR?)

Senter syndrome (SN)

Vitiligo, congenital deafness, muscle wasting, and achalasia (AR)

Waardenburg syndrome (SN) (AD)

Metabolic and endocrinologic diseases

Alport syndrome (progressive renal impairment and deafness)

Diabetes mellitus, optic atrophy, and perceptual hearing loss

Goiter, increased protein-bound iodine, stippled epiphyses, and deafness (AR)

Hunter syndrome (SN and/or C) (SL)

Hurler syndrome (SN and/or C) (AR)

Hypoglycemia

Hypoproteinemia

Hypothyroidism (SN)

Kernicterus (SN)

Maroteaux-Lamy mucopolysaccharidosis (SN) (AR)

Morquio syndrome (SN) (AR)

Pendred disease (goiter and deafness) (AR)

Pyridoxine dependency

Refsum disease (AR)

Tay-Sachs disease (AR)

Thiamine dependency

(continued)

Table 3. *(continued)*

Metabolic and endocrinologic diseases *(continued)*

Wilson disease (AR)

Neoplastic

Leukemia

Neurofibromatosis

Neurologic

Acoustic neuromas (AD)

Photomyoclonus, hearing loss, diabetes, and nephropathy (AD)

Richards-Rundel disease (deafness, mental deficiency, ataxia, and hypogonadism) (AR)

Sensory radicular neuropathy (AD)

Other malformation syndromes

Camurati-Engelmann syndrome (SN) (AD)

Cleidocranial dysostosis syndrome (SN) (AD)

Diastrophic dysplasia syndrome (C) (AR)

Ectodermal dysplasia (SL)

EEC syndrome (AD)

18q syndrome (C)

Facioauriculovertebral spectrum (Goldenhar syndrome) (C)

Fanconi pancytopenia (SN) (AR)

Frontometaphyseal dysplasia syndrome (C and/or SN) (SL)

Frontonasal dysplasia sequence

Hag-Wells syndrome

Johanson-Blizzard syndrome (SN) (AR)

Killian/Teschler-Nicola syndrome (SN)

Langer-Giedion syndrome (SN)

Laurence-Moon-Biedl syndrome (AR)

Levy-Hollister syndrome (C and/or SN) (AD)

Melnick-Fraser syndrome (AD)

MURCS association (SN)

Nager syndrome (C)

Oculodentodigital syndrome (AD)

Progeria (SN)

Saethre-Chotzen syndrome (SN) (AD)

Scheie syndrome (SN) (AR)

Shprintzen syndrome (velocardiofacial syndrome) (C) (AD)

Townes (SN) (AD)

Trisomy 8S

Prenatal toxic syndromes

Fetal alcohol syndrome (SN)

Fetal iodine deficiency effect (SN)

Fetal methyl mercury effects (SN)

Fetal trimethadione effects

Renal

Alport disease (nephritis and hearing loss) (AD)

Branchio-otorenal (BOR) syndrome (C and/or SN) (AD)

Renal, genital, and middle ear anomalies

Urticaria amyloidosis, nephritis, and hearing loss (AD)

Skeletal disease

Absence of tibia and deafness (AR)

Albers-Schönberg disease (osteopetrosis) (SN) (AR)

Cranialmetaphyseal dysplasia (SN) (AD and AR)

Crouzon syndrome (SN) (AD)

Engelmann disease (progressive diaphyseal dysplasia) (AR)

Multiple synostoses syndrome (C) (AD)

Oralfaciodigital (OFD) syndrome II (Mohr syndrome) (C) (AR)

Otopalatodigital syndrome (C) (X-linked, semidominant)

Paget disease of bone (osteitis deformans) (AD)

Proximal symphalangism and hearing loss (AD)

Pyles disease (craniometaphyseal dysplasia) (AD)

Sclerosteosis (SN) (AR)

Split hand and foot syndrome (AR)

Treacher-Collins syndrome (C) (AD)

Van Buchen disease (hyperostosis corticolis glueralisata) (AR)

Trauma

Acoustic trauma

Hypoxia

Skull fracture

Visual system

Alstrom disease (SN) (AR)

Cockayne syndrome (SN) (AR)

Familial hearing loss, polyneuropathy, optic atrophy (AR and SL)

Marshall syndrome (SN) (AD)

Myopia and hearing loss (AR)

Myopia, hearing loss, peripheral neuropathy, and skeletal abnormalities (AD)

Optic atrophy, hearing loss, and juvenile diabetes (AR)

Retinal changes, deafness, muscular wasting, and mental retardation (AR)

Saddle nose, myopia, cataracts, and hearing loss (AD)

Stickler syndrome (C and/or SN) (AD)

Usher syndrome (SN) (AR)

Adapted from Hawkins (1977), Jones (1988), Konigsmark (1969a, 1969b, 1969c), Konigsmark and Gorlin (1976), and Northern and Downs (1974).

Key: AD, autosomal dominant; AR, autosomal recessive; C, conductive; SL, sex linked; SN, sensorineural.

lovirus (CMV), with congenital infection from herpes simplex, rubella, syphilis, and toxoplasmosis occurring less often. The neonatal period is the easiest time to diagnose congenital infection by available tests, but 90% of neonates infected with CMV, 50% infected with congenital herpes simplex, 50% infected with congenital rubella, 33%–66% infected with syphilis, and 90% infected with congenital toxoplasmosis are asymptomatic. Therefore, by the time the diagnosis of SNHL is established, the diagnosis of a congenital infection frequently cannot be documented. Occasionally, physical findings, such as choreoretinitis, are helpful. A more in-depth discussion of congenital infections is located in Chapter 8 (Volume I).

Cytomegalovirus infection occurs in 0.2%–2.2% of all newborns, making it the most common congenital infection. The fetus can acquire the infection when the mother becomes infected during the pregnancy or from the mother who is seropositive prior to the pregnancy. More than 85% of congenitally infected infants are asymptomatic in the neonatal period. Of the asymptomatic group, 5% will have SNHL as a complication of the infection. Of the children with symptomatic congenital CMV, 10%–15% will exhibit symptoms such as petechiae (79%), hepatosplenomegaly (74%), jaundice (63%), intrauterine growth retardation (41%), prematurity (34%), inguinal hernia (26%), and chorioretinitis (12%). Of children who are symptomatic as newborns, 61% develop a SNHL, with 70% of the losses being bilateral, 57% progressive, and more than 50% being greater than 50 dB.

SNHL is the most common permanent complication of congenital rubella. The classic congenital rubella syndrome is characterized by congenital heart disease, deafness, eye defects, intrauterine growth retardation, mental retardation, and microcephaly. The earlier in the pregnancy the fetus is infected, the greater the chance that it will develop defects. SNHL affects 68%–93% of children with congenital rubella and is most frequently bilateral and profound, affecting all frequencies evenly, and may be progressive in some cases. In 3%–19% of children, the hearing loss is associated with blindness. Complicating the evaluation of a possible SNHL is the increased incidence in the congenital rubella population of central auditory imperception. This is the inability at the cortical level to respond appropriately to sound.

Congenital infection of the fetus occurs in 0.4% of the children of mothers with syphilis. The signs and symptoms of congenital infection are divided into early manifestations, which emerge in the first 2 years, and late manifestations, which emerge anytime thereafter. In the first 2 years, symptoms include hepatosplenomegaly (91%), anemia (64%) and other hematologic aberrations, jaundice (49%), skin rashes (31%), bony changes (20%), and snuffles (12%). Late manifestations are the result of persistent, active disease that causes inflammation and scarring. In the 3% of children with hearing loss from congenital syphilis, the onset may be sudden and accompanied by vertigo, occurring at ages 8–40 years.

Rubeola, congenital toxoplasmosis, and congenital herpes infections can also be complicated by SNHL. Congential toxoplasmosis occurs between 1 in 4,000 and 1 in 40,000 births. At birth, 90% of the cases are asymptomatic. Of the 10% who are symptomatic, 20% develop SNHL. When treated with antibiotics, the percentage of children with SNHL decreases significantly.

Mumps is an acute contagious disease caused by a paramixovirus that has a predilection for glandular and nervous tissue. The clinical manifestations of mumps include salivary gland inflammation and, less commonly, epididymoorchitis, meningoencephalitis, and pancreatitis. A rare complication of mumps is irreversible, unilateral SNHL secondary to neuritis of the auditory nerve. The SNHL usually develops suddenly and is heralded by the onset of vertigo (48%), tinnitus (57.9%), ataxia, and vomiting.

Iatrogenic Factors in the Neonatal Intensive Care Unit

The development of a SNHL is one of the many recognized complications in a high-risk premature infant. The neonatal intensive care unit (NICU) experience accounts for the etiology of about 17% of children with SNHL, and between 2% and 10% of NICU graduates exhibit SNHL. The potential factors to be considered as contributing to a SNHL include apnea, central nervous system bleeding, congenital infections, hyperbilirubinemia, hypoxia, ototoxic drugs, meningitis, and noise pollution. The possibility of the synergistic effects of two or more of these factors is difficult to measure or analyze.

In studies of the factors most frequently found in NICU graduates with SNHL, hypoxia consistently appears as a major factor in predicting high risk for SNHL. A difficult delivery is found 3.8 times as often, and a 5-minute Apgar score of 6 or less is found 7.6 times as often, among NICU graduates with SNHL than among NICU graduates without SNHL. Fully one third of the children with SNHL are of low birth weight associated with hypoxia.

An increased incidence of hyperbilirubinemia appears in children with a NICU experience showing a course complicated by a SNHL. In the presence of hyperbilirubinemia, specific aberrations appear in ABRs that improve after exchange transfusion with the establishment of a normal bilirubin level. Most studies of NICU graduates find that premature babies with a total bilirubin increased to 14 mg/dl have an increased risk of SNHL 2.5 times greater than that of children without hyperbilirubinemia. In children with hyperbilirubinemia, adverse perinatal factors, such as a longer mean duration of hyperbilirubinemia (48 vs. 24 hours), acidosis, and lower birth weight, increased the association with SNHL.

The contribution of NICU ototoxic drug use to the development of SNHL is unclear. The ototoxic drugs used in the NICU associated with SNHL are aminoglycosides such as gentamycin and kanomycin and diuretics such as furosemide. However, studies that have examined the use of aminoglycosides in the NICU have not found it to be a significant neonatal predictor of SNHL (Bergman et al., 1985; Finitzo-Hieber, McCracken, & Brown, 1985; Simmons, 1980).

Concerns remain about the intensity of continuous noise levels produced in the incubators. The baseline continuous noise level in infant incubators is 50–68 dB. Slamming of incubator doors and infant crying raise the noise level to 90–100 dB. Animal studies have documented the potentiation of noise-induced hearing loss by the ototoxic aminoglycosides (Falk, 1972). A clinical study looking at this association in the NICU concluded that there was no evidence

that noise had affected the hearing of the very low birth weight infants (Abramovich, Gregory, Slemick, & Stewart, 1979).

Ototoxic Drugs

Hearing loss from ototoxic drugs is an infrequent but preventable cause of SNHL in children. These drugs (Table 4) may permanently injure or destroy the hair cells of the cochlea, creating SNHL. Exposure to some drugs causes irreversible SNHL, whereas other drugs cause hearing loss that is reversible once the drug is stopped. With drugs excreted by the kidney, increase of drug levels to the ototoxic range is more likely to be complicated by hearing impairment. There appears to be both idiosyncratic and genetic susceptibility to ototoxic drugs. The hearing impairment caused by drugs is usually bilateral, symmetrical, and of varying severity.

The ingestion of ototoxic drugs by pregnant women can result in hearing loss to the fetus of prenatal origin. The drugs most commonly associated with prenatal hearing impairment include chloroquine, quinine, streptomycin, salicylate, and thalidomide. The period in gestation when the use of ototoxic medications is most likely to cause damage to the auditory system is in the first trimester, especially in the sixth and seventh weeks. In hearing loss secondary to exposure to ototoxic drugs, otologic anomalies have included aplasia of the inner ear, outer and inner hair cell damage, middle ear anomalies, absence of the

Table 4. Ototoxic drugs and substances known to cause SNHL

Acetylsalicylic acid	Mercury
Alcohol	Neomycin
Aminoglycosides	Nitrogen mustard
Analine dyes	Nortryptaline
Arsenic	Pharmacetin
Carbon monoxide	Polybrene
Chloramphenicol	Polymixin B
Chloroquine phosphate	Quinine
Cisplatin	Ristocetin
Deferoxamine	Salicylates
Dihydrostreptomycin	Streptinomycin
Ethacrynic acid	Thalidomide
Furosemide	Vancomycin
Gold	Viomycin
Lead	

Adapted from Hawkins (1977) and Northern and Downs (1974).

VIIth and VIIIth nerves, dysplasia of the organ of Corti, and decreased number of ganglion cells. Prenatal use of ototoxic medications has been believed to cause conductive hearing loss as a result of ossicular malformation of the middle ear.

Noise-Induced Hearing Loss

Noise-induced hearing loss (NIHL) is a preventable cause of SNHL. In children, NIHL tends to be asymmetrical and high frequency (3,000–6,000 Hz) and begins in a notched audiologic pattern that evolves with continuous noise exposure to a high-frequency sloping pattern. How commonly NIHL occurs is unknown, but boys account for 90% of the cases. The most frequent cause of NIHL is fireworks and firearms, followed by loud music, recreational vehicles, and power tools and equipment. Children who live on farms are especially vulnerable in light of the noisy heavy machinery (Brookhouser, Worthington, & Kelly, 1992).

Hereditary Hearing Impairment

Hereditary hearing loss accounts for 40%–60% of hearing losses. Several characteristic elements distinguish one type from another. The means of transmission can be autosomal recessive, as with Usher syndrome; autosomal dominant, as with Waardenburg syndrome; or sex linked, as with Parker syndrome. The onset can be congenital, as in Waardenburg syndrome; occur in the teens, as in Alport syndrome; or occur in adult life, as in otosclerosis. The specific hearing frequencies involved can be genetically determined but are not pathognomonic. A hearing loss can be progressive or nonprogressive and unilateral or bilateral (see Table 3).

Autosomal recessive hearing loss accounts for as much as 40% of childhood hearing loss. Most children with autosomal recessive hearing loss will have no associated anomalies. Approximately one person in eight is a carrier of a recessive form of hearing loss. More than six different sites for autosomal recessive hearing loss have been identified. Thus, the risk among couples with autosomal recessive hearing loss of parenting children with this deficit is low. Autosomal dominant hearing impairment accounts for 15% of childhood deafness. Sex-linked syndromes account for 10% of childhood deafness.

A simple way to organize these syndromes is based on associated anomalies. The systems included would be as follows: cardiac, endocrine, external ears, integumentary, nervous, skeletal, urinary, and visual. Several types are not associated with anomalies.

Two syndromes involve cardiac anomalies and hereditary deafness. The most important of these syndromes to diagnose is Jervell and Lange-Nielsen disease, an autosomal recessive disease consisting of a prolonged QT interval and congenital neurosensory hearing loss that accounts for less than 1% of deafness in children. The hearing loss is bilateral, congenital, and sensorineural, with low frequencies preserved. The prolonged QT interval often presents in the 2- to 6-year-old group as syncopal attacks, sometimes provoked by physical or mental stress. As the child ages, the rhythm disturbances lead to loss of consciousness, convulsions, and incontinence of urine, which frequently leads to a mistaken diagnosis of epilepsy. Mortality is 33% for 3- to 13-year-olds. Diagnosis can improve the prognosis by identifying the associated cardiac defect, which is treatable. Treatment of Jervell and Lange-Nielsen disease includes decreasing stress, relieving the cardiac anomaly with digitalis or propranolol, and, if needed, performing a left cervical thoracosympathectomy–ganglionectomy. This latter procedure changes conduction patterns so that syncopal attacks become less frequent.

Of the two endocrine syndromes, the more important is Pendred syndrome, which is recessive goiter and congenital deafness. Pendred syndrome accounts for 1%–10% of hereditary deafness. Children with Pendred syndrome are born with a severe hearing loss. At puberty, a diffuse goiter usually develops with euthyroid function.

Five diseases are characterized by external ear malformations and hearing loss. Four of the five are autosomal dominant and four of the five are conductive. Congenital external ear malformations include preauricular pits, brachial fistulas, thickened ears, and flabby ears.

Eighteen syndromes involve childhood hearing loss and the integumentary system (Konigsmark, 1972). The most common of all these syndromes is Waardenburg syndrome, which is autosomal dominant and accounts for 2.3% of congenital deafness. In Waardenburg syndrome, the most common features are a widely placed medial canthus and flat nasal root with confluent eyebrows (dystrophia canthorum). Other features of Waardenburg syndrome include vestibular hypofunction (75%), congenital mild to severe bilateral or unilateral hearing loss (50%), a white forelock (20%), heterochromia iridium and loss of the epithermal pigment of the optic fundus (15%), and skin pigmentation aberrations (<10%), including vitiligo, spotting, and hypopigmentation.

Waardenburg syndrome is included in the eight syndromes that involve hearing loss and skin pigmentary changes. The other seven include dominant albinism and congenital deafness, dominant lentigines and congenital deafness, hereditary piebaldness and congenital deafness, sex-linked pigmentary abnormalities and congenital deafness, and central neurofibromatosis. In four syndromes, atopic dermatitis, keratopachydermia, digital constrictions, hydrosis, and ichthyosis are found. In five syndromes there is a combination of hearing loss and abnormalities of the fingernails and toenails, such as knuckle pads, pilitorti, leukonychia, onychodystrophy, and coniform teeth.

Three diseases are characterized by deafness associated with nervous system disease: dominant sensory radicular neuropathy; dominant photomyoclonus, hearing loss, diabetes, and neuropathy; and recessive deafness, mental retardation, ataxia, and hypogonadism (Richards-Rundel disease).

Twelve hereditary diseases link hearing impairment and disease of the skeletal system: Crouzon disease, dominant proximal symphalangism, Treacher-Collins disease, Mohr syndrome, otopalatodigital syndrome, recessive absence of tibia and deafness, recessive split hand and foot syndrome, Engelmann disease, Paget disease of bone, Albers-Schönberg disease, Van Buchen disease, and Van der Hoeve disease.

The three diseases with an association between renal disease and deafness include Alport disease; dominant urticaria with amyloidosis, nephritis, and hearing impairment; and recessive renal, genital, and middle ear anomalies. The most frequent of these, Alport disease, is autosomal dominant. The hearing impairment in this condition is associated with progressive nephritis characterized by hematuria and proteinuria that begins in the first or second decade of life. The SNHL begins at about 10 years of age. Hearing loss with this syndrome tends to progress more quickly in boys, and they are more likely to die of uremia. Ocular lens anomalies, including severe spherophakia, cataracts, and lenticonus, are found in about 10% of patients with Alport disease.

There are nine hereditary diseases in which hearing impairment and the visual system are affected. Three of these—Usher syndrome, Alstrom disease (deafness, retinitis pigmentosa, obesity, and diabetes), and Refsum disease (retinitis pigmentosa, polyneuropathy, ataxia, and hearing loss)—include retinitis pigmentosa. Three groups of hereditary diseases include myopia: myopia (dominant saddle nose, myopia, cataracts) and hearing loss; dominant myopia, hearing loss, peripheral neuropathy, and skeletal abnormalities; and recessive myopia and hearing loss. Two heredity diseases include optic atrophy: recessive optic atrophy, hearing loss, and juvenile diabetes; and familial hearing loss, polyneuropathy, and optic atrophy. One syndrome includes recessive retinal changes, deafness, muscular wasting, and mental retardation.

Usher syndrome, which consists of congenital deafness and progressive blindness caused by retinitis pigmentosa, is one of the most frequent causes of hereditary hearing loss, with a prevalence of 4.4 per 100,000 in the United States. Usher syndrome accounts for 3%–6% of children who are congenitally deaf and 1.8% of deaf school-age children, and constitutes a large percentage of deaf-blind children. Usher syndrome has at least two types, with one type having vestibular dysfunction that results in a delay in walking to 22–29 months. The first symptom after congenital deafness is blindness associated with abnormalities on electroretinogram. Usher disease, which is autosomal recessive, has no treatment, but for genetic counseling and educational planning purposes it is important to diagnose it as early as possible.

Twelve different types of hearing losses are not associated with anomalies (Konigsmark, 1969a). The six autosomal dominant types include dominant unilateral deafness, dominant low-frequency hearing loss, dominant midfrequency hearing loss, and otosclerosis. Otosclerosis is autosomal dominantly transmitted with 25%–40% penetrance, with a slow progressive, conductive, symmetrical hearing loss with onset in the second or third decade. In one survey, otosclerosis accounted for 47% of 2,000 patients attending a hearing aid distribution center. The three syndromes that are autosomal recessive include recessive congenital severe deafness, recessive early-onset neural deafness, and recessive congenital moderate hearing loss. The three sex-linked syndromes include sex-linked congenital neural deafness, sex-linked early-onset neural deafness, and sex-linked moderate hearing loss.

Heredity accounts for more cases of SNHL in children than any other etiology. Hereditary hearing loss always should be considered when a clear-cut cause for the SNHL is not apparent. Medical history, family history, and a careful physical examination that pursues associated findings as described will enable the physician to identify some of these syndromes. An ophthalmologic consultation is necessary to rule out Usher syndrome. It also has the potential of providing information to rule out or confirm other diagnoses (e.g., congenital rubella or toxoplasmosis, Alstrom disease, Refsum disease). A urinalysis to look for protein and red blood cells can rule out Alport syndrome. An electroencephalogram to look for prolonged QT interval can rule out Jervell and Lange-Nielsen syndrome. A thyroxine uptake or perchlorate discharge test can diagnose Pendred syndrome in the presence of a goiter. Negative TORCH titers can rule out specific intrauterine infections; however, positive TORCH titers are inconclusive. Most often the child with hereditary SNHL will have no associated anomalies, no family history of SNHL, and normal growth and development for a deaf child. After appropriate laboratory evaluation and consultations have been pursued, genetic counseling is indicated.

TYPES OF HEARING LOSS

Unilateral Hearing Loss

In school-age children, the prevalence of unilateral hearing loss of greater than 40 dB is 3 per 1,000; for milder losses (26–40 dB), the rate increases to 13 per 1,000. Unilateral hearing loss occurs more commonly in boys (62.3%) and in the left ear (52.5%). The most common etiology for congenital unilateral hearing impairment is heredity. The most common etiology for acquired unilateral hearing loss is mumps, with other less common etiologies including hypoxia and infections, such as cytomegalovirus, meningitis, and rubella. Although rare, a unilateral neurofibroma of the VIIIth nerve always must be considered and evaluated if no clear etiology exists. The etiology is unknown in 42%–66% of the cases examined.

The lack of a binaural auditory advantage affects children with unilateral hearing loss in several ways. First, there is a decrease in auditory threshold of 3 dB in the better ear when speech is presented monaurally as opposed to binaurally. Second, the "squelch effect" (ability of two ears to suppress background noise) is lacking. Third, binaural hearing provides the ability to localize sounds in space. How clinically significant these effects are is controversial.

Indirect evidence indicates that a longstanding unilateral hearing loss can present some educational problems. In one study of 60 children with a unilateral hearing loss of greater than 50 dB, 35% had failed one or more grades compared to 3.2% of the control population (Bess & Tharpe, 1984). Teachers considered 22.2% of the students with unilateral hearing loss to be above average academically, compared to 47.3% of the students with normal hearing. Although there were no significant differences between the two groups on the Weschler Intelligence Scale for Children–Revised (WISC–R), the WISC–R Full-Scale IQ was significantly lower in children with unilateral hearing impairment greater than 60 dB. Thus children with a unilateral hearing loss may be at risk for academic difficulties.

High-Frequency Hearing Loss

High-frequency hearing loss occurs in 14% of cases of bilateral SNHL (Matkin, 1986). Children with high-frequency hearing loss often exhibit a delay in speech development but exhibit auditory behavior unlike that usually encountered in children with hearing loss. Children with high-frequency hearing losses respond inconsistently to sound and exhibit speech and language delays that often lead to the mistaken diagnosis of mental retardation or emotional disturbance. Identification of the high-frequency hearing loss has the pattern of a bimodal time frame at either 3 or 6 years of age. Although both groups have parents who are concerned about a speech deficit at about 2 years of age, children whose hearing loss is identified at 3 years have had pure-tone testing done with a speech evaluation. Children with a hearing loss identified at 6 years have undergone informal testing and were identified by hearing screening conducted at age 6 in the school. Once the diagnosis of high-frequency hearing loss is made, two new problems are encountered. Because of the relatively good hearing in the low frequencies, the effectiveness of conventional hearing aids is limited, and fewer classes are available for children with high-frequency hearing loss. The most frequently identified specific etiologies include heredity, hypoxia, and hyperbilirubinemia. Thirty-one percent of cases have an unknown etiology.

Conductive Hearing Loss

Middle ear anomalies, and most commonly middle ear effusion, cause conductive hearing loss. Middle ear anomalies and middle ear effusion may coexist with congenital SNHL. Although the conductive hearing loss may be less severe than the SNHL, the conductive loss may muffle the sounds that are detected and, therefore, must be treated and reversed. Middle ear anomalies most often are found in children with craniofacial anomalies such as Apert syndrome, cleft plate, Crouzon syndrome, hemifacial atrophy, and Treacher-Collins syndrome, and with generalized skeletal anomalies such as Fanconi anemia. Rubella is associated with stapes fixation. Conductive hearing loss is associated with a loss of less than 60 dB, with middle ear effusion generally causing the mild-to-moderate high-frequency losses and structural anomalies causing the more severe losses in the spectrum of conductive losses. SNHL can cause a hearing loss of from 0 to 100 dB (Stewart & Downs, 1993).

Fluctuating Hearing Loss

Audiologists are expressing more concerns about the effects of hearing loss in children with chronic or recurrent otitis media with effusion. Although studies examining the long-term effects of fluctuating hearing loss in infancy are inconclusive, professionals are recommending early identification of hearing loss associated with middle ear effusion. Audiologists recommend screening of hearing, middle ear function, and communication development in children with otitis media at less than 6 months of age, in child care settings with many children, with cleft palate, and with Down syndrome. The audiologists recommend audiologic screening twice annually, once before the school year commences and a second time in the winter months.

EDUCATIONAL CONSIDERATIONS

The child with hearing loss has delayed acquisition of both expressive and receptive language skills. The normal 4-year-old has an estimated vocabulary of between 2,000 and 3,000 words, whereas the prelingually deaf child (deaf before the age of 3 years) of this age has fewer than 25 words. Deaf children who have been exposed to educational programs as infants and who have deaf parents have considerably larger vocabularies.

Deaf children usually obtain scores within the normal range on nonverbal intelligence tests (Meadow, 1975). A national sample of 1,228 deaf children obtained a mean IQ of 95.70 on the WISC–R Performance Scale (Sisco & Anderson, 1978). However, the general level of academic achievement was much below that which would be expected based on such performance. Fifty percent of children with a hearing loss of greater than 85 dB have no reading comprehension, and average reading achievement for 16-year-olds with a hearing loss is at the third or fourth grade level. Verbal tests are useful in measuring the language ability of children with hearing impairment but are inappropriate for measuring their intelligence.

How best to educate the deaf child is an area of controversy. The debate rages between the supporters of the "oral system" and the "manual system." Currently, there are several schools in deaf education. The oral school includes the auditory–verbal approach, the oral-ocular approach, and the oral–tactile approach. Included in the manual school are finger spelling, Seeing Essential English, Signing Exact English, and American Sign Language. The third approach, which integrates these approaches, is total communication.

Within the oral school, the auditory-verbal approach relies on the learning of speech through hearing alone. Through early identification (before age 2), early use of binaural aids, and intense parent participation, the use of residual hearing is optimized. This method offers the best opportunity for the acquisition of speech, better voice quality, and verbal language. However, not all children with SNHL have the appropriate home environment, are identified early enough, and are intelligent enough to make the best use of this approach. The oral-ocular approach uses limited auditory input supplemented with lip reading. A major drawback to this method is that approximately 40% of English speech sounds have the same visual characteristics but different formative and auditory characteristics. Lip reading is an art mastered by few. Because of the visual similarity of sounds, cued speech is used with the oral approach to speech and language development. Cornett (1967) at Gallaudet College developed eight cues presented to the face simultaneously with oral speech so that both forms of information could be used to interpret communication. The oral-tactile approach uses feeling the vibration of the larynx and is especially helpful for individuals with a visual loss as well as a hearing loss.

In the manual school, the finger spelling system uses a manual alphabet and duplicates spoken English by spelling each word precisely. This method takes more time but exposes the student to the correct syntax of language. Seeing Essential English (SEE–I) is a manual approach used to supplement lip reading and the auditory-verbal approach. This system attempts to make signs compatible with English by representing word parts such as prefixes, roots, or suffixes. Verb tenses are indicated by signs and grammatical endings. Signing Exact English (SEE–II) is signed as it is spoken and is thus an easier form for hearing parents. It is faster than finger spelling and easier to read. American Sign Language (Ameslan or ASL) is the manual system used most by deaf adults. It relies solely on the visual reception of the sign system. It omits articles of speech and verb tenses, making it the fastest manual method for communication. However, because the specific order does not necessarily agree with spoken English, the system does not transfer easily to writing.

Total communication uses all methods (manual communication, speech reading, and auditory training through amplification) to communicate with the child with hearing loss. The use of sign language along with speech is supposed to enhance the meaningfulness of receptive hearing and lip reading.

Educators have no accepted criteria for determining which deaf educational system is best for a particular child. Educators generally agree that children with severe hearing impairment will find it easier to learn to speak with their hands than to speak out loud. Supporters of the manual system believe that children learn more through the visual mode and thus develop a wider knowledge base. Supporters of the oral approach believe that the manual approach forces deaf children into deaf society because of their communication limitations. They point out that manual communication draws the child's attention to visual stimuli, resulting in the child's ignoring residual hearing potential and neglecting lip reading. The supporters of oral communication express concern that signing draws negative attention to the child's disability.

An educational placement evaluation should include the four areas of development (fine motor, gross motor, self-help, and language skills), as well as behavior, intelligence, and psychological testing. The choice of educational placement must take into consideration all of this information plus the age of the child, the motivation and availability of the parents, and the resources available locally. A survey of educational placements revealed that 62% of all educational programs for deaf children used the total communication approach, while the remaining 38% used the combined oral-aural approach.

Despite efforts to develop new educational techniques, deaf high school graduates consistently read at the fourth- to sixth-grade level. Several factors contribute to this low reading level. Ninety percent of deaf children have two hearing parents who are later to suspect the diagnosis, do not know sign language, and are not acquainted with the deaf community. With the increasing percentage of NICU graduates, the deaf population now has an increasing percentage of children with multiple disabilities. The educational potential of deaf children must be addressed with intensive educational efforts.

MEDICAL MANAGEMENT

The physician has two responsibilities with respect to the child with hearing loss. First, the physician should seek early identification of the hearing loss. Failure of the physician to listen to parents' concerns and not expeditiously refer the child for a definitive hearing evaluation results in many parents of deaf children harboring intense anger at their physicians. Children with hearing loss compensate for their loss by responding to visual cues and are easily missed with casual screening techniques. Only through a formal evaluation by a trained audiologist in a controlled environment can the presence of a hearing loss be determined.

The physician's second goal is to identify a likely etiology for the hearing loss. Because 40%–60% of hearing losses are genetic in etiology, early identification of a genetic etiology is important for genetic counseling. Although there are more than 150 etiologies for hearing loss, the majority fall into four groups: congenital infections (10%), meningitis (10%), NICU experiences (17%), and heredity (40%–60%). A careful history and physical, followed by indicated laboratory tests, would lead to the most likely etiology in many cases. The family history should focus on such factors as hearing loss and sudden death (Jervell and Lange-Nielsen syndrome), different colored eyes, and a white forelock (Waardenburg syndrome). Important in the prenatal history is the use of ototoxic medications and prenatal infections. The physical examination should focus on anomalies of the head and neck, goiters, skin and pigmentary aberrations, and ophthalmologic anomalies. Based on the information gained from the medical history, family history, and physical examination, laboratory exploration should be indicated. Because 40% of hearing impairment is of the autosomal recessive hereditary type, the majority of chil-

dren will exhibit no clues to the etiology from their medical history, family history, and physical examination. In this case, it is important to rule out congenital infections with TORCH titers and culture for CMV; obtain an electrocardiogram to rule out Jervel and Lange-Nielsen syndrome (prolonged QT interval); and perform an ophthalmologic evaluation, including an electroretinogram, to rule out Usher syndrome. If the results of the above evaluation indicate no specific etiology, an autosomal recessive genetic disease is the most likely etiology and a referral for genetic counseling is indicated.

The physician also needs to encourage the family to follow through on the multiple responsibilities related to the management of the child with hearing loss. This child needs hearing evaluations twice a year at least until the age of 3, followed by annual hearing evaluations throughout the child's life, to rule out a progression in the hearing loss that may be due to drugs or occult infections and may be preventable, and to identify any type of superimposed conductive loss. The parent needs to pursue an appropriate educational placement, learn sign language at a rate faster than the child, obtain follow-up for hearing aid adjustment, and seek aggressive treatment of serious otitis media that interferes with speech discrimination. The physician needs to watch for the adjustment problems that are more common in children with hearing loss and expeditiously refer for treatment. Children with hearing loss are generally behind their hearing peers in social maturity. The children most at risk are those with less adequate communication skills and those with hearing parents, both of which are factors that limit opportunities for social interaction.

ASSISTIVE DEVICES

Hearing Aids

A hearing aid is an instrument that amplifies sound to provide the listener with sufficient acoustics with which to develop speech perception ability. Hearing aids are of various kinds, including body vibrator aids, bilateral and unilateral aids, aids behind the ears, aids in eyeglasses, and aids in the ears. The hearing aid can be adjusted to select the appropriate frequency to amplify. The quality of sound and clarity perceived through a damaged hearing apparatus may be distorted, however.

The audiologist fits the child with hearing aids and provides ongoing evaluation and habilitation work to help the child use the aids most effectively. Determination of the appropriate kind of aid will depend on the home and educational environment, the configuration of the hearing loss, the degree of loss, and the age of the child. A close, ongoing relationship with an experienced audiologist must be developed to maximize the child's use of the hearing aid over time. The audiologist teaches the parents to care for and adjust the aid. The audiologist teaches the child to listen because this is not an automatic response. The child must be helped to link the sound to the source. Background noise from television sets and radios must be kept to a minimum. The child needs to focus on the silence as well as the voices that break the silence.

Cochlear Implants

A cochlear implant is a prosthetic device used to produce the sensation of sound by electrically stimulating the auditory system. Cochlear implants have two major components, the internal or implanted component and the external component, which is worn on the body. The internal component consists of one or more electrodes implanted into or on the cochlea and an external receiver embedded into the temporal bone. The external component consists of a microphone, an external transmitter, and a signal processor. The use of cochlear implants in children began experimentally in 1980, and in 1990 the U.S. Food and Drug Administration approved implants for general use in children. Cochlear implants are recommended for children who

1) demonstrate a lack of benefit with hearing aids; 2) exhibit on radiologic studies the inner ear anatomy needed for electrode placement; and 3) have the personal attributes, parental commitment, and educational setting that would make successful completion of the program likely (Kveton & Balkany, 1991). Cochlear implants have been used most frequently (60%) in children whose hearing loss is due to meningitis. The children with cochlear implants who have the most rapid and greatest improvement are those with postlingual onset of deafness, implantation during preschool years, a short period of auditory deprivation, and participation in an oral communication therapy program. Studies generally report that the gains in language skills are minimal during the first year but significant during the second year after transplant (Kennedy, 1991).

SUMMARY

One of the most important responsibilities a pediatrician has is early identification of hearing loss in a child. Early identification of hearing loss can be ensured by referral for hearing evaluation all children who fit the risk criteria for hearing loss as described by the Joint Committee on Infant Hearing (1995). Once a child is identified as having a hearing loss, the pediatrician is responsible for identifying its etiology. Finally, the pediatrician needs to support parents in following through on the extensive educational, communication, and audiologic commitments needed to optimize their child's functioning. The three most common pitfalls in this process are 1) delay in identification of the hearing loss, 2) an inadequate evaluation for identification of the etiology, and 3) missing a hearing loss in a child with developmental disabilities.

REFERENCES

Abramovich, S.J., Gregory, S., Slemick, M., & Stewart, A. (1979). Hearing loss in very low birthweight infants treated with neonatal intensive care. *Archives of Diseases in Childhood, 54,* 421–426.

Arnos, K.S., Israel, J., Devlin, L., & Wilson, M.P. (1992). Genetic counseling for the deaf. *Otolaryngologic Clinics of North America, 25,* 953–971.

Bergman, I., Hirsch, R.P., Fria, T.J., Shapiro, S.M., Holzman, I., & Painter, M.J. (1985). Cause of

hearing loss in the high-risk premature infant. *Journal of Pediatrics, 106,* 95–101.

Bess, F.H., & Tharpe, A.M. (1984). Unilateral hearing impairment in children. *Pediatrics, 74,* 206–216.

Brookhouser, P.E., Worthington, D.W., & Kelly, W.J. (1992). Noise-induced hearing loss in children. *Laryngoscope, 102,* 615–655.

Cornett, R.O. (1967). Cued speech. *Annals of the Deaf, 112,* 3–13.

Dodge, P.R., Davis, H., Feigin, R.D., Holmes, S.J., Kaplan, S.L., Jubelirer, D.P., Stechenberg, B.W., & Hirsh, S.K. (1984). Prospective evaluation of hearing impairment as a sequela of acute bacterial meningitis. *New England Journal of Medicine, 311*, 869–874.

Education for All Handicapped Children Act of 1975, PL 94-142. (August 23, 1975). Title 20, U.S.C. 1401 et seq: *U.S. Statutes at Large, 89*, 773–796.

Falk, S.A. (1972). Combined effects of noise and ototoxic drugs. *Environmental Health Perspectives, 2*, 5.

Finitzo-Hieber, T., McCracken, G.H., & Brown, K.C. (1985). Prospective controlled evaluation of auditory function in neonates given netilmicin or amikacin. *Journal of Pediatrics, 106*, 129–136.

Fortnum, H.M. (1992). Hearing impairment after bacterial meningitis: A review. *Archives of Diseases of Childhood, 67*, 1128–1133.

Hawkins, J.E., Jr. (1977). Ototoxicity in the infant and fetus. In F.A. Bess (Ed.), *Childhood deafness: Causation, assessment, and management* (pp. 37–52). New York: Grune & Stratton.

Hotchkiss, D. (1989). *Demographic aspects of hearing impairment: Questions and answers* (2nd ed.). Washington, DC: Gallaudet University Press.

Individuals with Disabilities Education Act of 1990 (IDEA), PL 101-476. (October 30, 1990). Title 20, U.S.C. 1400 et seq: *U.S. Statutes at Large, 105*, 587–608.

Joint Committee on Infant Hearing. (1982). Position statement. *Pediatrics, 70*, 496–497.

Joint Committee on Infant Hearing. (1990). Position statement. *ASHA, 33*(Suppl. 5), 3–6.

Joint Committee on Infant Hearing. (1995). 1994 position statement. *Pediatrics, 95*, 152–156.

Jones, K.L. (1988). *Smith's recognizable patterns of human malformation.* Philadelphia: W.B. Saunders.

Kaplan, S.L., Catlin, E.I., Weaver, R., & Feigin, R.D. (1984). Onset of hearing loss in children with bacterial meningitis. *Pediatrics, 73*, 575–578.

Kemp, D.T. (1988). Developments in cochlear mechanics and techniques for non-invasive evaluation. *Advances in Audiology, 5*, 27–45.

Kennedy, C., Kimm, L., Dees, D., Evans, P., Hunter, M., Lenton, S., & Thorton, A. (1991). Otoacoustic emissions and auditory brainstem responses in the newborn. *Archives of Disease in Childhood, 66*, 1124–1129.

Konigsmark, B.W. (1969a). Hereditary deafness in man (first of three parts). *New England Journal of Medicine, 281*, 713–720.

Konigsmark, B.W. (1969b). Hereditary deafness in man (second of three parts). *New England Journal of Medicine, 281*, 774–778.

Konigsmark, B.W. (1969c). Hereditary deafness in man (third of three parts). *New England Journal of Medicine, 281*, 827–832.

Konigsmark, B.W. (1972). Hereditary childhood hearing loss and integumentary system. *Journal of Pediatrics, 80*, 909–919.

Konigsmark, B.W., & Gorlin, R.J. (1976). *Genetic and metabolic deafness.* Philadelphia: W.B.Saunders.

Kveton, J., & Balkany, T.J., American Academy of Otolaryngology–Head and Neck Surgery Subcommittee on Cochlear Implants (1991). Status of cochlear implantation in children. *Journal of Pediatrics, 118*, 1–7.

Lincoln, E.M., Sordillo, S.V.R., & Davies, P.A (1960). Tuberculous meningitis in children. *Journal of Pediatrics, 57*, 807–823.

Lorber, J. (1961). Long-term follow-up of 100 children who recovered from tuberculous meningitis. *Pediatrics, 28*, 778–791.

Matkin, N.D. (1986). The child with a marked high-frequency hearing impairment. *Pediatric Clinics of North America, 15*, 677–690.

Meadow, K.P. (1975). The development of deaf children. In E.M. Heatherington (Ed.), *Review of child development research* (vol. 5, pp. 481–508). Chicago: University of Chicago Press.

Nadol, J.B. (1993). Hearing loss. *New England Journal of Medicine, 329*, 1092–1102.

NIH Consensus Development Conference. (1993, March). *Early identification of hearing impairment in infants and children.* Washington, DC: National Institutes of Health.

Northern, J.L., & Downs, M.P. (1974). *Hearing in children.* Baltimore: Williams & Wilkins.

Paparella, M.M., Fox, R.Y., & Schachern, P.A. (1989). Diagnosis and treatment of sensorineural hearing loss in children. *Otolaryngologic Clinics of North America, 22*, 51–73.

Simmons, F.B. (1980). Patterns of deafness in newborns. *Laryngoscope, 90*, 448–454.

Sisco, F.H., & Anderson, R.J. (1978). Current findings regarding the performance of deaf children on the WISC–R. *American Annals of the Deaf, 123*, 115–121.

Stewart, J.M., & Downs, M.P. (1993). Congenital conductive hearing loss: The need for early identification and intervention. *Pediatrics, 91*, 355–359.

U.S. Department of Health and Human Services. (1990). *Healthy people 2000.* Washington, DC: Author.

Vienny, H., Despland, P.A., Lütschg, J., Deonna, T., Dutoit-Marco, M.L., & Gander, C. (1984). Early diagnosis and evolution of deafness in childhood bacterial meningitis: A study using brainstem auditory evoked potentials. *Pediatrics, 73*, 579–586.

White, K.R., & Behrens, T.R. (Eds.). (1993). The Rhode Island Hearing Assessment Project: Implications for universal newborn hearing screening. *Seminars in Hearing, 14*, 1–119.

White, K.R., Vohr, B.R., & Behrens, T.R. (1993). Universal newborn hearing screening using transient evoked otoacoustic emissions: Results of the Rhode Island Hearing Assessment Project. *Seminars in Hearing, 14*, 30–45.

Chapter 33

Tourette Syndrome

Harvey S. Singer, M.D.

The Gilles de la Tourette syndrome and related tic disorders represent a spectrum of involuntary motor and/or vocal tics and comorbid neuropsychiatric problems (Singer & Walkup, 1991). The first medical description of a patient with the disorder now known as Tourette syndrome was given in 1825, when Itard reported on his patient the Marquise de Dampierre, a noblewoman who developed persistent body tics, barking sounds, and uncontrollable utterances of obscenities (Itard, 1825). In 1885, the French physician George Gilles de la Tourette, for whom this disorder is named, made reference to Itard's extraordinary patient and reviewed eight additional cases with multiple tics, involuntary movements, coprolalia (obscene language), and echolalia (repeating a last heard sound). Despite its prolonged history with frequent descriptions in the pediatric, developmental, neurologic, psychiatric, and lay literature, physicians are reluctant to make the diagnosis of Tourette syndrome, fail to appreciate the diversity of associated features, and often misdirect therapy. This chapter reviews the clinical features, epidemiology, genetics, and therapy of tic disorders.

TICS

The presence of tics is the cardinal symptom in all tic disorders. Readily observed but vaguely defined, tics are involuntary, sudden, usually rapid, brief, repetitive, nonrhythmic stereotyped movements or vocalizations. The two major categories of tics, motor and phonic, are each subdivided into a simple and a complex category. Simple motor tics are those that involve only one muscle group, resulting in an instantaneous eye blink, eye jerk, head twitch, head thrust, or shoulder shrug. A more complex motor tic is one that involves either a cluster of simple motor tics or a more coordinated sequence of movements, such as facial grimacing, touching, jumping, smelling, or copropraxia (obscene gesturing). Phonic (or vocal) tics, produced by moving air through the nose or mouth, may be simple sounds such as grunting, barking, sniffing, snorting, or throat clearing or more complex vocalizations, including syllables, words, phrases, sentences, palilalia (repeating one's own words), echolalia (repeating other people's words), or coprolalia (using obscene words). Dystonic (tonic) tics, slow and temporary twisting, pulling, or squeezing movements, may also be part of the normal spectrum of Tourette syndrome (Elston, Grenje, & Lees, 1989; Jankovic & Stone, 1991). Fifty-seven percent of Jankovic and Stone's patients demonstrated one or more dystonic tics, usually oculogyric deviations, blepharospasms, and dystonic neck movements. Dystonic tics may be differentiated from torsion dystonia by the accompaniment of other features of Tourette syndrome, including lack of persistent abnormal (usually twisting) postures, their occurrence in abrupt bursts, and their brevity and voluntary suppressibility (Stone & Jankovic, 1991).

Premonitory (sensory) experiences have been described with varied frequencies. Initially thought to be an uncommon phenomenon, these previously labeled "sensory tics" include uncomfortable sensations (tickle, irritation, temperature change, unusual feeling) that cause the patient to produce voluntary movements or sounds (Shapiro, Shapiro, Young, & Feinbert, 1988). More recently, Kurlan (1989) found that 41% of his patients experience a localizable sensation, whereas Leckman and colleagues reported that 92% of 135 subjects (ages 8–71 years) describe tics as a voluntary response to a premonitory sensation most often in palms, shoulders, midabdomen, and throat regions (Leckman, Walker, & Cohen, 1993). In these instances, patients characterize their tics as intentionally produced but not truly voluntary, because the patient has little control over the need to perform the movement. An unusual case of "signing" tics occurred in a young woman with Tourette syndrome who incorporated sign language into her tic behavior (Lange, Consky, & Sandor, 1993). In this individual, swearing, echoing what others said, and repeating her own phrases were expressed in sign language, emphasizing a complex association between purposeful and automatic execution of movements in Tourette syndrome.

In general, tics have several defining characteristics that assist in the diagnosis. Tics typically wax and wane, and there is gradual replacement of old symptoms with new ones. Tics are increased by anxiety, emotional stress, anger, excitement, and fatigue, and are usually less noticeable during sleep or during periods of relaxation, distraction, or concentration on complex tasks. Tics are briefly suppressible, although attempts to inhibit the movements frequently result in a buildup of "inner" (emotional) tension. This ability to suppress tics for various lengths of time is different from that in most other hyperkinetic movement disorders, in which tics can, at best, be suppressed for only very short periods of time (Koller & Biary, 1989). Individuals will often attempt to mask their tics by converting them to pseudovoluntary sounds or noises. Tics are usually easily identifiable, although it is common to observe fewer tics in the office setting than described by history. In those instances in which movement/vocalizations are not observed in the office, we often request that the patient be videotaped in a more natural setting.

CLASSIFICATION OF TIC DISORDERS

In October 1993, a committee of the Tourette Syndrome Association published a detailed outline of research definitions for various tic disorders (Tourette Syndrome Classification Study Group, 1993) (Table 1). A simplified version of that classification divides tic disorders into those that are transient (duration of tics less than 1 year) and those that are chronic (history of tics for more than 1 year). *Transient tic disorder*

Table 1. Classification of tic syndromes

Transient tic disorder (< 1 year duration)
  By history[a]
  Definite
Definite tic disorder, diagnosis deferred
  Meets all criteria for chronic disorder except required duration of illness for 1 year
Chronic tic disorder (> 1 year duration)
  a. Chronic single tic
  b. Chronic multiple motor tic or phonic tic
     By history[a]
     Probable[b]
     Definite
  c. Tourette syndrome
     By history[a]
     Probable[b,c]
     Definite
Nonspecific tic disorder
  Does not meet criteria for a specific tic disorder (e.g., onset in adulthood or onset in association with another neurologic disorder)
     By history[a]
     Definite

Adapted from Tourette Syndrome Classification Study Group (1993).

[a]Diagnosis "by history" is used when tics have not been witnessed by a knowledgeable observer.

[b]Diagnosis of "probable" disease is used when an individual fulfills all the criteria for a definite syndrome except for an ill-defined age of onset, fulminant appearance of tics, or a nonfluctuating course.

[c]"Probable Tourette syndrome" may also include an individual with a single motor tic and vocalization, or with multiple motor tics and a possible vocal tic.

(TTD) is the mildest and most common of tic disorders, with an estimated occurrence in about 5%–24% of schoolchildren. Because TTD requires a duration of tics for less than 1 year, the diagnosis is strictly retrospective. There is no accurate way to predict whether an individual will have resolution of tics within months, add others to the repertoire, or have persistent tics that will become chronic. For the diagnosis of *chronic multiple (motor or phonic) tic disorder* (CMTD), the tics must be present for more than 1 year. Individuals in this category must have either entirely motor or, less commonly, solely vocal tics. Several studies have documented that CMTDs represent a variant of Tourette syndrome, and both are transmitted as inherited traits in the same family. Kurlan, Behr, Medved, and Como (1988) have suggested that TTD may also be a manifestation of the putative gene.

The *Gilles de la Tourette syndrome* is characterized by the presence of both motor and vocal tics and is a fluctuating disorder of variable severity. The current recommended essential diagnostic criteria include onset before 21 years of age, multiple involuntary motor tics, one or more vocal tics, a waxing and waning course, a gradual replacement of old symptoms with new ones, the absence of any other medical explanation for the tics, and the presence of tics for more than 1 year. Tics must be also witnessed directly by a reliable observer or be recorded by videotape or cinematography. The correct diagnosis of Tourette syndrome often is delayed for many years because of numerous misconceptions, including a tendency to associate unusual symptoms with psychological problems, incorrect attribution of vocal tics to respiratory disorders or eye blinking and ocular tics to ophthalmologic abnormalities, and an inclination to await the appearance of coprolalia, which occurs in only about 15% of patients. Even with greater awareness of Tourette syndrome throughout the medical and lay community, the mean delay between onset of the disorder and its correct diagnosis is still about 5 years (Park, Como, Cui, & Kurlan, 1993).

Tourette syndrome is more common in males than females (3:1 to 4:1). The mean age of onset is typically between 6 and 7 years, with most patients developing tics before age 13. Eye blinking, facial grimacing, and head jerking are the most common initial tics. In many cases, motor tics progress in a rostral–caudal fashion, involving the face, head, or shoulders before other body parts. Because the severity of tics can vary widely in families, as well as in monozygote twins (Hyde, Aaronson, Randolph, Rickler, & Weinberger, 1992), it is difficult to prognosticate about long-term severity. In a study of 47 women, 26% had a premenstrual exacerbation of their tics (Schwabe & Konkol, 1992). Drugs that may exacerbate tics include psychomotor stimulants (methylphenidate, amphetamines, pemoline, cocaine), anticholinergics (scopolamine), antihistaminics (diphenhydramine, dexchlorpheniramine), antidepressants (imipramine, fluoxetine, fluvoxamine, lithium), antiepileptics (carbamazepine, phenytoin), and opioids (see Sanchez-Ramos & Weiner, 1993).

Goetz, Tanner, Stebbins, Leipzig, and Carr (1992) have suggested that the presence of only mild tics in early and late adolescence is a good predictor of mild tics in adulthood. Neither severe tics in childhood nor the presence of coprolalia was an adverse indicator.

Although Tourette syndrome was originally proposed to be a lifelong disorder, several studies indicate that many individuals have a spontaneous remission or marked improvement, independent of the use of medications. In a study following the course of tics in 58 teenagers/young adults, tics had almost disappeared in 26%, lessened considerably in 46%, remained unchanged in 14%, and worsened in 14% (Erenberg, Cruse, & Rothner, 1987). Significant reductions in the severity of tics occurring over time have also been noted by other investigators; for example, in 136 patients the occurrence of moderate to severe tics decreased from 41% to 9% (Bruun, 1988), and in 58 adults the occurrence of moderate to severe tics decreased from 60% to 24% and coprolalia from 22% to 4% (Goetz et al., 1992).

Nonspecific tic disorder includes those tic syndromes that do not meet the criteria for a more specific tic disorder. For example, an individual may have a syndrome with multiple motor and vocal tics, but have had its onset either in adulthood or associated with other medical conditions. This entity, previously designated "tourettism," was first observed following an epidemic of encephalitis lethargica around 1920. It has subsequently been reported in association with a variety of other acute and chronic neurologic disorders, such as after head injury, stroke, or infectious disease, as well as in degenerative disorders such as neuroacanthocytosis, Huntington disease, and Creutzfeld-Jakob disease (Fahn, 1982a, 1982b; Sacks, 1982; C. Singer, Sanchez-Ramos, & Weiner, 1989). We have identified a Tourette-like syndrome that began with the acute fulminant onset of motor and phonic tics in a 6-year-old girl following presumed herpes encephalitis (Northam & Singer, 1991). *Tardive tourettism* is the de novo appearance of motor and vocal tics in patients being withdrawn from chronic neuroleptic treatment (Karagianis & Nagpurkar, 1990; Klawans, Falk, Dausieda, & Wiener, 1978).

PHYSICAL EXAMINATION
AND LABORATORY TESTS

A neurologic examination in Tourette syndrome typically shows no focal or lateralizing signs. "Soft" signs, including abnormalities of coordination and fine motor performance, synkinesis, and motor restlessness, are often observed in affected children, especially those with symptoms of attention-deficit/hyperactivity disorder (ADHD). Despite the presence of oculogyric deviations and blepharospasm, we and others have found no abnormalities of saccadic eye movement, fixation, or pursuits (Lasker, Zee, Hain, Folstein, & Singer, 1987, 1988). We have also been unable to confirm a report of inherited paracentral kinetic visual deficits in patients with Tourette syndrome (Repka & Singer, 1992).

There is no diagnostic laboratory test for tic syndromes, and the diagnosis is based solely on clinical features. Electroencephalography (EEG), computed EEG topography (brain mapping), evoked responses, and brain imaging with computerized tomography or magnetic resonance imaging are generally not helpful, nor are they routinely indicated in the evaluation of Tourette syndrome (Drake, Hietter, Padamadan, & Bogner, 1991; Drake et al., 1992; Harcherik et al., 1985; Krumholz, Singer, Neidermeyer, Burnite, & Harris, 1983; Robertson, 1989). Auditory and long latency event-related potentials are abnormal in some patients with Tourette syndrome (Van de Wetering, Martana, Fortgens, Slasta, & Van Woerkom, 1985; Van Woerkom, Fortgens, Rompel-Martana, & Van de Wetering, 1988; Van Woerkom, Fortgens, Van de Wetering, & Martana, 1988), but are influenced by comorbid conditions such as obsessive–compulsive disorder (OCD) and ADHD (Drake et al., 1992).

EPIDEMIOLOGY AND GENETICS

Tourette syndrome has been reported to occur worldwide. In the United States, it is more common in Caucasians than in African Americans or Hispanics, although this may represent the demographics of populations attending specific clinics. The prevalence (total number of cases at a specific time in a specific place) of Tourette syndrome has been quantified in several geographic areas by different ascertainment methods (see Tanner, 1993). Prevalence estimates based on individual or physician identification range from 2.9 in 10,000 children in Monroe County, New York, to 5.2 in 10,000 North Dakota schoolchildren (Burd, Kerbeshian, Wikenheiser, & Fisher, 1986; Caine, McBride, Chiverton, Bamford, & Rediess, 1988). Because methodologic problems (insufficient precision in inquiry about symptoms, missed diagnosis in mild cases, or affected individuals being unaware of their symptoms) may lead to underestimation of the number of affected individuals, some investigators have suggested a lifetime prevalence rate of 1–10 in 1,000 (Shapiro et al., 1988, pp. 45–59).

Although in his original monographs Gilles de la Tourette commented on the hereditary nature of Tourette syndrome, this aspect remains controversial, and attempts to isolate the gene or genes have been unsuccessful. The most widely accepted hypothesis, based on segregation analyses of family and twin studies, suggests a sex-influenced, autosomal dominant mode of inheritance with variable expressivity as either Tourette syndrome, CMTD, or OCD (see Pauls, Leckman, & Cohen, 1993). More specifically, a boy who inherits the *Gts* gene has a 100% chance of expressing the gene either as Tourette syndrome, CMTD, or OCD; a 99% chance of having either Tourette syndrome or CMTD; and a 45% possibility of having Tourette syndrome alone. In contrast, a girl inheriting the same gene has a 71% chance of phenotypically having either Tourette syndrome, CMTD, or OCD; a 56% chance of having either Tourette syndrome or CMTD; and a 17% likelihood of having Tourette syndrome alone (Pauls & Leckman, 1986; Pauls et al., 1990). The hypothesis that OCD represented a variant manifestation of the syndrome stemmed from studies that documented increased frequency of obsessive–compulsive symptoms among persons with Tourette syndrome (Pauls, Towbin, Leckman, Zahner, & Cohen, 1986). In a 1995 family study and segregation analysis on 53 children with Tourette syndrome and their nuclear families performed at Johns Hopkins, results suggested that this syndrome is inherited by an additive major locus in conjunction with a polygenic background (H. Singer, 1995).

ADHD also commonly co-occurs in probands and families with Tourette syndrome, but the possibility of a genetic relationship between the two also remains controversial (see Comings & Comings, 1993). A study by Pauls et al. (1993) suggested that there may be two types of individuals with Tourette syndrome and ADHD; in one type ADHD is independent of Tourette syndrome and in the other ADHD is secondary to the occurrence of Tourette syndrome. In the former, the onset of ADHD symptomatology precedes the appearance of tics and in the latter both symptomatologies appear simultaneously. Other investigators have suggested that Tourette syndrome represents a common, broad-based neuropsychiatric disorder with manifestations of numerous behavioral disturbances, such as obsessive–compulsive behaviors, ADHD, learning disabilities, sleep problems, speech problems, and other psychopathologies (conduct disorder, oppositional disorder, multiple phobias, panic attacks, anxiety disorders, depression, mania, inappropriate sexual behaviors, addictive behaviors, and paranoid tendencies) (Comings & Comings, 1987a, 1987b, 1987c, 1987d, 1987e). On the assumption that Tourette syndrome is a spectrum disorder, Comings and Comings (1992) have postulated a "semidominant semirecessive" mode of inheritance—more severe patients are homozygotes for the putative *Gts* gene, but heterozygotes could have tics or other behavior manifestations of the spectrum.

The postulated autosomal dominant inheritance pattern and the availability of several large kindreds segregating Tourette syndrome, CMTD, and OCD has led to an intense search to identify a genetic marker linked to this disease. Vigorous attempts to map and clone the responsible *Gts* gene(s) have to date been unsuccessful. Among the explanations for this lack of success are locus heterogeneity, incorrect assumptions of inheritance, an ambiguous phenotype, mild cases that escape detection, and the inclusion of genetically unrelated but highly associated traits. In contrast, our recent identification of a mixed model for inheritance (unpublished data) would suggest the necessity of performing genetic studies on independent families with affected sib-pairs. In view of pathophysiologic hypotheses that suggest an abnormality of the dopaminergic system, investigators have specifically studied markers relating to this neurotransmitter in several kindreds. No evidence has been found to support linkage in Tourette syndrome to the dopamine-1 or dopamine-2 receptor or the dopamine transporter locus (Brett, Curtis, Robertson, & Gurling, 1995; Devor et al., 1990; Gelernter et al., 1990, 1993; Vandenbergh et al., 1993).

Twin studies also support a genetic factor in the etiology of Tourette syndrome. The possibility of noninherited tics was also proposed because, in a questionnaire-based study, concordance in monozygotic twins for either Tourette syndrome, or CMTD was only 77% (Price, Kidd, Cohen, Pauls, & Leckman, 1985). In a follow-up evaluation designed to evaluate this question further, each subject or his or her parents were interviewed directly (J.T. Walkup, unpublished data). The results of this reevaluation (19 of 30 of twins in the original study) demonstrated that 89% of monozygotic twins were now concordant for Tourette syndrome, and 100% were concordant for either Tourette syndrome or CMTD. These data have shifted a potential role of nongenetic factors from a purely etiologic one to a role in which they may mediate the form or severity of the phenotype. For example, in monozygotic twins the severity of tics is extremely variable (Hyde et al., 1992; Price, Kidd, Cohen, Pauls, & Leckman, 1985). Several prenatal factors have been hypothesized to explain differences in Tourette syndrome severity in twin pairs. Because more severely affected twins had lower birth weights, determinants that influence intrauterine growth, including sex-specific hormones and maternal stress during pregnancy, have been proposed to be nongenetic factors influencing tic severity (see Leckman & Peterson, 1993). One hypothesis is that normal surges of androgenic steroids acting in the intrauterine period influence various aspects of brain development, which, in the genetically vulnerable individual, leads to the subsequent appearance of tics (Peterson et al., 1992). Other possibilities include exposure to drugs/toxins, hypothermia, or streptococcal infection.

COMORBID DISORDERS

Gilles de la Tourette, in his descriptions of this disorder in the 1880s, noted the presence of comorbid psychopathologies, including obsessive–compulsive symptoms, anxieties, and phobia. Since that time an increasing variety of concomitant behavioral problems have been identified in individuals with Tourette syndrome. Although obsessive–compulsive phenomena and ADHD are the two most prevalent problems, other disruptive behaviors, learning difficulties, school problems, and sleep abnormalities are commonly observed. The magnitude of these disorders is indicated by studies showing that more than half of persons with Tourette syndrome have sought counseling for behavioral difficulties (Stefl, 1984) and by use of the Child Behavior Checklist (CBCL) to evaluate behavior in Tourette syndrome probands. In the latter, we have shown that, for each of the 10 behavioral categories, 27%–57% of adolescents with Tourette syndrome scored more than 2 standard deviations above the mean (Singer & Rosenberg, 1989).

Obsessive–Compulsive Problems

In groups of persons with Tourette syndrome, the reported incidence of obsessive–compulsive symptoms is generally about 40%–50%, although some studies report incidences as high as 89% (see Leonard et al., 1992). Some of these discrepancies may be related to a failure to distinguish clearly between complex tics and compulsive rituals and the lack of consistently applied diagnostic criteria. The diagnosis of OCD requires recurrent obsessions or compulsions (or both) that are distressing and interfere with social or occupational functioning. Using structured interviews and American Psychiatric Association (1987) *Diagnostic and Statistical Manual of Mental Disorders*, third edition (revised) (DSM-III-R) criteria to identify OCD, investigators have shown an association of OCD with Tourette syndrome ranging from 28% to 62%. Using the obsessive–compulsive subscale of the CBCL Parent Form to evaluate Tourette syndrome probands, we have shown that 43% of 6- to 11-year-old children (9 of 21) and 40% of 12- to 16-year-olds (12 of 30) had obsessive–compulsive symptoms (Singer & Rosenberg, 1989). Furthermore, Park et al. (1993) showed that, if OCD was absent on initial evaluation in children with Tourette syndrome (mean age 12 years), it was usually not present several years later (mean follow-up of 1.6 ± 1.3 years). In twin studies of persons with Tourette syndrome, it and OCD co-occurred in 83% of individuals (43 pairs); concordance rates for OCS approximated those for Tourette syndrome and were 53% for monozygotic versus 15% for dizygotic twins (Price et al., 1985). As mentioned, it has been suggested that OCD is an alternative phenotype of the putative Tourette syndrome gene. Acceptance of an association between obsessive–compulsive symptoms/OCD and Tourette syndrome is not unanimous, and Shapiro and Shapiro (1992) continue to express concerns that essential well-characterized experimental studies have not been performed.

Attention-Deficit/Hyperactivity Disorder

Components of ADHD, including short attention span, restlessness, poor concentration, and diminished impulse control, with or without hyperactivity, are noted in 50%–60% of children with Tourette syndrome (Comings & Comings, 1987a, 1988; Nee, Caine, Polinsky, Eldridge, & Ebert, 1980; Park et al., 1993; Pauls, Kruger, Leckman, Cohen, & Kidd, 1984). The symptoms of ADHD usually precede the onset of motor and phonic tics by 2–3 years, although there may be a subgroup in whom ADHD begins simultaneously with tics (Pauls et al., 1993). In our referral-oriented Tourette syndrome clinic at Johns Hopkins, about 80% of children with Tourette syndrome also have ADHD. This overrepresentation is consistent with reports that referrals of persons with Tourette syndrome for medical attention is increased when ADHD is present (Caine et al., 1988; Pauls, Hurst, et al., 1986). In an open series, about 50 of 200 persons with Tourette syndrome required psychostimulant therapy for ADHD. The ability of stimulant (methylphenidate, dextroamphetamine, and pemoline) to exacerbate existing tics or to provoke tics in susceptible individuals has been documented, although the extent to which this phenomenon occurs is still under study.

Learning Difficulties

Children with Tourette syndrome often have difficulties in the classroom, and indeed many require special classes. In a California school district comprising about 3,000 students, a total of 28% of children in special education classes had a tic disorder, with 12% having Tourette syndrome (Comings, Himes, & Comings, 1990). Similar findings have been reported in Monroe County, New York, where examination of a randomly selected sample of full-time special education students identified 26% with definite or probable tics (Kurlan, Whitmore, Irvine, McDermott, & Como, 1994). In a survey of 200 children and adolescents by Erenberg, Cruse, and Rothner (1986), 36% experienced learning problems, including learning disabilities, poor grades, the need to repeat a grade, or the need to attend full- or part-time special education classes. School difficulties may be related to the Tourette syndrome symptoms themselves (e.g., when tics disrupt other classmates or interfere with handwriting or participation in class discussions); to the use of pharmacotherapies to suppress tics; to the presence of ADHD, OCD, or other psychopathologies; or to specific neuropsychoeducational problems (Singer, Schuerholz, & Denckla, 1995).

Although psychoeducational studies have not uncovered any impairments of general intellectual functioning, they have identified specific learning deficits, impaired visual–perceptual performance, reduced visual–motor skills, and discrepancies between verbal and performance IQ (Bornstein, Carroll, & King, 1985; Como, 1993; Ferrari, Mathews, & Barabas, 1984). On the basis of the Maryland State Department of Education criteria for learning disabilities, we identified discrepancies-based learning disabilities in 23% of 65 children with Tourette syndrome (Schuerholz, Baumgardner, Singer, Reiss, & Denckla, in press). Interestingly, learning disabilities were absent in a group with only Tourette syndrome (0 out of 21), but relatively common (15 out of 44) in a cohort with Tourette syndrome and ADHD. In another study using a 1.5–standard deviation IQ/specific academic skill discrepancy, 51% of 12 children with IQs above 70 met criteria for a learning disability in at least one academic area, and 21% met criteria in two or more areas (Burd, Kauffman, & Kerbeshian, 1992). In particular, impairments occur in reading skills, mathematics, and the use of written language (Burd & Hearle, 1992; Hagin & Kugler, 1988; Hagin, Beecher, Pagano, & Kreeger, 1982; Ludlow, Polinsky, Caine, Bassich, & Ebert, 1982).

Neuropsychological and executive functioning has also been analyzed in children with Tourette syndrome with and without ADHD (Schuerholz et al., in press). Executive function refers to a domain of cognitive abilities that include self-regulation, set maintenance, selective inhibition of responding, cognitive flexibility, planning, prioritizing, and organizing time and space, presumably mediated by pre-frontal regions of the brain and varied interconnecting structures/pathways. Children with Tourette syndrome alone were less impaired than those who also had ADHD on Wisconsin Card Sort Perservative Responses, Rey-Osterreith Copy Organization, Rey Osterreith Recall Organization, and Judgement of Line Orientation. Those with Tourette syndrome alone were deficient, but to a lesser extent, on Test of Variables of Attention (TOVA) reaction time and variability of reaction time. In general, children with Tourette syndrome alone show less executive dysfunction and have significantly better perceptual organization scores than do children with Tourette syndrome plus ADHD (Harris et al., in press; Schuerholz et al., in press). These findings suggest that many, but not all, of the neuropsychological impairments described in children with Tourette syndrome are related to an associated comorbid condition. A surprising finding in our studies was that bright, Tourette syndrome-only subjects with no learning disabilities performed significantly poorer on Letter Word Fluency tests, compared with a Tourette syndrome plus ADHD cohort (Schuerholz, et al., submitted). Since impairment on Letter Word Fluency occurred in the absence of abnormalities on Semantic Word Fluency testing, which identifies deficits of the posterior language system, we have interpreted our findings as a sign of frontal-subcortical circuit inefficiency. We have therefore hypothesized that "cognitive showing" is an important factor in understanding poor school performance in children with Tourette syndrome. This proposal is consistent with our clinical observations that children with Tourette syndrome have their greatest problems in completing timed-tests and finishing their homework.

Other Behavioral Disorders

A variety of other behavioral–emotional problems have been identified in persons with Tourette syndrome (Comings, 1990; Golden, 1984; Grossman, Mostofsky, & Harrison, 1986; H.S. Singer & Rosenberg, 1989; Stokes, Bawden, Camfield, Backman, & Dooley, 1991). Whether these additional behavioral problems are related to tic severity, are a direct consequence of having a stigmatizing disorder, are attributable to accompanying ADHD, or have nothing to do with tics remains to be determined. The CBCL has identified obsessive–compulsive behaviors, aggressiveness, hyperactivity, immaturity, withdrawal, and somatic complaints in association with Tourette syndrome (H.S. Singer & Rosenberg, 1989). Comings and Comings (1987a, 1987b, 1987c, 1987d, 1987e) have concluded that ADHD, anxiety, OCD, conduct disorders, depression, discipline problems, dyslexia, mania, panic attacks, phobias, and stuttering occur 5–20 times more commonly in clinically referred persons with Tourette syndrome than in controls. Social problems have been reported in Tourette syndrome irrespective of tic severity. Children with mild to moderate tics are more withdrawn, more aggressive, and less popular, and 35% were in the lowest class rating on peer relationship evaluations (Stokes et al., 1991). People with tic disorders tend to have more unexplained physical (somatic) complaints, but it is unclear whether these are a symptom of Tourette syndrome or an anxiety reaction as part of a chronic disorder (Frank, Sieg, & Gaffney, 1991). Robertson, Trimble, and Lees (1988) have suggested that affected individuals are more likely to be depressed and anxious, and to exhibit neuroses, hostility, and inappropriate sexual thoughts or behavior. Self-injurious (self-inflicted, nonaccidental) behavior occurs in persons with Tourette syndrome and usually correlates with the severity of Tourette syndrome or

the presence of obsessive–compulsive behaviors (see Robertson & Yakeley, 1993).

Sleep Abnormalities

Disturbed sleep patterns have been reported in people with Tourette syndrome, ranging from somnambulism (sleep walking), night terrors, and nightmares to less specific complaints such as talking in sleep, restlessness, and difficulty with falling asleep (Comings & Comings, 1987f). Polygraphic sleep studies have shown decreased rapid eye movement sleep, but whether delta sleep is increased or decreased is unclear (Glaze, Frost, & Jankovic, 1983; Mendelson, Caine, Goyer, Ebert, & Gillin, 1980). Tics in sleep are most likely to occur after awakening or during lightening of sleep, or in Stage 1 sleep (Fish, Sawyers, & Allen, 1991). Using a sleep behavior questionnaire with 146 children with Tourette syndrome, we confirmed the greater occurrence of insomnia, dreams, required bedtime rituals, and parasomnias (Allen, Singer, Brown, & Salam, 1992). Our data, however, did not support the postulate that Tourette syndrome is a disorder of arousal (impaired transition from Stage III-IV slow-wave sleep to lighter states), but suggested that the presence of ADHD may be a significant determinant for sleep problems in Tourette syndrome.

TREATMENT

In our referral-based population, only about 60% of children require medication for tic suppression. Moreover, in many children, associated problems such as attention deficit, hyperactivity, obsessive–compulsive symptoms, or other difficulties represent a greater disability. Therapy should be targeted to and reserved for those symptoms that are functionally disabling for the child. The treatment of tic and accompanying behavior problems requires comprehensive, multimodal individualized programs. After a complete assessment, the physician must educate the patient and family about tic disorders, define the target symptoms requiring treatment, choose the proper therapeutic modality, take an active role in the therapeutic plan, and provide long-term support. It is unreasonable to expect that a single visit or medication will completely resolve the many issues confronting the child and his or her family.

Tics

Pharmacotherapy for tic disorders is strictly symptomatic and is not curative. Hence, treatment should be reserved for those children with psychosocial or functionally disabling problems. The main goal of treatment is to reduce tics to a tolerable level. A variety of non-pharmacologic treatments (conditioning techniques, relaxation training, biofeedback, and hypnosis) have been proposed (Culbertson, 1989; Michultka, Blanchard, & Rosenblum, 1989; A.L. Peterson & Azrin, 1992; Robertson, Trimble, & Lees, 1989). In a study evaluating behavioral training as an alternative mode of treatment for children with Tourette syndrome, we showed that relaxation therapy improved tics in 7 of 7 children compared to only 5 of 8 children getting "minimal therapy" (H.S. Singer, Waranch, & Brown, 1993). This beneficial response was only short term and the treatment was insufficient as the sole therapy in young children and in those with more severe tics. Further studies are necessary to determine the value of relaxation training as an adjunctive therapy to medications for the suppression of tics. Hence, in most children with tics who require symptomatic therapy, pharmacotherapeutic agents should be prescribed, with consideration of several basic principles: use as little medicine as possible, follow the child closely, periodically determine whether continued treatment is required for tic suppression, and reinitiate medication only if significant symptoms recur.

At present, two classes of drugs to suppress tic are used primarily: α-adrenergic agonists and neuroleptics. Several other agents, including benzodiazepines, catecholamine-depleting agents, calcium channel blockers, nicotine, and opiate antagonists, have been advocated, but further investigation is required. Although the efficacy of clonidine (Catapres) to suppress motor tics and vocalizations has been questioned (Goetz et al., 1987), some have found it to be useful as an initial medication, especially in children with mild symptoms or those in whom behavior disturbances predominate. Sedation is the major complication, and tics may intensify if this drug is withdrawn abruptly.

Neuroleptics are the most effective tic-suppressing agents, although frequent side effects, including sedation, dysphoria, weight gain, movement abnormalities (acute dystonic reactions, bradykinesia, and akathisia), depression, poor school performance, and school phobias, limit the usefulness of these drugs. Studies have shown that these complications may occur even when low doses of drugs are given that result in low serum levels. Additionally, both individuals receiving stable doses and those being withdrawn from neuroleptics have been reported to suffer from tardive or withdrawal dyskinesia (Golden, 1985). Because, in my experience, pimozide (Orap) and fluphenazine (Prolixin) are equipotent to haloperidol (Haldol) but have fewer side effects, these are my primary drugs of choice. An electrocardiogram should be obtained routinely before initiation of pimozide because its use has led to prolongation of the QT interval. Detailed descriptions of pharmacotherapy in Tourette syndrome can be found elsewhere (Kurlan & Trinidad, 1995).

Surgical therapies (limbic leukotomy and stereotaxic thalamotomy) have been tried in individuals with severe tics plus other psychopathologies with limited success (Robertson, Doran, Trimble, & Lees, 1990). Persistent neurologic deficits following such surgical procedures have been documented (Leckman et al., 1993).

Attention-Deficit/Hyperactivity Disorder

The approach to the treatment of ADHD in children with Tourette syndrome is controversial because psychostimulant medications may provoke or intensify tics. In children with established tics, it has been estimated that psychostimulants exacerbate motor–vocal symptoms in about 27%–50% of those treated with stimulants (Comings & Comings 1987a; Erenberg, Cruse, & Rothner, 1985; Price, Leckman, Pauls, Cohen, & Kidd, 1986). In most studies, exacerbation of tics usually resolves when the inciting medication is withdrawn. In contrast, other investigators argue that the worsening of tics that occurs with these medications may be the result of the natural waxing phase of the Tourette syndrome. Some researchers have even suggested that methylphenidate might have a beneficial effect on Tourette syndrome symptoms. For example, Gadow, Nolan, and Sverd (1992) reported that methylphenidate reduced the occurrence of vocal tics in classroom and lunchroom settings. Hence, recommendations for use of stimulants in patients with tics range from careful monitoring for the exacerbation of tics to the avoidance of these drugs. If behavioral and educational approaches to ADHD fail, I currently recommend, on the basis of significant improvement shown in a double-blind, placebo-controlled study (Singer et al., 1995), a trial with desipramine (Norpramin). If this drug is ineffective, a brief trial with a psychostimulant is initiated. Other proposed nonstimulant agents for treatment of ADHD in children with Tourette syndrome include clonidine, deprenyl (Jankovic, 1993), and nortriptyline (Spencer, Biederman, Wilens, Steingard, & Geist, 1993). If the child improves with stimulants and tics are not exacerbated, the drug is maintained, whereas if ADHD improves but tics worsen, the drug is withdrawn and a trial with another stimulant begun. In the occasional situation in which a psychostimulant is required for attendance at school or performance at work and tics remain constant, stimulants and tic-suppressing medications are given simultaneously.

Obsessive–Compulsive Disorder

For children with Tourette syndrome with disabling obsessive–compulsive behaviors, serotonin reuptake inhibitors, clomipramine (Anafranil), fluoxetine (Prozac), and sertraline (Zoloft) have been used successfully. Fluoxetine has been linked to suicidal behavior in patients with major depression.

Other Behavioral Disorders

Although it is well established that behavioral, emotional, and other psychopathologies occur in children with Tourette syndrome, their relationship to the syndrome itself is unclear. By discussing and treating comorbid symptoms as separate entities from tics, families and health care specialists have been able to focus on individual needs more effectively. Appropriate interventions may include counseling for the family unit, behavior modification, educational intervention, pharmacotherapy, and psychiatric referral. A multidisciplinary team approach is strongly advocated.

REFERENCES

Allen, R.P., Singer, H.S., Brown, J.E., & Salam, M.M. (1992). Sleep disorders in Tourette syndrome: A primary or unrelated problem? *Pediatric Neurology, 8*, 275–280.

American Psychiatric Association. (1987). *Diagnostic and statistical manual of mental disorders* (3rd ed., rev.). Washington, DC: American Psychiatric Press.

Bornstein, R.A., Carroll, A., & King, G. (1985). Relationship of age to neuropsychological deficit in Tourette's syndrome. *Developmental and Behavioral Pediatrics, 6*, 284–286 .

Brett, P.M., Curtis, D., Robertson, M.M., & Gurling, H.M.D. (1995). The genetic susceptibility to Gilles de la Tourette syndrome in a large multiple affected British kindred-linkage analysis excludes a role for genes coding for dopamine D1, D2, D3, D4, D5 receptors, dopamine beta hydroxylase, tyrosinase, and tyrosine hydroxylase. *Biology Psychiatry, 37*, 533–540.

Bruun, R.D. (1988). Subtle and underrecognized side effects of neuroleptic treatment in children with Tourette's disorder. *American Journal of Psychiatry, 145*, 621–624.

Burd, L., & Hearle, T. (1992). Educational needs of children with Tourette syndrome. In L. Burd & T. Hearle (Eds.), *Children with Tourette syndrome: A parent's guide* (pp. 169–205). Rockville, MD: Woodbine House.

Burd, L., Kauffman, D.W., & Kerbeshian, J. (1992). Tourette syndrome and learning disabilities. *Journal of Learning Disabilities, 25*, 598–604.

Burd, L., Kerbeshian, J., Wikenheiser, M., & Fisher W. (1986). Prevalence of Gilles de la Tourette's syndrome in North Dakota adults. *American Journal of Psychiatry, 143*, 787–788.

Caine, E.D., McBride, M.C., Chiverton, P., Bamford, K.A., & Rediess, S. (1988). Tourette's syndrome in Monroe County school children. *Neurology, 38*, 472–475.

Comings, D.E. (1990). *Tourette syndrome and human behavior*. Duarte, CA: Hope Press.

Comings, D.E., & Comings, B.G. (1987a). A controlled study of Tourette syndrome: I. Attention deficit disorder, learning disorders and school problems. *American Journal of Human Genetics, 41*, 701–741.

Comings, D.E., & Comings, B.G. (1987b). A controlled study of Tourette syndrome: II. Conduct. *American Journal of Human Genetics*, *41*, 742–760.

Comings, D.E., & Comings, B.G. (1987c). A controlled study of Tourette syndrome: III. Phobias and panic attacks. *American Journal of Human Genetics*, *41*, 761–768.

Comings, D.E., & Comings, B.G. (1987d). A controlled study of Tourette syndrome: IV. Obsessions, compulsions, and schizoid behaviors. *American Journal of Human Genetics*, *41*, 782–803.

Comings, D.E., & Comings, B.G. (1987e). A controlled study of Tourette syndrome: V. Depression and mania. *American Journal of Human Genetics*, *41*, 804–821.

Comings, D.E., & Comings, B.G. (1987f). A controlled study of Tourette syndrome: VI. Early development, sleep problems, allergies, and handedness. *American Journal of Human Genetics*, *41*, 822–838.

Comings, D.E., & Comings, B.G. (1988). Tourette's syndrome and attention deficit disorder. In D.J. Cohen, R.D. Bruun, & J.F. Leckman (Eds.), *Tourette's syndrome and tic disorders* (pp. 119–135). New York: John Wiley & Sons.

Comings, D.E., & Comings, B.G. (1992). Alternative hypotheses on the inheritance of Tourette syndrome. *Advances in Neurology*, *58*, 189–200.

Comings, D.E., & Comings, B.G. (1993). Comorbid behavior disorders. In R. Kurlan (Ed.), *Handbook of Tourette syndrome and related tic and behavioral disorders* (pp. 111–150). New York: Marcel Dekker.

Comings, D.E., Himes, J.A., & Comings, B.G. (1990). An epidomiologic study of Tourette's in a single school district. *Journal of Clinical Psychiatry*, *51*, 463–469.

Como, P.G. (1993). Neuropsychological testing. In R. Kurlan (Ed.), *Handbook of Tourette's syndrome and related tic and behavioral disorders* (pp. 221–242). New York: Marcel Dekker.

Culbertson, F.M. (1989). A four-step hypnotherapy model for Gilles de la Tourette's syndrome. *American Journal of Clinical Hypnosis*, *31*, 252–256.

Devor, E.J., Grandy, D.K., Civelli, O., Litt, M., Burgess, A.K., Isenberg, K.E., van de Wetering, B.J., & Dostra, B. (1990). Genetic linkage is excluded for the D2-dopamine receptor lambda HD2G1 and flanking loci on chromosome 11q22-q23 in Tourette syndrome. *Human Heredity*, *10*, 105–108.

Drake, M.E. Jr., Hietter, S.A., Padamadan, H., & Bogner, J.E. (1991). Computerized EEG frequency analysis in Gilles de la Tourette syndrome. *Clinical Electroencephalography*, *22*, 250–253.

Drake, M.E. Jr., Hietter, S.A., Padamadan, H., Bogner, J.E., Andrews, J.M., & Weate, S. (1992). Auditory evoked potentials in Gilles de la Tourette syndrome. *Clinical Electroencephalography*, *23*, 19–23.

Elston, J.S., Grenje, F.C., & Lees, A.J. (1989). The relationship between eye-winking tics, frequent eye-blinking and blepharospasm. *Journal of Neurology, Neurosurgery and Psychiatry*, *52*, 477–480.

Erenberg, G., Cruse, R.P., & Rothner, A.D. (1985). Gilles de la Tourette's syndrome: Effects of stimulant drugs. *Neurology*, *35*, 1346–1348.

Erenberg, G., Cruse, R.P., & Rothner, A.D. (1986). Tourette syndrome: An analysis of 200 pediatric and adolescent cases. *Cleveland Clinic Quarterly*, *53*, 127–131.

Erenberg, G., Cruse, R.P., & Rothner, A.D. (1987). The natural history of Tourette syndrome: A follow-up syndrome. *Annals of Neurology*, *22*, 383–385.

Fahn, S. (1982a). A case of post-traumatic tic syndrome. In A.J. Friedhoff & T.N. Chase (Eds.), *Gilles de la Tourette syndrome* (pp. 349–350). New York: Raven Press.

Fahn, S. (1982b). The clinical spectrum of motor tics. In A.J. Friedhoff & T.N. Chase (Eds.), *Gilles de la Tourette syndrome*, (pp. 341–344). New York: Raven Press.

Ferrari, M., Mathews, W.S., & Barabas, G. (1984). Children with Tourette syndrome: Results of psychological tests given prior to drug treatment. *Developmental and Behavioral Pediatrics*, *5*, 116–119.

Fish, D.R., Sawyers, D., & Allen, P.J. (1991). The affect of sleep on the dyskinetic movements of Parkinson's disease, Gilles de la Tourette syndrome, Huntington's disease and torsion dystonia. *Achives of Neurology*, *18*, 210–214.

Frank, M.S., Sieg, K.G., & Gaffney, G.R. (1991). Somatic complaints in childhood tic disorders. *Psychosomatics*, *32*, 396–399.

Gadow, K.D., Nolan, E.E., & Sverd, J. (1992). Methylphenidate in hyperactive boys with comorbid tic disorder: II. Short-term behavioral effects in school settings. *Journal of the American Academy of Child and Adolescent Psychiatry*, *31*, 462–471.

Gelernter, J., Kennedy, J.L., Grandy, D.K., Zhou, Q.Y., Civelli, O., Pauls, D.L., Pakstis, A., Kurlan, R., Sumahara, R.K., & Niznik, H.B., O'Doud, B., Seeman, P., & Kidd, K.K. (1993). Exclusion of close linkage of Tourette's syndrome to D1 dopamine receptor. *American Journal of Psychiatry*, *150*, 449–453.

Gelernter, J., Pakstis, A.J., Pauls, D.L., Kurlan, R., Gancher, S.T., Civelli, O., Grandy, D., & Kidd, K.K. (1990). Gilles de la Tourette syndrome is not linked to D2-dopamine receptor. *Archives of General Psychiatry*, *47*, 1073–1077.

Gilles de la Tourette, G. (1885). Etude sur une affection nerveuse caracterisee par de l'incoordination motrice accompagnee de'echolalie et la copralalie. *Archives de Neurologie*, *9*, 19–42, 158–200.

Glaze, D., Frost, J.D., Jr., & Jankovic, J. (1983). Sleep in Gilles de la Tourette's syndome: Disorder of arousal. *Neurology*, *33*, 586–592.

Goetz, C.G., Tanner, C.M., Stebbins, G.T., Leipzig, G., & Carr, W.C. (1992). Adult tics in Gilles de la Tourette's syndrome: Description and risk factors. *Neurology, 12*, 784–788.

Goetz, C.G., Tanner, C.M., Wilson, R.S., Carroll, V.S., Como, P.G., & Shannon, K.M. (1987). Clonidine and Gilles de la Tourette syndrome: Double-blind study using objective rating methods. *Annals of Neurology, 21*, 307–310.

Golden, G.S. (1984). Psychologic and neuropsychologic aspects of Tourette's syndrome. *Neurology Clinics, 21*, 91–102.

Golden, G.S. (1985). Tardive dyskinesis in Tourette syndrome. *Pediatric Neurology, 1*, 192–194.

Grossman, H.Y., Mostofsky, D.I., & Harrison, R.H. (1986). Psychological aspects of Gilles de la Tourette syndrome. *Journal of Clinical Psychology, 42*, 228–235.

Hagin, R.A., Beecher, R., Pagano, G., & Kreeger, H. (1982). Effects of Tourette syndrome on learning. In A.J. Friedhoff & T.N. Chase (Eds.), *Gilles de la Tourette syndrome* (pp. 323–333). New York: Raven Press.

Hagin, R.A., & Kugler, J. (1988). School problems associated with Tourette's syndrome. In D.J. Cohen, R.D. Bruun, & J.F. Leckman (Eds.), *Tourette's syndrome and tic disorder* (pp. 223–236). New York: John Wiley & Sons.

Harcherik, D.F., Cohen, D.J., Ort, S., Paul, R., Shaywitz, B.A., Volkmar, F.R., Rothman, S.L.G., & Leckman, J.F. (1985). Computed tomographic brain scanning in four neuropsychiatric disorders of childhood. *American Journal of Psychiatry, 142*, 731–734.

Harris, E.L., Schuerholz, L.J., Singer, H.S., Readen, M.J., Brown, J.B., Cox, C., Mohr, J., Chase, G.A., & Denckla, M.B. (in press). Executive function in children with Tourette syndrome and/or attention deficit hyperactivity disorder. *Journal of International Neuropsychological Society.*

Hyde, T.M., Aaronson, B.A., Randolph, C., Rickler, W.C., & Weinberger, D.R. (1992). Relationship of birth weight to the phenotypic expression of Gilles de la Tourette's syndrome. *Neurology, 42*, 652–658.

Itard, J.M.G. (1825). Memoire sur quelques fonctions involontaires des appareils de la locomotion, de la prehension et de la voix. *Archives Generale de Medicine, 8*, 385–407.

Jankovic, J. (1993). Deprenyl in attention deficit associated with Tourette syndrome. *Archives Neurology, 50*, 286–288.

Jankovic, J., & Stone, L. (1991). Dystonic tics in patients with Tourette's syndrome. *Movement Disorders, 6*, 248–252.

Karagianis, J.L., & Nagpurkar, R. (1990). A case of Tourette syndrome developing during haloperidol treatment. *Canadian Journal Psychiatry, 35*, 228–232.

Klawans, H.L., Falk, D.K., Nausieda, P.A., & Weiner, W.J. (1978). Gilles de la Tourette's syndrome after long-term chlorpromazine therapy. *Neurology, 28*, 1064–1066.

Koller, W.C., & Biary, N.M. (1989). Volitional control of involuntary movements. *Movement Disorders, 4*, 153–155.

Krumholz, A., Singer, H.S., Neidermeyer, E., Burnite, R., & Harris, K. (1983). Electrophysiological studies in Tourette's syndrome. *Annals of Neurology, 14*, 638–641.

Kurlan, R. (1989). Tourette's syndrome: Current concepts. *Neurology, 39,* 1625–1630.

Kurlan, R., Behr, J., Medved, L., & Como, P. (1988). Transient tic disorder and the clinical spectrum of Tourette's syndrome. *Archives of Neurology, 45*, 1200–1201.

Kurlan, R., Lichter, D., & Hewitt, D. (1989). Sensory tics in Tourette's syndrome. *Neurology, 39*, 731–734.

Kurlan, R., & Trinidad, K.S. (1995). Treatment of tics. In R. Kurlan (Ed.), *The treatment of movement disorders* (pp. 365–406). Philadelphia: J.B. Lippincott.

Kurlan, R., Whitmore, D., Irvine, C., McDermott, M.P., & Como, P.G. (1994). Tourette's syndrome in a special education population: A pilot study involving a single school district. *Neurology, 44*, 699–702.

Lang, A.E., Consky, E., & Sandor, P. (1993). "Signing-tics" . . . insights into the pathophysiology of symptoms in Tourette syndrome. *Annals of Neurology, 33*, 212–215.

Lasker, A.G., Zee, D.S., Hain, T.C., Folstein, S.J., & Singer, H.S. (1987). Saccades in Huntington's disease: Initiation defects and distractibility. *Neurology, 37*, 364–370.

Lasker, A.G., Zee, D.S., Hain, T.C., Folstein, S.J., & Singer, H.S. (1988). Saccades in Huntington's disease: Slowing and dysmetria. *Neurology, 38*, 427–431.

Leckman, J.F., de Lotbiniére, A.J., Marek, K., Gracco, C., Scahill, C., & Cohen, D.J. (1993). Severe disturbances in speech, swallowing, and gait following stereotactic infrathalamic lesions in Gilles de la Tourette's syndrome. *Neurology, 43*, 890–894.

Leckman, J.F., & Peterson, B.S. (1993). The pathogenesis of Tourette's syndrome: Epigenetic factors active in early CNS development. *Biological Psychiatry, 34*, 425–427.

Leckman, J.F., Walker, D.E., & Cohen, D.J. (1993). Premonitory urges in Tourette's syndrome. *American Journal of Psychiatry, 150*, 98–102.

Leonard, H.L., Lenane, M.C., Swedo, S.E., Rettew, D.C., Gershon, E.S., & Rapoport, J.L. (1992). Tics and Tourette syndrome: A 2 to 7 year follow up of 54 obsessive-compulsive children. *American Journal of Psychiatry, 148*, 1244–1247.

Ludlow, C.L., Polinsky, R.J., Caine, E.D., Bassich, C.J., & Ebert, M.H. (1982). Language and speech abnormalities in Tourette's syndrome. In A.J. Friedhoff & T.N. Chase (Eds.), *Gilles de la Tourette syndrome* (pp. 351–361). New York: Raven Press.

Mendleson, W., Caine, E.D., Goyer, P., Ebert, M., & Gillin, J.C. (1980). Sleep in Gilles de la Tourette syndrome. *Biological Psychiatry, 15*, 339–343.

Michultka, D.M., Blanchard, E.B., & Rosenblum, E.L. (1989). Stress management and Gilles de la Tourette's syndrome. *Biofeedback and Self Regulation, 14*, 115–123.

Nee, L.E., Caine, E.D., Polinsky, R.J., Eldridge, R., & Ebert, M.H. (1980). Gilles de la Tourette syndrome: Clinical and family study of 50 cases. *Annals of Neurology, 7*, 41–49.

Northam, R.S., & Singer, H.S. (1991). Postencephalitic acquired Tourette-like syndrome in a child. *Neurology, 41*, 592–593.

Park, S., Como, P.G., Cui, J., & Kurlan, R. (1993). The early course of Tourette's syndrome clinical spectrum. *Neurology, 43*, 1712–1715.

Pauls, D.L., Hurst, C.R., Kruger, S.D., Leckman, J.F., Kidd, K.K., & Cohen, D.J. (1986). Gilles de la Tourette's syndrome and attention deficit disorder with hyperactivity: Evidence against a genetic relationship. *Archives of General Psychiatry, 43*, 1177–1179.

Pauls, D.L., Kruger, S.D., Leckman, J.F., Cohen, D.J., & Kidd, K.K. (1984). The risk of Tourette's syndrome and chronic multiple tics among relatives of Tourette's syndrome patients obtained by direct interviews. *Journal of the American Academy of Child and Adolescent Psychiatry, 23*, 134–137.

Pauls, D.L., & Leckman, J.F. (1986). The inheritance of Gilles de la Tourette's syndrome and associated behaviors: Evidence for autosomal dominant transmission. *New England Journal of Medicine, 315*, 993–997.

Pauls, D.L., Leckman, J.F., & Cohen, D.J. (1993). The familial relationship between Gilles de la Tourette's syndrome, attention deficit disorder, learning disabilities, speech disorders and stuttering. *Journal of the American Academy of Child and Adolescent Psychiatry, 32*, 1044–1050.

Pauls, D.L., Pakstis, A.J., Kurlan, R., Kidd, K.K., Leckman, J.F., Cohen, D.J., Kidd, J.R., Como, P., & Sparkes, R. (1990). Segregation and linkage analysis of Tourette's syndrome and related disorders. *Journal of the American Academy of Child and Adolescent Psychiatry, 29*, 195–203.

Pauls, D.L., Towbin, K.E., Leckman, J.F., Zahner, G.E.P., & Cohen, D.J. (1986). Gilles de la Tourette's syndrome and obsessive-compulsive disorder: Evidence supporting a genetic relationship. *Archives of General Psychiatry, 43*, 1180–1182.

Peterson, A.L., & Azrin, N.H. (1992). An evaluation of behavioral treatments for Tourette syndrome. *Behaviour Research and Therapy, 30*, 167–174.

Peterson, B., Leckman, J.F., Scahill, L., Naftolin, F., Keefe, D., Charest, N.J., & Cohen, D.J. (1992). Steroid hormones and CNS sexual dimorphisms modulate symptom expression in Tourette's syndrome. *Psychoneuroendocrinology, 6*, 553–563.

Price, R.A., Kidd, K.K., Cohen, D.J., Pauls, D.L., & Leckman, J.F. (1985). A twin study of Tourette syndrome. *Archives of General Psychiatry, 42*, 815–820.

Price, R.A., Leckman, J.F., Pauls, D.L., Cohen, D.J., & Kidd, K.K. (1986). Gilles de la Tourette syndrome: Tics and central nervous system stimulants in twins and non-twins. *Neurology, 26*, 232–237.

Repka, M.X., & Singer, H.S. (1992). Gilles de la Tourette syndrome and the afferent visual system. *Neuro-ophthalmology, 6*, 367–374.

Robertson, M.M. (1989). The Gilles de la Tourette syndrome: The current status. *British Journal of Psychiatry, 154*, 147–169.

Robertson, M.M., Doran, M., Trimble, M., & Lees, A.J. (1990). The treatment of Gilles de la Tourette syndrome by limbic leucotomy. *Journal of Neurology, Neurosurgery and Psychiatry, 53*, 691–694.

Robertson, M.M., Trimble, M.R., & Lees, A.J. (1988). The psychopathology of the Gilles de la Tourette syndrome: A phenomenological analysis. *British Journal of Psychiatry, 152*, 383–390.

Robertson, M.M., Trimble, M.R., & Lees, A.J. (1989). Self-injurious behavior and the Gilles de la Tourette syndrome: A clinical study and review of the literature. *Psychological Medicine, 19*, 611–625.

Robertson, M.M., & Yakeley, J.W. (1993). Obsessive compulsive disorder and self injurious behavior. In R. Kurlan (Ed.), *Handbook of Tourette's syndrome and related tic and behavioral disorders* (pp. 45–87). New York: Marcel Dekker.

Sacks, O.W. (1982). Acquired tourettism to adult life. In A.J. Friedhoff & T.N. Chase, (Eds.), *Gilles de la Tourette syndrome* (pp. 89–92). New York: Raven Press.

Sanchez-Ramos, J.R., & Weiner, W.J. (1993). Drug induced tics. In R. Kurlan (Ed.), *Handbook of Tourette's syndrome and related tic and behavioral disorders* (pp. 183–197). New York: Marcel Dekker.

Schuerholz, L.J., Baumgardner, T.L., Singer, H.S., Reiss, A.L., & Denckla, M.B. (in press). Neuropsychological status of children with Tourette syndrome with and without attention deficit hyperactivity disorder. *Neurology.*

Schwabe, M.J., & Konkol, R.J. (1992). Menstrual cycle–related fluctuations of tics in Tourette syndrome. *Pediatric Neurology, 9*, 43–46.

Shapiro, A.K., & Shapiro, E. (1992). Evaluation of the reported association of obsessive-compulsive symptoms or disorder with Tourette's disorder. *Comparative Psychiatry, 33*, 152–165.

Shapiro, A.K., Shapiro, E.S., Young, J.G., & Feinbert, E. (1988). *Gilles de la Tourette syndrome.* (2nd ed.). New York: Raven Press.

Singer, C., Sanchez-Ramos, J., & Weiner, W.J. (1989). A case of post-traumatic tic disorder. *Movement Disorders, 4,* 342–344.

Singer, H.S. (1995). [Children with Tourette syndrome and their families]. Unpublished raw data.

Singer, H.S., Brown, J.E., Quaskey, S., Rosenberg, L.A., Mellits, B.D., & Denckla, M.B. (1995). The treatment of attention-deficit hyperactivity disorder in Tourette syndrome: A double blind placebo controlled study with clonidine and desipramine. *Pediatrics, 95,* 74–81.

Singer, H.S., & Rosenberg, L.A. (1989). The development of behavioral and emotional problems in Tourette syndrome. *Pediatric Neurology, 5,* 41–44.

Singer, H.S., Schuerholz, L.J., & Denckla, M.B. (1995). Learning difficulties in children with Tourette syndrome. *Journal of Child Neurology, 10*(Suppl. 1), S58–S61.

Singer, H.S., & Walkup, J.T. (1991). Tourette syndrome and other tic disorders: Diagnosis, pathophysiology, and treatment. *Medicine, 70,* 15–32.

Singer, H.S., Waranch, H.R., & Brown, J. (1993). Relaxation therapy: An alternative treatment for Tourette's syndrome? *Annals of Neurology, 34,* 439.

Spencer, T., Biederman, J., Wilens, T., Steingard, R., & Geist, D. (1993). Nortriptyline treatment of children with attention-deficit hyperactivity disorder and tic disorder or Tourette's syndrome. *Journal American Academy of Child and Adolescent Psychiatry, 32,* 205–210.

Stefl, M.E. (1984). Mental health needs associated with Tourette syndrome. *American Journal of Public Health, 74,* 1310–1313.

Stokes, A., Bawden, H.N., Camfield, P.R., Backman, J.E., & Dooley, J.M. (1991). Peer problems in Tourette's disorder. *Pediatrics, 87,* 936–942.

Stone, L.A., & Jankovic, J. (1991). The coexistence of tics and dystonia. *Archives of Neurology, 48,* 862–865.

Tanner, C.M. (1993). Epidemiology. In R. Kurlan (Ed.), *Handbook of Tourette's syndrome and related tic and behavioral disorders* (pp. 337–347). New York: Marcel Dekker.

Tourette Syndrome Classfication Group. (1993). Definition and classification of tic disorders. *Archives of Neurology, 50,* 1013–1016.

Van de Wetering, B.J.M., Martana, C.M.C., Fortgens, C., Slasta, J.P.J., & Van Woerkom, T.C.A.M. (1985). Late components of the auditory evoked potentials in Gilles de la Tourette syndrome. *Clinical Neurology and Neurosurgery, 87,* 181–186.

Van Woerkom, T.C.A.M., Fortgens, C., Rompel-Martana, C.M.S., & Van de Wetering, B.J.M. (1988). Auditory event-related potentials in adult patients with Gilles de la Tourette's syndrome in the oddball paradigm. *Electroencephalography and Clinical Neurophysiology, 71,* 443–449.

Van Woerkom, T.C.A.M., Fortgens, C., Van de Wetering, B.J.M., & Martana, C.M.C. (1988). Contingent negative variation in adults with Gilles de la Tourette syndrome. *Journal of Neurology, Neurosurgery and Psychiatry, 51,* 630–634.

Vandenbergh, D.J., Persico, A.M., Gelernter, J., Bird, G.S., Crowe, R., Surratt, C., Kurlan, R., Singer, H., Kidd, K.K., & Uhl, G.R. (1993). Dopamine and vesicular transporter gene markers in neuropsychiatric disorders. *Society for Neuroscience Abstracts, 19,* 201.

Chapter 34

Epilepsy and Developmental Disabilities

Eileen P.G. Vining, M.D., and John M. Freeman, M.D.

Every physician working with children and adolescents who have disabilities should be able to recognize seizures; should be able to separate seizures from other episodic events such as reflux, syncope, or behavioral manifestations that may mimic seizures; and should be able to initiate appropriate evaluation and therapy. Epilepsy is common in children and eminently treatable, even curable, and is more prevalent in children with developmental disabilities. If the developmental pediatrician is to be the center of a management team for children with disabilities, he or she must avoid unwarranted referrals while recognizing the limitations of his or her expertise.

EPIDEMIOLOGY

A *seizure* is an alteration of motor or sensory function, behavior, or consciousness caused by a discharge of electrical activity in the brain. *Epilepsy* is recurrent seizures. Febrile seizures occur in 3%–5% of all children. Nonfebrile seizures occur in 0.5%–2% of children; epilepsy occurs in 0.5%–1%. In contrast, seizures and epilepsy are far more common in children with other disabilities.

There are many ways to attempt an analysis of the frequency of epilepsy in children with developmental disabilities, and it is clearly dependent on the nature/extent of the disability. In children with mental retardation, including those who have mild mental retardation (IQ<70), about 5%–10% will have epilepsy (Hauser & Hesdorffer, 1990). If there is evidence of additional central nervous system damage (i.e., cerebral palsy), then a larger percentage is usually found to have epilepsy (approximately 40%–50%). The likelihood of developing epilepsy also is influenced by the cause of the mental retardation; those children who acquired mental retardation as the result of a postnatal brain injury had a much higher incidence of epilepsy (70%) than did those with mental retardation caused by a genetic syndrome (trisomy 21, etc.) (Figure 1) (Goulden, Shinar, Koller, Katz, & Richardson, 1991). Focusing on those individuals with IQs less than 50, approximately 30% have epilepsy, although many cases may be inactive. If a child has cerebral palsy without mental retardation, the risk of epilepsy is about 30%. Studies attempting to define the percentage of children with autism who also have epilepsy are more ambiguous, perhaps reflecting difficulties in determining autism, and incidence estimates range from 10% to 35% (Figure 2) (Hauser & Hesdorffer, 1990).

From a developmentalist's point of view, another important question is what percentage of those with epilepsy also will have other developmental problems. Sillanpaa (1992), utilizing

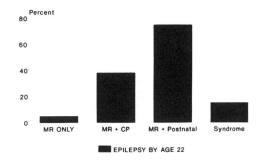

Figure 1. Epilepsy in mental retardation. (MR, mental retardation; CP, cerebral palsy.) (Adapted from Goulden, Shinar, Koller, Katz, & Richardson, 1991.)

511

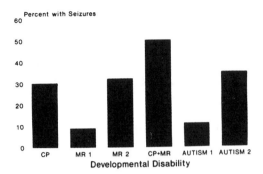

Figure 2. Seizures in developmental disabilities. (CP, cerebral palsy; MR 1, Isle Of Wight Study (general population); MR2, London Study (severe MR); Autism 1, New York Study; Autism 2, Swedish Study. (Adapted from Hauser & Hesdorffer, 1990.)

World Health Organization definitions, suggested that, in a population of children with epilepsy, about 30% will have mental retardation, 27% will have a speech disorder, 23% will have specific learning disabilities, 10% will have minimal brain dysfunction, and about 27% will have other neurologic impairments (Figure 3). It is clear that, in a clinical setting dealing with children with developmental disabilities, there will be many children with epilepsy, a neurologic condition that is readily amenable to intervention.

CLASSIFICATION OF SEIZURES

It is important to understand the classification of seizures because this information affects understanding of etiology, prognosis, and treatment. Seizures continue traditionally to be divided

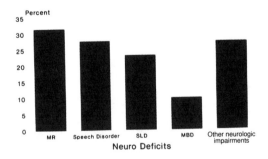

Figure 3. Accessory neurologic deficits in children with epilepsy. (MR, mental retardation; SLD, specific learning disability; MBD, minimal brain dysfunction.) (Adapted from Sillanpaa, 1992; epilepsy prevalence 0.68%.)

into those believed to have a partial (focal) onset and those that appear to start all over the brain simultaneously (generalized). Partial seizures may remain very localized (motor, sensory, autonomic) or they may spread and impair consciousness (complex) or become secondarily generalized, with loss of consciousness and alterations in motor function (Dreifuss, 1989).

Generalized seizures have a variety of manifestations, ranging from absence seizures (petit mal) to generalized tonic–clonic seizures (grand mal). Infantile spasms and akinetic seizures are also forms of generalized seizures. An abbreviated classification scheme is shown in Table 1.

The importance of these distinctions lies in recognizing a potential focal abnormality of the brain that might be amenable to surgery and in identifying seizure types that might require specific antiepileptic drug therapy.

EPILEPSY SYNDROMES

In addition to classifying according to seizure type, an attempt is made to determine if a particular epilepsy syndrome exists. An epilepsy syndrome is a specific epileptic disorder characterized by a cluster of signs and symptoms customarily occurring together. The distinction is again made whether seizures are generalized or partial *and* whether they are considered symptomatic or secondary to an identifiable neurologic

Table 1. Classification of seizure types

I. Partial (focal, local) seizures
   A. Simple partial seizures (consciousness not impaired)
   B. Complex partial seizures (with impairment of consciousness)
   C. Partial seizures secondarily generalized
II. Generalized seizures (convulsive or nonconvulsive)
   A. 1. Absence seizures
      2. Atypical absence seizures
   B. Myoclonic seizures
   C. Clonic seizures
   D. Tonic seizures
   E. Tonic–clonic seizures
   F. Atonic seizures
III. Unclassified epileptic seizures

Adapted from Commission on Classification and Terminology of the International League Against Epilepsy (1981).

process or are idiopathic, cryptogenic, or of un-known origin. There is also a group of epilep-sies that are considered undetermined as to whether they are focal or generalized (neonatal seizures, etc). Finally, there are special syn-dromes that include febrile seizures and very unique, rare seizure disorders (Table 2) (Drei-fuss, 1989).

There are several epilepsy syndromes that de-serve emphasis for developmental pediatricians because of their prevalence and need for addi-tional understanding. These are listed here in or-der according to the International Classification.

Benign Childhood Epilepsy with Centrotemporal Spikes (BECTS, benign rolandic epilepsy)

This syndrome occurs between 3 and 12 years of age, predominantly in the early school years. The seizures generally occur during the night

Table 2. International classification of epilepsies and epilepsy syndromes

1. Localization-related (focal, local, partial) epilepsies and syndromes
    1.1 Idiopathic (with age-related onset)
        Benign childhood epilepsy with centrotem-poral spike
    1.2 Symptomatic (includes the partial seizures)
    1.3 Unknown as to whether syndrome is idio-pathic or symptomatic
2. Generalized epilepsies and syndromes
    2.1 Idiopathic (with age-related onset)
        includes juvenile myoclonic epilepsy
    2.2 Cryptogenic or symptomatic
        includes West syndrome, Lennox-Gastaut syndrome
    2.3 Symptomatic
3. Epilepsies and syndromes undetermined whether focal or generalized
    3.1 With both generalized and focal seizures
        includes neonatal seizures, epilepsy with continuous spike–waves during slow-wave sleep, acquired epileptic aphasia (Landau-Kleffner syndrome)
    3.2 Without unequivocal generalized or focal features
4. Special syndromes
    4.1 Situation-related seizures
        includes febrile seizures

Adapted from Commission on Classification and Terminology of the International League Against Epilepsy (1985).

and typically involve the face; spread may occur and the seizure can generalize. This onset is in keeping with the electroencephalo-graphic abnormalities of spikes over the central–midtemporal region, seen especially during light non–rapid eye movement (non-REM) sleep. These seizures often do not need to be treated because they are usually infrequent and occur only at night, not disrupting the child's daily ac-tivities. When more frequent or disruptive, they almost always respond to carbamazepine. They are benign not only because of the nature of the seizure but because they are virtually always outgrown by puberty.

Juvenile Myoclonic Epilepsy (of Janz)

This syndrome typically begins in young people ages 12–19 and involves a variety of seizures, including myoclonic, tonic–clonic, and absence. Seizures are exacerbated by sleep deprivation and classically are myoclonic on awakening. The electroencephalogram (EEG) shows a fast spike–wave pattern (3.5–6 Hz) and multiple spike–wave complexes, especially during sleep. Therapy with valproic acid is usually successful but generally needs to be maintained throughout life. Family history is often positive, and early work appears to suggest that the genetic marker for some forms of this syndrome may lie on the short arm of chromosome 6 (Greenberg & Delgado-Escueta, 1993).

West Syndrome (Infantile Spasms)

This is an age-related syndrome rarely occur-ring after 2 years of age and accounting for 35%–52% of all afebrile seizures occurring in the first year of life (Chevrie & Aicardi, 1977). The seizures involve a sudden flexion of the body and extension of the arms recurring in clusters. They often occur on awakening. Ap-proximately two thirds of cases of infantile spasms are *symptomatic*, caused by develop-mental, metabolic, or genetic abnormalities, and one third are *cryptogenic*, occurring in a child who appeared normal neurologically prior to the onset of the seizures. With advanced neu-roimaging techniques, increasing numbers of children with structural abnormalities are being identified. Hypsarrhythmia, an EEG pattern usually seen in association with this disorder, is very high voltage with a multifocal spike pattern. It is completely disorganized and chaotic, often showing periods of burst–suppression. Therapy remains difficult and generally involves the use of adrenocorticotropic hormone or steroids (Snead, 1990). More than two thirds of these children, perhaps as many as 95%, ultimately are shown to have mental retardation. Even when seizures have been well controlled, children generally do not develop normally. A child who has the typical infantile spasms, a hypsarrhythmic EEG, and mental retardation is said to have West's syndrome.

Lennox-Gastaut Syndrome

Forty percent of children with infantile spasms develop Lennox-Gastaut syndrome, a combination of seizure types (tonic, atonic, absence, myoclonic) with a very abnormal EEG with slow-spike waves and runs of rapid spikes in sleep. Mental retardation occurs in up to 90% of children with this syndrome. These seizures are exceedingly difficult to control and often require multiple medications. The most effective therapy has been valproic acid and the ketogenic diet, although new medications, including felbamate, and lamotrigine may be promising. Attempts at palliating the atonic (drop) spells with corpus callosotomy have been marginally successful.

Neonatal Seizures

Neonatal seizures occur in the first month of life and are almost always symptomatic of a central nervous system disturbance such as chemical or metabolic imbalance, trauma, hemorrhage, hypoxia, or developmental abnormalities of the brain. The seizures are often fragments of those seen in older children and adults, often manifesting as "subtle" seizures involving reflexive movements such as sucking, swimming, or "bicycling" movements. The outcome certainly depends on the cause of the seizures. Early-onset seizures, beginning in the first days of life, are regarded as a marker for potential central nervous system dysfunction with an increased chance of neurologic abnormality, including cerebral palsy, mental retardation, and epilepsy (Painter & Gaus, 1991).

Epilepsy with Continuous Spike Waves During Slow-Wave Sleep (Electrical Status Epilepticus During Sleep)

This syndrome involves a pattern of electrical status epilepticus in the EEG with continuous slow-spike–wave activity during non-REM sleep. It generally occurs in school-age children and is associated with a variety of seizure types, including myoclonic, tonic–clonic, and absence. There is often intellectual as well as behavioral dysfunction.

Acquired Epileptic Aphasia (Landau-Kleffner Syndrome)

Landau-Kleffner syndrome is a childhood epilepsy syndrome involving progressive aphasia and epilepsy. Onset is usually between 4 and 6 years, with gradually deteriorating expressive and receptive language. These children may become mute and have many autistic characteristics because they are unable to understand language. Multiple seizure types are reported, and the EEG often shows more marked abnormality maximal over the left temporal regions. Medical therapy is often ineffective; various surgical interventions, including temporal lobectomy and multiple subpial resections, are controversial because spontaneous recovery has occurred (Paquier, VanDongen, & Loonen, 1992).

EVALUATION

Differential Diagnosis of "Episodes"

First, it must be clear that the episode or episodes in question are actually seizures. This may be particularly difficult in children who have significant neurologic dysfunction on a chronic/underlying basis. In addition, there are a number of entities seen in childhood that are often difficult to distinguish from epilepsy, especially for parents and caregivers (Rothner, 1989; Stephenson, 1993). A brief review of these other paroxysmal disorders follows.

Breathholding Spells Breathholding spells occur in about 5% of children. The symptoms may relate to an apparently immature central nervous system. In *cyanotic breathholding*, something precipitates the child's crying and then he or she stops breathing in expiration, becomes progressively cyanotic and stiff, and loses consciousness. It truly appears as though the child is having a tonic seizure, although a concomitant EEG would show the slowing and then flattening associated with cerebral hypoxia. This "tonic" phase may be followed by some minor clonic activity. The child then becomes limp and begins breathing again. He or she may be tired or fussy momentarily. The spells usually begin between 6 and 18 months of age. Family history is frequently positive. Development is usually normal, and the EEG normal as well. The seizurelike component is simply a reaction to the hypoxia the child is experiencing and, therefore, antiepileptic medications are useless. Phenobarbital may make the situation worse because the child may become more irritable. The family needs education about the process, as well as about the fact that these episodes are not harmful and that the child will grow out of them before school begins. The best approach may well be quickly to manipulate the child's attention away from the source of crying.

The *pallid* form of breathholding appears vagal in nature and usually occurs after pain or fright. The vagal slowing of the heart may even result in a brief asystole. The child may fall or seem to faint and, if the asystole is long enough, the child will experience a brief period of cerebral ischemia and become tonic or have a tonic–clonic seizure. The child then becomes limp, regains consciousness, and resumes baseline functioning. An EEG during one of these episodes would show slowing, not epileptiform activity. Antiepileptic drugs are not useful and generally one does not need to consider using a vagal blocking agent such as atropine.

Syncope Fainting, or syncope, is also due to cerebral hypoperfusion and is often precipitated by heat, illness, phlebotomy, and pain (even as mild as haircombing). There is usually a warning of lightheadedness, dizziness, or visual obscuration. The child then becomes limp and sometimes, again because of hypoperfusion, may occasionally experience an apparent generalized convulsion. The episode is brief and

consciousness is resumed quickly. The EEG is not helpful, and treatment should involve avoidance of behaviors or situations that might precipitate fainting. Evaluation perhaps should include an electrocardiogram; occasionally more aggressive investigation would proceed to Holter monitoring or tilt table testing.

Migraine Migraines are also paroxysmal episodes of the central nervous system, and some symptoms may overlap with those seen in seizures, such as an aura. Conversely, a headache sometimes may be seen postictally. A positive family history of migraines is often important in making the diagnosis. An EEG may be helpful because clearly epileptogenic changes are more suggestive of a seizure disorder.

Movement Disorders Paroxysmal choreiform and dystonic disorders may mimic seizures; however, the EEG usually does not show epileptiform disturbances. A careful history and observation usually will make the diagnosis clear, even in children with cerebral palsy. Paroxysmal movements in the setting of cerebral palsy usually do not interfere with consciousness, and posturing can be eliminated by changes in position of the child. Tics are sometimes mistaken for seizures but are usually quicker and more stereotyped in nature than seizures. They also can usually be brought under voluntary control, whereas seizures cannot be stopped.

Disorders of Sleep Many children experience night terrors (pavor nocturnus) during the toddler and early preschool years. They usually are seen in the early hours of sleep, arising from deep slow-wave sleep. Typically the child screams, sits up, crying as if terrified and making thrashing movements, and is virtually inconsolable. This may last several minutes and the child then spontaneously quiets and returns to sleep without any memory of this event (Thorpy & Glovinsky, 1987).

Psychological Phenomena

Pseudoseizures Although probably less common in young children, pseudoseizures are seen with some frequency in adolescents. The phenomena/changes in behavior described are usually less stereotyped than those seen in epileptogenic seizures. The more generalized episodes are easier to differentiate because the movements are usually more violent, thrashing, and less "controlled" and rhythmic than a tonic–clonic seizure. There is usually no postictal period. The EEG during the episode, although often obscured by artifact, does not show epileptiform activity and will usually show normal rhythms immediately before and subsequent to the episode. Episodes that involve alterations in consciousness, or more limited "partial" phenomenology, are often more difficult to interpret. An attempt to induce one of these episodes under EEG monitoring is often helpful in determining the exact nature of the episode.

Episodic Dyscontrol   Episodic dyscontrol is attacks of seemingly uncontrolled rage. The history is absolutely critical because it indicates that there is *always* some form of precipitating event. There is usually no aura and the rage is often directed, unlike the occasional anger or hostility that is unfocused in a patient experiencing a seizure, wherein confusion and inability to interpret intervention correctly are often the cause of the apparently violent behavior. After a seizure, the patient is usually confused, unlike episodic dyscontrol, in which the child quickly returns to baseline function. Episodic changes in behavior *in the absence of other clearly definable seizures* are virtually never seizures, even when abnormalities on the EEG are detected.

Daydreaming   Children, especially those with attention-deficit/hyperactivity disorder, may appear to have alterations in consciousness, posing the question of whether absence seizures are occurring. Generally careful observation, along with mild physical stimulation (touching, tickling, gentle pinching), will differentiate a seizure from attentional problems. Just as children with attention-deficit/hyperactivity disorder sometimes have difficulty focusing attention, they may have difficulty shifting or manipulating their attention, which can be just as dysfunctional.

Other Disorders   Perhaps the most poorly understood and recognized entity affecting children with significant motor problems (cerebral palsy) is *gastroesophageal reflux* (Sandifer syndrome). This is generally seen in young children and consists of tonic stiffening that may or may not be related to feeding. Appropriate study will reveal gastroesophageal reflux, and treatment consists of appropriate management.

Another problem that must be included in any differential diagnosis involving change in function or behavior is *intoxication*. Unfortunately, this must be recognized on an acute basis so that appropriate confirmatory testing can be done.

Workup

Evaluation must be situational, depending on when a child has had the seizure. Obviously, if the seizure is occurring in an emergency room, acute problems must be appropriately evaluated including metabolic, infectious, and toxic problems. If the seizure has occurred and the child has returned to baseline, the evaluation should be pertinent. In general, it would include a complete history and physical examination.

Electroencephalogram   An EEG may delineate focality, clarify the nature of paroxysmal activity (if any), and be helpful in prognosticating and choosing medication. The EEG may be normal in children who have seizures, and it may quickly revert to normal after a seizure. Its stability over time therefore may be limited. It is more likely to be abnormal (slow) in children with developmental disabilities, especially those with structural abnormalities. The EEG may be abnormal in children who have never had a seizure. In fact, abnormalities may be seen in 5%–15% of children who have no history of seizures (Tsuboi, 1978). Physicians should make certain that the EEGs they request include both an awake and a sleep tracing. Sleep is one of the best provocateurs of abnormal activity, and a sleep EEG should be obtained even if it is necessary to sedate the child with chloral hydrate. Conversely, an awake EEG is important in assessing the normalcy of background function. In addition, photic stimulation and well-performed hyperventilation for 4 minutes are important adjuncts in EEG assessment.

An EEG should be repeated *only* when additional information is being sought. It is useful when seizures have not been controlled, when seizure phenomenology has changed, when there are questions concerning the child's development, and when there is the possibility of discontinuing medication (Shinnar et al., 1985).

Imaging Studies A computerized tomography (CT) scan or magnetic resonance imaging (MRI) is rarely useful after a single seizure. Such imaging studies should be obtained only when there is great concern over focality either because of the seizure, residual neurologic dysfunction, or evidence of significant focality on the EEG. When done in the presence of epilepsy (recurring seizures), approximately 40% of studies will be abnormal, but only a small percentage show abnormalities that actually lead to therapeutic intervention. Yang and colleagues reported that, if the neurologic examination and EEG were normal, abnormal CT scans were found in only 5% of children. The yield was 50% if the seizures were simple partial in nature and 30% when the seizures were complex partial (Yang, Berger, Cohen, & Duffner, 1979). MRI is clearly a superior technique when there is ongoing concern about possible focal abnormalities or when more subtle changes of cortical development are being sought (Brodtkorb, Nilsen, Smevik, & Rinck, 1992; Holmes, 1989).

Biochemical/Metabolic Testing The use of various tests seeking etiology (organic acids, metabolic screening, chromosome analysis, etc.) should be placed in the context of the child's abnormalities and the history.

SEIZURES IN THE CHILD WITH MILD DEVELOPMENTAL DISABILITIES

Recurrent seizures may or may not constitute a disability. Occasional seizures that occur at night may not interfere with a child's function. Even seizures that are focal, occurring frequently during the day, may not constitute a substantial disability. It is critical to think of how a particular child's seizures interfere with *that* particular child's abilities. Seizures should not be treated merely because they are there, but rather if, and only if, the treatment causes less dysfunction than the seizures. The concept of delineating and discussing the risk–benefit analysis for a particular child is dealt with in de-

tail in *Seizures and Epilepsy in Childhood: A Guide for Parents* (Freeman, Vining, & Pillas, 1990). The following case discussions illustrate some of these concepts.

    Case 1 Jamel is 8 years old. He has a congenital left hemiparesis. He is ambulatory, has mild learning impairments, and twice a day has a brief focal seizure involving his arm. Will medication, if successful in abolishing these brief seizures, improve his well-being? Or will medication further increase his learning disability?

    Case 2 Elizabeth is 9 years old and has an attention-deficit disorder. She has just had her second generalized tonic–clonic seizure during sleep. Because by definition she now has epilepsy, should she be treated?

    Case 3 Lorenzo, age 7, is daydreaming in school. His mother has seen a single episode during dinner when he stopped and stared, picking at his food. Does he need further workup and treatment?

Jamel (Case 1) has a mild to moderate disability because of his hemiparesis. His learning disability might be exacerbated by medication used to prevent seizure recurrence. Unless the seizures are frequent or are clearly interfering with his daily function, they may not need treatment. If not, then they do not need an extensive workup either. The EEG is likely to be abnormal, with slowing and spike activity over the right hemisphere. (Does that help in making a decision about therapy?) MRI may show underlying porencephaly, but not a lesion which requires specific surgical therapy. Therefore, if it is decided that the seizures do not require medical therapy, they probably require little evaluation either. Obviously, the child and the parents must concur in this assessment or the anxiety involving the possibility of recurring seizures may limit the child's confidence and abilities.

In Case 2, it is unclear that the two nocturnal seizures have any relationship to the attention-deficit disorder. If the chance of having a third seizure is 60%–75%, should Elizabeth be treated? Possibly. If this young lady has a very abnormal (spike–wave) EEG, her chances of additional seizures may be even higher. A relatively normal EEG may be a good prognostic feature. In this case, evaluation with an EEG may help in decision making. MRI is unlikely to be useful unless there is evidence of a new neurologic deficit. The correct answer regarding therapy for Elizabeth lies in a frank discussion with the family.

In Case 3, Lorenzo's mother has probably seen the tip of the iceberg. Staring spells are virtually never isolated events. Hyperventilation for 3 or 4 minutes may precipitate a seizure in the office and confirm that the daydreaming is an ictal event. An EEG with hyperventilation may document that there are many brief alterations in electrical activity that may interfere with attention and learning. We are far more likely to treat this youth who has had one brief witnessed event because of the likelihood that the even more frequent electrical events are playing a role in his dysfunction. Lorenzo does not need an MRI unless his seizures prove difficult to control (Freeman & Vining, 1992).

TREATMENT

Treatment of epilepsy should be initiated when the benefits are believed to outweigh the risks. Once the decision to treat has been made, several principles should be followed.

1. *Choose the medication that is most effective for a particular type of seizure disorder and that has the least likelihood of producing side effects.* The choice of medication is based on

particular seizure types, and medications in the order in which we usually prefer using them are shown in Figure 4. A list of recommended doses, therapeutic ranges, and common side effects is presented in Table 3. Considering possible side effects involves knowledge of a child's age and baseline function. Phenobarbital is not a good choice in a child who already is perceived to have attention-deficit/hyperactivity disorder. Phenytoin might be a poor first choice in a rapidly growing 6-year-old girl who might be prone to gingival hyperplasia and hirsutism. It is often difficult to achieve stable therapeutic levels of phenytoin in young children.

2. *The medication should be increased until seizures are controlled or until clinical toxicity is seen in the child.* Serum levels of anticonvulsants can be helpful in assessing compliance and in unravelling concerns about toxicity. The fact that a child has a blood level that is at the high end of the "therapeutic range" does not mean that medication cannot be increased if seizures have not been controlled. It can be increased as long as careful questioning and examination shows no evidence of toxicity. In addition, if a child's seizures are controlled and there is no evidence of clinical toxicity, finding that the serum level is above the "therapeutic

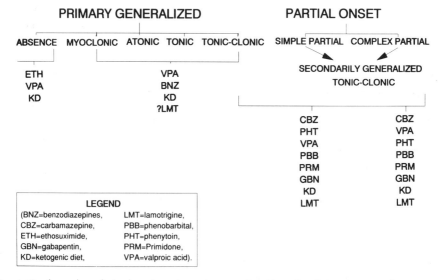

Figure 4. Antiepilepsy drug choice by seizure type; drugs are listed in order of our current preference.

Table 3. Antiepileptic drugs in children

Drug	Dose (mg/kg/day)	Side effects	Therapeutic range (mg/l)
Carbamazepine	10–40	Headache, drowsiness, dizziness, diplopia, blood dyscrasias	8–12
Clonazepam	0.05–0.3	Drowsiness, ataxia, increased secretion	
Ethosuximide	20–40	Gastrointestinal distress, rash, drowsiness, dizziness, systemic lupus erythematosos	40–80
Felbamate	15–45	Nausea, weight loss, insomnia, headache, increased infection	
Gabapentin	15–30	Drowsiness, dizziness, headache, hypotonia, cardiac arrhythmia	
Phenobarbital	2–8	Drowsiness, rash, ataxia, behavior changes	15–40
Phenytoin	4–8	Drowsiness, gingival hyperplasia, rash, anemia, ataxia, hirsutism	10–20
Primidone	12–25	Drowsiness, dizziness, rash, anemia, ataxia	8–12
Valproic acid	10–60	Gastrointestinal distress, thrombocytopenia, liver dysfunction, alopecia, drowsiness, ataxia	50–100
Lamotrigine	2–10	Rash, dizziness, diplopia, ataxia, nausea, vomiting	

range" should not lead to decreasing the child's dose and increasing the likelihood of seizure recurrence. The child who is being treated with phenytoin and whose seizures have been almost completely controlled might have a serum level of 18 mg/l (therapeutic range 10–20 mg/l). After carefully ascertaining that there are no side effects (e.g., school is going well, the child is the high scorer on the soccer team), it is appropriate to increase the dose slightly to see if seizures can be controlled completely without toxicity. When the child returns to the clinic with the seizures completely controlled with a serum level of 22 mg/l, again without any clinical toxicity, it is appropriate to maintain the current dose of phenytoin. It would be therapeutically incorrect to lower the dose and expose the child to recurrent seizures simply because the level was "supratherapeutic."

3. *The child should be monitored.* Monitoring involves more than just assessing control of seizures, the presence or absence of side effects, and whether the child is continuing to develop and function in an expected fashion. Monitoring often means obtaining information from school and questioning the child and family about outside activities, relationships, and behavior. Problem areas must be addressed and outside assistance sought. Routine blood work is unnecessary and is not a substitute for this comprehensive monitoring. Families should be told that routine blood counts, liver function tests,

and blood levels are not substitutes for assessing whether the child is doing well. They should be told that, if the child is having problems (medical, psychological, or educational) and they do not know why, the question of a problem related to the medication should be raised. Several studies have indicated that routine blood work cannot predict problems and is prohibitively expensive (Pellock & Willmore, 1991).

4. *If a child's seizures have not been controlled after a single medication, or at most two, have been tried, referral to an epilepsy center is warranted.* This is potentially useful from the point of view of reexamining seizure type and cause, considering alternative medications, providing access to new medications and finally providing access to consideration of possible surgical intervention.

CONCLUSIONS

Children with developmental disabilities have a higher incidence of seizures. The seizure types are frequently very difficult to control. However, the goal of therapy should be the complete control of seizures without intolerable side effects. The thoughtful clinician, working with the child, the family, and other health/education providers, should be able to make this goal a reality for most children with developmental disabilities.

REFERENCES

Brodtkorb, E., Nilsen, G., Smevik, O., & Rinck, P.A. (1992). Epilepsy and anomalies of neuronal migration: MRI and clinical aspects. *Acta Neurologica Scandinavica, 86,* 24–32,.

Chevrie, J.J., & Aicardi, J. (1977). Convulsive disorders in the first year of life: Etiologic factors. *Epilepsia, 18,* 489–498.

Commission on Classification and Terminology of the International League Against Epilepsy. (1981). *Epilepsia, 22,* 489–501.

Commission on Classification and Terminology of the International League Against Epilepsy. (1985). *Epilepsia, 26,* 268–278.

Dreifuss, F.E. (1989). Classification of epileptic seizures and the epilepsies. *Pediatric Clinics of North America, 36,* 265–279.

Freeman, J.M., & Vining, E.P. (1992). Decision making and the child with afebrile seizures [Review]. *Pediatrics in Review, 13,* 305–310.

Freeman, J.M., Vining, E.P.G., & Pillas, D.J. (1990). *Seizures and epilepsy in childhood: A guide for parents.* Baltimore: Johns Hopkins University Press.

Goulden, K.J., Shinnar, S., Koller, H., Katz, M., & Richardson, S.A. (1991). Epilepsy in children with mental retardation: A cohort study. *Epilepsia, 32,* 690–697.

Greenberg, D.A., & Delgado-Escueta, A.V. (1993). The chromosome 6p epilepsy locus: Exploring mode of inheritance and heterogeneity through linkage analysis. *Epilepsia, 34*(Suppl. 3), S12–S18.

Hauser, W.A., & Hesdorffer, D.C. (1990). *Epilepsy: Frequency, causes and consequences.* Landover, MD: Epilepsy Foundation of America.

Holmes, G.L. (1989). Electroencephalographic and neuroradiologic evaluation of children with epilepsy. *Pediatric Clinics of North America, 36,* 395–420.

Painter, M.J., & Gaus, L.M. (1991). Neonatal seizures: Diagnosis and treatment [Review]. *Journal of Child Neurology, 6,* 101–108.

Paquier, P.F., VanDongen, H.R., & Loonen, C.B. (1992). The Landau-Kleffner syndrome or "acquired aphasia with convulsive disorder": Long-term follow-up of six children and a review of the recent literature. *Archives of Neurology, 49,* 354–359.

Pellock, J.M., & Willmore, L.J. (1991). A rational guide to routine blood monitoring in patients receiving antiepileptic drugs [Editorial]. *Neurology, 41,* 961–964.

Rothner, A.D. (1989). "Not everything that shakes is epilepsy": The differential diagnosis of paroxysmal nonepileptiform disorders. *Cleveland Clinical Journal of Medicine, 56*(Suppl. 2), S206–S213.

Shinnar, S., Vining, E.P., Mellits, E.D., D'Souza, B.J., Holden, K. Baumgardner, R.A., & Freeman, J.M. (1985). Discontinuing antiepileptic medication in children with epilepsy after two years without seizures: A prospective study. *New England Journal of Medicine, 313,* 976–980.

Sillanpaa, M. (1992). Epilepsy in children: Prevalence, disability, and handicap. *Epilepsia, 33,* 444–449.

Snead, O.C. (1990). Treatment of infantile spasms [see comments] [Review]. *Pediatric Neurology, 6,* 147–150.

Stephenson, J.B.P. (1990). *Fits and faints.* Clinics in Developmental Medicine, Vol. 109. London: MacKeith.

Thorpy, M.J., & Glovinsky, P.B. (1987). Parasomnias. *Psychiatric Clinic of North America, 10,* 623–639.

Tsuboi, T. (1978). Correlation between EEG abnormality and age in childhood. *Neuropadiatrie, 9,* 229–238.

Yang, P.J., Berger, P.E., Cohen, M.E., & Duffner, P.K. (1979). Computer tomography and childhood seizure disorders. *Neurology, 29,* 1984–1988.

Index

Page numbers followed by "f" indicate figures; those followed by "t" indicate tables.